HIGH ROYDS HOSPITAL
MEDICAL LIBRARY
WITHDRAWN

WM 21   STO

D0297357

LCUH6305
NS H901
14/8/96.

WITHDRAWN

MEDICAL-PSYCHIATRIC PRACTICE

Volume 3

Editorial Advisory Board

Jimmie C. Holland, M.D.
Frits J. Huyse, M.D., Ph.D.
Donald S. Kornfeld, M.D.
Norman B. Levy, M.D.
Don R. Lipsitt, M.D.
George B. Murray, M.D.
Robert O. Pasnau, M.D.
Miriam B. Rosenthal, M.D.
James J. Strain, M.D.
Troy L. Thompson II, M.D.
Gary J. Tucker, M.D.
Thomas N. Wise, M.D.

MEDICAL-PSYCHIATRIC PRACTICE

Volume 3

Edited by

Alan Stoudemire, M.D.
*Professor, Department of Psychiatry
and Behavioral Sciences
Emory University School of Medicine
Atlanta, Georgia*

Barry S. Fogel, M.D.
*Professor, Department of Psychiatry
and Human Behavior
Brown University School of Medicine
Providence, Rhode Island*

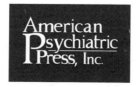

Washington, DC
London, England

Note: The authors have worked to ensure that all information in this book concerning drug dosages, schedules, and routes of administration is accurate as of the time of publication and consistent with standards set by the U.S. Food and Drug Administration and the general medical community. As medical research and practice advance, however, therapeutic standards may change. For this reason and because human and mechanical errors sometimes occur, we recommend that readers follow the advice of a physician who is directly involved in their care or the care of a member of their family.

Books published by the American Psychiatric Press, Inc., represent the views and opinions of the individual authors and do not necessarily represent the policies and opinions of the Press or the American Psychiatric Association.

Copyright © 1995 American Psychiatric Press, Inc.
ALL RIGHTS RESERVED
Manufactured in the United States of America on acid-free paper.
First Edition

98 97 96 95   4 3 2 1

American Psychiatric Press, Inc.
1400 K Street, N.W., Washington, DC 20005

ISSN 1054-4712
ISBN 0-88048-427-6

*The editors dedicate this book to their students,
many of whom will form the next generation of
medical-psychiatric practitioners.*

Contents

Contributors ix

Preface xiii
    Alan Stoudemire, M.D.
    Barry S. Fogel, M.D.

Acknowledgments xvii

1 Psychopharmacokinetics:
   Clinical Applications in Medical Illnesses 1
   Karen E. Beliles, M.D.
   Alan Stoudemire, M.D.

2 Psychopharmacology in Medical Patients:
   An Update 79
   Alan Stoudemire, M.D.
   Barry S. Fogel, M.D.

3 Treatment of Psychosis in Parkinson's Disease 151
   Stuart S. Rich, M.D.
   Joseph H. Friedman, M.D.

4 Neuropsychiatric Aspects of
   Systemic Lupus Erythematosus 183
   Martin J. Kelly, M.D.
   Malcolm P. Rogers, M.D.

5 Diagnostic Assessment of Chronic Fatigue Syndrome . . 215
   Theodore J. Anfinson, M.D.

6 Psychiatric Aspects of HIV Infection and AIDS:
   An Overview and Update 257
   Joel J. Wallack, M.D.
   Philip A. Bialer, M.D.
   Steven L. Prenzlauer, M.D.

7 Neuropsychiatric Sequelae of
   Mild Traumatic Brain Injury 307
     John G. Tierney, M.D.
     Barry S. Fogel, M.D.

8 Psychiatric Aspects of
   "Chemical Sensitivity" Syndromes 347
     Donald W. Black, M.D.
     Patricia J. Sparks, M.D., M.P.H.

9 Vulvodynia: Chronic Vulvar Pain Syndromes 381
     Marilynne McKay, M.D.
     Julie Farrington, M.D.

10 Psychiatric Aspects of Bone Marrow Transplantation . . 415
     Lynna M. Lesko, M.D., Ph.D.

Index 467

Cumulative Index for Volumes 1–3 507

Contents to Volume 1 611

Contents to Volume 2 615

Contributors

Theodore J. Anfinson, M.D.
Assistant Professor, Department of Psychiatry
  and Behavioral Sciences
Emory University School of Medicine
Atlanta, Georgia

Karen E. Beliles, M.D.
Assistant Professor, Departments of Medicine,
  Surgery, and Psychiatry
Vanderbilt University
Nashville, Tennessee

Philip A. Bialer, M.D.
Assistant Professor, Department of Psychiatry
Albert Einstein School of Medicine
New York, New York

Donald W. Black, M.D.
Associate Professor, Department of Psychiatry
University of Iowa College of Medicine
Iowa City, Iowa

Julie Farrington, M.D.
Assistant Professor, Department of Psychiatry
  and Behavioral Sciences
Emory University School of Medicine
Atlanta, Georgia

Barry S. Fogel, M.D.
Professor, Department of Psychiatry and Human Behavior
Brown University School of Medicine
Providence, Rhode Island

Joseph H. Friedman, M.D.
Professor, Department of Clinical Neuroscience
Brown University School of Medicine
Providence, Rhode Island

Martin J. Kelly, M.D.
Associate Professor, Department of Psychiatry
Harvard Medical School
Boston, Massachusetts

Lynna M. Lesko, M.D., Ph.D.
Adjunct Professor, Department of Psychiatry
Cornell University Medical College
New York, New York

Marilynne McKay, M.D.
Associate Professor, Departments of Dermatology
  and Gynecology
Emory University School of Medicine
Atlanta, Georgia

Steven L. Prenzlauer, M.D.
Clinical Instructor, Department of Psychiatry
Albert Einstein School of Medicine
New York, New York

Stuart S. Rich, M.D.
Assistant Professor, Department of Psychiatry
  and Human Behavior
Brown University School of Medicine
Providence, Rhode Island

Malcolm P. Rogers, M.D.
Associate Professor, Department of Psychiatry
Harvard Medical School
Boston, Massachusetts

Patricia J. Sparks, M.D., M.P.H.
Clinical Assistant Professor, Department
  of Environmental Health
University of Washington
Seattle, Washington

Alan Stoudemire, M.D.
Professor, Department of Psychiatry
  and Behavioral Sciences
Emory University School of Medicine
Atlanta, Georgia

John G. Tierney, M.D.
Assistant Professor, Department of Psychiatry
  and Behavioral Sciences
Emory University School of Medicine
Atlanta, Georgia

Joel J. Wallack, M.D.
Clinical Associate Professor,
  Department of Psychiatry
New York University
New York, New York

Preface

This textbook comes to press at a time of great irony for American psychiatry. Although the potential ability of psychiatrists to accurately diagnose and effectively treat symptoms of patients with disorders of mood, thought, and behavior has never been greater, interest of American medical students in psychiatry residency training has declined substantially over the past 5 years. Continued advances in neuroscience and clinical psychopharmacology are bringing rigor and precision to understanding the pathophysiology and treatment of mental illness. Research findings are also providing a scientific basis for matching focused psychotherapeutic and psychopharmacological treatments to specific disorders. Nevertheless, psychiatry has come under great duress as a result of the phenomenon of managed care that has, in a relatively short time, radically altered many components of psychiatric practice. Insurance companies define "coverage" in terms of arbitrary numbers of treatment sessions in the effort to contain costs and decrease overall use of mental health services. Psychiatrists have also seen increased competition from other mental health professionals to provide psychotherapy. Some health plans relegate psychiatrists to providing psychopharmacological treatment, while psychotherapy is provided by other professionals at a lower price. Particularly in health maintenance organizations, referrals to specialists by primary care providers are discouraged. Primary care physicians with very limited, if any, formal training in psychiatric diagnosis and psychopharmacology are expected to provide drug treatment of mental disorders. Because of these changes in the provision of mental health services, psychiatry in the United States is undergoing radical changes, and the future of the profession is uncertain.

Although these ironic conditions may someday become fascinating social history, at present, they have resulted in considerable numbers of underserved patients and distressed psychiatrists. Our society already has many patients with psychiatric disorders, and evidence suggests that prevalence rates are increasing. The expert services of psychiatrists are greatly needed, even if this need is not reflected in the priorities of our current system of health care. Meeting this need will require modification and improvement in psychiatry's morale, recruitment, reimbursement, training programs, identity, and practice patterns. We believe that such improvements are more likely to result from a revised positive and highly specific view of psychiatry as a medical specialty.

In several previous publications that we have edited together, we have endorsed the view that psychiatry has a bright future if it focuses on the diagnosis and treatment of symptoms of mental disorders within the framework of a medical model. Such a model emphasizes precise clinical diagnosis and the focal application of specific psychotherapeutic and psychopharmacological interventions in an integrated manner. A medical model of treatment is especially practical in treating patients with psychiatric disorders who also have medical or neurological diseases. Diagnosing and treating psychiatric conditions in patients who have combined psychiatric and medical or neurological illness takes full advantage of the psychiatrist's dual identity as a physician and a specialist in the treatment of patients with mental disorders. Psychiatrists are the professionals who are optimally trained to integrate diagnostic information and treatment modalities that comprise biological, psychological, and sociological factors.

We believe that the continued evolution of psychiatry as a well-defined clinical specialty that consistently applies a medical model will ensure an appropriate and respected place for psychiatry among the medical specialties and with the general public. It is no longer productive for psychiatrists to claim superiority in performing psychotherapy to professionals of other disciplines who are well-trained therapists. Psychiatrists should emphasize their highly varied skills in treating patients with complex medical-psychiatric conditions.

We believe that the future of psychiatry will necessitate substantial changes in residency training programs. Specifically, we recommend that these programs refocus to address our society's future needs for mental health services, as well as the survival and prosperity of psychiatry as a medical specialty. Developmental psychology and psychodynamic psychotherapy should remain in the psychiatrists' repertoire of knowledge and skill, but training programs should also systematically teach the appropriate use of short-term psychotherapeutic and cognitive-behavioral interventions. The field of neuropsychiatry should also be emphasized, including the ability to critically evaluate and appropriately use brain imaging in psychodiagnostic assessment. Increased expertise in geriatric psychiatry will be needed to serve an aging population.

Continued emphasis should be placed on psychopharmacology, but psychiatrists will more often manage refractory psychiatric conditions and complex multiple drug regimens, because most "routine" treatment of anxiety and mood disorders will be handled in the primary care sector. It will become increasingly important for psychiatrists to understand the interaction of psychotropic medications with drugs used in internal medicine and neurology and to thoroughly comprehend the pharmacokinetics of psychotropic medications in patients with medical illness. The identity of the psychiatrist as a physician must be maintained by stressing the importance of performing physical and neurological examinations and administering and interpreting basic laboratory and neuroendocrine tests.

With the emphasis on the treatment of patients with psychiatric conditions in the primary care setting, the liaison role of the psychiatrist as a consultant and educator of primary care physicians and other mental health professionals should be emphasized in residency training. This may require a revitalization and an increasingly important role of the educational mission of consultation-liaison psychiatry.

We believe that psychiatrists who are trained in this way will be in great demand regardless of the outcome of contemporary political, economic, and interdisciplinary conflicts about health care organization and financing. Such psychiatrists would be versatile, pragmatic, and well-grounded in developmental psychology, psychotherapy, psychopharmacology, and neuroscience.

This third volume in our series entitled *Medical-Psychiatric Practice* addresses several specific clinical problems that require an integrated medical-psychiatric approach to their diagnosis and treatment. These populations include patients with systemic lupus erythematosus, Parkinson's disease, traumatic brain injury, chronic fatigue syndrome, and chronic vulvar pain and recipients of bone marrow transplants. This volume also includes an in-depth discussion of psychopharmacokinetics in medically ill patients and our third update on psychopharmacology in medically ill patients. This textbook is meant to be used as a reference for timely and important topics in medical psychiatry; it complements our comprehensive textbook *Psychiatric Care of the Medical Patient* (Oxford University Press 1993). As with our previous volumes, we emphasize practical aspects of diagnosis and treatment for the busy practicing physician.

We have both benefited from undergoing personal psychoanalysis. We continue to practice psychodynamic psychotherapy, and we believe that both psychoanalysis and long-term dynamic psychotherapy modalities are invaluable personal and professional options for psychiatrists and their patients who are interested in, or clinically require, an in-depth exploration of their inner lives. Present and future realities, however, indicate that training in general psychiatry should not be *primarily* based on a practice model in which these techniques predominate. Although it is essential that psychiatry retain its humanistic focus and its traditional emphasis on the importance of developmental experiences in personality and susceptibility to mental illness, the psychiatrist of the future will primarily practice within a medical model and will treat patients who have complex and refractory mental disorders or psychiatric disorders, combined with medical or neurological disease. Like other medical specialists, psychiatrists must increasingly focus their careers on meeting the needs of patients who require their unique knowledge and special skills. This will ensure their successful transition to new models of medical care, as well as continued emotional satisfaction and unlimited intellectual challenges.

Alan Stoudemire, M.D.
Barry S. Fogel, M.D.

Acknowledgments

As with our previous publications, the editors would like to thank the contributors to this volume, who have been so resilient and cooperative with our strenuous editorial demands. The editors would also like to acknowledge and thank our superbly dedicated administrative assistants, Lynda Mathews and Rita St. Pierre, for their excellent help and tireless support over the years.

Chapter 1

Psychopharmacokinetics: Clinical Applications in Medical Illnesses

Karen E. Beliles, M.D.
Alan Stoudemire, M.D.

Important factors that influence the pharmacokinetics of psychotropic drugs include age, gender, race, genetic phenotype, and, in particular, the presence of disease. The influence of somatic illness on the pharmacokinetics of many psychiatric medications, however, has not been extensively studied. In this chapter, we discuss practical pharmacokinetic principles that should guide the selection and dosage of psychotropic drugs in the context of physical illness. First, we discuss basic pharmacokinetic principles and parameters. We then review several general categories of disease (gastrointestinal, cardiac, hepatic, and renal) commonly encountered in medical-surgical settings for their potential impact on the pharmacokinetics of psychotropic drugs. Emphasis is placed on practical considerations in dose adjustment for various psychotropic drugs in the presence of disease. Readers are also referred to Chapter 2 in this textbook and other sources that discuss clinical aspects of psychotropic drug use in medically ill patients (Fogel and Stoudemire 1993; Stoudemire et al. 1991, 1993).

ABSORPTION

Absorption of a drug is influenced by many factors, including the physicochemical properties of the drug itself and certain characteristics of the absorption site, such as 1) surface area, 2) ambient pH at the site(s) of dissolution and absorption, 3) mucosal integrity and function, and 4) local blood flow (Table 1–1). Conditions that possibly influence drug absorption from the gastrointestinal (GI) tract include GI motility, diseases of the stomach, GI surgery, diseases of the small and large intestine, GI infections, and interactions with other substances (e.g., other drugs, food) (Brater and Vasko 1988; Welling 1984). Clinically significant alterations of drug absorption might be expected in surgical GI resection (particularly of the stomach and proximal small intestine), short bowel syndromes, exacerbations of celiac disease, and in situations in which treatment modalities include drugs that alter GI motility (e.g., metoclopramide, propantheline) (Welling 1984). Furthermore, gastroparetic conditions (e.g., diabetes mellitus, pancreatitis, gastric ulcer, and anticholinergic drug-induced states of decreased gastric motility) may slow drug absorption rates and, thus, theoretically cause clinically important delays in time to onset of medication effect (Leipzig 1990) (Table 1–2).

Orally administered drugs are absorbed from the GI tract into the portal circulation. Thus, some agents may be extensively metabolized in the liver *before* reaching the systemic circulation. This phenomenon is referred to as the *first-pass effect*. The first-pass effect can be minimized by use of sublingual and topical preparations. The effect is reduced by use of rectal suppositories (about 50% of a rectal dose can be assumed to bypass the liver) (Benet and Massoud 1984; de Boer et al. 1982) and by intravenous administration. The fact that the required intravenous dose is significantly less than the oral (but not the sublingual) dose of equivalent efficacy demonstrates that first-pass metabolism plays an important kinetic role (Benet and Massoud 1984). For example, haloperidol undergoes extensive first-pass metabolism; it is generally given orally at two to four times the parenteral dose to achieve an equivalent blood level.

Lag time for absorption is defined as the time it takes for an orally administered drug to enter the systemic circulation. The most important determinants of lag time for absorption of an enterally administered agent are the specific formulation of the drug and gastric motility (including emptying time). Anticholinergic activity of certain psychotropic drugs may delay gastric emptying and therefore further lengthen lag time for absorption, beyond any disease-induced changes in absorption. *Absorption rate* refers not only to the lag time, but also to the time course of a drug's serum concentration after its initial appearance in the systemic circulation. Absorption rate is determined by drug formulation, drug interactions, and characteristics of the absorptive surface, including ambient pH and local blood flow (Brater and Vasko 1988) (Table 1–1). Solubilization processes usually result in delays of 30 minutes or more (DeVane 1990a). In general, rank order from most rapidly to most slowly absorbed formulations is solution, suspension, capsule, tablet, enteric-coated tablet. Thus, an elixir formulation of antipsychotic medication may be preferred over a tablet when fast onset of action is desired, as in a case of extreme psychotic agitation. Many antipsychotic drugs, with the exception of pimozide, are available in elixir or concentrated solution formulations (Table 1–3).

Parenteral administration of psychotropic agents may be preferable when rapid onset of action is desired (e.g., acute agitation), when coadministration with other drugs or food is expected to affect psychopharmacokinetic parameters unfavorably (e.g., decreased extent of absorption), or when patients are unable to tolerate oral medication (Santos et al. 1992) (Table 1–3). Absorption of drugs administered by the intramuscular route is usually faster than for enteral preparations (DeVane 1990a), especially if the injection site is a well-perfused muscle such as the deltoid. The benzodiazepines midazolam and lorazepam are available in formulations for intramuscular administration. However, some drugs, such as the benzodiazepines chlordiazepoxide and diazepam, precipitate when injected into muscle and thus are incompletely or erratically absorbed via this parenteral route (Brater and Vasko 1988). Other obvious disadvantages of intramuscular dosing include pain on administration and local muscular damage.

Clorazepate and prazepam are long-acting benzodiazepines that are not active in their original form, but they share the same active metabolite, N-desmethyldiazepam. Nevertheless, different lipid solubilities of the parent drugs result in different times for onset of action of these two drugs. For example, clorazepate (more lipophilic) produces high blood levels within 1 hour, whereas prazepam takes effect more slowly. After 4 hours, however, the concentration of desmethyldiazepam is essentially the same for these two drugs (Greenblatt 1980). This example illustrates how pharmacokinetics may influence the clinician's choice of benzodiazepine to be used as a hypnotic agent. When rapid sedation is desired, agents such as clorazepate, diazepam, lorazepam, or alprazolam may be preferable (Cassem et al. 1988).

Although absorption rate is important when rapid onset of action is required, the extent of absorption is more important when a drug is

Table 1–1. Pharmacokinetic terms and parameters

Terms	Definition	Determinants	Clinical significance
Absorption		Surface area Ambient pH at site(s) of dissolution and absorption Mucosal integrity and function Local blood flow	Diseases affecting specific sites of absorption may influence clinician to choose alternate route of administration
Bioavailability (F)	Fraction of a drug dose that reaches systemic circulation as unchanged drug after administration by a specified route	Rate of absorption Extent of absorption Drug distribution and first-pass metabolism	$F = 1.0$ indicates 100% bioavailability $F < 1$ when there is 1) incomplete absorption; 2) metabolism of enterally administered drug in gut, gut-wall portal blood, or liver before entry into systemic circulation; or 3) enterohepatic cycling with incomplete reabsorption after elimination into bile
Lag time for absorption	Time for an orally administered drug to enter systemic circulation	Drug formulation Gastric motility	Influences time to onset of pharmacologic activity
Absorption rate	Rate at which drug is delivered to the systemic circulation via absorption from a specified site of administration	Drug formulation Drug-food interactions Ambient pH Local blood flow Gastrointestinal motility	Influences time to onset of pharmacologic activity and time to peak activity

Term	Definition	Factors	Significance
Distribution	Delivery of drug to sites throughout the body	Lipid solubility Blood pH Plasma protein binding Tissue perfusion	Affects pharmacologic activity, metabolism, and excretion
Volume of distribution (Vd)	Conceptual volume that would be necessary to contain total amount of drug in the body if it were at the same concentration throughout the body as measured in plasma	Lipid solubility Plasma protein binding Tissue binding	Determines loading dose; relates plasma drug concentration to the total amount of drug in the body
Clearance (Cl)	Volume of blood or other fluid from which drug is irreversibly removed per unit of time	Body weight and surface area Plasma protein binding Extraction ratio Renal function Hepatic function Cardiac output	Determines maintenance dose; determines magnitude of steady-state concentration
Half-life ($T\frac{1}{2}$)	Time required for an amount of drug in the body or drug concentration to fall by $\frac{1}{2}$	Volume of distribution Clearance	Reflects time to achieve steady-state concentration after initiating drug administration, changing dosage, or discontinuing drug administration
Steady state	When rate of drug administration equals rate of drug elimination	Rates of absorption, distribution, metabolism, excretion	See Half-life

Source. Brater and Vasko 1988; DeVane 1990a; Rowland and Tozer 1989; Winter 1988a.

Table 1–2. Disease states and pharmacokinetic disruptions

Kinetic phase primarily affected	Disease examples
Absorption	Gastrointestinal motility changes
	Decreased
	• Mechanical obstruction, metabolic abnormalities (e.g., diabetes mellitus, hypothyroidism), muscular or connective tissue disorders (e.g., scleroderma), neurologic abnormalities (e.g., autonomic neuropathy, multiple sclerosis), trauma, and pain
	Increased
	• Celiac disease; duodenal ulcer, gastroenterostomy; pancreatic cholera syndrome
	Gastrointestinal mucosal integrity/function disruptions
	Surgical resection (e.g., J-tube, jejunoileal bypass), graft versus host of gut, Crohn's disease
	Diversion of blood flow away from absorptive site
	Congestive heart failure, acute stress, or trauma
Distribution	Blood pH changes
	Metabolic disruptions, food or drug ingestion
	Binding proteins
	Decreased
	• Cirrhosis, malnutrition, nephrotic syndrome, burns
	Increased
	• Hypothyroidism, celiac disease, Crohn's disease, stress- or disease-induced increase of acute-phase reactants including α_1-acid glycoprotein (e.g., myocardial infarction, renal failure, trauma)

Circulatory changes
  Cardiovascular disease, portosystemic shunting associated with liver disease, diseases reducing renal blood flow

Hepatic metabolism
  Alterations in hepatic blood flow
    Decreased
      •Cirrhosis, congestive heart failure
    Increased
      •Chronic respiratory disease, viral hepatitis, severe diarrhea
  Changes in protein binding and fluid shifts
    Disrupted hepatic synthetic function, bilirubin displacement of drugs from binding proteins, ascites
  Pericentral liver disease
    Acute viral hepatitis, alcoholic liver disease
  Periportal liver disease
    Chronic hepatitis without cirrhosis, early primary biliary cirrhosis

Renal excretion
  Fluid shifts
    Ascites, edema, dehydration, surgery, trauma, nephrotic syndrome
  Retained protein binding inhibitors
    Uremia
  Changes in renal blood flow
    Vascular glomerular disease, shock, hepatorenal syndrome
    Acute and chronic renal failure

Table 1–3. Available psychotropic drug formulations

Anxiolytics
  Alprazolam T
  Buspirone T
  Chlordiazepoxide T,C,V
  Clorazepate T,C
  Diazepam T,C$_{ER}$,E,S,V
  Estazolam T
  Flurazepam C
  Halazepam T
  Lorazepam T,S,M,V
  Midazolam M,V
  Oxazepam T,C
  Prazepam T,C
  Quazepam T
  Temazepam C
  Triazolam T

Antidepressants
  Amitriptyline T,M,(V)
  Amoxapine T
  Bupropion T
  Clomipramine C,(V)
  Desipramine T,C
  Doxepin C,E
  Fluoxetine C,E
  Imipramine T,C,M,(V)
  Maprotiline T
  Nortriptyline C,E
  Paroxetine T
  Protriptyline T
  Sertraline T
  Trazodone T

  Trimipramine T
  Venlafaxine T

Stimulants
  Methylphenidate T,T$_{DR}$,(V)
  Pemoline T

Mood stabilizers
  Carbamazepine T,E
  Divalproex sodium C,T$_{DR}$
  Lithium carbonate T,T$_{SR}$,C
  Lithium citrate E
  Valproate sodium E
  Valproic acid C

Antipsychotics
  Chlorpromazine T,C$_{ER}$,E,S,M,R
  Chlorprothixene T,E,M
  Droperidol T,E,M,V
  Fluphenazine T,E,S,M,D
  Haloperidol T,E,M,(V),D
  Loxapine C,S,M
  Mesoridazine T,S,M
  Molindone T,S
  Perphenazine T,S,M
  Pimozide T
  Prochlorperazine T,C$_{ER}$,E,M,V,R
  Risperidone T
  Thioridazine T,E,S
  Thiothixene C,E,M
  Trifluoperazine T,S,M

Note. T = tablet; T$_{DR}$ = tablet, delayed release; T$_{SR}$ = tablet, sustained release; C = capsule; C$_{ER}$ = capsule, extended release; E = elixir; S = "concentrated" solution; R = rectal suppository; M = intramuscular formulation; V = intravenous formulation; (V) = intravenous use described but not FDA approved; D = depot formulation.

administered chronically. **Bioavailability (F)** is a pharmacokinetic parameter determined by both rate and extent of absorption and the magnitude of first-pass metabolism, which is dependent on drug distribution (Brater and Vasko 1988; DeVane 1990a). Bioavailability is influenced by the inherent dissolution and absorption characteristics of a drug, the dosage form (e.g., tablet, liquid), the route of administration, the stability of the active ingredient in the GI tract, and the extent of first-pass metabolism (Winter 1988a). For parenterally administered drugs, $F = 1.0$ (100% bioavailable). However, for drugs administered in a pharmacologically inactive form, $F < 1$ (Winter 1988a) (Tables 1–1 and 1–4). Bioavailability of an orally administered drug may be less than 100% as a result of 1) incomplete absorption; 2) metabolism in the gut, gut wall, portal blood, or liver before entry into the systemic circulation; and 3) enterohepatic cycling with incomplete reabsorption after elimination into the bile (Benet and Massoud 1984).

DISTRIBUTION

Distribution is influenced by a drug's lipid solubility, blood pH, and plasma protein binding. Acidemia favors the nonionized form of

Table 1–4. Psychotropic drug metabolism

Extensively metabolized by phase I reactions (before phase II metabolism):	
Tricyclic antidepressants	Clonazepam[a]
Heterocyclic antidepressants	Diazepam
Selective serotonin reuptake inhibitors	Estazolam[a]
	Flurazepam
Antipsychotic agents	Halazepam
Carbamazepine	Midazolam
Valproate	Prazepam[b]
Alprazolam[a]	Quazepam
Clorazepate[b]	Triazolam[a]
Chlordiazepoxide	Buspirone
Primarily metabolized by phase II reactions:	
Lorazepam[a]	Temazepam[a]
Oxazepam[a]	

[a]No major active metabolites.
[b]Pharmacologically inactive prodrug.

weakly acidic drugs (e.g., phenytoin, valproate), thus increasing their lipid permeability and their distribution to the central nervous system (CNS) (Brater and Vasko 1988). The major drug-binding proteins are albumin and α_1-acid glycoprotein (AAGP). In general, "acidic" drugs (e.g., barbiturates, valproate [Benet and Massoud 1984]) bind primarily to albumin; "basic" drugs (e.g., phenothiazines, tricyclic antidepressants, amphetamines, nicotine, most benzodiazepines [Benet and Massoud 1984]) bind primarily to the globulins (Winter 1988a). For most psychotropic agents (with the exception of venlafaxine), the percentage bound to plasma proteins is in the range of 80%–95%. Frequently, the extent of protein binding of a particular drug is determined by processes that do not discriminate between the specific proteins involved. Thus, simply knowing that a specific disease may change binding protein concentration(s) does not allow extrapolation of specific drug dosage adjustments.

The degree of binding depends on the specific drug as well as the physical configuration of the binding proteins and their plasma concentrations (DeVane 1990a). Thus, disease may affect binding affinities of plasma proteins and concentrations. For example, albumin binding may be decreased in conditions such as cirrhosis, bacterial pneumonia, severe malnutrition, acute pancreatitis, renal failure, surgery, trauma, and burns. Albumin-bound drugs with low therapeutic indexes (e.g., valproate, phenytoin, barbiturates) are most likely to display clinically significant alteration(s) of their pharmacokinetics and resultant toxicity when disease affects protein binding. Both albumin and AAGP concentrations may be decreased by the nephrotic syndrome.

Increased albumin binding might be expected in hypothyroidism and with some benign tumors. Plasma concentrations of AAGP (not routinely measured in clinical settings) may be increased by celiac and Crohn's diseases and by other conditions such as myocardial infarction, renal failure, rheumatoid arthritis, stress, surgery, and trauma (Leipzig 1990; Piafsky et al. 1978; Tozer 1984; Winter 1988a) (Table 1–5).

Both endogenous (e.g., bilirubin) and exogenous (e.g., various medications) substances can interfere with the plasma protein binding of a specific drug. In general, only the free portion of drug can diffuse to its site of pharmacologic activity. One must recall that absorption, distribution, metabolism, and excretion are not sequential but simultaneous processes. A drug that has been freed from its binding protein is available not only to its desired site of action but also to tissues in which

Table 1–5. Disease states affecting drug binding by albumin and AAGP

Albumin binding of drugs *increased:*	Albumin and AAGP binding of drugs *decreased:*
Hypothyroidism	
Benign tumors	Nephrotic syndrome
Albumin binding of drugs *decreased:*	AAGP binding of drugs *increased:*
Cirrhosis	Bacterial infection
Bacterial pneumonia	Cancer
Severe malnutrition	Celiac disease
Acute pancreatitis	Myocardial infarction
Renal failure	Renal failure
Surgery	Rheumatoid arthritis
Trauma	Stress
Burns	Surgery
	Trauma

Note.   AAGP = α_1 acid glycoprotein.
Source.   Leipzig 1990; Piafsky et al. 1978; Tozer 1984; Winter 1988a.

it is not therapeutically active and those responsible for its metabolism and excretion. In other words, the initial increase in drug availability due to decreased protein binding may be followed by decreases in volume of distribution and half-life.

In the absence of metabolic or excretory compromise after steady state has been achieved, the clinical result of drug displacement from binding proteins is virtually identical to the unperturbed condition— that is, the plasma concentration of free (pharmacologically active) drug is the same. However, the total drug concentration, as measured by most laboratory assays of plasma or serum drug concentration, is less than it was before displacement. Two situations illustrating this phenomenon follow:

> Although drug displaced from binding proteins is initially "free," attainment of steady state includes metabolism and excretion of that free portion of the drug. For example, in the normal (disease-free) state, approximately 90% of valproate is protein bound. Disease affecting protein synthetic function of the liver could cause a significant decrease in serum albumin, thus initially increasing the free portion of valproate in blood. This portion of the valproate would be available to sites of pharmacologic activity but also to sites of metabolism and

excretion. When a new steady state is achieved, the total (laboratory-determined) valproate concentration is lower (free drug displaced has been metabolized and excreted), but the plasma concentration of the pharmacologically active free valproate is virtually the same as in the unperturbed condition.

Chlorpromazine kinetics also illustrate the importance of understanding the clinical consequences of disease-induced changes in protein binding. In vitro studies (Piafsky et al. 1978) indicate that chlorpromazine binding by AAGP is significantly increased in plasma from patients with Crohn's disease and that the free drug concentration is inversely correlated to AAGP concentration. In this situation, measured chlorpromazine concentrations are increased, but they reflect increased bound drug, not pharmacologically active free drug.

When a drug's therapeutic margin is narrow (e.g., valproate, carbamazepine), displacement from binding proteins and the resultant transient increase in free drug concentration are more likely to be clinically significant. Laboratory assays generally quantitate total drug concentration. So-called therapeutic ranges for laboratory-determined drug levels are statistically generated with the assumption that the measured total drug concentration reflects a fixed percentage of free drug. Thus, when protein binding of a specific drug is decreased (as in various disease states or as a result of drug interaction), the reported (total) serum drug level actually reflects a lower free (active) drug concentration than initially assumed. In other words, when protein binding of a psychotropic drug is decreased by disease, a high blood level does not necessarily reflect increased free drug. If this is not taken into account when considering the laboratory-reported value, a naive clinician may make an unnecessary reduction in drug dosage (DeVane 1990a). When disease compromises drug metabolism and excretion in addition to protein binding, an increase in free drug is more likely to be sustained and may therefore be clinically significant (Brater and Vasko 1988).

Volume of distribution (Vd) is another pharmacokinetic parameter that is used to assess the importance of the dynamic factors discussed earlier in this chapter. Vd is a function of a drug's lipid solubility and its plasma- and tissue-binding properties (Table 1–1). A Vd larger than the plasma compartment (approximately 3 L) indicates that a drug is also present in tissues or fluids outside that compartment. Drugs with relatively high lipid solubility (e.g., diazepam) may be more quickly distributed to the brain. However, extensive extracerebral adipose stores make rapid redistribution of diazepam theoretically possible; this redistribution (away from brain and to lipid stores that are not sites of diazepam's psychopharmacologic activity) may shorten this drug's clinical therapeutic activity.

It is helpful to conceptualize the body in a two-compartment model, particularly when the administered drug is initially distributed in one volume (e.g., blood and those organs or tissues with high blood flow) and then rapidly redistributed to a second compartment that equilibrates over a relatively long period. The two-compartment model has particular applicability to lithium. Plasma samples obtained less than 12 hours after an oral lithium dose may be misleading because the end organ (brain) is a more slowly equilibrating tissue compartment than is plasma. Thus, plasma lithium concentrations measured during the initial (plasma) distribution phase (i.e., before equilibrium with the brain is complete) are higher and the observed pharmacologic response is less than this plasma lithium concentration would normally predict (Winter 1988a).

Most psychotropic medications are fairly lipid soluble but are also extensively bound to proteins in plasma. The larger a drug's Vd, the more likely that its tissue binding is greater than plasma protein binding (Brater and Vasko 1988; DeVane 1990a). Drugs such as imipramine (Vd 14 L/kg), nortriptyline (Vd 20 L/kg), and propranolol (Vd 4 L/kg) have high Vds, although more than 90% of these drugs in blood are bound to plasma proteins. This indicates that these drugs are more extensively bound to tissue than to plasma proteins and/or are more soluble in peripheral adipose tissues than in blood (Benet and Massoud 1984). For such drugs (with relatively large Vds despite a high protein-bound fraction in plasma), disease-induced decreases in plasma concentration of bound drug will likely result in clinically insignificant increases in the plasma concentration of free drug; the free drug released as a result of decreased plasma proteins will easily equilibrate with the tissue compartments (Winter 1988a). Valproate (Vd 0.14 L/kg), chlordiazepoxide (Vd 0.30 L/kg), oxazepam (Vd 0.65 L/kg), lithium (Vd 0.80 L/kg), midazolam (Vd 0.90 L/kg), diazepam (Vd 1.2 L/kg), and lorazepam (Vd 1.2 L/kg) are examples of psychotropic medications with relatively low Vds. A table of psychotropic drug Vds is not included in this chapter because this pharmacokinetic parameter is so frequently altered by disease in an unpredictable manner.

Vd determines the loading dose required to achieve a chosen initial plasma concentration:

IV loading dose = Vd × desired initial plasma concentration[*]

Note again that Vd is not a unique or unvariable characteristic of a given drug; a drug's Vd can be altered by disease via changes in its plasma or tissue binding. Required loading dose, as indicated above, is independent of a drug's clearance or half-life (Brater and Vasko 1988; DeVane 1990a; Winter 1988a).

An additional parameter, S, must be introduced to understand the relationship of Vd to the loading dose for a drug given by a nonintravenous route. S represents the portion of an administered dose that is pharmacologically active drug; therefore, it depends on drug formulation. When a drug is administered entirely in active form, $S = 1.0$.

$$\text{Loading dose} = \frac{\text{Vd} \times \text{desired plasma concentration}}{F \times S}$$

The product $F \times S$ is the fraction of an administered dose that reaches systemic circulation (Winter 1988a). Recall that Vd is not a measured parameter; thus, the equations above are infrequently used to determine doses in the clinical setting. We cited them to illustrate the relationship of route of administration and drug formulation to Vd.

ELIMINATION (METABOLISM AND EXCRETION)

The major pathways of psychotropic drug elimination are hepatic metabolism and renal excretion. The liver converts drugs to more polar compounds that are then excreted primarily by the kidney. The microsomal P_{450} system, which can be induced or inhibited by various drugs and disease processes, is responsible for oxidative (phase I) reactions (dealkylation, deamination, and desulfuration), as well as glucuronide synthesis and conjugation. Most psychotropic drugs (e.g., antidepressants, antipsychotics, and benzodiazepines other than lorazepam, ox-

---

[*] This concentration is that which exists immediately after administration, before significant elimination of drug.

azepam, and temazepam) undergo significant metabolism by phase I reactions. On the other hand, the hepatic nonmicrosomal metabolic system is responsible for processes including acetylation, methylation, conjugation with glycine and sulfate, hydrolysis, and reduction reactions (Table 1–4). (Conjugation reactions are also referred to as phase II reactions.)

Clorazepate and prazepam are long-acting benzodiazepines that are not pharmacologically active in their original forms, but they share the same active metabolite (N-desmethyldiazepam). The benzodiazepines oxazepam, lorazepam, and temazepam are primarily metabolized by conjugation. Many hepatically formed drug metabolites are pharmacologically active. In general, hydroxylated or demethylated metabolites are pharmacologically and/or toxicologically active. For tricyclic antidepressants and carbamazepine, currently available data do not support routine measurement of hydroxylated metabolites, but these metabolite levels may be useful in understanding toxicity occurring in the context of "therapeutic" parent drug levels (Stoudemire et al. 1991). Thus, most cyclic antidepressants, antipsychotics, and some anxiolytics have pharmacologically active metabolites (Table 1–4). Hepatic metabolism is influenced by 1) liver blood flow, 2) competitive inhibition at the enzymatic site, and 3) induction (or deactivation) of metabolic enzymes (Brater and Vasko 1988).

Clearance (Cl) is a pharmacokinetic concept that quantitates the intrinsic ability of the body, primarily the liver and kidneys, to remove a drug from the plasma compartment. Factors influencing Cl include 1) body weight, 2) body surface area, 3) plasma protein binding, 4) extraction ratio (fraction of drug presented to the primary organ of elimination that is cleared from the blood after a single pass through that organ), 5) renal function, 6) hepatic function, and 7) cardiac output (Winter 1988a). For a drug that does not undergo significant first-pass metabolism, the maximum hepatic Cl is equal to liver blood flow (approximately 1500 ml/min in a healthy adult) (Table 1–1).

Using the plasma concentration versus time curve for a drug after a single dose, Cl is calculated by dividing that dose by the area under the curve (AUC). If the AUC is small after a single dose, the Cl of that drug is high (DeVane 1990a). The magnitude and shape of a drug's AUC are dependent on how rapidly it is eliminated or cleared from the body (Figure 1–1).

The following equation demonstrates the relationship of Cl to maintenance dose:

$$\text{Maintenance dose} = \frac{\text{Steady-state plasma concentration}^{**} \times \text{dosing interval} \times \text{Cl}}{F}$$

In the clinical setting, the Cl of a specific drug is determined infrequently, but serial plasma drug levels may be useful in gauging disease-induced alterations of pharmacokinetics and making necessary dose adjustments.

A drug's **half-life (T½)** is a reflection of the time required to achieve steady-state plasma concentration (Table 1–1). Approximately

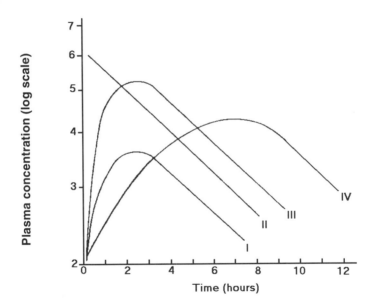

Figure 1–1. Predicted plasma concentration time course after single doses of a drug in an intravenous formulation (II), a totally absorbed oral formulation (III), a more slowly absorbed oral formulation (IV), and an incompletely absorbed dose (I). Because absorption does not alter elimination rate, the terminal half-lives are similar, as indicated by parallel decline. *Source.* Reprinted from DeVane CL: "Principles of Pharmacokinetics," in *Fundamentals of Monitoring Psychoactive Drug Therapy.* Edited by DeVane CL. Baltimore, MD, Williams & Wilkins, 1990, p 42. Used with permission.

** The steady-state plasma concentration value must be used in this calculation (Brater and Vasko 1988; DeVane 1990a; Winter 1988a).

four to five T½s are necessary to achieve steady state at a constant dose or to achieve a new steady state when dosing is changed. T½ can thus also be used to estimate how long it will take to eliminate a drug from the body after discontinuation. This pharmacokinetic parameter is determined by plotting drug concentration on a semi-log scale versus time. The slope is $-k/2.303$, and the drug's T½ is equal to 0.693 divided by k. T½ is influenced by the extent of drug distribution within the body (i.e., Vd) and by Cl of the drug from the body:

$$T½ = \frac{0.693 \times Vd}{Cl}$$

Benzodiazepine pharmacokinetics illustrate this relationship between T½, Vd, and Cl. For instance, diazepam and lorazepam have similar Vds (1.2 L/kg) but markedly different Cls (28 and 53 ml/min, respectively). Their T½s, 45 hours for diazepam and 12 hours for lorazepam, reflect this difference in Cl. On the other hand, chlordiazepoxide and lorazepam have similar T½s (12 hours), but their Cls (20 ml/min for chlordiazepoxide, 53 ml/min for lorazepam) and Vds (0.4 L/kg for chlordiazepoxide, 1.3 L/kg for lorazepam) differ significantly (Arris et al. 1988).

The selective serotonin reuptake inhibitors (SSRIs) also demonstrate the clinical importance of drug T½s. Fluoxetine has as its principal active metabolite, norfluoxetine, which has a T½ of more than 10 days. Thus, 3 to 4 weeks may be required to achieve steady state after initiation or change of dosing. In contrast, paroxetine (T½ 24 hours) and sertraline (T½ 24 hours) may reach steady-state concentration much more rapidly, thus allowing the clinician to make dose adjustments (according to assessment of therapeutic and toxic responses) more quickly (Fogel and Stoudemire 1993).

Although T½ determines the time required to achieve steady state, Cl of the drug from the body determines the magnitude of steady-state concentration (Brater and Vasko 1988; DeVane 1990; Winter 1988a). Thus, for the benzodiazepine examples in the preceding paragraph, chlordiazepoxide and lorazepam require similar times to reach steady state after a single oral dose (40–60 hours), but the magnitudes of concentration achieved at steady state will be different (i.e., chlordiazepoxide higher than lorazepam). Moreover, long-acting (long-T½) benzodiazepines such as diazepam (T½ 20–50 hours) administered chronically can accumulate and thus cause problematic toxicity, partic-

increasing doses, their T½s increase and their Cls decrease. For example, increasing phenytoin dose from 200 to 300 mg/day may increase the steady-state blood level from 10 to 15 µg/ml. However, when metabolic enzymes are saturated by a further increase in dose from 300 to 400 mg/day, the blood concentration may rise from 15 to 30 µg/ml or more. Therefore, increases in dosage above the "usual normal dose" (i.e., that generally found to be clinically effective) should be made in very small increments, particularly in medically ill patients who may have disease-induced loss of metabolic capacity (Brater and Vasko 1988).

Theoretically, all drugs are capable of saturating their metabolic sites, thus shifting from first- to zero-order kinetics. However, plasma concentrations high enough to accomplish this transition are rarely attained. Nevertheless, when several drugs are coadministered (e.g., carbamazepine and a tricyclic antidepressant [TCA]), they may compete for the same metabolic sites, thus reducing the individual concentrations necessary for saturation (and a switch from first- to zero-order kinetics) (DeVane 1990a; Rowland and Tozer 1989). A complete discussion of drug interactions and alteration of pharmacokinetic parameters is not within the scope of this chapter, but a number of excellent reviews are available elsewhere (Glassman and Salzman 1987; Pond 1984; Vasko and Brater 1988; Watsky and Salzman 1991).

DISEASE AND PSYCHOPHARMACOKINETICS

Disease can affect absorption, distribution, metabolism, and excretion of drugs. Often, several pharmacokinetic parameters are altered and vary over time. Few medically ill patients are unmedicated; both the pharmacodynamic and pharmacokinetic effects of individual drugs and drug combinations must be considered when selecting medications and determining appropriate dosages. Although many diagnostic procedures and laboratory values help to establish the presence of organ system dysfunction, few are useful in predicting the extent of pharmacokinetic disruption. Psychiatric symptomatology and side-effect profiles will generally guide the clinician in selection of drug class, but familiarity with psychopharmacokinetics must play an important role in selection of a drug and dosage. Route of administration, an important determinant of pharmacokinetics, may also be dictated by patients' medical conditions.

GASTROINTESTINAL DISEASE

Most orally administered psychotropic drugs are absorbed by the proximal ileum (Brater and Vasko 1988; DeVane 1990a). As discussed earlier in this chapter, disease can alter drug absorption in various ways, including changing GI motility or pH, decreasing functional absorptive surface area (e.g., when disease necessitates surgical resection), disrupting mucosal function, or diverting blood flow to other organ systems. In general, slowed GI motility results in better absorption of poorly soluble drugs and decreased rate or extent of absorption of others. Various drugs (e.g., metoclopramide, narcotics) alter gastric emptying time and thus change the rate of drug absorption (Brater and Vasko 1988). Absorption of drugs, particularly enteric-coated and slow-release formulations, may be inhibited by rapid intestinal transit time because of diarrhea (Welling 1984). Changes in GI motility are difficult to quantitate; the clinician must rely on plasma drug concentration measurements to select the dosage.

Routine serial measurements of gastric acidity are not clinically feasible. Moreover, no useful guidelines exist to employ such data in making dose adjustments when pH changes have altered pharmacokinetics. However, changes in gastric acidity may affect absorption of orally administered psychotropic agents. Weak bases (e.g., phenothiazines, TCAs, most benzodiazepines) would dissolve best in an acidic environment where they are ionized, but they are not well absorbed. Most psychotropic drugs will be absorbed in the more alkaline environment of the small intestine (Cassem et al. 1988). The absorption of some psychotropic drugs (e.g., chlordiazepoxide) is unaffected by concomitant antacid administration, but absorption of others (e.g., chlorpromazine) appears to be decreased by antacids (Johnson and Cattau 1988). However, it is not possible to predict the effects of concomitant antacid administration knowing only a psychotropic drug's pKa. Histamine (H_2) blockers such as cimetidine and ranitidine inhibit all phases of gastric secretion, including that of pepsin, mucus, and acid (Johnson and Cattau 1988). Aside from cimetidine's influence on P_{450} metabolism, little evidence supports consistently predictable, clinically significant kinetic changes for psychotropics coadministered with cimetidine. Plasma drug levels, when available, are the most easily used tools for adjustment of psychotropic drug dosages when disease has altered GI pH.

Likewise, there are no easily applied indices of altered drug absorption when disease has changed mucosal surface area or function.

Surgical procedures (e.g., jejunoileal bypass, J-tube placement) may alter drug absorption by reducing epithelial surface area or by changing motility or secretory patterns. On the other hand, psychotropic drug absorption is minimally affected by GI disease localized to the large intestine, because absorption of most psychotropic drugs occurs in the proximal small intestine, as previously mentioned (Welling 1984). Some drugs may be well absorbed after sublingual or rectal administration; this may be helpful when the clinician wants to restrict the number of drugs an "NPO" (nothing by mouth) patient receives by intramuscular and intravenous routes (Tables 1–2 and 1–3). (Rectal administration of doxepin and carbamazepine is discussed in Chapter 2.)

Anxiolytic Drugs in GI Disease

Kinetic parameters are of primary importance in the selection of antianxiety agents, in contrast to other classes of psychotropic agents for which potencies govern side-effect profiles (Santos et al. 1992). All benzodiazepines are lipid soluble, so that they are nearly totally absorbed from the GI tract, despite different rates of dissolution and absorption. The rapidity of pharmacologic effect after a single benzodiazepine dose is well correlated with absorption rate (DeVane 1990a). Most drugs are best absorbed on an empty stomach. Food may alter the rate of benzodiazepine absorption but usually does not affect the extent (Cassem et al. 1988). Rate of absorption governs rapidity of onset of action; this must be remembered when selecting benzodiazepines (and doses) for patients with GI disease. The preferred route of administration may also limit benzodiazepine choice.

Clorazepate is a benzodiazepine whose pharmacologic activation is dependent on gastric pH. It is administered in an inactive form that is converted to desmethyldiazepam in the stomach before absorption. A lower gastric pH allows faster hydrolysis. When gastric pH is increased by disease (or other medications), the clinical effects of clorazepate are attenuated (DeVane 1990a).

Antipsychotic Drugs in GI Disease

Antipsychotic drugs are generally well absorbed from the GI tract (primarily the jejunum), but they undergo extensive presystemic elimination via biotransformation by the gut wall and liver. As previously mentioned, parenteral administration not only circumvents problems of GI absorption but also avoids first-pass hepatic metabolism. Thus, a lower dose is usually required for parenteral administration.

Several antipsychotic drugs are available for parenteral administration (Table 1–3). Despite the availability of these formulations, the clinician may want to avoid use of chlorpromazine in patients with GI disease; this drug undergoes extensive metabolism by enzymes in the gut wall (Cassem et al. 1988), thus rendering disease-induced pharmacokinetic changes unpredictable. Moreover, Crohn's disease, which is associated with elevated AAGP levels, may increase circulating chlorpromazine concentrations (Piafsky et al. 1978). The overall pharmacokinetic effect of GI disease on chlorpromazine disposition has not been closely studied in a clinically applicable format. Unfortunately, there has been little study of disease-induced changes in absorption of antipsychotic drugs other than chlorpromazine, which is now rarely employed in medical-surgical settings.

Antipsychotic drug formulation may affect absorption, as illustrated by the more complete absorption of liquid-concentrate preparations. However, liquid concentrates can form insoluble precipitates when these drugs are given with milk, fruit juice, coffee, or tea (DeVane 1990a). One must also remember the anticholinergic effect of slowing gastric motility when antipsychotic drugs are given to patients with GI disease.

Antidepressant and Mood-Stabilizing Drugs in GI Disease

TCAs, monoamine oxidase inhibitors (MAOIs), and SSRIs are all generally well absorbed after an oral dose (Aronoff et al. 1984; DeVane 1990a; Lemberger et al. 1985; Roerig 1992; Schenker et al. 1988; SmithKline Beecham Pharmaceuticals 1992; Wernicke 1985). Administration with food seems to have little effect on absorption of the TCAs, although this issue has not been extensively studied for any of these medications. Some TCAs (e.g., nortriptyline) and fluoxetine are available in liquid forms (Table 1–3). As noted earlier in this chapter, solutions and suspensions are more quickly absorbed than their solid equivalents. The slowing of GI motility by very anticholinergic TCAs (e.g., amitriptyline, protriptyline, domipamine) must be kept in mind for patients with GI disease. Fluoxetine (Wernicke 1985), sertraline (Roerig 1992), paroxetine (SmithKline Beecham Pharmaceuticals 1992), and trazodone may cause GI distress.

Several groups of investigators (Brunswick et al. 1979; Cooper and Simpson 1978; Montgomery et al. 1979) reported methods for dosage adjustment using blood levels of imipramine, desipramine, or nortriptyline after a single dose of drug. However, studies on which these methods are based generally used medically healthy subjects. In the complex setting of medical illness and polypharmacy, individual patient response and steady-state drug levels are likely to be more useful clinical guides.

Lithium. Conventional lithium carbonate tablets and capsules are usually 95%–100% absorbed via the GI tract. Although capsules usually require more time than tablets to dissolve, the dissolution differences do not appear to be clinically significant. Peak serum lithium concentrations after administration of lithium carbonate capsules or tablets occur within 0.5 to 3 hours. Lithium citrate oral solutions are essentially 100% absorbed; peak serum lithium concentration occurs within 15 to 60 minutes after lithium citrate administration (McEvoy 1993). Extended- and sustained-release lithium preparations have wide variability (i.e., 60%–90%) in completeness of absorption (Amidsen and Carson 1986). Peak serum lithium concentrations occur within 4 to 12 hours of administration of extended-release formulations (McEvoy 1993). Some studies indicate that once-daily lithium may reduce lithium-induced tubular dysfunction and resultant polyuria (Bowen et al. 1991). Plenge and co-workers (1982) have demonstrated that urine volume is positively correlated with the trough lithium serum concentration during a 24-hour period. To minimize the risk of lithium-associated renal dysfunction, theoretically at least, the clinician should use a sustained-release lithium preparation, especially in patients with existing medical illnesses. GI disease may disrupt lithium absorption in an unpredictable manner. Thus, regular monitoring of serum lithium concentrations is the best way to select the proper lithium formulation and to adjust the dose. Furthermore, when switching lithium preparations, the serum lithium concentration and its variation over time must be reassessed.

In cases of gastroenteritis or other diarrheal disease, lithium absorption by the small intestine may be decreased, most significantly when a slow-release formulation is used (Erlich and Diamond 1983). Lithium has been administered to humans via parenteral routes, but this is a rare and unproven practice at this time (Santos et al. 1992). Cooper and Simpson (1976) developed a method to predict individual lithium dose requirements with a single test dose (600 mg) of lithium and a blood level drawn 24 hours later. A nomogram reveals the expected daily dose requirement for a healthy adult. More conservative initial dosing is recommended for medically ill or elderly patients, however. Careful monitoring of blood levels and patient response is always advisable.

Carbamazepine. Not unexpectedly, carbamazepine (with its structural resemblance to the TCAs) is well absorbed when given orally (DeVane 1990a; Ellenhorn and Barcelous 1988). Tegretol suspension is available. Studies in healthy individuals indicate that both suspension and tablet forms deliver equivalent amounts of drug to the systemic circulation, but the suspension is absorbed faster than the tablet. Following a twice-a-day dosage regimen, the suspension had higher peak levels and lower trough levels than those obtained from the tablet formulation (given by the same dosage regimen). However, three-times-a-day dosing of the suspension afforded steady-state plasma levels comparable to Tegretol tablets given twice a day, administered at the same total milligram daily dose (Physicians' Desk Reference 1991). In general, careful monitoring of plasma concentrations of mood-stabilizing and antidepressant drugs is recommended for patients with altered GI function.

Valproate. The formulation of valproate determines its rate of absorption. However, in general, it is fully absorbed—the bioavailability approaches 100% with all preparations (Levy and Shen 1989; Wilder 1992). Rapid-release formulations, including syrup, capsule, and tablet, are absorbed by healthy subjects with peak times of less than 2 hours. Enteric-coated tablets are more variable in rate of absorption, but these times are often delayed by 3 hours or more. A sprinkle capsule has been developed to avoid GI side effects, which are generally dose-related and tend to occur during the rapid rise in serum valproate level. The sprinkle pellets' release is slow and sustained over 4 to 6 hours (Wilder 1992). As a result of the favorable absorption characteristics of the sprinkle valproate formulation, it may be preferred in medically ill patients with increased susceptibility or sensitivity to nausea. Indeed, some of the CNS side effects such as lethargy and lassitude may be alleviated by using a valproate formulation with a more sustained, slow rate of absorption. On the other hand, if disease (e.g., surgical GI alterations, syndromes with increased GI motility) alters

confused" patients. There are few published studies of the effects CHF has on delivery of psychotropic agents to the brain. Therefore, the clinician must rely on subjective and objective indices of response when selecting psychotropic drugs and making dose adjustments.

Antipsychotic and Antidepressant Drugs in Cardiac Disease

When treating patients with existing cardiovascular disease, clinicians must recall that TCAs and antipsychotic drugs have anticholinergic, antiadrenergic, and quinidine-like effects. These side effects can include alterations of heart rate, rhythm, electrical conduction, blood pressure, and myocontractility (Stoudemire et al. 1993). Heart rate may increase (10 to 20 beats/minute) when TCA therapy is initiated. In some patients, this chronotropic effect may be beneficial, but in others, the increased heart rate may worsen CHF and require discontinuation of the TCA (Vrobel 1989).

Animal studies (Cairncross and Gershon 1962; Sigg et al. 1963) have attributed a negative inotropic effect to TCAs, but clinical studies employing radionuclide ventriculograms of patients with CHF have failed to demonstrate any significant change in ventricular ejection fractions after starting antidepressant drugs (Glassman et al. 1983; Jefferson 1975; Veith et al. 1982; Vrobel 1989). However, Dalack and associates (1991) reported a case of worsened CHF when a patient with preexisting cardiovascular disease (e.g., ejection fraction less than 25%) was given nortriptyline and, later, doxepin. Dalack and co-workers point out that unusually high levels of hydroxy metabolites (of TCAs) may have been responsible. A separate study comparing the cardiovascular effects of the TCA imipramine and another antidepressant, bupropion, showed that bupropion does not affect ejection fraction or other indices of left ventricular function in patients with CHF (Roose et al. 1987). Furthermore, depressed patients with CHF, when treated with imipramine, are at relatively high risk for developing orthostatic hypotension, compared with depressed patients who are otherwise "medically" healthy (Glassman et al. 1983). Glassman and colleagues (1979) also produced evidence suggesting that CHF patients with preexisting orthostatic hypotension are more susceptible to exacerbation of this symptom by imipramine.

Some antidepressants such as the SSRIs (Roerig 1992; SmithKline Beecham Pharmaceuticals 1992; Wernicke 1985) and trazodone (Feighner 1981; Vrobel 1989) have been reported to have less anticholinergic and quinidine-like activity than TCAs. The SSRI paroxetine is weakly anticholinergic (Caley and Weber 1993) but less so than many of the TCAs (Jenner 1992), including imipramine (Feighner et al. 1993). Rarely, ventricular and supraventricular arrhythmias have been attributed to antidepressant drugs (Janowsky et al. 1983; Zavodnick 1981). An SSRI or bupropion may therefore be preferable in cardiovascularly compromised individuals. The antipsychotic drugs thioridazine (Risch et al. 1982) and pimozide (Fulop et al. 1987) have been shown to be particularly arrhythmogenic; thus, they are generally not used in patients with severe cardiac disease (Arana and Hyman 1991). Overall, little information is available about how CHF influences the pharmacokinetics of psychotropic agents. Recent controversy over the use of tricyclics in the post–myocardial infarction period is discussed in Chapter 2 of this volume.

Mood-Stabilizing Drugs in Cardiac Disease

Electrocardiographic changes (T-wave flattening or inversion, most commonly), arrhythmias (sinus node dysfunction, most commonly), and sudden death have been associated with lithium use (DasGupta and Jefferson 1990; Tilkian et al. 1976). However, lithium appears to have few adverse effects on the inotropic state of the heart and on blood pressure (Eisenberg et al. 1960; Jefferson and Greist 1977; Levenson et al. 1986; Lydiard and Gelenberg 1982; Lyman et al. 1984; Vrobel 1989). Although reversible repolarization changes have been attributed to lithium, they are not considered indicators of significant cardiotoxicity nor of the need to reduce lithium dosage. Recent studies of lithium's effects on cardiac conduction are also discussed in Chapter 2.

Lithium has been suggested as both a precipitant and ameliorator of CHF (DasGupta and Jefferson 1990). A 900-mg lithium carbonate dose is equivalent to a "salt load" of approximately 24 mEq (DeVane 1990a). Lithium kinetics are similar to those of sodium; the kidney handles both elements in a similar manner. Many clinicians are aware of the possibility of enhanced lithium toxicity in cases of serum sodium restriction or depletion. Nevertheless, no systematic studies have demonstrated a consistent association between lithium dose and exacerbation of CHF.

CHF theoretically affects lithium pharmacokinetics via reduction of lithium Cl mediated by a decrease in the GFR (Vrobel 1989). However, the preponderance of data argues against clinical significance in this regard (Bendz 1983; Boton et al. 1987; DasGupta and Jefferson 1990; Schou 1988; Vaamonde et al. 1986). The effects of diuretics and dietary sodium chloride restriction on lithium pharmacokinetics are more well known. (The interested reader is referred to DasGupta and Jefferson [1990] for a synopsis of the literature on the effects of various diuretics on serum lithium levels.) Clinical response and serial plasma lithium levels are the best guide to lithium dose adjustment in patients with CHF.

HEPATIC DISEASE

Liver disease is associated with many psychiatric symptoms. Clinicians must become familiar with effects of disease-associated alterations of pharmacokinetics to select appropriate psychotropic agents and dose adjustments for patients with liver disease. Absorption, distribution, metabolism, and excretion may change in patients with compromised liver function. The liver has significant reserve and repair capacities; thus, it is often difficult to determine the extent of liver damage and to predict its effect on the pharmacokinetics of a specific drug at a particular time. Pharmacologic agents vary in their sensitivity to disease-induced alterations of liver function.

Hepatic Blood Flow

Cirrhosis is characterized by distortion of liver architecture and resultant changes in the pattern of blood flow through the organ. As resistance to blood flow through the liver increases, portal venous blood pressure rises. In response to this disruption, blood is shunted around the liver through collateral channels into the systemic circulation. This portosystemic shunting can affect the absorption of an orally administered drug (Arris et al. 1988; Grossman et al. 1972; Secor and Schenker 1987; Syrota et al. 1976, 1981; Wilkinson and Branch 1984) (Table 1–2). In severely cirrhotic patients, portosystemic shunting may involve 60% or more of the total portal vein flow.

Bioavailability of drugs whose disposition is determined primarily by effective HBF—*flow limited* (e.g., propranolol, verapamil, TCAs)—is altered by portosystemic shunting; peak blood concentration following a single oral dose is expected to be significantly higher in patients with cirrhosis (and associated portosystemic shunting) versus healthy individuals. Drugs whose dispositions are determined primarily by hepatic metabolic rates—*enzyme limited*—would be expected to show comparatively little change in their bioavailabilities as a result of liver blood flow shunting (Secor and Schenker 1987). Drugs that are normally rapidly extracted by the liver (i.e., those that are flow limited) will be handled more like enzyme-limited drugs in patients with cirrhosis-associated blood flow shunting. Moreover, intrahepatic shunts route drugs around functioning hepatocytes and thereby reduce drug metabolism (Huet and Villeneuve 1983; Secor and Schenker 1987). Peak blood concentrations of enzyme-limited drugs (e.g., chlordiazepoxide, lorazepam, oxazepam, chlorpromazine) following a single oral dose are essentially the same in patients with cirrhosis and in healthy people (Arris et al. 1988). This feature of enzyme-limited drugs is clinically relevant only when a single dose is to be used, as in an emergent need to sedate an agitated patient. More commonly, however, psychotropic therapy is achieved by repeated (chronic) dosing; thus, the distinction between enzyme- and flow-limited drugs is less clinically meaningful.

HBF may be increased by chronic respiratory problems, viral hepatitis, severe diarrhea, and drugs such as clonidine and low-dose dopamine (Wilkinson 1976; Wilkinson and Branch 1984) (Table 1–2). Pharmacokinetic complications (see previous paragraph for examples) arising from disease-associated changes in liver blood flow may be partially circumvented by the use of parenteral psychotropic agents. HBF is most commonly reduced by severe cirrhosis; therefore, a psychotropic agent with less liver-dependent excretion is preferable (e.g., lithium favored over carbamazepine; oxazepam favored over diazepam). When all members of the indicated psychotropic class undergo significant hepatic metabolism (e.g., antipsychotics, antidepressants), parenteral administration to patients with severe cirrhosis may be preferred, theoretically avoiding HBF-induced reduction in the drug's first-pass metabolism.

Quantitation of disease-induced HBF changes is not feasible for the purpose of calculating alterations of other pharmacokinetic parameters. (Please refer to "Cardiac Disease" section for a discussion of experimental indices of changes in local blood flow.) Hepatic disease rarely affects HBF in isolation; usually, there are associated changes in plasma protein binding, hepatic metabolic activity, and bile secretion. Thus, parenteral administration of psychotropic agents with easily monitored efficacy and toxicity and easily measured clinically meaningful serum levels may simplify psychopharmacology in patients with liver disease.

Protein Binding

Hepatic disease affects drug distribution via changes in quantities and affinities of binding proteins (Table 1–2). Hepatocytes synthesize plasma proteins such as albumin and AAGP. Infectious and inflammatory diseases of the liver (e.g., celiac and Crohn's diseases), surgery, and trauma result in substantial increases of the acute-phase reactant AAGP. Production of AAGP may be increased in some patients with cirrhosis (Winter 1988a). However, albumin levels are generally decreased in hepatic diseases such as cirrhosis and liver abscess (Leipzig 1990). (For clinical examples, please refer to the explanation of the clinical implications of altered protein binding in the "Distribution" section.)

Damaged hepatocytes may produce defective plasma proteins. These altered proteins may have decreased binding affinities for their usual ligands. Patients with cirrhosis have markedly increased free fractions of both acidic and basic drugs. In contrast, patients with acute viral hepatitis have smaller increases (Blaschke 1977; Leipzig 1990; Reidenberg and Affrime 1973; Wilkinson and Branch 1984). Theoretically, a cirrhosis-induced decrease in plasma protein binding affinity may result in a heightened therapeutic or toxic response (despite an unchanged steady-state measurement of total drug concentration in plasma). Specific psychotropic drugs affected by these conditions are discussed in the following sections.

Acute viral hepatitis and primary biliary cirrhosis may elevate serum bilirubin levels. Bilirubin has a strong affinity for binding sites on albumin and thus may displace acidic drugs (e.g., valproate, phenytoin) normally bound by this protein. Liver disease often results in accumulation of both endogenous and exogenous substances that can displace drugs from their usual protein binding sites (Blaschke et al. 1975; Leipzig 1990). Again, the clinician must be cognizant of possible heightened drug response (therapeutic or toxic) during unchanged total drug concentrations. Dose reductions may be preferable or necessary for patients with liver disease and associated hyperbilirubinemia.

A drug's apparent Vd is increased when its protein binding is decreased. Recall the equation relating T½ to Vd: $T\frac{1}{2} = 0.693Vd/Cl$. As previously noted, T½ can be very misleading in the determination of the effect of liver disease on drug elimination. An increase in apparent Vd may lead to a prolongation of elimination T½ in the absence of any significant change in metabolic elimination. In general, enzyme-limited drugs (e.g., chlordiazepoxide, lorazepam, oxazepam, chlorpromazine) are more likely to be sensitive to changes of elimination caused by decreased protein binding. Increases in free drug fraction associated with decreases in protein binding result in increased availability of free drug to metabolic enzymes that at least partially offsets disease-associated decreases in hepatocyte metabolic capability. In such situations, total drug Cl may be minimally affected. However, changes in drug binding and metabolism are not always clinically insignificant; the increased free (pharmacologically active) fraction may cause an exaggerated clinical response that requires dose reduction (Leipzig 1990).

The significance of disease-induced changes in protein binding depends on two issues: 1) the resultant change in free fraction of the specific drug and 2) the drug's therapeutic index. In general, the degree of liver damage is reflected by the extent of change in drug binding to plasma proteins. Cirrhosis tends to cause more significant change in the binding of drugs than does acute viral hepatitis. More extensively bound (greater than 60%) drugs—the vast majority of psychotropic agents—are affected more than poorly bound drugs (e.g., lithium). No practical methods are available to predict drug binding changes that result from altered protein binding. Thus, serum drug (bound + free) concentrations must be interpreted in the context of observed therapeutic effects and toxicity. A drug with a narrow therapeutic margin (e.g., carbamazepine or valproate) is more likely to be significantly affected by changes in protein binding than is a drug with a large therapeutic index (e.g., a benzodiazepine). Altered drug binding should not be the sole influence on clinical decisions regarding dose adjustments, because liver disease most often results in multiple pharmacokinetic parameter changes (Blaschke et al. 1975).

Ascites

Hepatic disease also influences drug distribution via formation of ascites (Table 1–2). Ascitic fluid contains albumin and other plasma proteins. If protein synthetic function is also compromised, the development of ascites may reduce serum proteins and binding of drugs. Drugs are then less confined to the vascular space; their apparent Vds change (Blaschke et al. 1975). The volume of ascites is usually greater than 3 L before it becomes clinically apparent. Massive ascites may exceed 20 L (Blaschke et al. 1975; Wilkinson and Williams 1979).

Hepatic Metabolism

Drug metabolism is often affected by liver disease, but not all metabolic pathways within the liver are equally influenced by a given disease entity (Table 1–2). Water-soluble drugs (e.g., lithium, conjugated drugs/metabolites) are usually excreted by the kidney, requiring little or no modification by disease-altered hepatic metabolism. Lipid-soluble drugs (most psychotropic agents), on the other hand, are generally metabolized to more polar, water-soluble forms before elimination. Phase I oxidation reactions, affecting psychotropics such as TCAs, SSRIs, antipsychotics, and some benzodiazepines (Table 1–4), which may result in either pharmacologic activation or inactivation, occur primarily in the smooth endoplasmic reticulum of the cytochrome P_{450} (CyP_{450}) system localized in the pericentral regions of the liver. Reductases and hydrolases are cytoplasmic. Phase II reactions (such as those primarily responsible for metabolism of phase I products and the benzodiazepines lorazepam, temazepam, and oxazepam; Table 1–4) transform agents to more polar metabolites by attaching hydrophilic moieties such as glucuronyl, acetyl, and sulfate groups. Glucuronyl transferases are most highly concentrated in the periportal regions, whereas acetylases are more localized to the pericentral regions (Secor and Schenker 1987). (Other phase II reactions include conjugation to glycine, glutamine, or glutathione. Few psychotropic agents are known to be significantly metabolized in this manner.)

Distinct subfamilies of CyP_{450} enzymes have been identified; each is subject to independent genetic control and has relatively specific affinity for certain subgroups of drugs. CyP_{450}-2D6 mediates the biotransformation of the psychotropic drugs desipramine, nortriptyline, perphenazine, and thioridazine (von Moltke et al. 1994). Quinidine is a highly potent inhibitor of P_{450}-2D6 (Otton et al. 1988; von Moltke et al. 1994). The SSRI antidepressants are also inhibitors of this cytochrome 450 subfamily. Fluoxetine, norfluoxetine, and paroxetine are more potent inhibitors of P_{450}-2D6 than are sertraline and its principal metabolite desmethylsertraline (Crewe et al. 1992) (Table 1–7).

Another cytochrome subfamily, P_{450}-3A4, mediates the biotransformation of some psychotropic drugs including triazolam, alprazolam, and midazolam (Kronbach et al. 1989). CyP_{450}3A4 metabolizes the antidepressants nefazodone and sertraline. In addition, the initial demethylation of imipramine and amitriptyline has been attributed to P_{450}-3A4 (Lemoine et al. 1993; Ohmori et al. 1993). Ketoconazole (Gascon and Dayer 1991) and cimetidine (von Moltke et al. 1994) have been identified as important inhibitors of P_{450}-3A4. The SSRIs inhibit the P_{450}-3A4 subfamily as well as the P_{450}-D26 subfamily, but SSRI inhibition potency for the P_{450}-3A4 subfamily is less than that for the latter (von Moltke et al. 1994).

The clinical relevance of the cytochrome subfamilies, their substrates, and their inhibitors is highlighted by the following examples. If a patient is being treated with the antiarrhythmic agent quinidine, the biotransformation of nortriptyline by P_{450}-2D6 may be inhibited, thus causing an increased serum nortriptyline level to exceed the "therapeutic window" and extend into the toxic range. Moreover, when fluoxetine (an inhibitor of P_{450}-2D6 and P_{450}-3A4) is coadministered with clonazepam (metabolized primarily by nitro-reduction rather than by P_{450} oxidation), the SSRI is not likely to increase serum levels of clonazepam, in contrast to its tendency to increase levels of P_{450}-2D6 substrates (e.g., desipramine) and P_{450}-3A4 substrates (e.g., alprazolam). On the other hand, if a transplant patient taking cyclosporine is given midazolam as a sedative for a brief diagnostic procedure, the cyclosporine might compete more effectively for enzyme metabolic sites, thus prolonging biotransfomation (inactivation) of midazolam and extending the sedative effect. The clinical relevance for psychotropic serum levels of various medications inhibiting or competing for CyP_{450} enzymes is extensively discussed in Chapter 2 of this volume.

Disease may characteristically affect a particular anatomic region of the liver and alter some metabolic processes more than others. For example, acute viral hepatitis and alcoholic liver disease have a more pronounced effect on the pericentral regions where oxidative metabolic reactions are concentrated. Therefore, these diseases may be expected to affect metabolism of most psychotropic agents (with notable exceptions including lithium and the benzodiazepines lorazepam, oxazepam, and temazepam). In the absence of cirrhosis, chronic hepatitis predominantly affects periportal regions, thus sparing some hepatic oxidative function (Pauwels et al. 1982; Secor and Schenker 1987). In its early stages, primary biliary cirrhosis primarily affects periportal regions (Kraus et al. 1978; Secor and Schenker 1987).

Acute and chronic liver disease tends to spare glucuronidation reactions (Hoyumpa and Schenker 1982; Kraus et al. 1978; Levi et al. 1968; Secor and Schenker 1987). This relative preservation of function is attributed to a large reserve of glucuronidating enzymes that may be activated by liver disease and to the existence of extrahepatic (gut,

Table 1–7. Partial listing of cytochrome P_{450} enzyme biotransformations

Subfamily	Psychotropic drugs biotransformed	Nonpsychiatric drugs biotransformed	Inhibitors
P_{450}-2D6	Desipramine Nortriptyline Clomipramine Perphenazine Thioridazine Paroxetine Fluoxetine	Encainaide Mexiletine Codeine Dextromethorphan Propranolol	Quinidine Fluoxetine, norfluoxetine, paroxetine, sertraline, and desmethylsertraline
P_{450}-3A4	Triazolam Alprazolam Midazolam Imipramine Amitriptyline Sertraline	Cyclosporine Terfenadine Lidocaine Nifedipine Quinidine Carbamazepine	Ketoconazole Cimetidine SSRIs, but less potently than P_{450}-2D6 Nefazodone Erythromycin

Source. Crewe et al. 1992; Gascon and Dayer 1991; Kronbach et al. 1989; Lemoine et al. 1993; Ohmori et al. 1993; Otton et al. 1988; von Moltke et al. 1994.

kidney) glucuronidation systems. Many psychotropic agents require phase I metabolism before phase II glucuronide conjugation. However, drugs that are primarily metabolized by glucuronide conjugation (e.g., lorazepam, temazepam, oxazepam) are less likely to be pharmacokinetically affected by liver disease. Thus, clinicians often prefer to administer drugs with minimal requirements for hepatic metabolism to patients with liver disease; dose reductions may not be necessary when such drugs are used.

Hepatic clearance (Cl_H) is a pharmacokinetic parameter that indicates the efficiency with which the liver irreversibly removes a drug from the blood. Cl_H is determined by 1) the fraction of drug removed from the blood during passage through the liver (**E**) and 2) liver blood flow (**Q_H**). The equation relating these parameters is

$$Cl_H = Q_H E$$

The liver's extraction ability is dependent on 1) intrinsic activity of metabolic enzymes and transport processes within the liver that irreversibly remove drug from the blood, 2) the fraction of total drug that is free to interact with eliminative enzymes, and 3) the rate at which drug passes through the liver (Arris et al. 1988; Rowland et al. 1973; Wilkinson and Shand 1975) (Table 1–2).

Systemic availability is defined as the ratio of plasma drug concentration after oral versus intravenous administration. This depends on the degree to which a drug's metabolism is dependent on liver blood flow. Bioavailability of the drug is the portion of drug left in the circulation after its first pass through the liver. This equation defines bioavailability:

$$\text{Bioavailability} = 1 - \text{extraction ratio}$$

The classification of drugs into flow-limited and enzyme-limited categories (see "Hepatic Blood Flow" section earlier in the chapter for a discussion of this concept) can be misleading because cirrhosis often disrupts both blood flow and metabolic capacity of the liver. Drugs that are normally highly extracted by the liver (e.g., TCAs) are generally given to patients without liver disease in relatively high oral doses to compensate for hepatic removal to achieve adequate blood levels. In patients with cirrhosis, however, these drugs may behave more like enzyme-linked agents (e.g., benzodiazepines), and dose reductions may be required. This concept is significant because when extraction of a psychotropic agent is markedly reduced by liver disease, the drug's systematic availability and toxicity may be enhanced (Secor and Schenker 1987); dose reduction is thereby indicated.

General Considerations

Ultimately, the clinician's practical concerns are selecting a psychotropic agent and deciding whether dose adjustments are required for a specific patient with a particular type of liver disease. Drug selection depends on indications for its use and assessment of its benefits and risks. These pharmacodynamic considerations are not within the scope of this review. In general, however, the pertinent questions are 1) Can the drug cause liver damage even in healthy subjects? 2) Will the drug further compromise disrupted function in individuals with liver disease? 3) Is the drug likely to exacerbate extrahepatic complications of liver disease (e.g., encephalopathy)? It is often wise to select drugs that are extensively eliminated by the kidneys or that utilize metabolic pathways that are spared by the disease (Arris et al. 1988). However, note that liver disease can be associated with renal impairment, as we discuss later in this chapter.

An indicator of the severity of liver damage would be extremely helpful in determining whether dose adjustment is necessary. Commonly available laboratory liver function tests (e.g., serum glutamic-oxaloacetic transaminase [SGOT], serum glutamic-pyruvic transaminase [SGPT], bilirubin, prothrombin time [PT], activated partial thromboplastin time [APTT]) reflect liver damage but do not necessarily indicate its extent (Arris et al. 1988). CyP_{450} levels of liver biopsies have been measured in experimental settings. P_{450} levels are essentially normal in fatty liver, mild viral hepatitis, and early primary biliary cirrhosis. Under these conditions, P_{450}-related drug metabolism appears relatively undisturbed. However, alcoholic hepatitis and active cirrhosis have been associated with 30%–50% reductions in CyP_{450} levels, correlating with decreased P_{450} drug metabolism in patients with these diseases (Farrell et al. 1979; Secor and Schenker 1987). P_{450} levels are not generally clinically available. Their practical application in guiding dose adjustment requires further study (Homeida et al. 1979; Pirttiaho et al. 1978).

In general, minimal dosage adjustments are required for patients with "compensated cirrhosis," i.e., with essentially normal albumin, bilirubin, and prothrombin levels and absence of ascites or prior encephalopathy (Child's class A). However, patients with decompensated cirrhosis or alcoholic hepatitis, characterized by albumin less than 3.0 g/dl, bilirubin greater than 3.0 mg/dl, PT greater than 3 seconds over control, and the presence of ascites or encephalopathy (Child's class C), usually require significant dose adjustment of hepatically metabolized drugs. Patients with Child's class C liver disease are also more likely to exhibit alteration of renal drug Cl. A good rule of thumb is to reduce the initial dose of a psychotropic agent by 50% when it is to be administered to a patient with severe (Child's class C) liver disease. Such dose reductions are particularly important when a primarily hepatically metabolized drug with a relatively low therapeutic index (e.g., TCA, carbamazepine) is used. When liver disease decreases the Cl of a psychotropic drug, its dosage can be proportionally decreased, or its dosing interval can be lengthened (Secor and Schenker 1987). Increasing the dosing interval might be necessary or preferable in patients who regularly undergo dialysis (e.g., when the drug's hepatic metabolite is ultimately excreted by the kidney, in a healthy subject, as for most TCAs and antipsychotic drugs).

Associated Renal Disease

As mentioned earlier in this chapter, renal handling of drugs may be disturbed in liver disease. Mechanisms responsible for these changes in renal pharmacokinetics include 1) alterations in renal hemodynamics (Anderson et al. 1986; Laffi et al. 1986; Wilkinson and Williams 1979), 2) competition between coadministered drugs, and 3) impairment of the tubular secretion of organic cations (Bunke et al. 1983; Secor and Schenker 1987; Villeneuve et al. 1983). Patients with cirrhosis may have altered renal function despite a normal serum creatinine value. Creatinine Cl is a more useful marker in this setting (Secor and Schenker 1987). Because most drugs are cleared by hepatic and renal mechanisms, systemic Cl is generally equal to the sum of the fractions of drug eliminated by these two organs:

Systemic Cl = hepatic Cl + renal Cl

Hepatic Cl is often calculated (rather than measured) because renal Cl, derived from urine measurements, is more easily determined than hepatic Cl, which requires hepatic vein sampling (Secor and Schenker

1987). As renal function approaches zero, the importance of nonrenal Cl increases (Rowland and Tozer 1989). (See the following section, "Renal Disease," for further discussion of appropriate drug selection and dose adjustment.)

In summary, many factors must be considered in the selection and dosage of psychotropic agents for patients with liver disease. These factors include severity of liver damage, alterations in blood flow and associated changes in drug absorption and distribution, effects on protein binding, route of administration, need for single-dose or chronic therapy, and other individual variables such as patient age, smoking, and genetics. Management of these patients' symptoms includes frequent monitoring of blood drug levels and close observation for signs of drug toxicity.

Anxiolytic Drugs in Hepatic Disease

Most benzodiazepines are extensively protein bound (Vozeh et al. 1988); thus, their distribution may be altered by liver disease. Overall, impaired liver function has been associated with increases in benzodiazepine T½s (Cassem et al. 1988; Klotz et al. 1975; Roberts et al. 1978). Benzodiazepine metabolism in liver disease has been extensively studied. Cl of benzodiazepines by phase I reactions (e.g., diazepam, nitrazepam, triazolam, alprazolam, and chlordiazepoxide) has been shown to be decreased by 30%–60% in patients with cirrhosis or acute viral hepatitis (Jochemsen et al. 1983; Juhl et al. 1984; Klotz et al. 1975; Kroboth et al. 1987; Leipzig 1990; Ochs et al. 1983; Sellers et al. 1979; Wilkinson 1978). In contrast, benzodiazepines metabolized by phase II reactions (e.g., oxazepam, lorazepam, and temazepam) show little change in Cl despite the presence of cirrhosis or acute viral hepatitis (Andreasen et al. 1976; Ghabrial et al. 1986; Leipzig 1990; Ochs et al. 1986; Shull et al. 1976). Lorazepam is the only benzodiazepine principally metabolized by phase II reactions that is available in both parenteral and intravenous forms. Other agents such as clorazepate, prazepam, halazepam, and flurazepam, which undergo oxidative metabolism, would be expected to show decreased Cl in patients with liver disease (Secor and Schenker 1987). Alprazolam is metabolized by hydroxylation and has been shown to have a 50% decrease in Cl and a 50% increase in elimination T½ in stable cirrhosis (Secor and Schenker 1987). Like alprazolam, triazolam has a short T½ and its first-pass hepatic metabolism is primarily hydroxylation. Triazolam has not been extensively studied in patients with liver disease. Not unexpectedly, recovery from acute viral hepatitis appears to be related to improvement of drug Cl (Leipzig 1990; Roberts et al. 1978; Wilkinson 1978). Most pharmacokinetic studies in medically ill patients involve single benzodiazepine doses. Further study is required to better delineate changes in kinetics with chronic dosing. For practical purposes, if a benzodiazepine is administered to a patient with chronic liver disease, dose reduction is indicated, especially if it is a drug with oxidatively formed active metabolites (DeVane 1990b).

Midazolam is a benzodiazepine that is approved for parenteral use and frequently used as a sedative for short diagnostic or therapeutic procedures. Unlike many other drugs in its class, midazolam is rapidly and well absorbed intramuscularly (Matson and Thurlow 1988). Its onset of action is rapid after parenteral administration. Midazolam's short T½ and the associated reduction in risk of cumulation suggests that this benzodiazepine should be used in pharmacokinetically complex medical situations (Ritz 1991).

Buspirone is a nonbenzodiazepine drug for chronic generalized anxiety that undergoes extensive presystemic metabolism. It has a large apparent Vd and a high plasma Cl (Mayol et al. 1985). The pharmacokinetics of a single oral dose have been studied in 12 patients with cirrhosis and compared with 12 healthy subjects (Dalhoff et al. 1987). The time until maximum concentration attained was similar in the two groups, but in the patients with cirrhosis, the mean maximum concentration was significantly higher and the mean elimination T½ was also greater.

Antipsychotic Drugs in Hepatic Disease

In general, the antipsychotic drugs have high hepatic Cls, low renal Cls, and high Vds. Most of these agents undergo significant first-pass metabolism. Their hepatic extraction ratios are high (0.5 to 0.9) (Wilkinson and Williams 1979). The pharmacokinetic profile of chlorpromazine is somewhat distinct. It is a low-Cl drug, but undergoes extensive biotransformation in the gut wall and the liver (Curry et al. 1971; DeVane 1990c). Two studies of chlorpromazine in patients with cirrhosis demonstrated no significant alteration of Cl (Maxwell et al. 1972; Read et al. 1969). Hepatotoxicity and cholestasis attributed to chlorpromazine have been associated with impairment of sulfoxidation (DeVane 1990c; Elias et al. 1984; Watson et al. 1988). In a study of patients with primary biliary cirrhosis (Olomu et al. 1988) (inflammation of interlobular bile ducts, associated with cholestasis and progression to cirrhosis), 80% of cases had impaired sulfoxidation. Leipzig (1990) demonstrated that this condition may specifically contraindicate the use of chlorpromazine. Additional in vitro studies have demonstrated that sulfoxidation of chlorpromazine produces metabolites that are less cholestatic than hydroxylated ones. General clinical practice is to avoid use of chlorpromazine in patients with liver disease.

Haloperidol, in contrast to chlorpromazine, is often used to treat medically ill patients because of its side-effect profile and its availability in parenteral form. It has a high Vd and is highly metabolized by the liver. Overall, elimination pathways for haloperidol are characteristically less complex than those of the other antipsychotic drugs. Leipzig (1990) suggested that, for patients with liver disease, the initial dose of neuroleptic drug should be reduced to one-third to one-half of the usual dose for healthy subjects.

Benztropine is an anticholinergic agent often used as an adjunct to antipsychotic agents when extrapyramidal symptoms may be problematic. Its pharmacokinetic profile has not been completely studied, and its use in medically ill patients has not been extensively investigated. Under normal circumstances, it appears to be rapidly distributed. It is excreted in the urine as 30%–50% unchanged drug (Cedarbaum 1987; DeVane 1990c). One study of serum concentrations showed 8- to 10-fold variability of effective steady-state concentrations. However, benztropine levels and their use in guiding dose adjustment are not established. No specific recommendations for dosing of patients with hepatic disease are available, but because medically ill patients are often more sensitive to drug side effects, it is wise to begin with conservative doses and to monitor closely for therapeutic and toxic effects (DeVane 1990c; Tune and Coyle 1980).

Antidepressant and Mood-Stabilizing Drugs in Hepatic Disease

TCAs are structurally similar to the phenothiazines and share many of their pharmacokinetic properties. They have high hepatic and low renal clearances. They are extensively bound by plasma proteins and have high Vds (DeVane 1990d). Primary metabolic pathways for TCAs are oxidation and glucuronidation (Preskorn and Irwin 1982). Hydroxylation is the predominant oxidative modification of the secondary amines, including protriptyline, desipramine, and nortriptyline (Ellenhorn and Barcelous 1988; Gram 1974; Ziegler et al. 1978a). Initially, the hydroxylated metabolites were thought to have little pharmacological significance, but more recent evidence (Baldessarini et al. 1988; McCue et al. 1989a, 1989b; Nelson et al. 1988a, 1988b; Nordin et al. 1987; Young et al. 1985) suggests that they may be important determinants of toxicity, particularly cardiotoxicity (conduction changes). In addition, Baldessarini and associates (1988) proposed that the hydroxy metabolites help to determine drug interactions. (Although carbamazepine usually lowers serum levels of the parent TCAs, hydroxylated metabolites of TCAs may be elevated by carbamazepine.)

Demethylation plays a major role in elimination of tertiary amines such as amitriptyline, imipramine, and doxepin (Ellenhorn and Barcelous 1988; Gram et al. 1983; Ziegler et al. 1978b). In general, primary monodemethylation of these compounds produces active metabolites, but further demethylation results in loss of pharmacological activity (Ellenhorn and Barcelous 1988).

Use of TCAs in patients with hepatic disease has not been extensively studied. In one uncontrolled, nonblinded study (Morgan and Read 1972), amitriptyline was administered to patients with cirrhosis, but blood levels were not reported. Because TCAs undergo significant hepatic metabolism, TCA dose reduction is recommended when liver disease potentially affects drug absorption, distribution, and elimination. Drug-level monitoring is widely available and should guide dose adjustments.

Trazodone. Trazodone is an antidepressant with a unique triazolopyridine structure. It is highly sedating but has relatively little anticholinergic activity. Its Vd is lower than that of the TCAs; this is reflected in its longer elimination T½. Trazodone is excreted primarily (75%) unchanged in the urine, but some hepatic metabolism occurs (Coccaro and Siever 1985). Prolonged Cl of trazodone from patients with compromised hepatocellular function is to be expected. Dose reduction is appropriate in these cases; however, the profound sedative effects must be considered a relative contraindication to use in encephalopathic patients.

Fluoxetine. Fluoxetine is a bicyclic antidepressant that is highly (94%) bound to plasma proteins. It is demethylated to a pharmacologically active metabolite, norfluoxetine. The elimination T½s for the parent and metabolite are long (average 4 and 7 days, respectively) (Lemberger et al. 1985). Fluoxetine pharmacokinetics have been studied in patients with cirrhosis. In the investigation by Schenker and co-workers (1988), fluoxetine elimination T½s were significantly reduced in the cirrhotic group compared with control subjects with normal liver function. Plasma Cl was reduced for the patients with cirrhosis. Moreover, the formation of norfluoxetine and its Cl were reduced in cirrhotic patients. Routine laboratory liver function tests (SGOT, alkaline phosphatase, bilirubin level) and indocyanine green Cls did not predict individual elimination parameters for fluoxetine. Inferring from these results, the investigators recommended dose reduction for patients with cirrhosis. Fluoxetine inhibits CyP_{450} and is highly protein bound; thus, it may alter kinetics of concomitantly administered drugs. Because of the long T½ of its primary metabolite norfluoxetine (greater than 10 days) at any given dose, steady-state serum levels are not reached for 3 to 4 weeks, as we discussed earlier in the chapter.

Sertraline. Sertraline is less potent than fluoxetine and paroxetine in its inhibition of CyP_{450} (Heym and Koe 1988). Crewe and associates (1992) examined in vitro inhibition of CyP_{450}-2D6-catalyzed metabolism by the SSRIs fluoxetine, sertraline, and paroxetine. Of the three parent SSRIs, paroxetine was the most potent inhibitor of CyP_{450}-2D6-catalyzed oxidation (of sparteine), followed by fluoxetine, and then sertraline. These investigators also studied SSRI-metabolite P_{450} inhibition and found that norfluoxetine (the principal metabolite of fluoxetine) was more potent than its parent, although not approaching paroxetine, in CyP_{450}-2D6 inhibition (Table 1–7). Sertraline's elimination T½ (approximately 24 hours) is significantly shorter than that of fluoxetine; thus, steady-state levels of sertraline are attained more rapidly. However, sertraline has been reported rarely as the cause of reversible elevations in SGOT and alkaline phosphatase values (Cohn et al. 1990). Despite this minor risk, sertraline's short T½ (relative to fluoxetine) and less potent inhibition of P_{450} metabolism (relative to fluoxetine and paroxetine) may render it most preferable in cases of liver disease with associated complex pharmacokinetic alterations.

Lithium. Lithium is unique among the psychotropic drugs in that it is polar and distributed in total body water. It is not protein bound (Jusko and Gretch 1976). Thus, its distribution is altered by the presence of ascites. In this situation, higher doses of lithium are required to produce desired plasma levels (Leipzig 1990). Lithium does not undergo hepatic metabolism, but its pharmacokinetics can be altered by liver disease when associated with renal failure. (Pharmacokinetic disturbances resulting from renal failure and the appropriate lithium dose adjustments are discussed in the "Renal Disease" section.)

Carbamazepine. Carbamazepine is structurally similar to the TCAs. It is a neutral compound that is primarily bound to albumin; changes in its distribution would be expected in liver disease (Hooper et al. 1975; Jusko and Gretch 1976). This drug is a potent inducer of the CyP_{450} system; it influences the metabolism of drugs relying on this system, including itself. Carbamazepine also can be hepatotoxic. The benign form of its hepatic effects (seen in no more than 5% of all patients, according to Jeavons [1983]) is characterized by mild elevations in serum SGOT and SGPT, usually less than twice the upper limit of normal range. However, the more serious form of its liver toxicity (with an incidence less than 1 in 10,000) is an idiosyncratic acute hepatic necrosis with resultant liver failure (Jeavons 1983).

Liver disease is a relative contraindication to the use of carbamazepine because 1) potential drug-induced hepatotoxicity will be superimposed on already disease-impaired liver function, and 2) carbamazepine relies on hepatic metabolism that may be impaired by liver disease, thus leading to accumulation of the parent drug. Consultation with a hepatologist is recommended before initiation of a carbamazepine trial. Furthermore, for alcoholic patients (who may have subclinical liver disease not revealed by physical examination or routine laboratory liver function tests), carbamazepine should be started more slowly than usual, with frequent monitoring of liver enzymes, PT, and serum drug levels. The clinician should also be aware of carbamazepine's antidiuretic action and possible resultant pharmacokinetic changes, in addition to hyponatremia.

Specific alterations of carbamazepine kinetics in liver disease have not been well studied, nor has carbamazepine's induction of the P_{450} metabolism of other drugs—in the setting of liver disease. Thus, when carbamazepine is to be used concomitantly with another psychotropic agent in a patient with liver disease, the clinician should select a second agent that undergoes less extensive P_{450} metabolism (e.g., the benzodiazepines lorazepam, temazepam, oxazepam; secondary versus tertiary TCAs; haloperidol versus a phenothiazine antipsychotic agent). Moreover, the choice of a second agent may be influenced by the availability of clinically meaningful drug levels (Winter 1988b). Lastly, electrocardiograms are indicated for patients at risk for cardiac conduction delays on both carbamazepine and a TCA because both possess quinidine-like properties.

Valproic acid. Valproic acid has widely variable reported Vds, likely associated with interindividual variations in plasma protein binding. It is bound primarily by albumin (Blaschke 1977) and is almost entirely eliminated from the body through hepatic metabolism. Less than 5% is eliminated by the kidneys (Klotz and Rappt Muller 1978). Decreased valproate T½s have been attributed to increased Vds secondary to plasma binding decreases. Valproic acid elimination is also decreased in patients with liver disease (Klotz and Rappt Muller 1978). Like carbamazepine, valproate has been associated with hepatic toxicity. In adults, the incidence of valproate-induced hepatic necrosis is estimated at 1/10,000 (Eadie et al. 1988; Jeavons 1983). Valproate inhibits urea synthesis and, thus, may increase serum ammonia levels (Cotairu and Zaidman 1988; Hjelm et al. 1986; Kugoh et al. 1986). Although this phenomenon may not produce symptoms in healthy patients, it may precipitate or exacerbate hepatic encephalopathy in patients with underlying liver disease. Thus, liver disease is a relative contraindication to valproate use. As with carbamazepine, hepatological consultation is recommended before starting valproate therapy for a patient with liver disease. Furthermore, valproate should be started more slowly in alcoholic patients. In addition to the toxic effects of valproate discussed above, this drug can increase PT, decrease fibrinogen levels, and reduce the platelet count—these effects may be of particular concern in patients with liver disease–associated coagulopathy. Before initiating valproate in any patient, a full coagulation panel (platelet count, PT, and PTT) is indicated. Close observation for signs of valproate toxicity should be reinforced with frequent serum valproate measurements in patients with liver disease.

Valproate competitively inhibits the oxidative metabolism of concomitantly administered drugs (e.g., carbamazepine). In light of their individual hepatotoxic risks and their opposing effects on P_{450} metabolism, concomitant use of carbamazepine and valproate should be avoided in patients with liver disease. If this drug combination would potentially greatly benefit the patient (e.g., treatment-refractory mania), the clinician must remember that valproate raises the concentration of the carbamazepine 10,11-epoxide metabolite (Pisani et al.

1986) whose toxicity is greater than that of carbamazepine (Bourgeois 1988; Bourgeois and Wad 1984). The 10,11-epoxide carbamazepine metabolite is generally not measured; therefore, when valproate is given concurrently, carbamazepine toxicity may occur despite apparently "therapeutic" measured serum carbamazepine levels (Stoudemire et al. 1991). In addition, valproate influences the kinetics of other drugs, such as diazepam and phenytoin, by displacing them from their protein binding sites, thus increasing their risk of toxicity (Janicak 1993). However, salicylates may displace valproic acid from its binding protein, which decreases valproate Cl and leads to increased pharmacologic and/or toxic effects of valproate (Janicak 1993).

Felbamate. Felbamate is an antiepileptic agent for treatment of refractory partial seizures. It is structurally similar to meprobamate. Felbamate induces and inhibits hepatic CyP_{450} enzymes, thus contributing to clinically important interactions with coadministered drugs. For instance, felbamate decreases plasma concentrations of carbamazepine by about 30% but increases concentrations of the pharmacologically active (and, perhaps toxic—see preceding discussion) 10,11-epoxide metabolite (Wagner et al. 1993). Felbamate increases serum concentrations of phenytoin and valproate (Sachdeo et al. 1992; Wagner et al. 1991). For healthy adults, a 20%–30% reduction in the dosage of concomitant phenytoin, valproate, or carbamazepine is recommended to minimize adverse effects from drug interactions (Palmer and McTavish 1993). However, until more information regarding felbamate use in patients with liver disease is available, concurrent use of felbamate and another anticonvulsant cannot be recommended.

RENAL DISEASE

The kidney's primary pharmacokinetic role is the elimination of drugs from the body. However, renal disease affects not only drug excretion but may also influence absorption, distribution, and metabolism (Reidenberg 1977). Renal failure can affect drug absorption by raised gastric pH caused by ammonia buffering (Anderson et al. 1976; Maher 1988). Passive reabsorption of some drugs (e.g., TCAs, amphetamine, phenobarbital) is affected by urinary pH and flow rate. However, disease-induced changes of pH and urine flow are rarely significant in clinical pharmacokinetics (Brater and Chennavasin 1984).

Fluid Shifts and Protein Binding

When acute renal failure results from ischemia, hepatic perfusion (and thus drug distribution to the liver) may also be reduced. Uremia may be associated with increased capillary permeability that can also alter drug distribution. Body water volume is generally increased in uremic patients (Maher 1988). Edema is reflected by an increased apparent Vd (Table 1–2). In these cases, larger doses of water-soluble drugs (e.g., lithium) or protein-bound drugs (e.g., most other psychotropics including TCAs) may be required to achieve a chosen serum drug concentration. The inverse is true for patients who are dehydrated or who have profound muscle wasting and therefore have decreased apparent Vds (Levy 1990). Plasma protein binding of drugs is frequently lower in uremic patients. This is attributed to a decrease in the affinity of albumin for drugs, as a result of retained binding inhibitors and decreased albumin concentrations (Levy 1990; Maher 1988). Displacement of highly bound (> 90%) drugs (e.g., most psychotropic drugs, with the notable exception of lithium) from plasma proteins may increase the fraction available for renal filtration and elimination via the urine. Nephrotic syndrome may cause hypoalbuminemia, which decreases drug binding. However, drug bound to albumin is also filtered by glomeruli whose integrity is disrupted during hypoalbuminemia (Gambertoglio 1984), which results in extremely difficult theoretical prediction of associated pharmacokinetic effects. In cases of nephrotic syndrome, psychotropic drug therapy should be initiated at a lower dose (e.g., 50% reduction from usual initial dose), and upward titration should proceed more slowly.

Renal Blood Flow

RBF influences filtration, secretion, and reabsorption of drugs by the kidney. RBF may be changed by pathological vascular glomerular processes, decreased effective circulation (e.g., abdominal ascites without cirrhosis, severe dehydration, rapid hemorrhage, shock), and disease primary processes affecting other organ systems (e.g., hepatorenal syndrome in liver failure, severe cirrhosis resulting in redistribution of blood from the renal cortex to the medulla, and cardiac failure) (Brater and Chennavasin 1984) (Table 1–2). No routine measurements of RBF are available to make clinical dose adjustments for drugs that are significantly excreted by the kidney (e.g., lithium, conjugated metabolites of most other psychotropic agents—see Table 1–4). In such complex disease-induced pharmacokinetic disruptions, the simplest and most conservative approach is to reduce initial dosage and to titrate upward more slowly if chronic psychotropic therapy is indicated.

Dialysis

Further pharmacokinetic perturbations result from dialysis. Drug removal rates or Cls are determined by concentration gradients and are inversely proportional to molecular mass. Hemodialysis involves higher flow rates than does peritoneal dialysis; thus, solute removal is more efficient in hemodialysis. Protein binding limits the transport rate of many drugs (Maher 1988). In general, drugs with a molecular weight of 500 Daltons or less (specifically, lithium) are removed by dialysis (dialyzable). Protein binding usually reduces dialyzability (Levy 1990). Drugs that are highly protein bound (> 90%—most psychotropic agents) are not significantly removed by dialysis (Gambertoglio 1984). Lipid-soluble drugs (i.e., pharmacologically active psychotropic drugs and metabolites) have larger Vds, are relatively less concentrated in blood, and thus are not substantially hemodialyzed from the patient (Gambertoglio 1984).

General Considerations

An applicable indicator of renal function would be of significant importance in guiding dose adjustments, particularly for drugs that are eliminated primarily by the kidney. Serum creatinine may be less helpful than measurements of creatinine Cl in this regard. One study indicated that serum β_2-microglobulin may be even more clinically relevant to pharmacokinetic alterations resulting from renal failure (Samiy and Rosnick 1987). Currently, however, this measurement is not widely available.

Dose adjustment for renal failure generally requires that drug dosage be reduced or that the dosing interval be lengthened. In some cases, tablet fractionation is not practical, so the interval must be changed. More often, dosing is planned according to established guidelines by use of indicators of renal function such as creatinine Cl. A comprehensive table of recommended adjustments for psychotropic drugs is available for psychotropic drug adjustment in patients with renal failure (Surman 1987) (Table 1–8). Knowledgeable use of these tables requires familiarity with the pharmacokinetic alterations resulting from kidney disease and dialysis. Serum creatinine relates correctly to renal function only during steady state with a stable serum creatinine (Traub and Johnson 1980). When renal function declines, creatinine T½ increases proportionally. A lag time (4–5 T½s) occurs before the change in serum creatinine correctly reflects the GFR. Serum creatinine changes occur frequently in medically ill patients, thus confounding the accurate calculation of creatinine Cl (Brater and Chennavasin 1984). For practical purposes, a "stable" serum creatinine can be assumed when two separate determinations (preferably obtained 24 hours apart) have values within 0.2 mg/dl of each other (Brater and Chennavasin 1984; Lott and Hayton 1978).

Anxiolytic Drugs in Renal Disease

Some benzodiazepines are metabolized by hepatic microsomal enzymes to form demethylated, hydroxylated, and other oxidized pharmacologically active products (Table 1–4). (As previously discussed, lorazepam, oxazepam, temazepam, alprazolam, triazolam, and clonazepam are exceptions.) The active metabolites are then conjugated with glucuronic acid, resulting in formation of pharmacologically inactive agents. Glucuronidated products are more water soluble and thus are excreted in urine. Lorazepam, oxazepam, and temazepam are metabolized only by glucuronidation and then are eliminated by the kidney (Arana and Hyman 1991). Impaired renal excretory function results in retention of glucuronidated (generally presumed pharmacologically inactive) benzodiazepine metabolites. Renal dysfunction is sometimes associated with impairment of hepatic metabolism, thus resulting in accumulation of parent drug and intermediate metabolites.

Measurement of serum benzodiazepine concentrations is less helpful than observation for pharmacological effects. This class of drugs is characterized by relatively high therapeutic indices, implying that toxicity is associated with serum concentrations significantly higher than those producing therapeutic benefits. Nevertheless, drug selection for patients with renal disease should be careful, and dose adjustment should be guided by an appropriate measure of renal function impairment. In general, benzodiazepines with few hepatic metabolites and relatively short T½s (e.g., lorazepam, oxazepam, alprazolam) are preferred for this group of patients (Gambertoglio 1984; Kraus et al. 1978; Surman 1987).

Plasma buspirone concentration measurements are not generally available, nor have they been shown to correlate with clinical effects. Gammans and co-workers (1986) have reported prolonged buspirone T½s in patients with renal impairment. Thus, dose reduction is recommended for patients with kidney failure (DeVane 1990b).

Antipsychotic Drugs in Renal Disease

The phenothiazines bind to plasma protein, and pharmacokinetics may be altered by renal disease. Uremic patients appear to have increased susceptibility to extrapyramidal and CNS effects of phenothiazines. Vds of these drugs are often quite high, so dialysis does not remove appreciable amounts of these drugs (Maher 1988). No specific dose adjustments are recommended for use of chlorpromazine in patients with isolated renal disease (Bennett et al. 1983)

In contrast to the phenothiazines, laboratory measurements of haloperidol are clinically available and may be useful adjuncts for making dose adjustments in patients with renal impairment. However, dose adjustments are generally unnecessary in patients with renal disease without accompanying hepatic impairment. Haloperidol is highly lipid soluble; no dose adjustment is specifically indicated for patients undergoing hemodialysis (DeVane 1990c).

Antidepressant and
Mood-Stabilizing Drugs in Renal Disease

Cyclic antidepressants are characterized by low renal Cls and high Vds. Their large Vds reflect significant drug penetration to tissues and predict poor dialyzability. Despite their small molecular weights, TCAs are relatively insoluble in water and are thus poorly dialyzable by conventional hemodialysis (as opposed to resin or charcoal hemoperfusion) (Brater and Vasko 1988). Less than 5% of an imipramine dose is excreted in an unchanged form in the urine. Most metabolites are expected to undergo relatively more renal excretion. In renal dysfunction, imipramine metabolites may accumulate (Lieberman et al. 1985). Plasma concentration monitoring is recommended for patients with kidney disease, but clinical signs of therapeutic and toxic effects are more reliable guides to dose adjustment.

Hydroxylated TCA metabolites have been studied in patients with chronic renal failure. Lieberman and co-workers (1985) demonstrated that conjugated hydroxylated metabolites of TCAs were markedly ele-

Table 1–8. Drug therapy in renal disease[a]

	Pharmacokinetic parameters				
		Half-life			
Drug	Elimination and metabolism	Normal (hour)	ESRD (hour)	Plasma protein binding (%)	Volume of distribution (L/kg)
Antidepressants					
Amoxapine	Hepatic	8–30	?	90	?
Bupropion	Hepatic	9.6–20.9	?	75–85	75–85
Fluoxetine	Hepatic	1–10	Unch	94.5	94.5
Maprotiline	Hepatic	48	?	?	?
Barbiturates*					
Hexobarbital	Hepatic	3.5–4.0	?	40–50	1.1
Pentobarbital**	Hepatic	18.48	Unch	60–70†	1
Phenobarbital	Hepatic (renal 30%)	60–150	117–160	40–60	0.7–1.0
Secobarbital	Hepatic	20–35	?	44	1.5–2.5
Thiopental	Hepatic	3.8	?	72–86	1.0–1.5
Benzodiazepines*					
Alprazolam	Hepatic	10–19	?	70–80	0.9–1.5
Brotizolam	Hepatic	4–8	7–9	90–95	0.4–0.7

Note. T½ = biologic half-life; ESRD = end-stage renal disease; GFR = glomerular filtration rate; I = interval extension method of dosage adjustment (data units are hours between maintenance doses); D = dose reduction method of dosage adjustment (data units are percentage of usual maintenance dose); H = hemodialysis; P = peritoneal dialysis; Unch = unchanged; GI = gastrointestinal.

	Adjustment for renal failure				
	GFR (ml/min)			Removed	
Method	>50	10–50	<10	by dialysis	Toxic effects and remarks
D	Unch	Unch	Unch	?	—
D	Unch	Unch	Unch	?	—
D	Unch	Unch	Unch	No (H)	—
D	Unch	Unch	Unch	?	—
					*Group remarks: may increase osteomalacia in hemodialysis patients; T½ decreases with chronic therapy because of hepatic microsomal enzyme induction; hemodialysis more effective than peritoneal dialysis in overdoses; charcoal hemoperfusion best for massive overdoses; all agents in this group may cause excessive sedation
D	Unch	Unch	Unch	No (H)	Group remarks
D	Unch	Unch	Unch	No (H)	Group remarks **Pharmacokinetics of amobarbital are similar †Decreased in ESRD
I	Unch	Unch	12–16	Yes (H,P)	Group remarks; up to 50% of drug excreted unchanged in alkaline diuresis
D	Unch	Unch	Unch	No (H,P)	Group remarks
D	Unch	Unch	75	?	Group remarks
					*Group toxicity: all agents in group may cause excessive sedation or encephalopathy, or both, in chronic hemodialysis patients
D	Unch	Unch	Unch	?	Group toxicity
D	Unch	Unch	Unch	?	Group toxicity
					(continued)

aFootnote symbols within the body of the table refer to footnotes in "Toxic effects and remarks" column at extreme right.
Source. Reprinted from Bennett WM, Singer I, Coggins CJ: "A Guide to Drug Therapy in Renal Failure." *Journal of the American Medical Association* 230:1544–1553, 1974. Copyright 1974, American Medical Association. Used with permission.

Table 1–8. Drug therapy in renal disease[a] *(continued)*

Drug	Elimination and metabolism	Half-life Normal (hour)	Half-life ESRD (hour)	Plasma protein binding (%)	Volume of distribution (L/kg)
		Pharmacokinetic parameters			
Chlordiazepoxide	Hepatic (renal)[**]	5–30[†]	?	94–97	0.3–0.5[‡]
Clonazepam	Hepatic	5–30	?	47	1.5–4.5
Clorazepate	Hepatic (renal)	36–200	?	?	?
Diazepam	Hepatic (renal,[*] GI[†])	20–90[‡]	?	94–98[§]	0.7–2.6[¶]
Flurazepam	Hepatic (renal)[*]	47–100	?	?[†]	3.4[‡]
Lorazepam	Hepatic	9–16	32–70	90	1.3

Note. T½ = biologic half-life; ESRD = end-stage renal disease; GFR = glomerular filtration rate; I = interval extension method of dosage adjustment (data units are hours between maintenance doses); D = dose reduction method of dosage adjustment (data units are percentage of usual maintenance dose); H = hemodialysis; P = peritoneal dialysis; Unch = unchanged; GI = gastrointestinal.

	Adjustment for renal failure				
	GFR (ml/min)			Removed	
Method	>50	10–50	<10	by dialysis	Toxic effects and remarks
D	Unch	Unch	Unch	No (H)	Group toxicity **Active metabolite excreted by kidney †Large variability; chronic therapy prolongs T½ ‡Excessive protein binding leads to underestimation of volume of distribution
D	Unch	Unch	Unch	?	Group toxicity
D	Unch	Unch	Unch	?	Group toxicity
D	Unch	Unch	Unch	No (H)	Group toxicity *Active metabolite desmethyl diazepam excreted by kidney †Enterohepatic circulation exists ‡Increased metabolism with prolonged therapy; extreme variability §Variably decreased to about 92% in ESRD; binding higher in males than in females ¶Increased in ESRD
D	Unch	Unch	Unch	No (H)	Group toxicity *First-pass hepatic metabolism; excretion routes and T½ pertain to active metabolites †Protein binding weaker than that of other benzodiazepines ‡Animal data
D	Unch	Unch	50	No (H)	Group toxicity

(continued)

aFootnote symbols within the body of the table refer to footnotes in "Toxic effects and remarks" column at extreme right.
Source. Reprinted from Bennett WM, Singer I, Coggins CJ: "A Guide to Drug Therapy in Renal Failure." *Journal of the American Medical Association* 230:1544–1553, 1974. Copyright 1974, American Medical Association. Used with permission.

Table 1–8. Drug therapy in renal disease[a] *(continued)*

Drug	Elimination and metabolism	Half-life Normal (hour)	Half-life ESRD (hour)	Plasma protein binding (%)	Volume of distribution (L/kg)
Midazolam	Hepatic	9–16	32–70	90[*]	1.3
Nitrazepam	Hepatic	21–40	—	83–88	2.4–4.8
Oxazepam	Hepatic	6–25	25–90	90	1.6[*]
Prazepam	Hepatic (renal)	36–200	?	?	?
Triazolam	Hepatic	1.4–3.3	—	85–95	—
Bromperidol	Hepatic	24–36	?	90	?
Buspirone	Hepatic	2–5	5–6	?	?
Chloral hydrate	Hepatic	7–14	Unch	35–40	1.6
Ethchlorvynol	Hepatic (renal)[*]	19–32	Unch	35–50	3–4
Glutethimide	Hepatic (renal)[*]	5–22[†]	Unch[‡]	54	2.7

Note. T½ = biologic half-life; ESRD = end-stage renal disease; GFR = glomerular filtration rate; I = interval extension method of dosage adjustment (data units are hours between maintenance doses); D = dose reduction method of dosage adjustment (data units are percentage of usual maintenance dose); H = hemodialysis; P = peritoneal dialysis; Unch = unchanged; GI = gastrointestinal.

Adjustment for renal failure

Method	GFR (ml/min)			Removed by dialysis	Toxic effects and remarks
	>50	10–50	<10		
D	Unch	Unch	Unch	No (H)	Group toxicity *Protein binding decreased in ESRD
D	Unch	Unch	Unch	?	Group toxicity
D	Unch	Unch	75	No (H)	Group toxicity; glucuronide metabolite increases in ESRD *Increased in ESRD, which accounts for increased T½
D	Unch	Unch	Unch	?	Group toxicity
D	Unch	Unch	Unch	?	Group toxicity
D	Unch	Unch	Unch	?	May cause hypotension, excessive sedation
D	Unch	Unch	50–75*	Yes (H)	*Active metabolite accumulates
D	Unch	Avoid	Avoid	Yes (H)	May cause excessive sedation or encephalopathy, or both, in chronic hemodialysis patients
D	Unch	Avoid	Avoid	No (H,P)	May cause excessive sedation; ?nephrotoxic; may be effectively removed by hemoperfusion *Proportion of hepatic and renal excretion uncertain
D	Unch	Avoid	Avoid	No (H,P)	May cause excessive sedation *Enterohepatic circulation exists; active metabolite excreted by kidney †T½ increases with dose and hypotension ‡Active metabolite 4-hydroxyglutethimide has long T½ in renal failure

(continued)

[a]Footnote symbols within the body of the table refer to footnotes in "Toxic effects and remarks" column at extreme right.
Source. Reprinted from Bennett WM, Singer I, Coggins CJ: "A Guide to Drug Therapy in Renal Failure." *Journal of the American Medical Association* 230:1544–1553, 1974. Copyright 1974, American Medical Association. Used with permission.

Table 1–8. Drug therapy in renal disease[a] *(continued)*

		Pharmacokinetic parameters			
	Elimina-	Half-life		Plasma protein	Volume of dis-
	tion and	Normal	ESRD	binding	tribution
Drug	metabolism	(hour)	(hour)	(%)	(L/kg)
Haloperidol	Hepatic (renal, GI)	10–36	?	90–92	14–21
Lithium carbonate	Renal	14–28[*]	Pro- longed	0	0.5–0.9
Meprobamate	Hepatic (renal 10%)[*]	6–17	Unch	0–20	0.75
Methaqualone	Hepatic	Biphasic: 0.9 and 16–42[*]	Unch	80	5–8

Note. T½ = biologic half-life; ESRD = end-stage renal disease; GFR = glomerular filtration rate; I = interval extension method of dosage adjustment (data units are hours between maintenance doses); D = dose reduction method of dosage adjustment (data units are percentage of usual maintenance dose); H = hemodialysis; P = peritoneal dialysis; Unch = unchanged; GI = gastrointestinal.

	GFR (ml/min)			Removed	
Method	>50	10–50	<10	by dialysis	Toxic effects and remarks
D	Unch	Unch	Unch	No (H,P)	May cause hypotension, excessive sedation
D	Unch	50–75	25–50	Yes (H,P)[†]	Nephrogenic diabetes insipidus; nephrotic syndrome; renal tubular acidosis; chronic interstitial fibrosis; toxicity when serum levels are > 1.2 mEq/L; serum levels 12 hr after a dose should be measured periodically; toxicity enhanced and drug clearance reduced by volume depletion, nonsteroidal antiinflammatory drugs, and diuretics; excretion enhanced by $NaHCO_3$, acetazolamide, aminophylline, and osmotic diuretics [*]Plasma T½ does not reflect extensive tissue accumulation [†]Plasma levels rise after dialysis as reequilibration with tissue stores occurs
1	6	9–12	12–18	Yes (N,P)[†]	May cause excessive sedation [*]Renal excretion may be increased by forced diuresis [†]Hemodialysis twice as efficient as peritoneal dialysis
D	Unch	Avoid	Avoid	No (H)	May cause excessive sedation; contaminant (*o*-toluidine) may cause hemorrhagic cystitis [*]Biexponential pharmacokinetics; longer T½ more important clinically

(continued)

[a]Footnote symbols within the body of the table refer to footnotes in "Toxic effects and remarks" column at extreme right.

Source. Reprinted from Bennett WM, Singer I, Coggins CJ: "A Guide to Drug Therapy in Renal Failure." *Journal of the American Medical Association* 230:1544–1553, 1974. Copyright 1974, American Medical Association. Used with permission.

Table 1–8. Drug therapy in renal disease[a] *(continued)*

	Pharmacokinetic parameters				
		Half-life		Plasma	Volume
	Elimina-			protein	of dis-
	tion and	Normal	ESRD	binding	tribution
Drug	metabolism	(hour)	(hour)	(%)	(L/kg)
Monoamine oxidase inhibitors[*]					
Phenelzine[*]	Hepatic	?	?	?	?
Phenothiazines[*]					
Chlorproma-zine	Hepatic	11–42	?	91–99	8–160[**]
Tricyclic antide-pressants[*]					

Note. T½ = biologic half-life; ESRD = end-stage renal disease; GFR = glomeru-lar filtration rate; I = interval extension method of dosage adjustment (data units are hours between maintenance doses); D = dose reduction method of dosage adjustment (data units are percentage of usual maintenance dose); H = hemodialysis; P = peritoneal dialysis; Unch = unchanged; GI = gastrointestinal.

Adjustment for renal failure

Method	GFR (ml/min) >50	10–50	<10	Removed by dialysis	Toxic effects and remarks
					*Group remarks: hypertensive crisis can be caused by interaction with tyramine in food and beverages or by interaction with sympathomimetics or levodopa
D	Unch	Unch	Unch	?	Group remarks
					*Group toxicity: all agents in this group are anticholinergic; may cause urinary retention, orthostatic hypotension, confusion, and extrapyramidal symptoms; characteristic acute toxic psychosis; > 800 mg/day thioridazine causes retinitis; prototype chlorpromazine
D	Unch	Unch	Unch[†]	No (H,P)	Group toxicity
					**Very large volume of distribution after oral dose
					[†]May need to decrease dose and increase interval if excessive sedation occurs
					*Group remarks: all agents in this group are anticholinergic and may cause urinary retention; may decrease hypotensive effects of guanethidine, clonidine, and methyldopa; enterohepatic circulation and genetic variation in metabolism exist; increased excretion in acid urine (total remains small), smoking, alcohol, and sedatives induce metabolism; neuro-

(continued)

[a]Footnote symbols within the body of the table refer to footnotes in "Toxic effects and remarks" column at extreme right.

Source. Reprinted from Bennett WM, Singer I, Coggins CJ: "A Guide to Drug Therapy in Renal Failure." *Journal of the American Medical Association* 230:1544–1553, 1974. Copyright 1974, American Medical Association. Used with permission.

Table 1–8. Drug therapy in renal disease[a] *(continued)*

Drug	Elimina-tion and metabolism	Half-life Normal (hour)	ESRD (hour)	Plasma protein binding (%)	Volume of dis-tribution (L/kg)
		Pharmacokinetic parameters			
Amitriptyline	Hepatic[*] (renal <5%)	32–40	?	96	6–36
Desipramine	Hepatic (renal <5%)	12–54	?	90	28–60
Doxepin	Hepatic	8–25	?	93–95	9–33
Imipramine	Hepatic[*] (renal <5%)	6–20	?	96	9–15
Nortriptyline	Hepatic (renal <5%)	18–93	15–66	95	15–23
Protriptyline	Hepatic	54–98	?	92	15–31

Note. T½ = biologic half-life; ESRD = end-stage renal disease; GFR = glomeru-lar filtration rate; I = interval extension method of dosage adjustment (data units are hours between maintenance doses); D = dose reduction method of dosage adjustment (data units are percentage of usual maintenance dose); H = hemodialysis; P = peritoneal dialysis; Unch = unchanged; GI = gastrointestinal.

	Adjustment for renal failure				
	GFR (ml/min)			Removed	
Method	>50	10–50	<10	by dialysis	Toxic effects and remarks
					leptics and advanced age inhibit metabolism; may cause excessive sedation; physostigmine indicated for life-threatening overdose
D	Unch	Unch	Unch[†]	No (H,P)	Group remarks [*]Metabolized to nortriptyline [†]Reported to stimulate weight gain and appetite in dialysis patients
D	Unch	Unch	Unch	No (H,P)	Group remarks
D	Unch	Unch	Unch	No (H,P)	Group remarks
D	Unch	Unch	Unch	No (H,P)	Group remarks [*]Metabolized to desipramine
D	Unch	Unch	Unch	No (H,P)	Group remarks
D	Unch	Unch	Unch	No (H,P)	Group remarks

[a]Footnote symbols within the body of the table refer to footnotes in "Toxic effects and remarks" column at extreme right.

Source. Reprinted from Bennett WM, Singer I, Coggins CJ: "A Guide to Drug Therapy in Renal Failure." *Journal of the American Medical Association* 230:1544–1553, 1974. Copyright 1974, American Medical Association. Used with permission.

vated (500%–1,500%) in hemodialysis patients compared with control subjects. The hemodialysis group had less profound increases of unconjugated hydroxylated metabolites. Apparently, differences in conjugated metabolite levels result from differences in elimination in patients undergoing dialysis. The bioactivity of conjugated hydroxylated TCAs is not well studied, but if these compounds are pharmacologically active, it might explain why dialysis patients seem to be hypersensitive to TCA side effects despite "therapeutic" serum levels of the parent drugs and their demethylated metabolites (Klotz et al. 1975).

Nortriptyline.   Single-oral-dose kinetics of nortriptyline and its two major metabolites, conjugated and unconjugated 10-hydroxynortriptyline, have been studied in patients with chronic renal failure (Dawling et al. 1982). The kinetics of the parent drug were not significantly different in renal failure patients compared with control patients. However, conjugated forms of 10-hydroxynortriptyline were higher in patients with kidney disease. Again, the phenomenon was attributed to decreased elimination of conjugated metabolites (Dawling et al. 1982; Morgan and Read 1972).

Fluoxetine.   Aronoff and co-workers (1984) studied fluoxetine kinetics and protein binding in renal disease. No correlations between the degree of renal dysfunction and the rate of elimination, Vd, or protein binding were found. These investigators also found that plasma concentrations of fluoxetine and norfluoxetine were not significantly changed by hemodialysis. More recent pharmacokinetic studies of fluoxetine as well as venlafaxine in renal disease are discussed further in Chapter 2.

Lithium.   Lithium is not metabolized; it is eliminated from the body almost exclusively by the renal route. Renal reabsorption of lithium is closely associated with sodium reabsorption and is influenced by changes in renal Cl of sodium (Winter 1988c). Use of lithium in patients with kidney disease has been influenced by conflicting evidence regarding lithium-induced impairment of urine concentrating ability and reduced glomerular function. Lithium distribution is affected by renal disease; this is reflected by changes in its apparent Vd, as previously discussed. As noted earlier in this chapter, because of its small molecular size, lithium is highly dialyzable. (This characteristic is particularly helpful in cases of serious overdose.) For patients with impaired renal function, frequent monitoring of serum lithium levels is useful in guiding dosage. Dose selection is generally determined by the severity of kidney damage (currently, as indicated by creatinine Cl or perhaps in the future by β_2-microglobulin measurements).

As previously noted, most psychotropic drugs are not removed from the blood by routine hemodialysis. Thus, dose reduction, as guided by some measure of renal function, is generally appropriate. Lithium, however, is eliminated from the body via the kidney, and it is removed by dialysis. Thus, the lithium dosing interval must be changed for patients on hemodialysis. Conventional practice is to give a single dose of lithium in the range of 300 to 600 mg after dialysis. No additional lithium is administered until after the next dialysis run. Obviously, careful monitoring of plasma lithium levels (postdosing and before the next dialysis) is recommended (Levy 1990; Lydiard and Gelenberg 1982).

SUMMARY

The pharmacokinetics of psychotropic agents are influenced by disease in various ways. Disease-induced changes in drug absorption, distribution, metabolism, and excretion can determine the nature and degree of therapeutic and toxic effects. Individuals who are medically ill often receive numerous nonpsychotropic agents that further disrupt psychopharmacokinetics via physiological effects and/or drug-drug interactions. In addition, medically ill patients may be particularly sensitive to CNS effects of their medications, and they are at risk for developing psychiatric symptoms that require pharmacological intervention. Knowledge of changes in pharmacokinetic parameters are useful in selection of drug and dose and subsequent dosage adjustment. Practical application of these concepts generally entails monitoring of measured serum drug concentrations and observing patient response and toxicity. Further study is needed to refine indicators of the severity of organ damage that correlate with specific changes in psychotropic drug kinetics.

REFERENCES

Amidsen A, Carson SW: Lithium, in Applied Pharmacokinetics: Principles of Therapeutic Drug Monitoring, 2nd Edition. Edited by Evans WE, Schentag JJ, Juskow J. San Francisco, CA, Applied Therapeutics, 1986, pp 978–1008

Anderson RJ, Gambertoglio JB, Schrier RW: Drugs used in neurology and psychiatry, in Clinical Use of Drugs in Renal Failure. Springfield, IL, CC Thomas, 1976, pp 194–208

Anderson SA, Brown-Cartwright D, Voelker JR: Acute renal ischemia from sulindac in patients with cirrhosis (abstract). Clin Res 34:212A, 1986

Andreasen PB, Hendel J, Grelden G, et al: Pharmacokinetics of diazepam in disordered liver function. Eur J Clin Pharmacol 10:115–120, 1976

Arana GW, Hyman SE (eds): Handbook of Psychiatric Drug Therapy, 2nd Edition. Boston, MA, Little, Brown, 1991, pp 32–33

Aronoff GR, Bergstrom RF, Pottratz ST, et al: Fluoxetine kinetics and protein binding in normal and impaired renal function. Clin Pharmacol Ther 36:138–144, 1984

Arris PA, Wedlund PJ, Branch RA: Adjustment of medications in liver failure, in The Pharmacologic Approach to the Critically Ill Patient, 2nd Edition. Edited by Chernow B. Baltimore, MD, Williams & Wilkins, 1988, pp 85–111

Baldessarini RJ, Teicher MH, Cassidy JW, et al: Anticonvulsant cotreatment may increase toxic metabolites of antidepressants and other psychotropic drugs (letter). J Clin Psychopharmacol 8:381–382, 1988

Bax NDS, Tucker GT, Woods HF: Lignocaine and indocyanine green kinetics in patients following myocardial infarction. Br J Clin Pharmacol 10:353–361, 1980

Bendz H: Kidney function in lithium-treated patients: a literature survey. Acta Psychiatr Scand 68:303–324, 1983

Benet LZ, Massoud N: Pharmacokinetics, in Pharmacokinetic Basis for Drug Treatment. Edited by Benet LZ, Massoud N, Gambertoglio JG. New York, Raven, 1984, pp 1–28

Bennett W, Aronoff G, Morrison G: Drug prescribing in renal failure: dosing guidelines for adults. Am J Kidney Dis 3:155–193, 1983

Benowitz NL: Effects of cardiac disease on pharmacokinetics: pathophysiologic considerations, in Pharmacokinetic Basis for Drug Treatment. Edited by Benet LZ, Massoud N, Gambertoglio JG. New York, Raven, 1984, pp 89–103

Benowitz NL, Meister W: Pharmacokinetics in patients with cardiac failure. Clin Pharmacokinet 1:389–405, 1976

Berkowitz D, Droll MN, Likoff W: Malabsorption as a complication of congestive heart failure. Am J Cardiol 11:43–47, 1963

Blaschke TF: Protein binding and kinetics of drugs and liver disease. Clin Pharmacokinet 2:32–44, 1977

Blaschke TF, Meffin PJ, Melmon KL, et al: Influence of acute viral hepatitis on phenytoin kinetics and protein binding. Clin Pharmacol Ther 17:685–691, 1975

Boton R, Gaviria M, Batlle DC: Prevalence, pathogenesis, and treatment of renal dysfunction associated with chronic lithium therapy. Am J Kidney Dis 10:329–345, 1987

Bourgeois BFD: Pharmacologic interactions between valproate and other drugs. Am J Med 84 (suppl 1A):29–33, 1988

Bourgeois BFD, Wad N: Individual and combined antiepileptic and neurotoxic activity of carbamazepine and carbamazepine 10,11-epoxide in mice. J Pharmacol Exp Ther 231:411–415, 1984

Bowen RC, Grof CM, Grof E: Less frequent lithium administration and lower urine volume. Am J Psychiatry 148:189–192, 1991

Brater DC, Chennavasin P: Effects of renal disease: pharmacokinetic considerations, in Pharmacokinetic Basis for Drug Treatment. Edited by Benet LZ, Massoud N, Gambertoglio JG. New York, Raven, 1984, pp 119–147

Brater DC, Vasko MR: Pharmacokinetics, in The Pharmacologic Approach to the Critically Ill Patient, 2nd Edition. Edited by Chernow B, Lake CR. Baltimore, MD, Williams & Wilkins, 1988, pp 1–20

Brunswick DJ, Amsterdam JD, Mendels J, et al: Prediction of steady-state imipramine and desmethyl-imipramine plasma concentrations from single dose data. Clin Pharmacol Ther 25 (5 pt 1):605–610, 1979

Bunke CM, Aronoff GR, Brier ME, et al: Mezlocillin kinetics in hepatic insufficiency. Clin Pharmacol Ther 33:73–76, 1983

Cairncross KD, Gershon S: A pharmacological basis for the cardiovascular complications of imipramine medication. Med J Aust 2:372–375, 1962

Caley CF, Weber SS: Paroxetine: a selective serotonin reuptake inhibiting antidepressant. Ann Pharmacother 27:1212–1222, 1993

Cannon PJ: The kidney in heart failure. N Engl J Med 296:26–32, 1977

Cassem EH, Lake CR, Boyer WF: Psychopharmacology in the ICU, in The Pharmacologic Approach to the Critically Ill Patient, 2nd Edition. Edited by Chernow B, Lake CR. Baltimore, MD, Williams & Wilkins, 1988, pp 491–510

Cedarbaum JM: Clinical pharmacokinetics of anti-parkinson drugs. Clin Pharmacokinet 13:141–178, 1987

Coccaro EF, Siever LJ: Second generation antidepressants: a comparative review. J Clin Pharmacol 25:241–260, 1985

Cohn CK, Shrivastava R, Mendels J, et al: Double-blind, multicenter comparisons of sertraline and amitriptyline in elderly depressed patients. J Clin Psychiatry 51 (12 suppl B):28–33, 1990

Cooper TB, Simpson GM: The 24-hour lithium level as a prognosticator of dosage requirements: a two-year follow-up study. Am J Psychiatry 133:440–445, 1976

Cooper TB, Simpson GM: Prediction of individual dosage of nortriptyline. Am J Psychiatry 135:333–335, 1978

Cotairu D, Zaidman JL: Valproic acid and the liver. Clin Chem 34:890–897, 1988

Crewe HK, Lennard MS, Tucker GT, et al: The effect of selective serotonin reuptake inhibitors on cytochrome P4502D6 (CYP2D6) activity in human liver microsomes. Br J Clin Pharmacol 34:262–265, 1992

Curry SH, D'Mello A, Mould GP: Destruction of chlorpromazine during absorption in the rat in vivo and in vitro. Br J Pharmacol 42:403–411, 1971

Dalack GW, Roose SP, Glassman AH: Tricyclics and heart failure (letter). Am J Psychiatry 148:1602, 1991

Dalhoff K, Paulsen HE, Garred P, et al: Buspirone pharmacokinetics in patients with cirrhosis. Br J Clin Pharmacol 24:547–550, 1987

DasGupta K, Jefferson JW: The use of lithium in the medically ill. Gen Hosp Psychiatry 12:83–97, 1990

Dawling S, Lynn K, Rosser R, et al: Nortriptyline metabolism in chronic renal failure: metabolite elimination. Clin Pharmacol Ther 32:322–329, 1982 de Boer AG, Moolenaar F, deLeede LGJ, et al: Rectal drug administration: clinical pharmacokinetic considerations. Clin Pharmacokinet 7:285–311, 1982

DeVane CL: Principles of pharmacokinetics, in Fundamentals of Monitoring Psychoactive Drug Therapy. Edited by DeVane CL. Baltimore, MD, Williams & Wilkins, 1990a, pp 27–49

DeVane CL: Drug therapy for anxiety and insomnia, in Fundamentals of Monitoring Psychoactive Drug Therapy. Edited by DeVane CL. Baltimore, MD, Williams & Wilkins, 1990b, pp 191–238

DeVane CL: Drug therapy for psychoses, in Fundamentals of Monitoring Psychoactive Drug Therapy. Edited by DeVane CL. Baltimore, MD, Williams & Wilkins, 1990c, pp 139–190

DeVane CL: Drug therapy for mood disorders, in Fundamentals of Monitoring Psychoactive Drug Therapy. Edited by DeVane CL. Baltimore, MD, Williams & Wilkins, 1990d, pp 82–138

Eadie MJ, Hooper WD, Dickinson RG: Valproate-associated hepatotoxicity and its biochemical mechanisms. Medical Toxicology and Adverse Drug Experience 3:85–106, 1988

Eisenberg S, Madison L, Sensenbach W: Cerebral hemodynamic and metabolic studies in patients with congestive heart failure, II: observations in confused subjects. Circulation 21:704–709, 1960

Elias E, Waring RH, Mitchell SC: Defective sulfoxidation combined with rapid carbon oxidation in the liver may predispose to chlorpromazine jaundice (abstract). Gut 25:A1130, 1984

Ellenhorn MJ, Barcelous DC (eds): Medical Toxicology: Diagnosis and Treatment of Human Poisoning. New York, Elsevier, 1988, pp 231–240, 401–420

Erlich BE, Diamond JM: Lithium absorption: implications for sustained-release lithium preparations (letter). Lancet 1:306, 1983

Farrell GC, Cooksley WGE, Powell LW: Drug metabolism in liver disease: activity of microsomal metabolizing enzymes. Clin Pharmacol Ther 26:483–492, 1979

Feighner JP: Clinical efficacy of newer antidepressants. J Clin Psychopharmacol 1:23–31, 1981

Feighner JP, Cohn JB, Fabre LF Jr: A study comparing paroxetine, placebo and imipramine in depressed patients. J Affect Disord 218:71–79, 1993

Fogel BS, Stoudemire A: New psychotropics in medically ill patients, in Medical-Psychiatric Practice, Vol 2. Edited by Stoudemire A, Fogel BS. Washington, DC, American Psychiatric Press, 1993, pp 69–111

Fulop G, Phillips RA, Shapiro AK: ECG changes during haloperidol and pimozide treatment of Tourette's disorder. Am J Psychiatry 144:673–675, 1987

Gambertoglio JG: Effects of renal disease: altered pharmacokinetics, in Pharmacokinetic Basis for Drug Treatment. Edited by Benet LZ, Massoud N, Gambertoglio JG. New York, Raven, 1984, pp 149–172

Gammans RE, Mayol RF, Labudde JA: Metabolism and disposition of buspirone. Am J Med 80:41–51, 1986

Gascon MP, Dayer P: In vitro forecasting of drugs which may interfere with the biotransformation of midazolam. Eur J Clin Pharmacol 41:573–578, 1991

Ghabrial H, Desmond PV, Watson KJR, et al: The effects of age and chronic liver disease on the elimination of temazepam. Eur J Clin Pharmacol 30:93–97, 1986

Glassman AH, Bigger JT, Giardina EV: Clinical characteristics of imipramine-induced orthostatic hypotension. Lancet 1:468–472, 1979

Glassman AH, Johnson LL, Giardina EGV, et al: The use of imipramine in depressed patients with congestive heart failure. JAMA 250:1997–2001, 1983

Glassman R, Salzman C: Interactions between psychotropic and other drugs: an update. Hosp Community Psychiatry 38:236–242, 1987

Gram LF: Metabolism of tricyclic antidepressants: a review. Dan Med Bull 21:218–231, 1974

Gram LF, Bjerre M, Kragh-Sorenson P, et al: Imipramine metabolics in blood of patients during therapy and after overdose. Clin Pharmacol Ther 33:335–342, 1983

Greenblatt DJ: Pharmacokinetic comparisons. Psychosomatics 21 (suppl):9–14, 1980

Grossman R, Kotelansk B, Khatril M, et al: Quantitation of portosystemic shunting from the splenic and mesenteric beds in alcoholic liver disease. Am J Med 53:715–722, 1972

Hackett TP, Rosenbaum JF, Tesar GE: Emotion, psychiatric disorders, and the heart, in Heart Disease, 3rd Edition. Edited by Braunwald E. Philadelphia, PA, WB Saunders, 1988, pp 1883–1900

Heym J, Koe BK: Pharmacology of sertraline: a review. J Clin Psychiatry 49 (suppl):40–45, 1988

Hjelm M, Oberholzer V, Seakins J, et al: Valproate-induced inhibition of urea synthesis and hyperammonaemia in healthy subjects (letter). Lancet 2:859, 1986

Homeida M, Roberts CJC, Halliwell M, et al: Antipyrine clearance per unit volume liver: an assessment of hepatic function in chronic liver disease. Gut 20:596–601, 1979

Hooper WD, Dubetz B, Bochner F, et al: Plasma protein binding of carbamazepine. Clin Pharmacol Ther 17:433–440, 1975

Hoyumpa AM, Schenker S: Influence of liver disease on the disposition and elimination of drugs, in Disease of the Liver. Edited by Schiff L, Schiff ER. Philadelphia, PA, JB Lippincott, 1982, pp 709–746

Huet PM, Villeneuve JP: Determinants of drug disposition in patients with cirrhosis. Hepatology 3:913–918, 1983

Janicak PG: The relevance of clinical pharmacokinetics and therapeutic drug monitoring: anticonvulsant mood stabilizers and antipsychotics. J Clin Psychiatry 54 (suppl 9):35–41, 1993

Janowksy D, Curtis G, Zisook S, et al: Ventricular arrhythmias possibly aggravated by trazodone. Am J Psychiatry 140:796–797, 1983

Jeavons PM: Hepatotoxicity in antiepileptic drugs, in Chronic Toxicity of Antiepileptic Drugs. Edited by Oxley J, Janz D, Meinardi H. New York, Raven, 1983, pp 1–46

Jefferson JW: A review of the cardiovascular effects and toxicity of tricyclic antidepressants. Psychosom Med 37:160–170, 1975

Jefferson JW, Greist JH (eds): Primer of Lithium Therapy. Baltimore, MD, Williams & Wilkins, 1977

Jenner PN: Paroxetine: an overview of dosage, tolerability, and safety. Int Clin Psychopharmacol 6 (suppl 4):69–80, 1992

Jochemsen R, VanBeuse Kom BR, Spoelstoa P, et al: Effect of age and liver cirrhosis on the pharmacokinetics of nitrazepam. Br J Clin Pharmacol 15:295–302, 1983

Johnson DA, Cattau EL: Pharmacologic approach to gastrointestinal disease in critical illness, in The Pharmacologic Approach to the Critically Ill Patient, 2nd Edition. Edited by Chernow B. Baltimore, MD, Williams & Wilkins, 1988, pp 322–345

Juhl RP, VanThiel DH, Dihert LW, et al: Alprazolam pharmacokinetics in alcoholic liver disease. J Clin Pharmacol 24:113–119, 1984

Jusko WJ, Gretch M: Plasma and tissue protein binding of drugs in pharmacokinetics. Drug Metab Rev 5:43–140, 1976

Klotz U, Rappt Muller WA: Disposition of valproic acid in patients with liver disease. J Clin Pharmacol 13:55–60, 1978

Klotz U, Avant GR, Hoyumpa A: The effects of age and liver disease on the disposition and elimination of diazepam in adult men. J Clin Invest 55:347–359, 1975

Kraus JW, Desmond PV, Marshall JP, et al: Effects of aging and liver disease on disposition of lorazepam. Clin Pharmacol Ther 24:411–419, 1978

Kroboth PD, Smith RB, VanThiel DH, et al: Nighttime dosing of triazolam in patients with liver disease and normal subjects: kinetics and daytime effects. J Clin Pharmacol 27:555–560, 1987

Kronbach T, Mathys D, Umeno M, et al: Oxidation of midazolam and triazolam by human liver cytochrome P450 III A4. Mol Pharmacol 36:89–96, 1989

Kugoh T, Yamamoto M, Hosokawa K: Blood ammonia level during valproic acid therapy. Jpn J Psychiatry Neurol 40:663–668, 1986

Laffi G, Daskalopoulos G, Kronborg I: Effects of sulindac and ibuprofen in patients with cirrhosis and ascites. Gastroenterology 90:182–187, 1986

Leipzig RM: Psychopharmacology in patients with hepatic and gastrointestinal disease. Int J Psychiatry Med 20:109–139, 1990

Lemberger L, Bergstrom RF, Wolen RL, et al: Fluoxetine: clinical pharmacology and physiologic disposition. J Clin Psychiatry 46:14–19, 1985

Lemoine A, Gautier JC, Azoulay D, et al: Major pathway of imipramine metabolism is catalyzed by cytochromes P-450 1A2 and P-450 3A4 in human liver. Mol Pharmacol 45:827–832, 1993

Levenson JL, Mishra A, Bauernfeind RA, et al: Lithium treatment in a patient with recurrent ventricular tachycardia. Psychosomatics 27:594–596, 1986

Levi AJ, Sherlock S, Walker D: Phenylbutazone and isoniazid metabolism in patients with liver disease in relation to previous drug therapy. Lancet 1:1275–1279, 1968

Levy NB: Psychopharmacology in patients with renal failure. Int J Psychiatry Med 20:325–334, 1990

Levy RH, Shen DD: Valproate absorption, distribution, and excretion, in Antiepileptic Drugs. Edited by Levy R, Mattson R, Meldrum B, et al. New York, Raven, 1989, pp 583–599

Lieberman JA, Cooper TB, Suckow RF: Tricyclic antidepressant and metabolite levels in chronic renal failure. Clin Pharmacol Ther 37:301–370, 1985

Lott RS, Hayton WL: Estimation of creatinine clearance from serum creatinine concentration. Drug Intelligence and Clinical Pharmacy 12:140–150, 1978

Lydiard RB, Gelenberg A: Hazards and adverse effects of lithium. Annu Rev Med 33:327–344, 1982

Lyman GH, Williams CC, Dinwoodie WR, et al: Sudden death in cancer patients receiving lithium. J Clin Oncol 2:1270–1275, 1984

Maher JF: Pharmacokinetic alterations with renal failure and dialysis, in The Pharmacologic Approach to the Critically Ill Patient, 2nd Edition. Edited by Chernow B. Baltimore, MD, Williams & Wilkins, 1988, pp 47–68

Matson AW, Thurlow AC: Hypotension and neurological sequelae following intramuscular midazolam (letter). Anesthesia 43:896, 1988

Maxwell JD, Carrella M, Parkes JD, et al: Plasma disappearance and cerebral effects of chlorpromazine in cirrhosis. Clin Sci 43:143–151, 1972

Mayol RF, Adamson DS, Gammans RE, et al: Pharmacokinetics and disposition of C-14 buspirone HCL after intravenous and oral dosing in man (abstract). Clin Pharmacol Ther 37:210, 1985

McCue RE, Georgotas A, Magachandan N, et al: Plasma levels of nortriptyline and 10-hydroxynortriptyline and treatment-related electrocardiographic changes in the elderly depressed. J Psychiatr Res 23:73–79, 1989a

McCue RE, Georgotas A, Suckow RF: 10-Hydroxynortriptyline and treatment effects in elderly depressed patients. J Neuropsychiatry 1:176–180, 1989b

McEvoy GK (ed): American Hospital Formulary Service Drug Information. Bethesda, MD, American Hospital Formulary Service, 1993, pp 1457–1464

Montgomery SA, McAuley R, Montgomery DB, et al: Dosage adjustment from simple nortriptyline spot level predictor tests in depressed patients. Clin Pharmacokinet 4:129–136, 1979

Morgan MH, Read AE: Antidepressants and liver disease. Gut 13:697–701, 1972

Nelson JC, Atillasoy E, Mazure C: Hydroxydesipramine in the elderly. J Clin Psychopharmacol 8:428–433, 1988a

Nelson JC, Mazure C, Jatlow PI: Antidepressant activity of 2-hydroxy-desipramine. Clin Pharmacol Ther 44:283–288, 1988b

Nordin C, Bertilsson L, Siwers B: Clinical and biochemical effects during treatment of depression with nortriptyline: the role of 10-hydroxy-nortriptyline. Clin Pharmacol Ther 42:10–19, 1987

Novack P, Goluboff B, Bortin L, et al: Circulation and metabolism in congestive heart failure. Circulation 7:724–731, 1953

Ochs HR, Greenblatt DJ, Eckard TB, et al: Repeated diazepam dosing in cirrhotic patients: cumulation and sedation. Clin Pharmacol Ther 33:471–476, 1983

Ochs HR, Greenblatt DJ, Verburg-Ochs B, et al: Temazepam clearance in unaltered cirrhosis. Am J Gastroenterol 81:80–84, 1986

Ohmori S, Takeda S, Rikihisa T, et al: Studies on cytochrome P450 responsible for oxidative metabolism of imipramine in human liver microsomes. Biological and Pharmaceutical Bulletin 16:571–575, 1993

Olomu AB, Vickers CR, Waring RH, et al: High incidence of poor sulfoxidation in patients with primary biliary cirrhosis. N Engl J Med 318:1089–1092, 1988

Otton SV, Crewe HK, Lennard MS, et al: Use of quinidine inhibition to define the role of the sparteine/debrisoquine cytochrome P450 in metoprolol oxidation by human liver microsomes. J Pharmacol Exp Ther 247:242–247, 1988

Palmer KJ, McTavish D: Felbamate: a review of its pharmacodynamic and pharmacokinetic properties, and therapeutic efficacy in epilepsy. Drugs 45:1041–1065, 1993

Pauwels S, Geubel AP, Dive C, et al: Breath $^{14}CO_2$ after intravenous administration of [^{14}C]aminopyrine in liver diseases. Dig Dis Sci 27:49–56, 1982

Physicians' Desk Reference: Tegretol Product Information. Oradell, NJ, Medical Economics Data, 1991, pp 1017–1018

Piafsky KM, Borga O, Odar-Cederlof I, et al: Increased plasma protein binding of propranolol and chlorpromazine mediated by disease-induced elevations of alpha-1-acid glycoprotein. N Engl J Med 299:1435–1439, 1978

Pirttiaho HI, Sotaniemi EA, Ahokas JT, et al: Liver size and indices of drug metabolism in epileptics. Br J Clin Pharmacol 6:273–278, 1978

Pisani F, Fazio A, Oteri G: Sodium valproate and valpromide: differential interactions with carbamazepine in epileptic patients. Epilepsia 27:548–552, 1986

Plenge P, Mellerup ET, Bolwig TG, et al: Lithium treatment: does the kidney prefer one daily dose instead of two? Acta Psychiatr Scand 66:121–128, 1982

Pond SM: Pharmacokinetic drug interactions, in Pharmacokinetic Basis for Drug Treatment. Edited by Benet LZ, Massoud N, Gambertoglio JG. New York, Raven, 1984, pp 195–200

Preskorn SH, Irwin HA: Toxicity of tricyclic antidepressants-kinetics, mechanisms, intervention: a review. J Clin Psychiatry 43:151–156, 1982

Read AE, Laidlaw J, McCarthy CF: Effects of chlorpromazine in patients with hepatic disease. Br Med J 3(669):497–499, 1969

Reidenberg MM: The biotransformation of drugs in renal failure. Am J Med 62:482–485, 1977

Reidenberg MM, Affrime M: Influence of disease on binding of drugs to plasma proteins. Ann N Y Acad Sci 226:115–126, 1973

Risch SC, Groom GP, Janowsky DS: The effects of psychotropic drugs on the cardiovascular system. J Clin Psychiatry 43:16–32, 1982

Ritz R: Benzodiazepine sedation in adult ICU patients. Intensive Care Med 17:511–514, 1991

Roberts RK, Wilkinson GR, Branch RA, et al: Effect of age and parenchymal liver disease on the disposition and elimination of chlordiazepoxide. Gastroenterology 75:419–485, 1978

Roerig, Division of Pfizer, Inc: Sertraline hydrochloride package insert. New York, 1992

Roose SP, Glassman AH, Giardina EGV, et al: Cardiovascular effects of imipramine and bupropion in depressed patients with congestive heart failure. J Clin Psychopharmacol 7:247–251, 1987

Routledge PA, Stargel WW, Wagner GS, et al: Increased alpha-1-acid-glycoprotein and lidocaine disposition in myocardial infarction. Ann Intern Med 93:701–704, 1980

Rowland M, Tozer TN: Disease, in Clinical Pharmacokinetics: Concepts and Applications, 2nd Edition. Edited by Rowland M, Tozer TN. Philadelphia, PA, Lea & Febiger, 1989, pp 238–254

Rowland M, Benet LZ, Graham GG: Clearance concepts in pharmacokinetics. J Pharmacokinet Biopharm 1:123–136, 1973

Sachdeo R, Kramer LD, Rosenberg A, et al: Felbamate monotherapy: controlled trial in patients with partial onset seizures. Epilepsia 32:386–392, 1992

Samiy AH, Rosnick PB: Early identification of renal problems in patients receiving chronic lithium treatment. Am J Psychiatry 144:670–672, 1987

Santos AB, Beliles KE, Arana GW: Parenteral use of psychotropic agents, in Medical-Psychiatric Practice, Vol 2. Edited by Stoudemire A, Fogel BS. Washington, DC, American Psychiatric Press, 1992, pp 113–137

Schenker S, Bergstrom RF, Wolen RL, et al: Fluoxetine disposition and elimination in cirrhosis. Clin Pharmacol Ther 44:353–359, 1988

Schou M: Effects of long-term lithium treatment on kidney function: an overview. J Psychiatr Res 22:287–296, 1988

Secor JW, Schenker S: Drug metabolism in patients with liver disease. Adv Intern Med 32:379–406, 1987

Sellers EM, Greenblatt DJ, Giles CA, et al: Chlordiazepoxide and oxazepam disposition in cirrhosis. Clin Pharmacol Ther 26:240–246, 1979

Sensenbach W, Madison L, Eisenberg S: Cerebral hemodynamics and metabolic studies in patients with congestive heart failure, I: observations in lucid subjects. Circulation 21:697–703, 1960

Shull HJ, Wilkinson GR, Johnson R, et al: Normal disposition of oxazepam in acute viral hepatitis and cirrhosis. Ann Intern Med 84:420–425, 1976

Sigg EB, Osborne M, Korol B: Cardiovascular effects of imipramine. J Pharmacol Exp Ther 141:237–243, 1963

SmithKline Beecham Pharmaceuticals: Paroxetine hydrochloride package insert. Philadelphia, PA, December 1992

Stenson RE, Constantino RE, Harrison DC: Interrelationships of hepatic blood flow, cardiac output, and blood levels of lidocaine in man. Circulation 43:205–211, 1971

Stoudemire A, Fogel BS, Gulley LR: Psychopharmacology in the medically ill: an update, in Medical-Psychiatric Practice, Vol 1. Edited by Stoudemire A, Fogel BS. Washington, DC, American Psychiatric Press, 1991, pp 29–97

Stoudemire A, Fogel BS, Gulley LR, et al: Psychopharmacology in the medical patient, in Psychiatric Care of the Medical Patient. Edited by Stoudemire A, Fogel BS. New York, Oxford University Press, 1993, pp 155–206

Surman OS: Hemodialysis and renal failure, in Massachusetts General Hospital Handbook of General Hospital Psychiatry, 3rd Edition. Edited by Cassem NH. Boston, MA, Mosby Year Book, 1987, pp 401–430

Syrota A, Vinot J-M, Paraf A, et al: Scintillation splenoportography: hemodynamic and morphological study of the portal circulation. Gastroenterology 7:652–659, 1976

Syrota A, Paraf A, Guadebout C, et al: Significance of intra- and extrahepatic portosystemic shunting in survival of cirrhotic patients. Dig Dis Sci 26:878–885, 1981

Tilkian AG, Schroeder JS, Jao JJ, et al: The cardiovascular effects of lithium in man: review of the literature. Am J Med 61:655–670, 1976

Tozer TN: Implications of altered plasma protein binding in disease states, in Pharmacokinetic Basis for Drug Treatment. Edited by Benet LZ, Massoud N, Gambertoglio JG. New York, Raven, 1984, pp 173–193

Traub SL, Johnson CE: Comparison of methods estimating creatinine clearance in children. Am J Hosp Pharm 37:195–201, 1980

Tune L, Coyle JT: Serum levels of anticholinergic drugs in treatment of acute extrapyramidal side effects. Arch Gen Psychiatry 37:293–297, 1980

Vaamonde CA, Milian NE, Magrinat GS: Longitudinal evaluation of glomerular filtration rate during long-term lithium therapy. Am J Kidney Dis 7:213–216, 1986

Vasko MR, Brater DC: Drug interactions, in The Pharmacologic Approach to the Critically Ill Patient, 2nd Edition. Edited by Chernow B. Baltimore, MD, Williams & Wilkins, 1988, pp 21–46

Veith RC, Kaskin MA, Caldwell JH, et al: Cardiovascular effects of tricyclic antidepressants in depressed patients with chronic heart disease. N Engl J Med 306:954–959, 1982

Villeneuve J-P, Fortunet-Fouin H, Arsene D: Cimetidine kinetics and dynamics in patients with severe liver disease. Hepatology 3:923–927, 1983

von Moltke LL, Greenblatt DJ, Harmatz JS, et al: Cytochromes in psychopharmacology (editorial). J Clin Psychopharmacol 14:1–4, 1994

Vozeh S, Schmidlin O, Taeschner W: Pharmacokinetic drug data. Clin Pharmacokinet 13:254–282, 1988

Vrobel TR: Psychiatric aspects of congestive heart failure: implications for consulting psychiatrists. Int J Psychiatry Med 19:211–225, 1989

Wagner ML, Graves NM, Marienau K, et al: Discontinuation of phenytoin and carbamazepine in patients receiving felbamate. Epilepsia 32:398–406, 1991

Wagner ML, Remmel RP, Graves NM, et al: Effect of felbamate on carbamazepine and its major metabolites. Clin Pharmacol Ther 53:536–543, 1993

Watsky EJ, Salzman C: Psychotropic drug interactions. Hosp Community Psychiatry 42:247–256, 1991

Watson RGP, Olomu A, Clements D, et al: A proposed mechanism for chlorpromazine jaundice-defective sulfoxidation combined with rapid hydroxylation. J Hepatol 7:72–78, 1988

Welling P: Effects of gastrointestinal disease on drug absorption, in Pharmacokinetic Basis for Drug Treatment. Edited by Benet LZ, Massoud N, Gambertoglio JG. New York, Raven, 1984, pp 29–48

Wernicke JF: The side effect profile and safety of fluoxetine. J Clin Psychiatry 46:59–67, 1985

Wilder BJ: Pharmacokinetics of valproate and carbamazepine. J Clin Psychopharmacol 12:645–675, 1992

Wilkinson GR: Pharmacokinetics in disease states modifying body perfusion, in The Effect of Disease States on Drug Pharmacokinetics. Edited by Benet LZ. Washington, DC, American Pharmaceutical Association, Academy of Pharmaceutical Sciences, 1976, pp 13–32

Wilkinson GR: The effects of liver disease and aging on the disposition of diazepam, chlordiazepoxide, oxazepam and lorazepam in man. Acta Psychiatr Scand Suppl 274:56–74, 1978

Wilkinson GR, Branch RA: Effects of hepatic disease on clinical pharmacokinetics, in Pharmacokinetic Basis for Drug Treatment. Edited by Benet LZ, Massoud N, Gambertoglio JG. New York, Raven, 1984, pp 49–62

Wilkinson GR, Shand DG: A physiological approach to hepatic drug clearance. Clin Pharmacol Ther 18:377–390, 1975

Wilkinson SP, Williams R: Ascites, electrolyte disorders and renal failure, in Liver and Biliary Disease Pathophysiology, Diagnosis, Management. Edited by Wright R, Alberti KGMM, Karran S, et al. Philadelphia, PA, WB Saunders, 1979, pp 1060–1086

Winter ME: Basic principles, in Basic Clinical Pharmacokinetics, 2nd Edition. Edited by Koda-Kimble MA, Young LY. Spokane, WA, Applied Therapeutics, 1988a, pp 7–99

Winter ME: Carbamazepine, in Basic Clinical Pharmacokinetics, 2nd Edition. Edited by Koda-Kimble MA, Young LY. Spokane, WA, Applied Therapeutics, 1988b, pp 139–146

Winter ME: Lithium, in Basic Clinical Pharmacokinetics, 2nd Edition. Edited by Koda-Kimble MA, Young LY. Spokane, WA, Applied Therapeutics, 1988c, pp 191–198

Young RC, Alexpopulos GS, Shamoian CA, et al: Plasma 10-hydroxy-nortriptyline and ECG changes in elderly depressed patients. Am J Psychiatry 142:866–868, 1985

Zavodnick S: Atrial flutter with amoxapine: a case report. Am J Psychiatry 138:1503–1504, 1981

Zelis R, Nellis SH, Longhurst J, et al: Abnormalities in the regional circulations accompanying congestive heart failure. Prog Cardiovasc Dis 18:181–199, 1975

Ziegler VE, Biggs JT, Wylie LT: Protriptyline kinetics. Pharmacol Ther 23:580–584, 1978a

Ziegler VE, Biggs JT, Wylie LT, et al: Doxepin kinetics. Clin Pharmacol Ther 23:573–579, 1978b

Zito RA, Reid PR: Lidocaine kinetics preceded by indocyanine green clearance. N Engl J Med 298:1160–1163, 1978

Chapter 2

Psychopharmacology in Medical Patients: An Update

Alan Stoudemire, M.D.
Barry S. Fogel, M.D.

For the past 8 years, we have periodically consolidated the literature on the use of psychotropic agents in medically ill patients. Comprehensive reviews of this subject appeared in our original textbook, *Principles of Medical Psychiatry* (Stoudemire and Fogel 1987), and more recently in *Psychiatric Care of the Medical Patient* (Stoudemire and Fogel 1993a). In this series of textbooks, *Medical-Psychiatric Practice,* approximately every 2 years we have published updated reviews of the psychotropic literature for the clinical care of medical patients (Fogel and Stoudemire 1993; Stoudemire et al. 1991b). We have also published interim review articles (Stoudemire et al. 1990, 1991a) and chapters in other textbooks (Stoudemire et al. 1993a; Stoudemire et al. 1995). In this chapter, we update the literature on the use of psychotropics in medically ill patients, with particular emphasis on newer drugs such as the selective serotonin reuptake inhibitors (SSRIs), venlafaxine, nefazodone, risperidone, tacrine, zolpidem, and clozapine, as well as lithium, carbamazepine, sodium valproate, psychostimulants, and the tricyclic antidepressants (TCAs). We encourage readers to read our comprehensive reviews on the use of these and other drugs (e.g., monoamine oxidase inhibitors [MAOIs]) in medically ill patients. This discussion presumes an extensive basic knowledge of general psychopharmacology as well as general pharmacodynamic and pharmacokinetic principles of the use of psychotropic agents in medically ill patients. Chapter 1 in this volume reviews in detail psychotropic pharmacokinetics in medically ill patients.

SELECTIVE SEROTONIN REUPTAKE INHIBITORS

Since the introduction of fluoxetine in the United States for the treatment of depression, several other SSRIs have been marketed including sertraline, paroxetine, and fluvoxamine. These drugs have been extraordinarily useful in the treatment of depression in medically ill patients because of their benign side-effect profiles, particularly their minimal quinidine-like properties, low or no anticholinergic effects, and lack of effects on blood pressure. Although bradycardia has been attributed to fluoxetine, reports of this effect have been extremely rare in relation to the widespread use of the drug. Reported adverse cardiac reactions in medically ill patients taking SSRIs are often in patients with extensive concomitant medical illness and those taking multiple medications. This suggests that the reported adverse effects may have resulted from drug interactions rather than direct effects of the SSRIs. In this chapter, we focus on drug interactions with the SSRIs relevant for medically ill patients. Particular attention is devoted to the effects of the SSRIs on the cytochrome P_{450} system, examining the potential for such effects to increase the likelihood of toxicity developing from both the SSRIs and other concurrently administered drugs.

CYTOCHROMES AND PSYCHOPHARMACOLOGY

Cytochromes are a family of hepatic enzymes that play a primary role in oxidative drug metabolism. At least 29 human forms of cytochrome P_{450} have been identified (isoenzymes) that are subject to genetic control. Each isoenzyme has relative specificity for the metabolism of various drugs, although considerable overlap exists. For many drugs, the specific P_{450} isoenzyme primarily responsible for their metabolism is not known. Cytochromes can be chemically inhibited by exogenous substances, including medications commonly used in both psychiatric and general medical practice (von Moltke et al. 1994).

Cytochrome P$_{450}$-2D6

The isoenzyme cytochrome P$_{450}$-2D6 (CyP$_{450}$-2D6) has received much recent attention because it is primarily involved in the metabolism of many psychotropic agents, including the TCAs and several neuroleptics, including haloperidol, perphenazine, and thioridazine. CyP$_{450}$-2D6 also is involved in the metabolism of β-adrenergic blocking agents (propranolol, metoprolol), antiarrhythmics (encainide, mexiletine), opiates (codeine, dextromorphan), and the stimulant methamphetamine and the oncologic agent vinblastine (Table 2–1).

The CyP$_{450}$-2D6 isoenzyme is lacking in about 5% of the Caucasian population, with varying degrees of inactivity in other ethnic groups (Caporaso and Shaw 1991). In patients who lack this isoenzyme, plasma concentrations of drugs preferentially metabolized by CyP$_{450}$-2D6 may be elevated to toxic levels even when relatively low doses of medication are used. The prototypical drug that has been studied in the assessment of CyP$_{450}$-2D6 activity is the antihypertensive debrisoquin. Debrisoquin, along with sparteine, is used as a model substrate for CyP$_{450}$-2D6 to study the metabolic activity of this isoenzyme, particularly with regard to experiments examining the activity of CyP$_{450}$-2D6 in connection with pharmacokinetic interactions.

Patients who have a genetically determined functional deficiency of CyP$_{450}$-2D6 (genetic polymorphism) show an exaggerated hypotensive reaction when given debrisoquin. CyP$_{450}$-2D6-deficient patients have been referred to as *poor metabolizers* (PMs), compared with *extensive metabolizers* (EMs), who have normal activity of this enzyme (Caporaso and Shaw 1991). Although deficiency of the isoenzyme is genetically determined in Caucasians and to varying degrees in other ethnic groups, activity of this enzyme can be inhibited pharmacologically, effectively converting an EM into a PM. A prototype drug that inhibits CyP$_{450}$-2D6 in this manner is quinidine. Quinidine is not metabolized by CyP$_{450}$-2D6, but quinidine binds to this isoenzyme and inhibits its metabolic activity. EMs who are given quinidine are pharmacologically converted to PMs, as noted above, by quinidine's inhibitory effects on CyP$_{450}$-2D6. Hence, they are prone to high serum levels and adverse side effects when concurrently given drugs primarily metabolized by this enzyme (e.g., TCAs). (Table 2–1 shows drugs metabolized by the CyP$_{450}$-2D6 isoenzyme and the potential clinical consequence of enzymatic deficiency or inhibition.)

Table 2–1. Drugs metabolized by CyP_{450}-2D6 isoenzyme and potential clinical consequences in poor metabolizers

Drug	Potential consequence
Antihypertensives	
Debrisoquin	Excessive hypotension
Guanoxan	Higher serum levels, hypotension
Indoramin	Increased side effects, sedation, nausea, dizziness
β-Blockers	
Timolol	Higher plasma concentration, greater β-blockade
Metoprolol	Excessive β-blockade, hepatitis, slow-release preparation not required, loss of cardioselectivity
Propranolol	4-Hydroxypropranolol level decreased, β-blockade little changed to slightly increased as measured by reduction in exercise-induced heart rate and prolongation of Q-T and P-R intervals
Bufuralol	Higher plasma levels
Propafenone	Long elimination half-life, debrisoquin metabolism inhibited, central nervous system toxic reaction (dizziness, paresthesia), greater β-blockade at lower doses associated with higher plasma levels
Tricyclic antidepressants	
Nortriptyline	Higher plasma concentrations and toxic side effects
Amitriptyline	Higher serum levels (of nortriptyline), hydroxylase-demethylase is induced in smokers; therefore, clinical effects may be more likely in nonsmokers
Clomipramine	Higher drug and metabolite levels
Desipramine	Higher serum levels, slow clearance
Imipramine	Higher serum levels, slow clearance
MAO inhibitors	
Amiflamine	Unknown
Methoxyphenamine	Higher serum levels
Neuroleptics	Increased toxic reaction, especially when used with tricyclic antidepressants
Perphenazine	Higher serum concentrations
Trifluperidol	Unknown, but competitive inhibition observed in vitro
Fluphenazine	Unknown, but competitive inhibition observed in vitro

(continued)

Table 2–1. Drugs metabolized by CyP_{450}-2D6 isoenzyme and potential
clinical consequences in poor metabolizers *(continued)*

Drug	Potential consequence
Thioridazine	In vitro inhibitor of debrisoquin-metabolizing enzymes and higher frequency of PM in treated subjects
Antiarrhythmics	
Encainide	High serum levels, inadequate suppression of arrhythmias
Flecainide	Increased side effects and competitive inhibition of CyP_{450}-2D6
Miscellaneous	
Codeine	Reduced therapeutic effect
Dextromethorphan	Lethargy, psychosis after overdose; uncertain effects after repeated administration at regular doses
Phenformin	Hypoglycemia, lactic acidosis
Vinblastine	Some inhibition of bufuralol hydroxylation (a prototype reaction for the debrisoquin polymorphism)
Perhexiline	Liver damage
Methamphetamine	Impaired metabolism
Dextropropoxyphene	Inhibits metabolism of debrisoquin and other substrates of CyP_{450}-2D6 (e.g., desipramine)

Note. PMs = poor metabolizers, EMs = extensive metabolizers, MAO = monoamine oxidase.
Source. Adapted from Caporaso NE, Shaw GL: "Clinical Implications of the Competitive Inhibition of the Debrisoquin-Metabolizing Isozyme by Quinidine." *Archives of Internal Medicine* 151:1985–1992, 1991.

SSRI Inhibition of CyP450-2D6

CyP_{450}-2D6 has received much attention in psychiatry because of the ability of the SSRIs to variably inhibit this isoenzyme. This effect was first manifested by reports that concurrent administration of SSRIs with TCAs and trazodone resulted in elevation of trazodone serum levels, sometimes to as much as four times the previous level.

There has been considerable recent discussion regarding the relative potencies of various SSRIs to differentially inhibit this enzyme system. It should be emphasized, however, that *all* of the SSRIs have the capacity to inhibit this isoenzyme to some extent. Paroxetine shows the most potent inhibition of this isoenzyme, but fluoxetine (including its metabolite norfluoxetine) and sertraline have inhibitory effects as well (Table 2–2). Note that thioridazine, a commonly used neuroleptic, has inhibitory effects similar to the SSRIs fluoxetine and sertraline. A general trend in most studies evaluating the effects of SSRIs on the CyP_{450}-

Table 2–2. Inhibition constants (K_i) for the inhibition of 2-dehydrosparteine metabolism in human liver microsomes

Compound	K_i (μm)
Paroxetine	0.15
M-I glucuronide*	> 200
M-I sulfate*	120
M-I	16
M-II	0.5
M-III	> 20
Fluoxetine	0.60
Norfluoxetine*	0.43
Sertraline	0.70
Citalopram	5.1
Fluvoxamine	8.2
Clomipramine	2.2
Desipramine	2.3
Amitriptyline	4.0
Quinidine	0.03
Thioridazine	0.52
Metoprolol	37
Lignocaine	200
Antipyrine	> 3,000

*Major metabolites.
Source. Reprinted from Crewe HK, Lennard MS, Tucker GT, et al: "The Effect of Selective Serotonin Re-uptake Inhibitors on Cytochrome P_{450}-2D6 (CYP2D6) Activity in Human Liver Microsomes." *British Journal of Clinical Pharmacology* 34:262–265, 1992. Copyright 1992, Blackwell Scientific Publications, Ltd. Used with permission.

2D6 system is that sertraline has relatively less inhibitory effects on CyP_{450}-2D6 than either fluoxetine or paroxetine. Thus, sertraline elevates desipramine serum levels less than fluoxetine (Preskorn et al. 1994). Moreover, the effects of fluoxetine on desipramine levels are much more persistent, lasting as long as 3 weeks, consistent with norfluoxetine's long elimination half-life.

Cytochrome P_{450}-3A4

A second isoenzyme system of relevance is the CyP_{450}-3A4. This isoenzyme metabolizes the triazolobenzodiazepines triazolam, alprazolam, and midazolam, as well as erythromycin, cyclosporine, lidocaine, nifedipine, quinidine, and terfenadine (Table 2–3). CyP_{450}-3A4 also participates in the demethylation of TCAs such as imipramine and amitriptyline (Lemoine et al. 1993; Ohmori et al. 1993; von Moltke et al. 1994). This enzymatic system is not subject to genetic variability (polymorphism) (i.e., all patients possess this isoenzyme), and it is present in both liver and gastrointestinal (GI) tissue.

Table 2–3. Substrates for and inhibitors of the CyP_{450}-3A4 isoenzyme

Drugs metabolized by CyP_{450}-3A4 isoenzyme
 Triazolam
 Alprazolam
 Midazolam
 Sertraline
 Terfenadine
 Astemizole
 Imipramine, amitriptyline (primary demethylation)
 Cyclosporine
 Lidocaine
 Nifedipine
 Quinidine
Inhibitors of CyP_{450}-3A4 activity
 Ketoconazole
 Itraconazole
 Erythromycin (and other macrolide antibiotics)
 Cimetidine
 Nefazodone
 Selective serotonin reuptake inhibitors (weak effect)

The antifungal agent ketoconazole is a potent inhibitor of the CyP_{450}-3A4 isoenzyme, as are erythromycin, cimetidine, and nefazodone. SSRIs can partially inhibit this enzyme but do so to a much lesser degree than they do CyP_{450}-2D6.

The major clinical impact of CyP_{450}-3A4 enzyme inhibition has been development of cardiotoxicity caused by prolonged Q-T syndrome, leading to the development of potentially lethal arrhythmias that occur when terfenadine's metabolism has been blocked by either ketoconazole or erythromycin. As noted above, ketoconazole, erythromycin, and nefazodone can inhibit CyP_{450}-3A4's activity, and this isoenzyme is primarily responsible for the metabolism of terfenadine. Unmetabolized terfenadine can potentially prolong the Q-T interval, possibly precipitating ventricular tachyarrhythmias (torsades de pointes). (This drug interaction is discussed in more detail later in this chapter.)

In contrast, fluconazole, a related antifungal agent, has 500 times less inhibitory activity on CyP_{450}-3A4 and therefore is a safer drug with regard to potential effects on both benzodiazepine and terfenadine metabolism (Gibaldi 1992). Only one case report thus far has suggested that concurrent use of fluoxetine may have contributed to an arrhythmia possibly caused by terfenadine via inhibition of terfenadine metabolism. The evidence for the proposed interaction was weak, and specific electrocardiogram (ECG) data to support prolonged Q-Tc (Q-T interval corrected for heart rate) conduction time were not presented (Swims 1993).

Space does not permit a detailed review of all of the reported drug interactions with the SSRIs. Table 2–4 summarizes drug interactions that have been reported over the past several years that appear to have the most clinical relevance. The mechanisms for these interactions vary; some may be related to direct metabolic effects on the cytochrome enzymatic systems, whereas others may be more related to pharmacodynamic interactions. Extensive details of side effects and drug interactions with fluoxetine can be found elsewhere (Messiha 1993).

SELECTIVE SEROTONIN REUPTAKE INHIBITORS AND IMIPRAMINE/DESIPRAMINE

When the SSRI fluvoxamine is added to the regimen of patients on steady doses of imipramine, imipramine levels may rise by factors of three to four. It is therefore likely that fluvoxamine inhibits the

Table 2–4. Reported drug interactions with selective serotonin reuptake inhibitors

Fluvoxamine

Drug	Effect	Reference
Propranolol	Five-time increase in propranolol levels	Benfield and Ward 1986; van Harten et al. 1992a
Warfarin	Increase in warfarin concentrations by 60%; increased prothrombin time	Benfield and Ward 1986
Theophylline	Increase in theophylline level by factor of three	Sperber 1991
Carbamazepine	Conflicting reports: increase in carbamazepine levels as well as stable carbamazepine levels reported when fluvoxamine added	Fritze et al. 1991 Spina et al. 1993b
Amitriptyline	Increase in tricyclic antidepressant serum levels	Bertschy et al. 1991
Atenolol	Some decrease in clinical effect of atenolol	Benfield and Ward 1986
Imipramine	Increased imipramine levels	Spina et al. 1993a, 1993c
Desipramine	Desipramine levels increase slightly when fluvoxamine added to patients with previously stable serum levels of desipramine	Spina et al. 1993a
Lorazepam	No effect	van Harten et al. 1992c

Fluoxetine

Drug	Effect	Reference
Imipramine	Increased levels	Bergstrom et al. 1992
Desipramine	Increased levels	Bergstrom et al. 1992
Nortriptyline	Increased levels	Ciraulo and Shader 1990
Haloperidol	Increased levels	Goff et al. 1991; Tate 1989
Perphenazine	Increased levels	Lock et al. 1990
Diazepam	Increased levels	Lemberger et al. 1988
Alprazolam	Increased levels	Lasher et al. 1991
Carbamazepine	Increase of both carbamazepine and carbamazepine 10,11-epoxide levels	Gidal et al. 1993; Grimsley et al. 1991

(continued)

Table 2–4. Reported drug interactions with selective serotonin reuptake inhibitors *(continued)*

Fluoxetine *(continued)*

Drug	Effect	Reference
Warfarin	No effect on half-life of warfarin or the prothrombin time	Rowe et al. 1978
Pimozide	Bradycardia when fluoxetine was added; delirium also reported, probably caused by increased pimozide levels	Ahmed et al. 1993; Hansen-Grant et al. 1993
Cyclosporine	No effect of fluoxetine on cyclosporine levels	Strouse et al. 1993
Valproic acid	Fluoxetine raises valproate serum levels	Sovner and Davis 1991
Clozapine	Clozapine levels increased by fluoxetine	Centorrino et al. 1994
Clonazepam	No effect by fluoxetine on clonazepam levels	Greenblatt et al. 1992
Phenytoin	May increase phenytoin levels	Woods et al. 1994
Metoprolol	Bradycardia when fluoxetine added	Walley et al. 1993

Paroxetine

Drug	Effect	Reference
Cimetidine	Paroxetine levels increased by 50%	Bannister et al. 1989
Phenobarbital	Paroxetine levels decreased by 25%	Greb et al. 1989
Carbamazepine, valproate, and phenytoin	No effect on carbamazepine, serum valproate, and phenytoin levels when paroxetine coadministered with these anticonvulsants	Andersen et al. 1991
Phenytoin, carbamazepine	May lower paroxetine levels	Andersen et al. 1991
Drugs metabolized via CyP_{450}-2D6	Elevated serum levels	See Table 2–1
Tolbutamide	Decreased levels of tolbutamide	Warrington 1991

(continued)

Table 2–4. Reported drug interactions with selective serotonin reuptake inhibitors *(continued)*

Sertraline		
Drug	Effect	Reference
Warfarin	Increased prothrombin time	Wilner et al. 1991
Atenolol	No effect on atenolol level	Warrington 1991
Tricyclics (including desipramine)	Elevated tricyclic anti-depressant levels	Barros and Asnis 1993
Drugs metabolized by CyP$_{450}$-2D6	Increased levels	See Table 2–1

demethylation pathway of imipramine. Fluvoxamine may also act as a competitive inhibitor for the same enzymatic systems with imipramine because fluvoxamine also undergoes oxidative demethylation. In the study by Spina (1993a), levels of desipramine were only slightly (insignificantly) raised by the addition of fluvoxamine to patients on stable doses of desipramine. This observation suggests that fluvoxamine affects TCA metabolism via inhibition of demethylation, and its effects on the hydroxylation of secondary amines such as desipramine are not clinically relevant.

However, it is well established that fluoxetine markedly raises both imipramine and desipramine levels similar to the effects of quinidine via inhibition of the CyP$_{450}$-2D6 system (Bergstrom et al. 1992; Suckow et al. 1992). Hence, it is now well established that fluoxetine can inhibit hydroxylation of desipramine in a concentration-dependent manner.

CLONAZEPAM AND PSYCHOTROPIC DRUG INTERACTIONS

It appears that SSRIs such as fluoxetine can alter the metabolism of benzodiazepines such as diazepam and alprazolam via interference with cytochrome oxidative mechanisms, but clonazepam metabolism does not appear to be affected by the SSRIs in this manner. The major metabolic pathway of clonazepam involves nitro-reduction, resulting in a 7-amino clonazepam metabolite (Greenblatt et al. 1992). Detailed pharmacokinetic studies of the effects of other drugs on clonazepam metabolism are not yet available; however, one may extrapolate from the studies of the 7-nitro benzodiazepine nitrazepam, which has a metabolic pathway essentially identical to clonazepam. Extrapolation suggests that clonazepam's metabolism would not be altered in a major way by either aging or liver cirrhosis, which decreases oxidative metabolic efficiency (Greenblatt et al. 1985; Jochemsen et al. 1983). Clonazepam's metabolism would also be predicted to be minimally affected by cimetidine (Ochs et al. 1983). In contrast, these factors (aging, cirrhosis) would impair the metabolism of benzodiazepines that are primarily oxidized (e.g., diazepam).

ADVERSE HEMATOLOGIC
EFFECTS OF FLUOXETINE

Continued reports have documented that fluoxetine may have significant hematologic effects. Fluoxetine diminishes granular storage of serotonin in platelets and has been reported to increase bleeding times. Other investigators have reported petechiae and ecchymoses and even melena with fluoxetine treatment. Some evidence suggests that these hematologic effects are dose related. Impaired platelet aggregation has been reported usually when fluoxetine was given in doses higher than 20 mg/day, with normalization of platelet activity within several days after the drug was discontinued (Alderman et al. 1992). This indicates that the parent drug (fluoxetine) was the culprit because the principal metabolite norfluoxetine would take much longer to be eliminated. It is not fully known the extent to which other SSRIs clinically affect platelet functioning. However, it would be prudent to obtain a bleeding time determination in a patient taking fluoxetine if elective surgery is planned.

Interactive effects between SSRIs and warfarin may alter coagulation time (prothrombin time or international normalized ratio [INR]). The potential interaction has been postulated to be based on the SSRIs displacing warfarin from protein-binding sites, thereby leaving more free warfarin to be biologically active. The best studies in this regard have been with fluoxetine, but fluoxetine does not appear to alter the pharmacologic effects of warfarin. Both fluvoxamine and sertraline, in contrast, have been reported to increase total warfarin levels and increase the prothrombin time. Fluvoxamine has been noted to increase warfarin levels by 60% and subsequently increase prothrombin times (Benfield and Ward 1986). There was no effect on the half-life of warfarin or the prothrombin time when fluoxetine was coadministered

(Rowe et al. 1978). Paroxetine has been reported to have no effect on total warfarin levels but nevertheless can lead to increased bleeding when the two drugs are coadministered, probably by displacing warfarin from protein-binding sites (Bannister et al. 1989). Sertraline coadministered with warfarin also has been noted to increase the prothrombin time (Wilner et al. 1991).

A question of significant clinical importance is whether any risk of increased bleeding is involved in patients being considered for prospective surgery who are being treated with SSRIs. As reviewed earlier, it appears that rapid normalization of platelet functioning occurs when fluoxetine is discontinued, because it has been postulated that fluoxetine, and not its primary long–half-life metabolite norfluoxetine, is responsible for effects on bleeding times (Alderman et al. 1992). If the bleeding time was elevated, fluoxetine could be discontinued temporarily; elective surgery could proceed when the bleeding time normalized. With other SSRIs, it would be advisable to check a prothrombin time and partial thromboplastin time before surgery as well, although if it were necessary to stop the SSRI, withdrawal symptoms could result after abrupt discontinuation—a problem less likely to occur with fluoxetine. Note, however, that if emergency surgery were necessary, an excessive clotting time could be reversed with fresh-frozen plasma or clotting factors.

SELECTIVE SEROTONIN REUPTAKE INHIBITORS AND EXTRAPYRAMIDAL SYMPTOMS

It is now well established that SSRIs can cause extrapyramidal side effects including akathisia, dyskinesias, dystonias, and drug-induced parkinsonism (Arya and Szabadi 1993; Baldwin et al. 1991; Nicholson 1992; Wils 1992). In our experience, extrapyramidal side effects other than akathisia are most likely to occur in older patients, particularly those whose histories or prior drug responses suggest preclinical Parkinson's disease (Dave 1994). The effect may be caused by inhibition of dopamine production by dopaminergic neurons, caused by increases in synaptic serotonin. Inhibitory effects of serotonin and SSRIs on dopamine systems have been demonstrated in animal models (Baldessarini and Marsh 1990).

Not surprisingly, SSRIs can exacerbate symptoms of preexisting Parkinson's disease (Steur 1993), although many neurologists believe that such effects rarely are clinically significant (Caley and Friedman 1992).

A number of the reported cases of SSRIs causing extrapyramidal side effects have occurred in patients treated concurrently with neuroleptics. In some of these cases, inhibition of neuroleptic metabolism by SSRIs may have been the mechanism of the observed interaction (Arya and Szabadi 1993; Nicholson 1992; Wils 1992).

Akathisia is the most common extrapyramidal symptom in patients treated with SSRIs. It is seen in patients of all ages and may be most often encountered in those treated with fluoxetine. This side effect can be managed by dose reduction or by treatment with low doses of propranolol.

FLUOXETINE IN HEPATIC AND RENAL DISEASE

In patients with mild, moderate, or severe renal dysfunction, the pharmacokinetics of fluoxetine and norfluoxetine are not meaningfully affected (Bergstrom et al. 1993). Daily administration of 20 mg of fluoxetine for 2 months to depressed patients on hemodialysis produced steady-state levels comparable to those in patients with normal renal function. These results indicate that renal disease is not an important consideration in fluoxetine dosage.

In patients with cirrhosis of the liver, the average clearance rates of fluoxetine and norfluoxetine were lower, and their elimination half-lives almost doubled compared with healthy control subjects. Thus, the steady-state level of drug and active metabolite might not be reached for months on a fixed daily dose (Bergstrom et al. 1993).

The elimination half-life of paroxetine has also been noted to be prolonged in the presence of liver disease (Dalhoff et al. 1991; Dechant and Clissold 1991). Similar reports exist for fluvoxamine (van Harten et al. 1993).

SELECTIVE SEROTONIN REUPTAKE INHIBITORS AND CARDIOVASCULAR DISEASE

We have recently reviewed the literature on SSRIs and cardiovascular disease (Levenson 1993; Stoudemire et al. 1993b). The benign cardiovascular profile of the SSRIs appears to be a consistent property of all of these drugs, including the newly introduced agents such as sertraline, paroxetine, and fluvoxamine (Laird et al. 1993; Warrington and Lewis 1992). However, almost all of the studies with the newer agents such as sertraline and fluvoxamine have been done in relatively healthy young to middle-aged adults generally free from cardiovascular disease (Fisch and Knoebel 1992). As with fluoxetine, there may be a propensity for the newer SSRIs to lower heart rate, an effect that has been observed in a few patients treated with sertraline. Clinically significant bradycardia with SSRIs alone is rare. Whether it may be more common in patients concomitantly receiving SSRIs and β-blockers or digoxin is not known.

VENLAFAXINE

Venlafaxine is a new antidepressant recently introduced into the United States. Venlafaxine exhibits both serotonergic and noradrenergic presynaptic reuptake inhibition. It has clinically relevant weak effects on dopamine reuptake at the high end of its dosage range. Neither venlafaxine nor its major metabolites exhibit significant binding at muscarinic, α-adrenergic, histaminergic, μ-opiate, or D_2-dopamine receptors. Venlafaxine lacks MAOI effects. In contrast to the SSRIs, which are highly protein bound, venlafaxine binds weakly to serum proteins (25%–30%). Its principal metabolite (O-desmethyl venlafaxine) has significant biological activity and retains reuptake inhibitory activity on both norepinephrine and serotonin uptake. Mean elimination half-life is 4.1 ± 1.3 hours for the parent compound and 10.4 ± 1.7 hours for the principal metabolite desmethyl-venlafaxine. No dose adjustments based on age appear necessary (Schweizer et al. 1994).

Venlafaxine and Side Effects

Venlafaxine appears to have a generally benign side-effect profile. No impairment of cognition has been observed in the therapeutic range, and it does not appear to interact with alcohol or benzodiazepines (Troy et al. 1992). The drug appears to have minimal to no effect on cardiac conduction.

The usual dose range is from 25 to 75 mg every 8 hours. Venlafaxine is generally well tolerated; the most common side effects are similar to those of the SSRIs—nervousness, sweating, nausea, sedation, anorexia, dry mouth, and dizziness. Like the SSRIs, patients may complain of insomnia or sedation and, occasionally, of both. Sexual dysfunction may occur but probably is less likely than with SSRIs; however, extensive assessment of its effects on sexual functioning has not yet been done. In preliminary trials, however, at doses at or near 375 mg/day, almost 13% of men reported orgasm or abnormal ejaculation, but at more routine doses (near 200 mg/day), this type of sexual dysfunction occurred in only 2% of patients. Women reported orgasmic dysfunction at a rate of about 2% when typical doses were used. A major potential drawback of the drug is the recommended three-times-a-day dosing regimen, although some evidence suggests that twice-a-day dosing may be just as effective (Mendels et al. 1993). One of us (B.S.F.) has had a number of patients do well with twice-a-day dosing, with most of the dose given at night in patients who experience substantial sedation from the drug.

This drug has also been associated with elevations in blood pressure, with an incidence of greater than 5% in doses above 200 mg/day (the average daily dose for most patients is between 150 and 225 mg/day). Sustained increase in blood pressure occurs in a dose-dependent fashion, with incidence rates of about 3% in doses below 100 mg/day, 5%–7% in doses between 100 and 300 mg/day, and 13% at doses above 300 mg/day. Because studies in patients with preexisting hypertension have not been conducted, blood pressure should be monitored weekly during upward dosage titration in patients with preexisting hypertension.

Half-life.   In the presence of hepatic cirrhosis, the elimination half-life of venlafaxine was increased by about one-third (30%), and clearance decreased by one-half as compared with control subjects. The half-life of its principal metabolite desmethyl-venlafaxine increased by 60%, and clearance decreased by 30%. With severe liver disease, clearance can be reduced by as much as 90% compared with healthy subjects (Wyeth Laboratories 1993).

In renal dysfunction (glomerular filtration rate [GFR] 10 to 70 ml/min), venlafaxine elimination half-life was prolonged by 50%, and clearance was reduced by 24% compared with control subjects. In dialysis patients, venlafaxine half-life was prolonged by 180%, and clearance was decreased by 57%. Desmethyl-venlafaxine half-life was increased by 40% in chronic renal failure patients (GFR 10 to 70 ml/min), and clearance appeared to be unchanged. In dialysis patients, desmethyl-venlafaxine was increased by 142%, and clearance was reduced by 56%. The clinical significance of these increases in elimination half-lives and decreases in clearance in venlafaxine and its principal metabolite is not entirely known but indicates reduced initial doses, slower dosage titration, and more frequent monitoring of blood pressure when the drug is used in patients with renal failure or insufficiency.

The prevalence of seizures with venlafaxine appears to be low (8 of 3,082 patients in clinical trials—0.26%), but five of the eight cases occurred at doses less than 150 mg/day. This seizure frequency is within range of that reported with the higher dose ranges of the TCAs.

Venlafaxine is metabolized by the isoenzyme CyP_{450}-2D6. Therefore, drugs such as thioridazine quinidine that inhibit this enzyme would result in higher levels of the parent venlafaxine compound when the two drugs are used concurrently. Venlafaxine itself is believed to have relatively weak inhibitory effects on CyP_{450}-2D6.

Venlafaxine appears not to affect the metabolism of diazepam or its principal metabolite desmethyl-diazepam. Cimetidine inhibits the metabolism of venlafaxine (clearance reduced by over 50%) but does not appear to affect desmethyl-venlafaxine in this manner.

In medically healthy individuals, there do not appear to be any significant effects of venlafaxine on the ECG. Experience with this agent in elderly and medically ill patients is quite limited, other than the pharmacokinetic studies noted above in patients with renal disease and hepatic cirrhosis. The major concern at this point would be its use in patients with a history of hypertension and the need for blood pressure monitoring in almost all patients, particularly those treated at the higher dose ranges and those with preexisting hypertension.

NEFAZODONE

Nefazodone is a new antidepressant that was introduced into the United States in 1995. The drug's primary effect is 5-HT_2-receptor inhibition, but it is also a weak inhibitor of norepinephrine reuptake. Presynaptically, nefazodone acutely increases 5-HT within synapses and increases the availability of 5-HT to interact with 5-HT_{1a} receptors. Postsynaptically, it acutely blocks 5-HT_2 receptors and downregulates them with chronic administration.

Nefazodone and Side Effects

Data from clinical trials indicate that nefazodone has a favorable side-effect profile for potential use in medically ill or elderly patients. The available information regarding its cardiac and other organ system effects and what is known regarding drug interactions is summarized below. The drug has been studied in more than 3,400 patients in clinical trials. More than 500 of these patients were older than age 65 years, but in relatively good general health (D. Jody, Bristol-Myers Squibb, personal communication, October 1994).

Nefazodone appears to have relatively benign effects on the ECG. Nefazodone has been associated with clinically asymptomatic bradycardia. In extensive clinical trials, only 13 patients were discontinued from nefazodone treatment due to ECG changes. These changes included three cases of nonspecific ST/T-wave changes, two cases of extrasystoles, two cases of first-degree atrioventricular block, two cases of ST/T-wave depression, two cases of bradycardia, one case of ventricular extrasystoles, one case of left ventricular hypertrophy, one case of angina pectoris, one case of sinus arrhythmia (with occasional premature ventricular contractions and premature atrial contractions), and one case of atrial fibrillation. According to information supplied by the manufacturer, these ECG findings were associated with few other signs and symptoms and generally occurred in patients with preexisting cardiovascular disease. One study by the manufacturer revealed that imipramine but not nefazodone produced orthostatic blood pressure changes, Q-Tc prolongation, and tachycardia. Modest decreases in supine (but not orthostatic) systolic and diastolic blood pressure, as well as decreases in resting pulse rates, have been observed.

In elderly patients, there does not appear to be a significant risk of orthostatic hypotension, even though patients treated with nefazodone had significantly lower supine systolic blood pressure than those given a placebo. Orthostatic hypotension, however, was reported in some patients in the drug's clinical trials, consistent with the drug's weak α_1-adrenergic blocking effects.

The drug has some mild GI side effects similar to those encountered with other predominantly serotonergic antidepressants. These include occasional reports of dyspepsia and abdominal pain, which appear to be more common in patients with a history of preexisting peptic ulcer disease. Mild dry mouth, nausea, and constipation have been reported. The drug does not appear to cause urinary retention. In contrast to other SSRIs (e.g., fluoxetine, sertraline, paroxetine), it is associated with a low rate of sexual dysfunction.

Other side effects that appear to occur more frequently than with placebo include somnolence, dizziness, weakness, lightheadedness, and blurred vision. The drug is therefore not totally devoid of anticholinergic, antihistaminic, or anti–α-adrenergic side effects, but they are much less problematic than those of the standard TCAs. No decrease in seizure threshold has been described.

Drug Interactions With Nefazodone

Nefazodone has been studied and found to have no clinically significant interactions with lorazepam, cimetidine, or warfarin. The drug does, however, appear to potentiate the psychomotor effects of alprazolam by increasing its serum levels. Therefore, reductions in the doses of alprazolam would be recommended if these two drugs were used together. Similar effects have also been described with triazolam. It has a relatively short elimination half-life (2 to 4 hours), and a steady state is reached in 3 to 4 days with twice-a-day dosing regimens. The pharmacokinetics of nefazodone are not altered by haloperidol.

Because nefazodone inhibits the CyP_{450}-3A4 isoenzyme, nefazodone should not be used with the antihistamines terfenadine or astemizole because of the risk of cardiac arrhythmias (see the subsection, "Terfenadine," later in this chapter for the mechanisms of this interaction).

It should be emphasized, however, that nefazodone has not been used in severely medically ill patients, so the usual conservative approach to dosage should be taken when using the drug in these patients. Likewise, with the exception of alprazolam and triazolam, drug interactions appear to be of minor clinical significance, but more extensive use of the drug in the medical-psychiatric population may lead to the identification of often clinically relevant interactions.

TRICYCLIC ANTIDEPRESSANTS

A significant emergent issue in the use of TCAs in medically ill patients has been the development of some concern that agents with certain antiarrhythmic properties may actually increase morbidity when used after myocardial infarction (MI). Until recently, it was generally believed that because of the quinidine-like effect of TCAs, with their type IA antiarrhythmic properties, depressed patients with cardiac arrhythmias might actually benefit from these agents. Results from the Cardiac Arrhythmia Suppression Trials (CASTs) have raised some concern regarding the use of antiarrhythmic agents after MI (Epstein et al. 1993). Less than 2 years into this study, which was designed to assess the prophylactic benefit of antiarrhythmics post-MI, the monitoring board of the study program recommended that two of the antiarrhythmics being studied—flecainide and encainide—be discontinued (Glassman et al. 1993). Rather than decreasing mortality, these two drugs appeared to be statistically associated with increased rates of mortality compared with placebo-treated patients. As noted in the review by Glassman and co-workers (1993), the increased mortality rates with these drugs were of even greater concern because use of antiarrhythmics in the CAST studies required an open-label, dose-titration phase to adequately demonstrate suppression of arrhythmias and to eliminate patients in whom proarrhythmic effects might occur.

Because both flecainide and encainide were class IC antiarrhythmics, it was initially hoped that the increased post-MI mortality would be confined only to this class of antiarrhythmics and that the remaining antiarrhythmic moricizine (a type IA antiarrhythmic) would possibly show a beneficial effect. Unfortunately, moricizine eventually also was associated with increased mortality and its use was discontinued as well (Epstein et al. 1993). A meta-analysis has also demonstrated an increased risk of mortality among patients with ventricular arrhythmias treated with the type IA antiarrhythmic quinidine (Morganroth and Goin 1991; Teo et al. 1993).

The studies discussed above were confined to patients with post-MI asymptomatic or minimally symptomatic ventricular arrhythmias. These results are not clear—and it is perhaps premature—to extend them to other populations, although the data indicate a trend for increased mortality with class I drugs (Na^+ channel blockers) when they are used post-MI.

One might question, however, to what extent (within their therapeutic dose range) the cardiac effects of TCAs can be compared with the cardiac effects of primary antiarrhythmic drugs such as moricizine. The primary question is whether TCAs and the antiarrhythmics used in the CAST study (as well as quinidine) are comparable in terms of their potential cardiac effects. More research is needed to resolve the question of whether TCAs pose any risk to patients prone to arrhythmias in the post-MI period.

It is therefore debatable as to whether clinicians treating depressed patients with cardiovascular disease should alter their prescribing habits based on these results. Although it is reasonable, based on the above data, to avoid TCAs with quinidine-like properties in the post-MI period—especially in patients with a history of ventricular arrhythmias—

there seems little reason to avoid their use in other patients, unless there is evidence of significant cardiac conduction disease. A conservative clinical stance would be to choose SSRIs, bupropion, or venlafaxine in the post-MI period to treat depression in patients with cardiovascular disease with cardiac conduction disturbances. Excessively conservative treatment based on overextrapolation from the CAST study results may also potentially result in inadequate treatment of patients with depression whose affective disorder might best respond to TCAs—particularly in the light of data that support major depression as a major risk factor negatively affecting survival post-MI (Frasure-Smith et al. 1993).

Imipramine and Chest Pain in Patients With Normal Coronary Angiograms

Ten to thirty percent of patients undergoing cardiac catheterization for chest pain have normal coronary angiograms. In a recent study, 60 patients who had chronic chest pain and normal angiograms were randomized to treatment with placebo, clonidine 0.1 mg bid, or imipramine 50 mg hs (Cannon et al. 1994). These patients underwent extensive pretreatment medical evaluations including treadmill exercise, testing, gated blood-pool scanning with technetium-99m radionuclide angiography at rest and during exercise, and cardiac catheterization. Patients also underwent esophageal motility testing. Patients were extensively evaluated for psychiatric illness with structured psychodiagnostic interviews.

The results showed that 22% (13/60) of the patients had evidence of ischemia on their exercise ECGs. Twenty-two of 54 patients (41%) who underwent esophageal motility testing had abnormal esophageal motility.

Sixty-three percent of this entire patient group had one or more lifetime psychiatric disorders (most commonly panic disorder 26/60, major depression 17/60, somatization disorder 11/60, current major depression 3/60, hypochondriasis 2/60, alcohol dependence 2/60, and other anxiety disorders 3/60). Patients with lifetime histories of psychiatric disorders, however, *were no more likely* to have esophageal dysmotility or cardiac pain sensitivity than patients *without* psychiatric histories. Eighty-seven percent (52/60) had their characteristic chest pain provoked by right ventricular electrophysiologic stimulation or intracoronary infusion of adenosine.

During treatment, the imipramine-treated group had a 52% reduction in episodes of chest pain and the clonidine group had a 39% reduction; the imipramine, but not the clonidine, effect was significantly greater than placebo. The response to imipramine did not appear to depend on the results of cardiac, esophageal, or psychiatric testing at baseline or on any changes in the psychiatric profile during the course of the study (which improved in all three groups over time). The authors proposed that the improvement in chest pain was possibly a result of a "visceral analgesic effect of imipramine." The ability of TCAs to improve cardiac perfusion, observed in animal models, may also be a possibility.

Thus, imipramine may have a primary analgesic effect on cardiac or esophageal pain, although the mechanism of action is not known. Effects mediated by decreasing anxiety and depression may contribute but are unlikely to be the whole explanation, because there was no significant correlation between improvement with imipramine and measured psychiatric symptoms (Cannon et al. 1994).

Tricyclics and Sudden Death in Children

Since 1990, five sudden deaths of children being treated with desipramine have been reported (Zimnitsky 1994). Clinical details of the cases are sparse, but at least three deaths occurred during or just after physical exertion. It has been proposed that desipramine's cardiotoxicity may be caused by its norepinephrine reuptake inhibition leading to sympathetic overstimulation (Popper 1994). Several recent studies have attempted to clarify whether children are more susceptible than adults to desipramine-induced ECG changes. Wilens and associates (1993) studied the ECG effects of desipramine and its primary metabolite 2-hydroxy-desipramine (2-OHD) in 50 children, 39 adolescents, and 30 adults. Moderate associations were observed between desipramine and 2-OHD serum levels and the length of the P-R, QRS, and Q-Tc intervals. When the children's ECG data were analyzed separately, no significant associations existed between desipramine or 2-OHD levels and ECG parameters. None of the patients studied experienced cardiac complications from desipramine treatment.

Another study utilized Holter monitoring and Doppler echocardiography in 35 children and 36 adolescents who had been taking desipramine for 0.1 to 5.3 years. The results were compared with a large control group of unmedicated healthy children. Desipramine-treated children had significantly lower rates of junctional rhythms and sinus pauses but significantly higher rates of premature atrial contractions and runs of supraventricular tachycardia. Three percent of the healthy children had episodes of ventricular tachycardia, compared with none of the desipramine-treated children. Conduction changes in the desipramine-treated children were considered benign, and, with the exception of an association between paired PACs and serum desipramine levels, there were no meaningful clinical effects between desipramine serum levels and abnormalities on Holter monitoring.

Although these reports are somewhat reassuring, the possibility remains that certain children may be vulnerable to desipramine-related arrhythmias because of intrinsic congenital cardiac disease (such as the prolonged Q-T syndrome) or possibly variant TCA metabolism. If clinicians use desipramine for the treatment of either depression or attention-deficit hyperactivity disorder in children, a pretreatment ECG is essential, with periodic ECGs until therapeutic serum levels are achieved. Some experts recommend a maximum upper limit of 0.425 to 0.450 seconds for the Q-Tc with tricyclic treatment (Tingelstad 1991). Although a prolonged Q-Tc interval is not necessarily pathologic, the presence of Q-Tc intervals in this range before treatment may indicate the presence of the congenital long Q-T syndrome (Weintraub et al. 1990). The development of Q-T intervals in this range with TCA treatment clearly warrants consultation with a pediatric cardiologist. Table 2–5 presents an outline for monitoring children treated with TCAs.

PSYCHOTROPICS AND TORSADES DE POINTES

Torsades de pointes is polymorphic ventricular tachycardia, an arrhythmia that occurs in the setting of a prolonged Q-T interval, which indicates prolonged cardiac repolarization. This arrhythmia is potentially fatal, because it can lead to ventricular fibrillation and cardiac arrest. A prolonged Q-T can result from congenital abnormalities in cardiac repolarization, although it is more commonly seen as a consequence of hypokalemia or the use of type IA antiarrhythmics such as quinidine or TCAs. Along with type IA drugs, type III antiarrhythmics and antianginal agents represent the most common medications associated with torsades de pointes. Women are more susceptible than men (Makkar et al. 1993).

Terfenadine

Earlier in this chapter, we pointed out that agents that inhibit CyP_{450}-3A4 lead to high levels of unmetabolized terfenadine. Terfenadine is equipotent to quinidine as a blocker of the delayed rectifier potassium current (Honig et al. 1993). Similar to quinidine, terfenadine is proarrhythmic at high serum levels, as may occur when terfenadine is given concurrently with potent inhibitors of the CyP_{450}-3A4 enzyme (e.g., ketaconazole, erythromycin, or nefazodone). When CyP_{450}-3A4 is not inhibited, the principal metabolite of terfenadine is terfenadine carboxylate, which does not inhibit the potassium current and therefore is not proarrhythmic (Woosley et al. 1993). Terfenadine should not

Table 2–5. Guidelines for monitoring for tricyclic cardiotoxicity in children

1. A thorough history should be obtained for cardiac arrhythmias, syncope, dizziness, hearing loss (congenital Q-T syndrome), and a family history of sudden cardiac death or arrhythmias.

2. A baseline 12-lead electrocardiogram (ECG) should be obtained. If significant arrhythmia is observed, the patient should receive a 2-minute rhythm strip to determine heart rate, P-R interval, QRS duration, and Q-Tc interval. Repeat ECG should be obtained during the drug "loading" period and maintenance phase of treatment.

3. Drug levels should be obtained when ECGs are performed. ECG changes typically occur at relatively higher plasma serum concentrations of tricyclics.

4. If the patient has a history of cardiac disease and/or significant baseline conduction delay, the risk and benefits of using tricyclic therapy should be seriously considered.

5. The optimal dose range of desipramine that should be given is 2.5 to 5.0 mg/kg for most children, although some children may not tolerate doses > 3.5 mg/kg.

6. Plasma desipramine levels should not exceed 300 ng/ml. P-R intervals should be < 0.20 second and the QRS duration < 0.12 second. The maximum limit of the Q-Tc (corrected for rate) should be no more than 0.45 second.

Source.   Reprinted from Tingelstad JB: "The Cardiotoxicity of the Tricyclics." *Journal of the American Academy of Child and Adolescent Psychiatry* 30:845–846, 1991. Used with permission.

be used with drugs that inhibit hepatic metabolism such as erythromycin, ciprofloxacin, cimetidine, or disulfiram ("Safety of Terfenadine," 1992). Astemizole is another nonsedating antihistamine similar to terfenadine that also can cause prolongation of the Q-T interval, potentially leading to torsades de pointes. A number of such arrhythmias have been reported in children. Dangerous prolongation of the Q-T interval also can occur when terfenadine is taken in overdose (with as little as 360 mg) and in the presence of significant hepatic dysfunction.

The second-generation H_1 blockers acrivastine and loratadine do not have cardiotoxic effects but are relatively nonsedating antihistamines equal in effectiveness to terfenadine and astemizole. They should be preferred to terfenadine or astemizole in patients at risk for overdose or in those likely (because of vulnerability to infections) to be treated with macrolides such as erythromycin or imidazole antifungal agents.

Intravenous Haloperidol

Intravenous haloperidol, which has gained increased popularity in the management of intensive care unit (ICU) agitation, has recently been reported to cause torsades de pointes (Metzger and Friedman 1993). This is not a new observation, because before 1993 there were at least five published cases of torsades de pointes or Q-T prolongation associated with haloperidol (Metzger and Friedman 1993). Two of these reported cases were associated with haloperidol overdoses of 420 mg and 1,000 mg. Other cases included a patient who took approximately 210 mg of haloperidol with 1,400 mg of the sympathomimetic orphenadrine, another schizophrenic patient who received "therapeutic" doses of 60 to 100 mg/day of haloperidol, and an elderly patient with sick sinus syndrome taking approximately 15 mg/day (Metzger and Friedman 1993).

In a small series of delirious, agitated ICU patients reported recently, two patients developed torsades de pointes, and one developed a dangerously prolonged Q-T interval apparently from intravenous haloperidol (Metzger and Friedman 1993). The patients who developed torsades de pointes received cumulative doses of 490 and 825 mg of haloperidol, and the patient who developed the prolonged Q-T interval received 115 mg. Possible risk factors for these patients included a history of alcoholism in all three patients and documented cardiac disease, in particular, cardiomyopathy.

Another series of four patients who developed torsades de pointes have been reported from the use of haloperidol in the following cumulative dose ranges: 580 mg/4-day period, 170 mg/24 hours, 489 mg/36 hours, and 10 mg/4 hours (Wilt et al. 1993). The patients had diagnoses of bacterial meningitis with congestive heart failure, status asthmaticus (two patients), and atrial fibrillation with congestive heart failure. The investigators noted, however, that these four patients were derived from a group of 1,100 ICU patients treated with combined haloperidol/lorazepam intravenously over a 3-year period, indicating an extremely low rate of this complication. These cases nevertheless suggest that ECG monitoring for prolonged Q-Tc is advisable when intravenous haloperidol is used in ICU patients with preexisting cardiac disease or in those taking other potentially cardiotoxic drugs. We advise against using intravenous haloperidol in patients with a prolonged Q-Tc interval. Prolongation of the Q-Tc interval beyond 0.45 seconds, or by greater than 25% over baseline, indicates an increased risk of ventricular arrhythmia.

Sotalol

Sotalol hydrochloride (Betapace in United States; Sotacor in Canada) is a newly introduced antiarrhythmic that prolongs repolarization. This class III antiarrhythmic medication also is a β-adrenergic blocker. It is used for the treatment of potentially lethal ventricular arrhythmias. Sotalol slows the heart rate and prolongs the Q-Tc interval but does not prolong QRS duration. Sotalol can cause torsades de pointes in 3%–5% of patients, particularly in the presence of hypokalemia. The risk is increased if sotolol is used with other drugs that prolong the Q-Tc interval, including terfenadine and astemizole, phenothiazines, and TCAs ("Sotalol for Cardiac Arrhythmias," 1993). In patients receiving sotalol, SSRIs or MAOIs would be preferred for depression, loratadine for allergy, and molindone for psychosis.

INCIDENTAL NOTES ON TRICYCLICS

Several incidental reports are of interest with regard to utilizing TCAs in medical patients. Storey and Trumble (1992) reported the novel use of rectal suppositories to deliver doxepin and carbamazepine to terminally ill cancer patients unable to take medication orally. The investigators prepared carbamazepine suppositories by crushing the tablets and compressing the drug compound into "00" gelatin capsules; 25-mg oral doxepin capsules were used without alteration. Rectal carbamazepine, 1,200 to 1,800 mg/day given in divided doses, yielded serum levels of 3.1 to 10.4 mg/L; 100 mg/day of rectal doxepin yielded doxepin and desmethyldoxepin levels of 204 to 573 ng/ml.

Another recent report of pharmacokinetic interest (Hermann et al. 1992) indicated that the calcium channel blockers verapamil and diltiazem and the β-blocker labetalol can increase the bioavailability (area under the curve) of single doses of imipramine. Verapamil and diltiazem increased the bioavailability of imipramine when a single oral dose of imipramine was administered to patients who had received one of these calcium channel blockers for 4 days before the imipramine. Theoretically at least, this enhanced bioavailability would result in 33% and 59% respective increases in steady-state imipramine levels if these drugs were given concurrently over a longer period. Two of the patients in this study developed second-degree heart block when treated with imipramine and verapamil. Both verapamil and imipramine can delay atrioventricular nodal conduction.

Labetalol slows imipramine metabolism, thus increasing bioavailability, by inhibiting the CyP_{450} enzymes. Labetalol inhibits the hydroxylation of both imipramine and desipramine to their 2-OH metabolites. Patients (usually with hypertension and/or angina) who are treated with any of these agents warrant an especially conservative approach to TCA dosage, using TCA levels to guide therapy if patients show neither benefit nor side effects on a modest dose.

Stewart (1992) reported that several patients who had been successfully treated with TCAs subsequently became refractory to treatment after beginning high-fiber diets. Presence of the high-fiber diets decreased TCA serum levels, presumably by impairment of absorption. Improvement in depression resulted when their high-fiber diets were discontinued, and therapeutic TCA serum levels were achieved. Raising TCA dosages with monitoring of blood levels would have been an alternative if the high-fiber diet were medically necessary.

Cholestyramine is an inert resin used in the treatment of hypercholesterolemia. Cholestyramine has also been reported to reduce the bioavailability of TCAs via impairment of GI absorption (Bailey et al. 1992).

Drug interactions with valproate are reviewed later in this chapter, but note that valproate has been reported to raise levels of concurrently administered TCAs. The primary reports to date have involved amitriptyline and nortriptyline, with serum levels of both increased by concomitant valproate treatment (Bertschy et al. 1990; Fu et al. 1994).

A 68-year-old man developed toxic levels of desipramine when desipramine 150 mg/day was added to his drug regimen consisting of 600 mg/day of the antiarrhythmic propafenone (Katz 1991). Even at 75 mg/day, his desipramine serum level was elevated. Both propafenone and desipramine are extensively metabolized through the CyP_{450} system. Propafenone also has been reported to elevate levels of propranolol, metoprolol, warfarin, and digoxin.

CLOZAPINE

Clozapine, the first atypical neuroleptic drug to be approved by the U.S. Food and Drug Administration (FDA), was introduced in the United States in February 1990. Its primary interest to psychiatrists working in medical settings has been its therapeutic advantage for patients with Parkinson's disease with concomitant psychosis, because all typical neuroleptics are associated with aggravation of parkinsonism. Risperidone, the second atypical neuroleptic to be released in the United States, has more extrapyramidal side effects than clozapine at doses equally effective for treatment of psychosis. The use of clozapine in patients with Parkinson's disease is reviewed in detail in Chapter 3 of this volume. In this section, we briefly update readers on recently reported medical complications of clozapine therapy and discuss its possible relation to the neuroleptic malignant syndrome (NMS).

Clozapine-Induced Agranulocytosis

The incidence of agranulocytosis with clozapine in the United States is approximately 0.80% at 1 year and 0.91% at 1.5 years (Alvir and Lieberman 1994; Alvir et al. 1993). The majority of cases of agranulocytosis (83%) have occurred within the first 3 months after the start of treatment, with the peak risk in the third month. In a recent extensive analysis of the incidence of clozapine-induced agranulocytosis, only 3 of 73 cases occurred after 6 months and 1 of 73 after 18 months. In the majority of cases, agranulocytosis was preceded by a relatively long period of neutropenia. In 16 of 73 patients, however, agranulocytosis developed within 8 days of white blood cell (WBC) counts above 3,500/mm^3 (Alvir et al. 1993).

The risk of agranulocytosis tends to increase with age, although the risk is slightly higher in patients below age 21 years than for patients between ages 21 and 40 years. Women are at higher risk than men. The general observation that agranulocytosis is rare after the first 3 to 6 months of treatment may not necessarily be true for higher-risk elderly patients with concomitant neuropsychiatric illness. Despite careful monitoring, 256 cases of clozapine-induced agranulocytosis were reported in the first 4 years of use of clozapine in the United States, with nine fatalities.

Recombinant granulocyte colony-stimulating factor (rG-CSF) has been used successfully in treating clozapine-induced agranulocytosis (Nielsen 1993). In a recently reported series of three patients who were treated with rG-CSF for clozapine-induced agranulocytosis, doses of rG-CSF were 300 μg sq, and the WBC count tended to rebound between 6 and 8 days of treatment. Treatment with rG-CSF appears to significantly reduce the duration of clozapine-induced agranulocytosis (Lamberti 1994).

Clozapine and Other Adverse Reactions

The most common side effects of clozapine, at doses used for schizophrenia, are drowsiness (40%), sialorrhea (30%), tachycardia (25%), dizziness (20%), and orthostatic hypotension (9%) ("Update on Clozapine," 1993). Generalized tonic-clonic seizures have occurred in about 3% of patients, with higher seizure rates (4.4%) occurring in patients taking more than 600 mg/day (Devinsky et al. 1991). Even if patients do experience seizures on clozapine, if clinically warranted, clinicians may consider continuing the medication. Therapeutic options in such patients, after a neurological evaluation, would be to concurrently treat the patient with an anticonvulsant, achieve therapeutic levels, and use clozapine at lower doses. The most commonly used anticonvulsants that have been used in this situation are phenytoin and phenobarbital (Devinsky et al. 1991). Because of potential drug interactions, serum levels of anticonvulsants must be carefully monitored until steady-state levels are achieved (see below).

Additional rare side effects of clozapine have included myoclonic seizures, acute pancreatitis, and priapism ("Update on Clozapine," 1993). Isolated cases have been reported of paradoxical hypertension (Gupta 1994), gastric outlet obstruction (Schwartz and Frisolone 1993), high fever (104°F) with profuse diarrhea (Patterson and Jennings 1993), and an acute (apparently allergic) asthmatic reaction (Stoppe et al. 1992). A case of polyserositis (with pleural and pericardial effusions) developed in a 39-year-old woman within 2 weeks of clozapine initiation (Daly et al. 1992). (The patient was also taking fluoxetine at the time, which could have raised the levels of clozapine—see below.) One 47-year-old female patient developed cardiorespiratory collapse within hours of clozapine initiation at a dose of 25 mg; she was successfully resuscitated (Friedman et al. 1991). The manufacturer has acknowledged the fact that other cases of respiratory arrest or suppression have occurred with clozapine; concurrent use of benzodiazepines appears to be a risk factor (Friedman et al. 1991). Because the autonomic side effects are dose related, a starting dose as low as 12.5 mg/day would be a reasonable precaution when treating elderly patients.

Eosinophilia associated with clozapine use occurred more often in women (23%) than in men (7%) in a recent series of 118 patients. Eosinophilia usually occurs early in therapy, spontaneously resolves, and is not known to be linked to any major complications (Banov et al. 1993).

Cimetidine can increase serum concentrations of clozapine (Szymanski et al. 1991) as can fluoxetine (Centorrino et al. 1994). In the study by Centorrino and colleagues, levels of clozapine in patients taking fluoxetine were 76% higher than in control patients on clozapine alone. Elevations of clozapine serum levels caused by fluoxetine or other SSRIs are predictable, because clozapine is metabolized by the CyP_{450}-2D6 isoenzyme (Fischer et al. 1992). In contrast, phenytoin can lower clozapine levels—for example, when phenytoin is given concurrently with clozapine to protect patients at increased risk for seizures (Miller 1991). Minor increases in clozapine metabolites are seen with concurrent use of valproate.

Clozapine and NMS

It was initially believed that clozapine would not cause NMS, because NMS is typically preceded or accompanied by severe extrapyramidal symptoms. Although a detailed review of all reported cases of purported clozapine-induced NMS is beyond the scope of this chapter, our examination of such cases supports the view that, despite a variety of potential confounding factors, NMS has likely occurred in association with clozapine therapy (DasGupta and Young 1991; Reddig et al. 1993; Thornberg and Ereshefsky 1993). Clozapine-related NMS is rare and differs from typical NMS in that hyperthermia and autonomic instability are more prominent than rigidity.

Before making the diagnosis of NMS in a patient on clozapine, it is important to distinguish NMS from the benign self-limited fever that occurs during the first month of therapy in 50%–60% of patients treated with clozapine. This fever may be as high as 103–104°F, but it is not accompanied by an elevated creatine phosphokinase or marked abnormality of other vital signs. Clozapine also can cause muscle stiffness with elevation in creatinine phosphokinase levels in 3%–4% of patients. About 25% of patients will develop tachycardia in the early phase of treatment with clozapine, and 10% will have a persistent tachycardia. Clozapine also may cause a toxic encephalopathy that can occur in the absence of extrapyramidal side effects (Viner and Escobar 1994).

Although some cases of NMS appear to be associated with clozapine, some clinicians have advocated use of clozapine as an alternative drug for patients who develop NMS on typical neuroleptics (Weller and Kornhuber 1992). Weller and Kornhuber reported that eight of nine patients who had developed NMS on typical neuroleptics were subsequently successfully treated with clozapine without recurrence of NMS. Other approaches, however, may be employed in treating patients with neuroleptics after NMS (such as waiting for several weeks after full recovery from NMS before neuroleptics are introduced, ensuring that patients are well hydrated, using "low-potency" typical neuroleptics that are less likely to cause NMS, using risperidone, or using concomitant low-dose bromocriptine [2.25 to 5 mg/day] when reintroducing neuroleptics). The "routine" use of clozapine in NMS-sensitive patients remains controversial (Buckley and Meltzer 1993).

Clozapine, Tardive Dyskinesia, and Tardive Dystonia

Clozapine can improve motor symptoms in some patients with tardive dyskinesia. In one relatively small series, clozapine was given to 30 patients with mild to severe tardive dyskinesia in doses of 500 to 900 mg for up to 3 years. Over time, the group experienced a 38% decline in tardive dyskinesia symptoms. The greatest improvement occurred in patients with severe tardive dystonia (Lamberti and Bellnier 1993; Lieberman et al. 1991). In one open, unblinded study, improvement in tardive dyskinesia and dystonia was demonstrated during clozapine therapy in a significant proportion of patients.

LITHIUM

In previous publications, including this textbook series, we have extensively reviewed the use of lithium in medically ill patients. In this section, we include several recent reports of interest regarding the medical complications of lithium and its use in medical patients.

Lithium and Renal Failure

Whether lithium leads to changes in GFR and chronic renal failure remains an unsettled issue despite more than two decades of study. Two major reviews concluded that it does neither (Schou 1988; Waller and Edwards 1989). One study examined renal function in patients, some of whom were treated for up to 17 years with lithium (mean 10 years) (Lokkegaard et al. 1985). Corrected for age-related decreases in GFR, this study found that creatinine clearance was not decreased after 7 years but was weakly decreased in the group of patients treated for 17 years. (Two patients from the original cohort stopped lithium treatment due to decreased GFR and were not studied.) Other studies involving follow-up periods averaging 6 and 14 years, respectively, have detected no significant changes in GFR (Christensen and Aggernaes 1990; Conte et al. 1989). These studies have been reviewed by Gitlin (1993), who concluded that most patients treated long term with lithium do not develop renal insufficiency. Although some patients have developed renal disease, such as tubulointerstitial nephritis (von Knorring et al. 1990) while taking lithium, it has not been proven that lithium therapy had a causal role. Case-control studies are needed to determine whether there is a higher incidence of renal disease in patients on long-term lithium treatment compared with control subjects. To our knowledge, such studies have not yet been done.

Reports incriminating lithium as a cause of nephrotoxicity continue to appear. In a series of 82 patients followed for an average of 4.3 years, 3 (3.7%) exhibited evidence of renal insufficiency (creatinine level > 2.0 mg/dl) (Gitlin 1993). Specific risk factors other than lithium use could not be identified. Creatinine levels should be monitored every 6 to 12 months for patients on lithium, and a creatinine clearance should be determined when a patient develops a creatinine level greater than 1.6 mg/dl.

When a patient taking lithium develops renal insufficiency, the therapeutic index of lithium drops, because even mild dehydration can lead to a sharp rise in lithium levels when the baseline GFR is low.

Thus, regardless of whether lithium causes renal failure, alternatives to lithium therapy should be considered. Moreover, clinicians should determine whether the patient might respond to low-dose lithium (i.e., < 1.0 mEq/L). The patient's primary care physician should be included in deliberations about continued lithium therapy, and the psychiatrist should ensure that the primary care physician is well aware of the early signs of lithium toxicity and of common interactions of medical drugs (e.g., nonsteroidal antiinflammatory drugs, diuretics) with lithium. The psychiatrist and primary care physician should jointly determine an appropriate schedule for monitoring of renal function and who will be responsible for the monitoring.

Lithium and Parathyroid Function

Taylor and Bell (1993) recently reviewed the long-known association of lithium therapy with hypercalcemia and hyperparathyroidism. Cross-sectional studies have revealed that as many as 10% of patients treated with lithium develop hypercalcemia and elevated parathyroid hormone (PTH) levels (Stancer and Forbath 1989), which may be associated with parathyroid hyperplasia (Nordenstrom et al. 1992). Discontinuation of lithium usually reverses the hypercalcemia. Although most cases of lithium-induced hyperparathyroidism are considered both benign and reversible, elevations in serum calcium may warrant discontinuation of lithium and a switch to alternative therapies. Taylor and Bell (1993) have offered clinical guidelines in this regard. They recommend that serum calcium levels should be monitored during lithium therapy; we would also periodically check serum albumin along with the usual thyroid-stimulating hormone (TSH) level and serum creatinine. PTH levels must be monitored when calcium is elevated and when patients have a history of parathyroid disease. Ionized calcium levels should be obtained in cases of low serum albumin, high serum levels of calcium, and renal insufficiency. A mildly elevated calcium level does not require that lithium be discontinued but does require more frequent monitoring for further elevation of calcium that would warrant lithium discontinuation. Thiazide diuretics should not be used in this setting, because they may cause hypercalcemia. In patients who have osteoporosis or who are at risk for it (i.e., postmenopausal women), elevated PTH levels with their effects on bone resorption are a significant issue. In such patients, alternative mood-stabilizing therapy is preferable.

Withdrawal of lithium almost always results in normalization of calcium and PTH levels, usually within 2 to 4 weeks. Patients with persistent elevation of calcium and PTH levels 1 month after lithium discontinuation should be evaluated for primary hyperparathyroidism and other causes of hypercalcemia. The pathophysiology of lithium-induced hypercalcemia and hyperparathyroidism have been discussed elsewhere (Kingsbury and Salzman 1993). Alternative mood stabilizers such as valproate should be considered for problematic clinical situations.

Lithium and Cardiac Function

Although lithium is generally considered to have low cardiotoxicity, a recent comparative study involving 45 patients on long-term lithium therapy suggested that ECG changes are not unusual (Rosenqvist et al. 1993). In this study, patients with a known history of cardiovascular disease on concomitant cardioactive medications and patients with metabolic disorders were excluded. Fifty-six percent of lithium-treated patients had sinus node pauses longer than 1.5 seconds, compared with 30% of a reference group not on lithium. Periods of bradycardia were seen in 28% of lithium-treated patients and 30% of the comparison group. Although lithium has been rarely reported to cause sinus node dysfunction leading to symptomatic sinus bradycardia, in this study of patients relatively free of preexisting heart disease, the measurable sinus arrests were not clinically significant. Nevertheless, at least 13 cases of lithium-induced bradycardia have been reported in patients who had no evidence of overt or latent sinus node disease (Rosenqvist et al. 1993). If patients have known sinus node dysfunction, however, lithium can cause bradyarrhythmia. If a prelithium ECG detects sinus node dysfunction (i.e., bradycardia, sinus arrest of > 1.5 seconds), then alternative mood stabilizers should be considered.

Lithium and Drug Interactions

There are relatively few new adverse drug interactions to report with lithium. One case suggested that synergistic effects occurred between lithium and diltiazem in causing delirium. A 66-year-old patient on a therapeutic dose of lithium became delirious when diltiazem was added to her medical regimen for hypertension. The delirium resolved with discontinuation of both diltiazem and lithium. Ultimately, a combination of lithium and carbamazepine stabilized the patient's mood without unacceptable side effects. Interestingly, during the acute confusional episode on lithium and diltiazem, the patient had severe extrapyramidal side effects even though her lithium levels were normal and she was not taking a neuroleptic (Binder et al. 1991). The basis of this apparent pharmacodynamic interaction may be that both lithium and calcium channel blockers attenuate the postsynaptic response to dopamine by different mechanisms.

Even though angiotensin-converting enzyme (ACE) inhibitors such as enalapril usually do not affect serum lithium levels (DasGupta et al. 1992), idiosyncratic elevations in lithium have been reported with ACE inhibitors (Shionoiri 1993). Lithium toxicity has been reported to develop when either lisinopril or enalapril was started in a patient on long-term lithium therapy (Correa and Eiser 1992). If ACE inhibitors are given to a patient on lithium, reasonable precautions would include reducing the lithium level to 0.6 to 1.0 mEq, beginning ACE inhibitor treatment, and checking the lithium level 2 to 3 days after each increase in the ACE inhibitor dose.

PSYCHOSTIMULANTS

There have been a few new studies of stimulants for treating depression in medically ill patients since these drugs were reviewed in our previous volumes (Fogel and Stoudemire 1993; Stoudemire et al. 1993b). Dextroamphetamine was useful in several cases of terminally ill patients with cancer (Burns and Eisendrath 1994). An open, uncontrolled study reported full or partial responses to methylphenidate in 8 of 10 patients with poststroke depression (Lazarus et al. 1992). Doses of methylphenidate were increased up to 40 mg/day, with an average dose of 17.0 mg/day. As has been usual for studies of this type in general hospital patients, no outcome was reported beyond 3 weeks, although the investigators did use the Hamilton Depression Rating Scale (Hamilton 1960) to measure the patients' improvement in mood. In the stroke patients, whose mean age was 73 years, no significant ECG changes were noted. Orally administered methylphenidate given in high test doses (e.g., 1 mg/kg) to drug-naive healthy adults resulted in an increase in heart rate averaging 12 bpm and increases in systolic blood pressure averaging 5 mmHg (Janowsky et al. 1978). With lower doses of 15 mg/day, no significant cardiovascular changes occurred (Gualtieri et al. 1986). No cardiac arrhythmias have been reported to be caused by methylphenidate, dextroamphetamine, or pemoline in customary oral doses in humans. Hence, there is little reason to be concerned about deleterious cardiovascular effects of these stimulants in normal dose ranges, although they have not been systematically studied in elderly medically ill patients with serious cardiovascular disease.

Risperidone

Risperidone is a novel benzisoxazole derivative antipsychotic that is characterized by potent central 5-HT_2–receptor antagonism at low doses and potent D_2-receptor antagonism at higher doses. It purportedly has therapeutic efficacy for the negative symptoms of schizophrenia, and it is an effective drug for the positive symptoms of this disorder as well. Risperidone's affinity for D_2 receptors is more than 100 times greater than for D_1 receptors. Risperidone tends to preserve normal small motor movements over a wide dose range. Compared with haloperidol, risperidone has very low cataleptic effects. Risperidone, together with its active metabolite 9-hydroxy-risperidone, has a terminal half-life of 24 hours (Chouinard et al. 1993). The drug's basic pharmacology and well-established efficacy in the treatment of patients with schizophrenia have been extensively reviewed recently by Ereshefsky and Lacombe (1993).

Effects of Risperidone

Risperidone does not show in vitro binding to β-adrenergic or muscarinic receptors (Kane 1993). It does show binding affinity for α_1- and α_2-noradrenergic receptors and has antihistaminic effects (Livingston 1994). Because of its α-blocking effects, it can lower blood pressure, although this effect is usually not clinically significant with gradual dosage titration. Symptomatic hypotension can occur when patients are treated acutely with doses of 4 mg/day or more. Risperidone can raise prolactin levels in a dose-related fashion with usual attendant side effects such as galactorrhea, gynecomastia, and decreased libido. Weight gain with the drug averages 2.3 kg. Reported central nervous system (CNS) side effects include sedation, agitation, anxiety, insomnia, and headache. One case of possible syndrome of inappropriate secretion of antidiuretic hormone has been associated with risperidone in an elderly patient; hyponatremia resolved after drug discontinuation (Berman 1994).

The major potential advantage of the drug for medical and neurologic patients is its relatively low propensity to cause extrapyramidal side effects—an advantage, however, that does not necessarily apply to elderly patients or patients with subclinical or clinically manifest Parkinson's disease. In clinical trials, the rate of extrapyramidal side effects did not differ from placebo when the risperidone dose was 6 mg/day or less. Chouinard and Arnott (1993) investigated the relationship between risperidone and parkinsonian symptoms and found no statistically significant difference from placebo in ratings of parkinsonian symptoms in doses of 2, 6, 10, or 16 mg of risperidone. Although risperidone can cause extrapyramidal side effects at higher doses, these side effects are unlikely within the usual therapeutic dose range in young to middle-aged physically healthy patients. No effects on the ECG have been noted (Remington 1993), although a heart rate–related decrease in the Q-T interval has been noted (Ereshefsky and Lacombe 1993).

Patients treated with risperidone for schizophrenia had significantly fewer dyskinesia symptoms than patients treated with placebo. Risperidone also can suppress symptoms of tardive dyskinesia. Its greatest benefit in reducing symptoms of tardive dyskinesia appears to be in patients who have the most severe symptoms. Suppression of tardive dyskinesia is maximal at doses of 6 to 10 mg/day. Risperidone's antidyskinetic effects occur without a concomitant increase in parkinsonian effects (Chouinard et al. 1993). Risperidone is metabolized by the CyP_{450}-2D6 isoenzyme, and therefore its metabolism will be inhibited by drugs such as SSRIs.

The low propensity of risperidone to cause extrapyramidal side effects may not hold true for elderly patients or those with latent or established Parkinson's disease. At least one of us (A.S.), however, has observed the development of severe extrapyramidal side effects in several elderly patients without evidence of pretreatment Parkinson's disease who were taking doses as low as 2 mg/day.

Although the drug can lower blood pressure, such effects appear to be minimal, particularly if low starting doses are used. No clinically significant effects have been noted on the ECG, and the drug is devoid of direct anticholinergic effects. Risperidone may be a good alternative to clozapine in patients with tardive dyskinesia who require antipsychotic treatment.

One of us (B.S.F.) recently reviewed early experience with the introduction of risperidone at a large public chronic disease hospital. Thirty elderly patients with either chronic psychosis or dementia with agitation or paranoia were switched from high-potency standard neuroleptics to risperidone, in doses ranging from 0.5 to 3 mg bid. Extrapyramidal side effects were less than with the standard neuroleptics used previously, and all patients showed moderate to good symptomatic improvement. Orthostatic hypotension was seen only in two patients who were receiving concomitant antihypertensive therapy. This early experience suggests that risperidone may find an important role as an alternative to haloperidol in the treatment of agitation and paranoid states in elderly patients with dementia and chronic medical illness.

ANTIEPILEPTIC (ANTICONVULSANT) DRUGS

In the past 2 years, two new antiepileptic drugs have been introduced in the United States, and the use of carbamazepine and valproate for psychiatric indications has continued to increase. Although the new antiepileptic drugs felbamate and gabapentin have yet to be tested for psychiatric indications, both have potential behavioral side effects of importance to psychiatrists, and felbamate is associated with a number of pharmacokinetic interactions with psychotropic agents. The increased use of carbamazepine and valproate has led to the broader recognition of side effects and interactions with other drugs. In this section, we review these issues.

Felbamate

Felbamate is a new antiepileptic drug indicated as add-on therapy for partial seizures, including complex partial seizures, and as add-on treatment for the Lennox-Gastaut syndrome (Schmidt 1993). The latter is characterized by atonic (astatic) postural lapses succeeded by various combinations of minor tonic-clonic and postural seizures, intellectual impairment (not part of typical petit mal), and a distinctive slow (1- to 2.5-per-second) spike-wave electroencephalogram (EEG) pattern. Felbamate's precise mechanism of antiepileptic action is not known but may be related to its ability to simultaneously inhibit neuronal responses to the excitatory neurotransmitter glutamate at the N-methyl-D-aspartate (NMDA) receptor and enhance neuronal responses to the inhibitory neurotransmitter γ-aminobutyric acid (GABA) (Rho et al. 1994). When felbamate is added to the regimen of patients with intractable complex partial seizures, approximately one-half will have a clinically significant reduction in seizure frequency, and some (probably < 10%) will become seizure free (Bourgeois et al. 1993; Fisher 1993; Graves 1993).

Side effects.   Felbamate is not sedating. In fact, insomnia is one of its most frequent side effects. Other common side effects are headache, nausea, and weight loss. Tolerance to headache, insomnia, or nausea may develop with continued use of the drug, although this may take several weeks. During the early period of side effects, patients may require symptomatic therapies, support, and reassurance. Fortunately, medically serious side effects are rare, and no routine monitoring of blood tests is necessary. Blood levels of felbamate are not helpful in adjusting dosage; the dose is raised gradually to a maximum of 1,200 mg tid or until seizures stop or unacceptable side effects develop. The manufacturer initially recommended a rapid dosage titration, but many neurologists are now attempting to minimize early side effects by starting with a low dose (e.g., 300 mg bid) and titrating in increments of 300 to 600 mg at weekly intervals.

In the summer of 1994, the FDA recommended that felbamate be reserved only for those patients who would experience a severe aggravation of seizures without the drug. The recommendation was based on several reports of agranulocytosis possibly associated with the drug. Based on those reports, the FDA estimated that the risk of agranulocytosis could be as high as 1:5,000. This rate is much higher than that seen with carbamazepine. The occurrence of agranulocytosis with felbamate is unpredictable and not dose related. Although the use of the drug is now greatly restricted, routine monitoring of blood counts is not required for those on the drug. Instead, patients on felbamate should be told to contact their physician for a blood count if they develop a fever or systemic symptoms.

Felbamate accelerates the metabolism of carbamazepine, decreasing carbamazepine levels while increasing the level of its 10,11-epoxide (toxic) metabolite (Wagner et al. 1993). (Valproate also increases relative levels of carbamazepine's epoxide metabolite.) Because carbamazepine's 10,11-epoxide can cause side effects but is less therapeutically effective than carbamazepine, the net effect is a reduction in the therapeutic index of carbamazepine for the patient on felbamate. A reasonable approach to handling the initiation of felbamate "add-on" therapy in a patient on carbamazepine is to slightly reduce the carbamazepine dosage if the level is high therapeutic and to leave it alone if it is not. Then, after 1 to 2 weeks on felbamate, the carbamazepine level is rechecked, and the carbamazepine dosage is adjusted if necessary. Carbamazepine increases the clearance of felbamate by 50%, resulting in a 40% decrease in steady-state trough concentrations of felbamate. Although this implies that patients on combined therapy will need higher felbamate dosages, it is not of great clinical relevance because felbamate usually is titrated to a clinical end point.

Felbamate increases valproate levels consistently enough so that valproate dosage should routinely be reduced by about one-third when felbamate add-on therapy is initiated. Subsequent adjustments in valproate dosage can be made according to blood levels. Clinical signs of sedation are also useful in identifying excessive valproate levels, because felbamate does not have sedative effects.

In addition to headache and insomnia, CNS side effects of felbamate include nervousness, agitation, and dizziness. Although they are usually transient, these CNS side effects may be poorly tolerated in patients with one of the psychiatric disorders associated with partial epilepsy. When felbamate is used in such patients, dosage titration should be especially slow. Benzodiazepines (e.g., clonazepam) can be used if drug treatment of insomnia or nervousness is necessary.

The reciprocal pharmacokinetic interactions of felbamate and antidepressant drugs have not been systematically studied, although the chemical similarity of the TCAs with carbamazepine suggests that felbamate may alter TCA metabolism. Monitoring of TCA blood levels during initiation of felbamate would be a reasonable precaution, and if signs of TCA toxicity were seen despite apparently therapeutic TCA levels, accumulation of TCA metabolites should be suspected. One of us (A.S.) observed loss of the antidepressant efficacy of sertraline when a 45-year-old female patient with a seizure disorder and a history of depression (in remission) had her maintenance phenytoin switched to felbamate. The patient had a precipitous relapse in her depression with profound anorexia and insomnia even though sertraline was continued at the maintenance dose (50 mg). Serum levels were not obtained of either sertraline or felbamate, although the patient's depression cleared completely within a week when she was switched back to phenytoin. Until more data are available regarding the interaction between felbamate and SSRIs, the combination is not recommended.

When felbamate add-on therapy is successful in reducing or eliminating seizures, many neurologists will attempt to convert the patient to monotherapy. If psychiatric symptoms arise in this setting, anti-epileptic drug withdrawal should be considered as a possible cause. A recent study of withdrawal of therapy with phenytoin, carbamazepine, and/or valproate in epileptic patients suggests that anxiety and/or depression frequently emerge, even when seizure frequency does not increase (Ketter et al. 1994). In that study, excess psychiatric symptoms resolved within 2 weeks of restarting the previous antiepileptic drug therapy. Reinitiation of the former antiepileptic drug should be seen as the initial treatment of choice in this situation, with felbamate being continued if it had been helpful as add-on therapy.

Gabapentin

Gabapentin is a GABA analogue indicated for add-on therapy in adults with partial seizures with or without secondary generalization. Although it is a GABA analogue, its mechanism of action does not appear to be related to GABA transmission (Goa and Sorkin 1993). It has modest efficacy and rarely makes a patient with intractable epilepsy seizure free, but either a decrease in seizure frequency or a lessening of seizure severity may warrant its continued use. In one double-blind study, the proportion of patients with at least a 50% reduction in seizure frequency ranged from 18% to 26%, depending on the gabapentin dose (U.S. Gabapentin Study 1993). A remarkable feature of gabapentin is that its clinical benefit may increase with long-term therapy, with greater reduction of seizure frequency at 12 and 24 months than at 3 months after starting therapy (Ojemann et al. 1992).

The main advantage of gabapentin is its very low systemic toxicity and the virtual absence of clinically significant drug interactions, including interactions with carbamazepine or valproate (Radulovic et al. 1994). It may therefore be added to an ongoing drug regimen without dosage adjustments.

Gabapentin is excreted by the kidney and does not undergo hepatic metabolism. Dosage reduction is therefore needed only for elderly patients or those with renal insufficiency but not for patients with liver disease. Patients with a creatinine clearance of 30 to 60 ml/min should receive 50% of the dose that would be planned for a patient without kidney disease, patients with a creatinine clearance of 15 to 30 ml/min should receive 25% of the dose, and those with more severe renal impairment should receive about 10% of the dose. Dosage is reduced by half in frail elderly patients.

Side effects.   Somnolence, fatigue, ataxia, or dizziness are seen in more than half of patients; these symptoms are usually mild (Goa and Sorkin 1993). More troublesome CNS side effects are infrequent, with tremor, the most common, being seen in approximately 7% of patients reported in the manufacturer's package insert. Anxiety was reported in more than 1% of the patients treated in initial clinical trials, and a few patients had symptoms of mood disorder or psychosis emerge on gabapentin therapy.

Carbamazepine

In other textbooks, we have extensively reviewed the use of carbamazepine in medical patients, including drug interactions (Fogel and Stoudemire 1993; Stoudemire et al. 1991b, 1993b). Carbamazepine has become established as a treatment of bipolar disorder, in both its manic and its depressed phases, with particular value in the treatment of rapid cycling, dysphoric mania, and mixed bipolar states (Dilsaver et al. 1993; Okuma 1993; Post et al. 1993; Zornberg and Pope 1993). It also may have a role in the treatment of depression refractory to conventional antidepressant drugs and in the maintenance of remission in patients with recurrent episodes of major depression (Stuppaeck et al. 1993; Varney et al. 1993). For example, Varney and colleagues reported improvement with carbamazepine in 11 of a series of 13 patients with refractory depression accompanied by partial seizurelike symptoms.

Side effects.   As carbamazepine is used increasingly in general psychiatric practice, its side effects and drug interactions will be encountered by psychiatrists with increasing frequency. As discussed in previous editions of *Medical-Psychiatric Practice* (Stoudemire and Fogel 1991, 1993b), agranulocytosis from carbamazepine is rare, and routine periodic monitoring of blood counts is not indicated. A number of other medically relevant side effects are far more common. In this section, we review recent literature on hematologic abnormalities, metabolic effects, and hypersensitivity syndromes associated with carbamazepine. We discuss new literature on carbamazepine overdose and on carbamazepine in pregnancy and some recently reported drug interactions. Finally, we mention some important considerations regarding the stability and bioavailability of carbamazepine.

It has become increasingly evident that the most common hematologic reactions to carbamazepine are neutropenia and thrombocytopenia. Regarding the former, O'Connor et al. (1994) reported on detailed hematologic assessments of seven patients with leukopenia due to antiepileptic drugs, of whom six were taking carbamazepine alone or as part of a combination. The average WBC in the sample was 3,000/μl, with 42% neutrophils. In all seven cases, the WBC increase with exercise was normal, antineutrophil antibodies were absent, and bone marrow aspirates were normal. The authors concluded that continued treatment with antiepileptic drugs in patients with chronic leukopenia was "probably safe" as long as the leukopenia was stable and the percentage of neutrophils was normal. A more conservative assessment is that therapy might be continued if it was necessary to prevent major symptoms and disability, and a consulting hematologist agreed on the relatively benign nature of the abnormality and assisted in planning a schedule of ongoing monitoring.

Several cases of clinically significant thrombocytopenia have been reported with carbamazepine (Kaneko et al. 1993; Shechter et al. 1993). In the case reported by Shechter and colleagues, an autoimmune mechanism was demonstrated. Platelet counts would be warranted in a patient on carbamazepine who developed easy bruising, but because the effect is rare, routine monitoring is not indicated.

Carbamazepine has been shown to have predictable effects on lipid metabolism, thyroid function, and sodium homeostasis. Isojarvi and co-workers (1993b) evaluated the effect of carbamazepine monotherapy on serum lipids in 36 previously untreated epileptic patients. They found that total cholesterol and high-density lipoprotein (HDL) cholesterol increased after 2 months and remained elevated at 1-year and 5-year follow-up. Low-density lipoprotein (LDL) cholesterol and triglycerides increased transiently but had returned to baseline within 1 year. Brown and associates (1992) found similar effects on total and HDL cholesterol in a series of 38 psychiatric patients treated with carbamazepine. The changes in cholesterol could potentially affect the risk of atherosclerosis, depending on whether the increase in cholesterol was offset by favorable changes in the HDL-LDL ratio. It would be conservative practice to check a lipid profile in patients on long-term carbamazepine therapy, particularly men and postmenopausal women with a personal or family history of atherosclerosis. If cholesterol levels were significantly elevated but carbamazepine was necessary to treat the patient's psychiatric disorder, dietary or pharmacological therapy for the hypercholesterolemia would be initiated.

Several reports have presented evidence that carbamazepine decreases levels of thyroxine (T_4) and sometimes triiodothyronine (T_3), without inducing a compensatory increase in TSH (Isojarvi et al. 1993a; Yuksel et al. 1993). In these reports, clinical hypothyroidism was not observed. However, the apparent downregulation of the pituitary-thyroid axis would place patients on carbamazepine at increased risk for hypothyroidism if they also had intrinsic thyroid disease. The key point is that in patients on carbamazepine, checking the level of TSH no longer suffices as a test for hypothyroidism in patients suspected of it on clinical grounds.

Hyponatremia due to carbamazepine was recently reviewed (Van Amelsvoort et al. 1994). In various case series, the rate of hyponatremia with carbamazepine therapy has varied from 4.8%–40%, depending on the population studied and the cutoff for diagnosis. In most cases, the hyponatremia is mild and asymptomatic and does not require discontinuation of the drug. Routine monitoring of electrolytes is not necessary for all patients on carbamazepine. However, patients with other risk factors for hyponatremia (e.g., congestive heart failure, thiazide diuretics) should have electrolytes checked periodically as carbamazepine is introduced.

Carbamazepine can cause a variety of hypersensitivity syndromes, including severe dermatologic reactions (Pagliaro and Pagliaro 1993), interstitial pneumonitis (King et al. 1994; Takahashi et al. 1993), an infectious mononucleosis-like illness (Scerri et al. 1993), and drug-induced lupus (Drory and Korczyn 1993; Kanno et al. 1992; Ohashi et al. 1993). These rare reactions involve both humoral and cell-mediated immunity (Horneff et al. 1992).

Two series of carbamazepine overdoses have been recently reported (Hojer et al. 1993; Seymour 1993). In Seymour's series, which included multiple-drug ingestions, the syndrome of overdose comprised a decreased level of consciousness, dilated pupils, abnormal muscle tone and reflexes, and ataxia, nystagmus, or ophthalmoplegia. Seizures occurred in about 25% of cases. Hyponatremia and transient hepatic dysfunction were frequent complications. In the other series, which was limited to single-drug ingestions, the life-threatening problems of respiratory failure and impaired cardiac conduction occurred only when the peak serum level was greater than or equal to 40 mg/L. Two of the 10 patients with levels this high died in the hospital. These reports suggest that carbamazepine overdose is not more dangerous than lithium overdose, so that concerns about potential overdose should not lead one to reject carbamazepine as an alternative to lithium for patients with mood disorders.

Carbamazepine and pregnancy.   Babies born to women who take carbamazepine during pregnancy have an increased risk of neural tube defects. This risk can be reduced by folate supplementation. Most significant neural tube defects can be detected by the end of the fourth month of gestation with a combination of amniotic fluid analysis and high-resolution ultrasound. Measurement of α-fetoprotein in maternal serum is insufficiently sensitive to be an adequate test for antenatal diagnosis of neural tube defects. Apart from an approximate 1% risk of neural tube defects, carbamazepine has relatively low teratogenic potential compared with phenytoin or phenobarbital (Waters et al. 1994). A recent study of pregnancy outcomes in 103 epileptic women found an 8.8% rate of major malformations. This rate, substantially lower than that seen in the previous decade, was attributed to the increased use of carbamazepine and valproate monotherapy. Among Canadian neurologists, carbamazepine currently is the antiepileptic drug of choice for pregnant women whose symptoms cannot safely be managed without medication (Morrison and Rieder 1993). Scolnik et al. (1994) compared pregnancy outcomes of 36 mother-child pairs exposed to carbamazepine monotherapy with those of 34 pairs exposed to phenytoin monotherapy and 70 mother-child pairs not exposed to teratogens. Control subjects were matched for maternal age, obstetrical history, and socioeconomic status. Outcomes were the children's global intelligence quotient (IQ) and language development scores. The offspring of mothers exposed to carbamazepine did not differ from the control subjects, and the children of mothers exposed to phenytoin had a mean global IQ 10 points lower than the control subjects. Thus, measures sensitive enough to detect behavioral teratogenicity of phenytoin detected no such problem with carbamazepine.

Drug interactions.   Several investigators have recently reported clinically significant increases in carbamazepine levels associated with simultaneous administration of drugs that inhibit one of the CyP_{450} enzymes or compete with carbamazepine for oxidative metabolism. Verapamil, erythromycin, and cimetidine are well-established examples (Patsalos and Duncan 1993). Recent additions to the list include diltiazem (Maoz et al. 1992), clarithromycin (Albani et al. 1993), and quinine (Amabeoku et al. 1993). Fluoxetine has been reported to raise carbamazepine levels (Gidal et al. 1993), but a systematic study of the effect of 20 mg/day of fluoxetine or 100 mg/day of fluvoxamine on carbamazepine levels found no significant changes after 3 weeks (Spina et al. 1993b). Clinical problems can arise both when the interacting drug is started and when it is stopped. For example, if carbamazepine dosage was titrated when a patient was on a calcium channel blocker and if the latter drug were subsequently discontinued, the carbamazepine level might drop below the threshold for therapeutic efficacy.

Carbamazepine is well known to induce hepatic oxidative enzymes, including those involved in its own metabolism and in the metabolism of TCAs, oral contraceptives, and warfarin (Patsalos and Duncan 1993). A recent report described a 73-year-old woman with bipolar depression maintained on nortriptyline whose nortriptyline level dropped by more than half when carbamazepine was added to her regimen (Brosen and Kragh-Sorensen 1993). One of us (B.S.F.) recently had a patient on warfarin rapidly lose anticoagulant efficacy when carbamazepine was started for neuropathic pain. A particularly important interaction for the psychiatrist is the potential of carbamazepine to accelerate the metabolism of opiate analgesics (Maurer and Bartkowski 1993). When this possibility is not recognized, the patient taking carbamazepine may be undertreated for acute pain, with adverse emotional consequences. The induction of oxidative enzymes by carbamazepine reverses rapidly after the drug is discontinued, with a half-time for deinduction of approximately 4 days (Schaffler et al. 1994). Therefore, if a patient discontinues carbamazepine therapy for as little as a week, the drug must be reintroduced slowly to avoid acute toxicity.

Whether the indication for carbamazepine is neurologic or psychiatric, a minimum serum level of carbamazepine usually is needed for a therapeutic response. Moreover, the therapeutic index of carbamazepine is low, with unacceptable side effects frequently occurring at levels as little as 25% greater than the level needed for clinical efficacy. Thus, differences in the bioavailability of carbamazepine preparations often are clinically relevant, leading either to toxicity or to a loss of therapeutic effect. Several recent reports have established that generic preparations of carbamazepine are not necessarily bioequivalent to Tegretol (Gilman et al. 1993; Meyer and Straughn 1993; Oles and Gal 1993). Switching preparations can thus lead to recurrent seizures (Jain 1993) or to toxicity due to increased levels (Gilman et al. 1993). The practical point is that patients should take the same carbamazepine preparation consistently. If a patient must switch from one brand to another, the switch should be gradual, levels should be checked at each step in the changeover, and the patient should be warned about the possibility of side effects or a breakthrough of symptoms.

Carbamazepine, regardless of the manufacturer, is not stable under conditions of high temperature and relative humidity (Wang et al. 1993). Patients on carbamazepine who live in warm, humid climates should be advised to keep the drug in the refrigerator until they are ready to take it.

Valproate

Valproate is rapidly gaining acceptance as a treatment for primary psychiatric disorders, perhaps more rapidly than did carbamazepine, the first antiepileptic drug to be widely recognized as psychotropic. The best established indication is bipolar disorder, especially the rapid cycling type (Calabrese et al. 1993; Keck et al. 1993a; Schaff et al. 1993). Recent reports suggest that it also may be efficacious for panic disorder (Keck et al. 1993b, 1993c), cyclothymia (Deltito 1993; Jacobsen 1993), and some behavior disorders in persons with dementia (Mellow et al. 1993) or mental retardation (Kastner et al. 1993). The last-mentioned report is of particular interest to psychiatrists who work with cognitively impaired or developmentally disabled populations. In their study, Kastner and co-workers identified 21 people with behavioral complications of mental retardation characterized by at least three of the following symptoms: irritability, sleep disturbance, aggressive or self-injurious behavior, and behavioral cycling. They administered valproate in an open-label trial to these patients, of whom 19 were followed for 2 years. One developed severe side effects; the remaining 18 continued on the drug for 2 years. Fourteen patients (78%) showed improvement; 9 of the 10 patients on neuroleptics were able to discontinue them.

Effects of valproate.   Initially, hepatic failure was the most feared complication of valproate therapy. However, this reaction is extremely rare in adults, and most psychiatrists regularly prescribing valproate have never seen a case. Far more often, they see hematologic side effects, drug interactions, and CNS toxicity of various kinds. In this section, we review recent literature on these issues and mention the recent association of valproate with pancreatitis and drug-induced lupus. We conclude with a comment on valproate dosing strategies.

The most common hematologic effect of valproate is an increase in red blood cell mean corpuscular volume and mean corpuscular hemoglobin (May and Sunder 1993; Ozkara et al. 1993). The effect may result from alteration of erythrocyte membrane phospholipids and is not associated with low B_{12} or folate levels or with liver disease. The next most common effect is thrombocytopenia, which occasionally is clinically significant. Platelet counts and bleeding times are indicated in patients on valproate before surgery or in the event of unusual bleeding or bruising.

Valproate in patients with liver disease.   As a drug with a significant potential for hepatic toxicity, valproate is relatively contraindicated in patients with advanced liver disease, such as those with chronic hepative encephalopathy or bleeding tendencies caused by clotting factor deficiencies. However, if the clinical indication for valproate is strong, the drug can be given to patients with less severe liver disease if reasonable precautions are followed. In general, an internist or gastroenterologist would collaborate with the psychiatrist in assessing risks and developing a plan for monitoring. We recommend the following steps at a minimum:

1. Dosage should be initiated at no more than 250 mg/day and slowly titrated upward, with frequent clinical reassessments and weekly monitoring of liver enzymes, prothrombin time, venous ammonia, and valproate levels during dosage titration.
2. A coagulation panel and bleeding time determination should be obtained before any invasive procedure or if the patient shows a tendency to bleed or bruise easily.
3. If the albumin level is low, the target valproate level should be reduced.

Valproate and coagulation.   The use of valproate is associated with increased bleeding tendencies, a problem that is rarely of clinical importance in patients in generally good physical health but one that is potentially serious in patients with medical conditions that predispose to hemorrhage or that will likely require surgery (Loiseau 1981). Drug-induced thrombocytopenia is an occasional cause; however, the more usual reason is qualitative dysfunction of platelets, as indicated by a prolonged bleeding time with normal prothrombin time, partial thromboplastin time, and platelet count. Kreuz and colleagues (1992) studied the effects of valproate on coagulation in 30 children. They found that von Willenbrand's factor (a plasma glycoprotein that facilitates platelet adhesion and carries factor VIII) was decreased in 25 of the 30 (83%) and that ristocetin cofactor was decreased in 20 (67%). Ten (33%) of the children had decreased levels of factor VIII complex. Overall, two-thirds of the subjects were diagnosed as having a drug-induced type I (i.e., mild to moderate) von Willenbrand's syndrome, of whom most had had episodes of bleeding or bruising. Seven of the patients (23%) had a prolonged bleeding time. The occurrence of bleeding problems was not related to dosage, duration of therapy, or symptomatic liver disease. The incidence of drug-induced platelet dysfunction in adults on valproate is not known, but it appears to be lower than in the children reported by Kreuz and colleagues.

The clinical implication is that bleeding time should be checked before surgery in patients on valproate; a prolonged bleeding time can be treated with cryoprecipitate or desmopressin (des-amino, des-arginine vasopressin [DDAVP]) if it is deemed an unacceptable surgical risk. Patients with recurrent bleeding from a medical condition should have coagulation parameters checked after beginning valproate therapy; substantial abnormality should trigger a reevaluation of the risks versus benefits of valproate treatment.

Valproate and lorazepam.   Lorazepam is frequently given to patients on valproate, either as an adjunct to antimanic therapy or for treatment of postictal agitation or flurries of seizures. Anderson and associates (1994) investigated the effect of chronic use of valproate on the metabolism of lorazepam by giving lorazepam to eight healthy volunteers before and after chronic dosing with valproate. Chronic valproate use decreased the formation of lorazepam glucuronide by the liver, leading to significantly decreased lorazepam clearance in six of the eight subjects. The results suggest that many, if not most, patients on valproate therapy will require smaller-than-usual doses of lorazepam.

Interactions with other psychotropics.   In addition to pharmacokinetic interactions related to its inhibition of hepatic enzymes, valproate is involved in pharmacodynamic interactions with other psychotropics including carbamazepine, neuroleptics, and lithium. The combination of valproate with lithium or with neuroleptics is therapeutically powerful, but it can be associated with neurotoxicity, such as tremor, confusion, or involuntary movements. A recent animal (rat) study by Li and co-workers (1993) sheds some light on this issue. They demonstrated that haloperidol, lithium, and valproate all affected the formation of inositol phosphate in response to agonists in various brain regions. Thus, their additive therapeutic and toxic effects might be related to common actions on a second-messenger system.

Other side effects.   Valproate is known to cause elevated ammonia levels, an effect that relatively contraindicates the drug in patients with hepatic insufficiency, such as those with cirrhosis of the liver. Stephens and Levy (1994) recently demonstrated in an animal model that lower ammonia levels were needed to produce coma in animals receiving valproate than in those not receiving the drug. When valproate appears to cause an unusual degree of sedation or other CNS side effects in patients with a history of liver disease, hepatic encephalopathy should be suspected even if "liver enzymes" are normal and ammonia is only mildly elevated. In exceptional cases, hyperammonemic coma can be induced by valproate without any history or evidence of hepatic disease (Duarte et al. 1993).

Administration of valproate increases serum amylase; this is usually asymptomatic, and the rise is not correlated with dose or serum levels (Jha et al. 1993). Overt clinical pancreatitis is relatively rare and appears to occur most often in younger patients, during the first year of treatment, and in association with multiple-drug therapy (Asconape et al. 1993). Although the pancreatitis usually resolves rapidly when valproate is discontinued, severe and even fatal cases have been reported. Currently, it is not clear what level of asymptomatic hyperamylasemia would warrant discontinuation of valproate or whether routine monitoring of amylase levels would be warranted in any specific patient group. We would advise checking an amylase level whenever a patient on valproate develops anorexia, nausea, vomiting, or abdominal pain. If the amylase is elevated by threefold or more, valproate should be discontinued. If the amylase is elevated to a lesser degree and the diagnosis is uncertain, the lipase level should be checked, and the amylase level should be repeated at weekly intervals until stable. Valproate would be discontinued if the amylase level rose progressively, if lipase were elevated, or if a typical clinical syndrome of pancreatitis developed.

Recent reports have confirmed that, like carbamazepine, valproate can cause the syndrome of drug-induced lupus (Asconape et al. 1994; Drory and Korczyn 1993). Antinuclear antibodies, together with anti-histone antibodies, strongly support the diagnosis of drug-induced lupus; treatment consists of drug discontinuation plus prednisone if warranted by the severity of the symptoms.

Benefits.   A particular benefit of valproate as a therapy for acute mania is that its onset of action is relatively rapid, so that neuroleptics with their associated risks can be minimized or avoided. Keck and others (1993a) recently reported on the safety and tolerability of rapid oral loading of valproate in 19 acutely manic patients who were given 20 mg/kg/day of valproate in divided doses, along with up to 4 mg/day of lorazepam. Fifteen patients remained in their study for at least 5 days, and all of them attained valproate levels of 50 mg/L. Ten of the 19 patients showed at least 50% improvement in a mania rating scale; side effects were "minimal." In contrast to carbamazepine, which regularly produces unpleasant neurologic side effects in patients started immediately on a full therapeutic dose, valproate appears to be suitable for rapid loading.

Other drug interactions with valproate.   Clinically significant drug interactions involving valproate are most easily understood by keeping three points in mind: 1) valproate is metabolized by hepatic oxidation, 2) valproate is an inhibitor of several hepatic enzymes, and 3) valproate is highly bound (80%–95%) to serum albumin, with a free fraction that increases nonlinearly with increasing total valproate levels (Mattson and Cramer 1989). The free fraction doubles from a total valproate level of 50 to 100 mg/L and doubles again from 100 to 150 mg/L.

Inhibition of hepatic glucuronidation by valproate is responsible for an interaction with lorazepam that at times may be clinically significant. Valproate can decrease lorazepam clearance by an average of 40%, by impeding the formation of lorazepam glucuronide (Anderson et al. 1994).

Inhibition of hepatic oxidation by valproate leads to increased levels of the relatively toxic metabolite carbamazepine 10,11-epoxide when valproate and carbamazepine are given together. The epoxide metabolite of carbamazepine, not routinely measured by many clinical laboratories, can contribute both to therapeutic and to toxic effects. The magnitude and relevance of the interaction is highly variable between patients (Cloyd et al. 1993; McKee et al. 1992). For example, McKee and colleagues gave valproate 500 mg bid to 16 patients established on therapeutic doses of carbamazepine. Carbamazepine epoxide levels after 5 days of valproate therapy varied from 25% decreased to 125% increased! When a patient receiving carbamazepine and valproate together develops ataxia, diplopia, sedation, or other signs of carbamazepine toxicity despite a carbamazepine level in the therapeutic range, a disproportionate elevation of carbamazepine epoxide should be considered as a cause. A serum sample can be sent to a reference laboratory to confirm the hypothesis.

The enzyme-inducing effects of carbamazepine will lower the valproate level attained at any given dose (Pisani 1992). However, the clinical effect of a lower level may be partially offset by an increase in free valproate, because carbamazepine and valproate compete for binding sites on serum albumin.

When valproate and carbamazepine are given together, relatively more of valproate's hepatotoxic 4-ene-valproic acid metabolite is formed as a result of carbamazepine's inducing enzymes responsible for this metabolite; this effect may account for the higher incidence of valproate liver toxicity with polytherapy (Levy et al. 1990).

Drugs that inhibit hepatic oxidative enzymes can increase valproate levels by decreasing its clearance. Antibiotics have been reported to precipitate valproate toxicity by this mechanism. Case reports have mentioned isoniazid (Jonville et al. 1991) and erythromycin (Redington et al. 1992). Psychiatrists may take some comfort from a report that paroxetine does not alter plasma concentrations of either valproate or carbamazepine (Andersen et al. 1991). However, it remains prudent to recheck antiepileptic drug levels periodically while titrating the dose of any SSRI, given the variability in pharmacokinetics among individual patients.

Aspirin is the most common example of a drug that can precipitate valproate toxicity by displacing the drug from serum albumin (Mattson and Cramer 1989; Yu et al. 1990). Aspirin also increases the relative amount of the hepatotoxic 4-ene-metabolite. Eventually, the increased free fraction of valproate, by causing increased clearance, leads to a lower total valproate level and an unchanged free valproate level. However, the free valproate level may be elevated to the toxic range for several hours after beginning aspirin, until the system comes into a new equilibrium.

Zolpidem

Zolpidem is a nonbenzodiazepine sedative hypnotic. It is an imidazopyridine that binds selectively to the type I benzodiazepine receptor. Compared with benzodiazepine hypnotics, it may have less tendency to cause tolerance, dependence, and withdrawal symptoms (Fillastre et al. 1993), although more widespread experience is needed with the drug to establish these speculations. However, it frequently causes GI symptoms, especially nausea and dyspepsia. In this section, we review features of zolpidem of particular relevance to its use in patients with medical illness.

Zolpidem is metabolized by the liver to entirely inactive metabolites. The half-life of the active parent compound is between 2 and 2.5 hours in most adults (Lavoisy et al. 1992). The pharmacokinetics and pharmacodynamics of zolpidem have been examined in patients on hemodialysis for end-stage renal failure; they have been found to be similar to those for healthy adults, suggesting that renal elimination of zolpidem metabolites is not relevant to termination of its clinical action (Fillastre et al. 1993). The half-life of zolpidem can be prolonged in some elderly patients because of a lower rate of hepatic metabolism of the drug, so a lower initial dose is suggested for older patients (5 mg compared to 10 mg). The half-life of zolpidem will be prolonged in virtually all patients with significant hepatic insufficiency.

At doses of 20 mg per night or less, zolpidem does not significantly suppress rapid eye movement (REM) sleep or slow-wave sleep (Blois et al. 1993). REM rebound does not occur when zolpidem is discontinued, a feature that may make it attractive for intermittent use in patients with posttraumatic stress disorder who have frequent nightmares.

Respiratory effects of zolpidem.   Zolpidem has minimal effect on respiratory drive in doses of 20 mg or less. Cohn (1993) tested and compared the respiratory effects of 10- and 20-mg doses of zolpidem in 12 healthy male volunteers with the effects of 60 mg of codeine and placebo. Measures were ventilatory responses to carbon dioxide and mouth occlusion pressure and mean inspiratory flow. Doses of 10 mg zolpidem did not differ from placebo in their effect on respiration; 20-mg doses produced minimal suppression of mean inspiratory flow only. Codeine, 60 mg, was the only treatment to significantly reduce the response to carbon dioxide. Steens and co-workers (1993) compared the respiratory effects of bedtime doses of zolpidem (5 or 10 mg) with those of triazolam (0.25 mg) and placebo in 24 patients with insomnia and mild to moderate chronic obstructive pulmonary disease (COPD)—forced expiratory volume (FEV_1) averaging 61% of predicted. Neither drug had any significant effect on oxygen saturation by hour or stage of sleep or on the apnea-hypopnea index for the night. The sleep-inducing effects of 10 mg of zolpidem and 0.25 mg of triazolam were comparable; the 5-mg dose of zolpidem was less efficacious for treating the patients' insomnia. Murciano and associates (1993) investigated the effects of single doses of 10 mg zolpidem, 0.25 mg triazolam, and 1 mg flunitrazepam in 12 patients with severe but stable COPD who were known to retain carbon dioxide at baseline. The mean baseline arterial carbon dioxide was 5.9 kPa (approximately 45 mmHg). Two hours after a 10-mg dose of zolpidem, there was no significant change in arterial carbon dioxide, minute ventilation, mouth occlusion pressure, ventilatory response to carbon dioxide stimulation, or mouth occlusion pressure increase in response to carbon dioxide stimulation. In contrast, both benzodiazepines decreased minute ventilation, and flunitrazepam was associated with a significant rise in arterial carbon dioxide.

Although these studies suggest that zolpidem is safer than benzodiazepine hypnotics for patients with COPD, it remains to be determined whether zolpidem aggravates sleep apnea in patients with severe COPD and whether respiratory parameters remain benign over an entire night's sleep in such patients. At this time, a conservative practice would be to use the drug for treatment of insomnia in outpatients with COPD who do not retain carbon dioxide and to consider it for carbon dioxide retainers only if it were first tested in the specific patient under close observation.

Other side effects.   Several studies of zolpidem in elderly populations, including elderly psychiatric inpatients receiving other psychotropics, suggest that it has a low rate of adverse CNS side effects such as confusion or ataxia. Roger and colleagues (1993) gave 5 mg of zolpidem, 10 mg of zolpidem, or 0.25 mg of triazolam to 221 patients with insomnia, aged 58 to 98 years. All three treatments were efficacious, but all were associated with nightmares, daytime drowsiness, and episodes of agitation in some of the patients treated. Confusion was mentioned as an adverse effect only in the triazolam group. Fairweather and others (1992) gave 5 mg zolpidem, 10 mg zolpidem, or placebo to 24 otherwise healthy elderly volunteers with prolonged sleep latency, in a three-way, double-blind, crossover study. Both doses of zolpidem improved subjective sleep, and neither impaired performance on cognitive tests the following morning, which included choice reaction time, critical flicker fusion threshold, word recognition, and a tracking task. Shaw and co-workers (1992) gave 10- or 20-mg doses of zolpidem or placebo to 119 elderly psychiatric inpatients in a double-blind, randomized trial. Both doses of zolpidem were superior to placebo in improving subjective measures of sleep quality. Three of the patients receiving 20 mg of zolpidem had daytime drowsiness, and 2 had ataxia. With the 10-mg dose, 1 patient had daytime drowsiness, and 1 had ataxia.

Taken together, these studies suggest that zolpidem is a relatively benign sedative hypnotic for elderly patients, particularly in doses of 10 mg or lower. It probably has fewer severe CNS side effects than triazolam, but it cannot be presumed to be totally benign. Hallucinations have been reported as a rare side effect (Ansseau et al. 1992; Iruela et al. 1993; Morselli 1993). Elderly patients who awaken at night after taking a bedtime dose of zolpidem are at increased risk for falling if they get out of bed. Berlin et al. (1993) demonstrated that a single dose of 10 mg of zolpidem significantly increased postural sway 1.5 hours after ingestion in 18 healthy volunteers. This effect of zolpidem would be especially relevant if other risk factors for falls, such as decreased vision and orthostatic hypotension, were also present.

As of this writing, no systematic studies on the use of zolpidem to treat insomnia or reversed day-night sleep cycles in patients with Alzheimer's disease or other dementias have been published. Because benzodiazepines are known to be a problematic treatment for this clinical problem, a safe and effective alternative would be a significant advance. The lack of such studies is in keeping with the general tendency of pharmaceutical companies to avoid undertaking studies of new drugs in populations in which side effects might be especially problematic.

Tacrine

The potential role of tacrine in the treatment of patients with Alzheimer's disease is gradually becoming better established by additional clinical trials and by the experience of clinicians since the drug was approved by the FDA in 1993. At this point, tacrine appears to be most helpful to patients with relatively mild dementia, in whom tacrine can improve memory, attention, and/or executive cognitive functions enough to measurably improve everyday function or caregiver burden. At least one-half of patients treated with tacrine will discontinue the drug because of side effects, and clinically meaningful benefits will be seen in less than one-half of those who are actually able to tolerate a dose of 80 to 160 mg/day. In this section, we discuss recent evidence that tacrine is efficacious, new work on its effects and side effects, and guidelines for selecting dementia patients for a therapeutic trial of tacrine.

The most important recent study on the efficacy of tacrine was the Tacrine Study Group's 30-week randomized, controlled trial of high-dose tacrine use in patients with Alzheimer's disease (Knapp et al. 1994). In this multicenter study, patients with Alzheimer's disease and Mini-Mental State Exam (MMSE) (Folstein et al. 1975) scores ranging from 10 to 26 were randomized to four groups: placebo; tacrine 40 mg/day for 6 weeks and 80 mg/day thereafter; tacrine 40 mg/day for 6 weeks, 80 mg/day for 6 weeks, and 120 mg/day thereafter; and tacrine 40 mg/day for 6 weeks, 80 mg/day for 6 weeks, 120 mg/day for 6 weeks, and 160 mg/day thereafter. Of 653 patients included in an intent-to-treat analysis, 384 dropped out before week 30, 74% of them because of adverse effects. Among those who did complete the study, 42% of those receiving tacrine showed improvement, as opposed to 18% who received placebo. The improvement rate for tacrine in the intent-to-treat population was 23%, as opposed to 17% in the placebo group. Thus, less than one-quarter of patients begun on tacrine both tolerated the drug and improved significantly.

The study did show a significant dose relationship for therapeutic effects. At 160 mg/day, 42% had at least a 3-point improvement in their MMSE score. Behavioral changes significant to the caregivers were noted in many of those who improved cognitively.

In the Tacrine Study Group population, 54% of all tacrine-treated patients had at least one elevated alanine aminotransferase (ALT) level; in 29%, the elevation was greater than three times the upper limit of normal. Ninety-four percent reported some adverse events, with nausea or vomiting in 35% and diarrhea in 18%. Ninety percent of ALT elevations requiring drug discontinuation occurred in the first 12 weeks of the study.

Attention versus memory improvements.   When tacrine does make a significant difference in a patient's function, the crucial factor may be improvement in attentional performance rather than improvement in memory. Sahakian and Coull (1993) gave tacrine to 89 patients with Alzheimer's disease in a placebo-controlled, crossover trial and evaluated their memory and attention with computerized cognitive tests. Attention, but not memory, improved in the patients with mild to moderate dementia who were given tacrine.

Based on the low rate of response to tacrine, and its high rate of adverse effects, investigators have attempted to predict which patients with Alzheimer's disease will respond and which will have severe hepatotoxicity. Alhainen and associates (1993a) reported that cognitive improvement 2 hours after a single 50-mg oral dose of tacrine predicted improvement after 4 weeks of treatment at 100 mg/day—improvement was defined as at least a 3-point improvement in MMSE. In their study of 14 patients, 8 who responded to tacrine showed improvement on Digit Span, Trail Making B, Clock Setting, and Clock Recognition tests when tested after 50 mg of tacrine was administered; the 6 nonresponders did not show acute improvement. Alhainen and associates remarked that tacrine seemed to help attentional and frontal lobe functions rather than memory.

The EEG has also been investigated as a predictor of response to tacrine. In a series of 17 patients, Minthon et al. (1993) found that a greater amount of high-frequency background activity on EEG was associated with a greater likelihood of response.

Watkins and co-workers (1994) evaluated predictors of adverse effects of tacrine treatment in a review of 2,446 patients enrolled in multicenter clinical trials of tacrine. They found that female gender, baseline hepatic ALT level, younger age, and larger body size were associated with a higher risk of ALT elevation to greater than three times normal. Drinking and smoking were not relevant risk factors. The total variance explained by the risk factors was, however, less than 3%, implying that clinically useful prediction of an individual's risk of tacrine toxicity is not currently possible.

Current recommendations are to discontinue tacrine if the ALT rises to greater than three times the upper limit of normal. After a drug-free interval for normalization of liver enzymes, rechallenge is acceptable. Studies of rechallenge reviewed by Watkins et al. showed that only one-third of patients rechallenged had a recurrence of ALT elevation to greater than three times normal. Monitoring of ALT levels may be done less frequently after the first 12 weeks of therapy at a given dose, because the conditional probability of developing clinically significant ALT elevation drops to 10% or less if that complication has not occurred in the first 12 weeks of therapy. Thus, there appears to be some tolerance to tacrine's hepatotoxicity (Watkins et al. 1994).

An important recent line of study of tacrine has emphasized its effect on multiple neurotransmitter systems. Tacrine increases the turnover of serotonin and dopamine by stimulating release and blocking reuptake (Nyback et al. 1993), and patients with better clinical responses to tacrine have higher increases in cerebrospinal fluid 5-hydroxyindoleacetic acid (5-HIAA) and homovanillic acid (HVA) after tacrine treatment (Alhainen et al. 1993b). Schneider and associates (1993) recently reported that adding 5 mg bid of selegiline to tacrine treatment enhanced improvements in patients' cognitive function.

To summarize, the ideal patient for a tacrine trial is a patient with relatively mild disease, beginning to lose one or more instrumental functions, a normal or mildly abnormal EEG, and a clinical situation in which a small increment in cognitive function might make a big difference in coping or caregiver burden. The patient would not have parkinsonian features or clinical depression; if the patient had one of these features at presentation, it should be adequately treated before trying tacrine. A positive response on cognitive tests after an acute dose would increase the likelihood of a successful outcome.

REFERENCES

Ahmed I, Dagincourt PG, Miller LG, et al: Possible interaction between fluoxetine and pimozide causing sinus bradycardia. Can J Psychiatry 38:62–63, 1993

Albani F, Riva R, Baruzzi A: Clarithromycin carbamazepine interaction: a case report. Epilepsia 34:161–162, 1993

Alderman CP, Moritz CK, Ben-Tovim DI: Abnormal platelet aggregation associated with fluoxetine therapy. DICP 26:1517–1519, 1992

Alhainen K, Helkala EL, Reikkinen P: Psychometric discrimination of tetrahydroaminoacridine responders in Alzheimer patients. Dementia 4:54–58, 1993a

Alhainen K, Helkala EL, Reinikainen K, et al: The relationship of cerebrospinal fluid monoamine metabolites with clinical response to tetrahydroaminoacridine in patients with Alzheimer's disease. J Neural Transm Park Dis Dement Sect 5:185–192, 1993b

Alvir JMJ, Lieberman JA: A reevaluation of the clinical characteristics of clozapine-induced agranulocytosis in light of the United States experience. J Clin Psychopharmacol 14:87–88, 1994

Alvir JMJ, Lieberman JA, Safferman AZ, et al: Clozapine-induced agranulocytosis: incidence and risk factors in the United States. N Engl J Med 329:162–167, 1993

Amabeoku GJ, Chikuni O, Akino C, et al: Pharmacokinetic interaction of single doses of quinine and carbamazepine, phenobarbitone and phenytoin in healthy volunteers. East Afr Med J 70:90–93, 1993

Andersen BB, Mikkelsen M, Vesterager A, et al: No influence of the antidepressant paroxetine on carbamazepine, valproate and phenytoin. Epilepsy Res 10:201–204, 1991

Anderson GD, Gidal BE, Kantor ED, et al: Lorazepam-valproate interaction: studies in normal subjects and isolated perfused rat liver. Epilepsia 35:221–225, 1994

Ansseau M, Pitchot W, Hansenne M, et al: Psychotic reactions to zolpidem (letter). Lancet 339(8796):809, 1992

Arya DK, Szabadi E: Dyskinesia associated with fluvoxamine (letter). J Clin Psychopharmacol 13:365–366, 1993

Asconape JJ, Penry JK, Dreifuss FE, et al: Valproate-associated pancreatitis. Epilepsia 34:177–183, 1993

Asconape JJ, Manning KR, Lancman ME: Systemic lupus erythematosus associated with use of valproate. Epilepsia 35:162–163, 1994

Bailey DN, Coffee JJ, Anderson B, et al: Interaction of tricyclic antidepressants with cholestyramine in vitro. Ther Drug Monit 14:339–342, 1992

Baldessarini R, Marsh E: Fluoxetine and side effects (letter). Arch Gen Psychiatry 47:191–192, 1990

Baldwin D, Fineberg N, Montgomery S: Fluoxetine, fluvoxamine and extrapyramidal tract disorders. Int Clin Psychopharmacol 6:51–58, 1991

Bannister SJ, Houser VP, Hulse JD, et al: Evaluation of the potential for interactions of paroxetine with diazepam, cimetidine, warfarin, and digoxin. Acta Psychiatr Scand 80 (suppl 350):102–106, 1989

Banov MD, Tohen M, Friedberg J: High risk of eosinophilia in women treated with clozapine. J Clin Psychiatry 54:466–469, 1993

Barros J, Asnis G: An interaction of sertraline and desipramine (letter). Am J Psychiatry 150:1751, 1993

Benfield P, Ward A: Fluvoxamine: a review of its pharmacodynamic and pharmacokinetic properties, and therapeutic efficacy in depressive illness. Drugs 32:313–334, 1986

Bergstrom RF, Peyton AL, Lemberger L: Quantification and mechanism of fluoxetine and tricyclic antidepressant interaction. Clin Pharmacol Ther 51:239–248, 1992

Bergstrom RF, Beasley CM, Levy NB, et al: The effects of renal and hepatic disease on the pharmacokinetics, renal tolerance, and risk-benefit profile of fluoxetine. Int Clin Psychopharmacol 8:261–266, 1993

Berlin I, Warot D, Hergueta T, et al: Comparison of the effects of zolpidem and triazolam on memory functions, psychomotor performances, and postural sway in healthy subjects. J Clin Psychopharmacol 2:100–106, 1993

Berman I: Risperidone in elderly psychotic patients, in New Research Program and Abstracts: American Psychiatric Association Annual Meeting, Philadelphia, PA, May 1994, p 183

Bertschy G, Vandel S, Jounet JM, et al: Valpromide-amitriptyline interaction. Encephale 16:43–45, 1990

Bertschy G, Vandel S, Bandel B, et al: Fluvoxamine-tricyclic antidepressant interaction. Eur J Clin Pharmacol 40:119–120, 1991

Binder EF, Cayabyab L, Ritchie DJ, et al: Diltiazem-induced psychosis and a possible diltiazem-lithium interaction. Arch Intern Med 151:373–374, 1991

Blois R, Gaillard JM, Attali P, et al: Effect of zolpidem on sleep in healthy subjects: a placebo-controlled trial with polysomnographic recordings. Clin Ther 15:807–809, 1993

Bourgeois B, Leppik IE, Sackellares JC, et al: Felbamate: a double-blind controlled trial in patients undergoing presurgical evaluation of partial seizures. Neurology 43:693–696, 1993

Brosen K, Kragh-Sorensen P: Concomitant intake of nortriptyline and carbamazepine. Ther Drug Monit 15:258–260, 1993

Brown DW, Ketter TA, Crumlish J, et al: Carbamazepine-induced increases in total serum cholesterol: clinical and theoretical implications. J Clin Psychopharmacol 12:431–437, 1992

Buckley PF, Meltzer HY: Clozapine and NMS (letter). Br J Psychiatry 162:566, 1993

Burns MM, Eisendrath SJ: Dextroamphetamine treatment for depression in terminally ill patients. Psychosomatics 35:80–83, 1994

Calabrese JR, Rapport DJ, Kimmel SE, et al: Rapid cycling bipolar disorder and its treatment with valproate. Can J Psychiatry 38 (suppl 2):S57–S61, 1993

Caley CF, Friedman JH: Does fluoxetine exacerbate Parkinson's disease? J Clin Psychiatry 53:278–282, 1992

Cannon RO, Quyyumi AA, Mincemoyer R, et al: Imipramine in patients with chest pain despite normal coronary angiograms. N Engl J Med 330:1411–1417, 1994

Caporaso NE, Shaw GL: Clinical implications of the competitive inhibition of the debrisoquin-metabolizing isozyme by quinidine. Arch Intern Med 151:1985–1992, 1991

Centorrino F, Baldessarini RJ, Kando J, et al: Serum concentrations of clozapine and its major metabolites: effects of cotreatment with fluoxetine or valproate. Am J Psychiatry 151:123–125, 1994

Chouinard G, Arnott W: Clinical review of risperidone. Can J Psychiatry 38 (suppl 3):S89–S95, 1993

Chouinard G, Jones B, Remington G, et al: A Canadian multicenter placebo-controlled study of fixed doses of risperidone and haloperidol in the treatment of chronic schizophrenic patients. J Clin Psychopharmacol 13:25–40, 1993

Christensen EM, Aggernaes H: Prospective study of EDTA clearance among patients in long-term lithium treatment. Acta Psychiatr Scand 81:302–303, 1990

Ciraulo DA, Shader RI: Fluoxetine drug-drug interactions, I: antidepressants and antipsychotics. J Clin Psychopharmacol 10:48–50, 1990

Cloyd JC, Fischer JH, Kriel RL, et al: Valproic acid pharmacokinetics in children, IV: effects of age and antiepileptic drugs on protein binding and intrinsic clearance. Clin Pharmacol Ther 53:22–29, 1993

Cohn MA: Effects of zolpidem, codeine phosphate and placebo on respiration: a double-blind, crossover study in volunteers. Drug Saf 9:312–319, 1993

Conte G, Vazzola A, Sacchetti E: Renal function in chronic lithium-treated patients. Acta Psychiatr Scand 79:503–504, 1989

Correa FJ, Eiser AR: Angiotensin-converting enzyme inhibitors and lithium toxicity. Am J Med 93:108–109, 1992

Crewe HK, Lennard MS, Tucker GT, et al: The effect of selective serotonin reuptake inhibitors on cytochrome P4502D6 (CYP2D6) activity in human liver microsomes. Br J Clin Pharmacol 34:262–265, 1992

Dalhoff K, Almdal TP, Bjerrum K, et al: Pharmacokinetics of paroxetine in patients with cirrhosis. Eur J Clin Pharmacol 41:351–354, 1991

Daly JM, Goldberg RJ, Braman SS: Polyserositis associated with clozapine treatment (letter). Am J Psychiatry 149:1274–1275, 1992

DasGupta K, Young A: Clozapine-induced neuroleptic malignant syndrome. J Clin Psychiatry 52:105–107, 1991

DasGupta K, Jefferson JW, Kobak KA, et al: The effect of enalapril on serum lithium levels in healthy men. J Clin Psychiatry 53:398–400, 1992

Dave M: Fluoxetine-associated dystonia (letter). Am J Psychiatry 151:149, 1994

Dechant KL, Clissold SP: Paroxetine: a review of its pharmacodynamic and pharmacokinetic properties, and therapeutic potential in depressive illness. Drugs 41:225–253, 1991

Deltito JA: The effect of valproate on bipolar spectrum temperamental disorders. J Clin Psychiatry 54:300–304, 1993

Devinsky O, Honigfeld G, Patin J: Clozapine-related seizures. Neurology 41:369–371, 1991

Dilsaver SC, Swann AC, Shoaib AM, et al: The manic syndrome: factors which may predict a patient's response to lithium, carbamazepine and valproate. J Psychiatry Neurosci 18:61–66, 1993

Drory VE, Korczyn AD: Hypersensitivity vasculitis and systemic lupus erythematosus induced by anticonvulsants. Clin Neuropharmacol 16:19–29, 1993

Duarte J, Macias S, Coria F, et al: Valproate-induced coma: case report and literature review. DICP 27:582–583, 1993

Epstein AE, Hallstrom AP, Rogers WJ, et al: Mortality following ventricular arrhythmia suppression by encainide, flecainide, and moricizine after myocardial infarction. JAMA 270:2451–2455, 1993

Ereshefsky L, Lacombe S: Pharmacologic profile of risperidone. Can J Psychiatry 38 (suppl 3):S80–S88, 1993

Fairweather DB, Kerr JS, Hindmarch I: The effects of acute and repeated doses of zolpidem on subjective sleep, psychomotor performance and cognitive function in elderly volunteers. Eur J Clin Pharmacol 43:597–601, 1992

Fillastre JP, Geffroy-Josse S, Etienne I, et al: Pharmacokinetics and pharmacodynamics of zolpidem following repeated doses in homodialyzed uraemic patients. Fundam Clin Pharmacol 7:1–9, 1993

Fisch C, Knoebel SB: Electrocardiographic findings in sertraline depression trials. Drug Investigation 4:305–312, 1992

Fischer V, Vogels B, Maurer G, et al: The antipsychotic clozapine is metabolized by the polymorphic human microsomal and recombinant cytochrome P450 2D6. J Pharmacol Exp Ther 260:1355–1360, 1992

Fisher RS: Emerging antiepileptic drugs. Neurology 43 (suppl 5):S12–S20, 1993

Fogel BS, Stoudemire A: New psychotropics in medically ill patients, in Medical-Psychiatric Practice, Vol 2. Edited by Stoudemire A, Fogel BS. Washington, DC, American Psychiatric Press, 1993, pp 69–111

Folstein MF, Folstein SE, McHugh PR: Mini-Mental State: a practical method for grading the cognitive state of patients for the clinician. J Psychiatr Res 12:189–198, 1975

Frasure-Smith N, Lesperance F, Talajic M: Depression following myocardial infarction: impact on 6-month survival. JAMA 270:1819–1825, 1993

Friedman LJ, Tabb SE, Sanchez CJ: Clozapine—a novel antipsychotic agent (letter). N Engl J Med 325:518, 1991

Fritze J, Unsorg B, Lanczik M: Interaction between carbamazepine and fluvoxamine. Acta Psychiatr Scand 84:538–584, 1991

Fu C, Katzman M, Goldbloom DS: Valproate/nortriptyline interaction (letter). J Clin Psychopharmacol 14:205, 1994

Gibaldi M: Drug interactions: part I. inhibition of drug metabolism. DICP 26:709–713, 1992

Gidal BE, Aderson GD, Seaton TL, et al: Evaluation of the effect of fluoxetine on the formation of carbamazepine epoxide. Ther Drug Monit 15:405–409, 1993

Gilman JT, Alvarez LA, Duchowny M: Carbamazepine toxicity resulting from generic substitution. Neurology 43:2696–2697, 1993

Gitlin MF: Lithium-induced renal insufficiency. J Clin Psychopharmacol 13:276–279, 1993

Glassman AH, Roose SP, Bigger JT: The safety of tricyclic antidepressants in cardiac patients: risk-benefit reconsidered. JAMA 269:2673–2675, 1993

Goa KL, Sorkin EM: Gabapentin. A review of its pharmacological properties and clinical potential in epilepsy. Drugs 46:409–427, 1993

Goff DC, Midha KK, Brotman AW, et al: Elevation of plasma concentrations of haloperidol after the addition of fluoxetine. Am J Psychiatry 148:790–792, 1991

Graves NM: Felbamate. DICP 27:1073–1081, 1993

Greb WH, Buscher G, Dierdorf H-D, et al: Effect of liver enzyme inhibition by cimetidine and enzyme induction by phenobarbitone on the pharmacokinetics of paroxetine. Acta Psychiatr Scand 80 (suppl 350):95–98, 1989

Greenblatt DJ, Abernethy DR, Locniskar A, et al: Age, sex, and nitrazepam kinetics: relation to antipyrine disposition. Clin Pharmacol Ther 38:697–703, 1985

Greenblatt DJ, Preskorn SH, Cotreau MM, et al: Fluoxetine impairs clearance of alprazolam but not of clonazepam. Clin Pharmacol Ther 52:479–486, 1992

Grimsley SR, Jann MW, Carter JG, et al: Increased carbamazepine plasma concentrations after fluoxetine coadministration. Clin Pharmacol Ther 50:10–15, 1991

Gualtieri T, Hicks RE, Levitt J, et al: Methylphenidate and exercise: additive effects on motor performance, variable effects on the neuroendocrine response. Neuropsychobiology 15:84–88, 1986

Gupta S: Paradoxical hypertension associated with clozapine (letter). Am J Psychiatry 151:148, 1994

Hamilton M: A rating scale for depression. J Neurol Neurosurg Psychiatry 23:56–62, 1960

Hansen-Grant S, Silk KR, Guthrie S: Fluoxetine-pimozide interaction (letter). Am J Psychiatry 150:1751–1752, 1993

Hermann DJ, Krol TF, Dukes GE, et al: Comparison of verapamil, diltiazem, and labetalol on the bioavailability and metabolism of imipramine. J Clin Pharmacol 32:176–183, 1992

Hojer J, Malmlund HO, Berg A: Clinical features in 28 consecutive cases of laboratory confirmed massive poisoning with carbamazepine alone. J Toxicol Clin Toxicol 31:449–458, 1993

Honig PK, Wortham DC, Zamani K, et al: Terfenadine-ketoconazole interaction. JAMA 269:1513–1518, 1993

Horneff G, Lenard HG, Wahn V: Severe adverse reaction to carbamazepine: significance of humoral and cellular reactions to the drug. Neuropediatrics 23:272–275, 1992

Iruela LM, Ibanez-Rojo V, Baca E: More on zolpidem side-effects (letter). Lancet 342(8885):1495–1496, 1993

Isojarvi JI, Airaksinen KE, Repo M, et al: Carbamazepine, serum thyroid hormones and myocardial function in epileptic patients. J Neurol Neurosurg Psychiatry 56:710–712, 1993a

Isojarvi JI, Pakarinen AJ, Myllyla VV: Serum lipid levels during carbamazepine medication. A prospective study. Arch Neurol 50:590–593, 1993b

Jacobsen FM: Low-dose valproate: a new treatment for cyclothymia, mild rapid cycling disorders, and premenstrual syndrome. J Clin Psychiatry 54:229–234, 1993

Jain KK: Investigation and management of loss of efficacy of an antiepileptic medication using carbamazepine as an example. J R Soc Med 86:133–136, 1993

Janowsky DS, Leichner P, Clopton P, et al: Comparison of oral and intravenous methylphenidate. Psychopharmacology 59:75–78, 1978

Jha S, Nag D, Shukla R, et al: Effect of sodium valproate on serum amylase in epileptics. J Indian Med Assoc 91:53–54, 1993

Jochemsen R, vanBeusekom BR, Spoelstra P, et al: Effect of age and liver cirrhosis on the pharmacokinetics of nitrazepam. Br J Clin Pharmacol 15:295–302, 1983

Jonville AP, Gauchez AS, Autret E, et al: Interaction between isoniazid and valproate: a case of valproate overdosage (letter). Eur J Clin Pharmacol 40:197–198, 1991

Kane JM: Newer antipsychotic drugs: a review of their pharmacology and therapeutic potential. Drugs 46:585–593, 1993

Kaneko K, Igarashi J, Suzuki Y, et al: Carbamazepine-induced thrombocytopenia and leucopenia complicated by Henoch-Schonlein purpura symptoms. Eur J Pediatr 152:769–770, 1993

Kanno T, Miyata M, Kazuta Y, et al: Carbamazepine-induced systemic lupus erythematosus–like disease. Internal Medicine 31:1303–1305, 1992

Kastner T, Finesmith R, Walsh K: Long-term administration of valproic acid in the treatment of affective symptoms in people with mental retardation. J Clin Psychopharmacol 13:448–451, 1993

Katz MR: Raised serum levels of desipramine with the antiarrhythmic propafenone (letter). J Clin Psychiatry 52:432–433, 1991

Keck PE Jr, McElroy SL, Tugrul KC, et al: Valproate oral loading in the treatment of acute mania. J Clin Psychiatry 54:305–308, 1993a

Keck PE Jr, Taylor VE, Tugrul KC, et al: Valproate treatment of panic disorder and lactate-induced panic attacks. Biol Psychiatry 33:542–546, 1993b

Keck PE Jr, McElroy SL, Tugrul KC, et al: Antiepileptic drugs for the treatment of panic disorder. Neuropsychobiology 27:150–153, 1993c

Ketter TA, Malow BA, Flamini R, et al: Anticonvulsant withdrawal-emergent psychopathology. Neurology 44:55–61, 1994

King GG, Barnes DJ, Hayes MJ: Carbamazepine-induced pneumonitis. Med J Aust 160:126–127, 1994

Kingsbury SJ, Salzman C: Lithium's role in hyperparathyroidism and hypercalcemia. Hosp Community Psychiatry 44:1047–1048, 1993

Knapp MK, Knopman DS, Solomon PR, et al: A 30-week randomized controlled trial of high-dose tacrine in patients with Alzheimer's disease. The Tacrine Study Group. JAMA 271:985–991, 1994

Kreuz W, Linde R, Funk M, et al: Valproate therapy induces von Willebrand disease type 1. Epilepsia 33:178–184, 1992

Laird LK, Lydiard RB, Morton WA, et al: Cardiovascular effects of imipramine, fluvoxamine, and placebo in depressed outpatients. J Clin Psychiatry 54:224–228, 1993

Lamberti JS: Treatment of clozapine-induced agranulocytosis, in New Research Program and Abstracts: American Psychiatric Association Annual Meeting, Philadelphia, PA, May 1994, p 143

Lamberti J, Bellnier T: Clozapine and tardive dystonia (letter). J Nerv Ment Dis 181:137–138, 1993

Lasher TA, Fleishaker JC, Steenwyk RC, et al: Pharmacokinetic pharmacodynamic evaluation of the combined administration of alprazolam and fluoxetine. Psychopharmacology 104:323–327, 1991

Lavoisy J, Zivkovic B, Benavides J, et al: Contribution of zolpidem in the management of sleep disorders. Encephale 18:379–392, 1992

Lazarus LW, Winemiller DR, Lingam VR, et al: Efficacy and side effects of methylphenidate for poststroke depression. J Clin Psychiatry 53:447–449, 1992

Lemberger L, Rowe H, Bosomworth JC, et al: The effect of fluoxetine on the pharmacokinetics and psychomotor responses of diazepam. Clin Pharmacol Ther 43:412–419, 1988

Lemoine A, Gautier JC, Azoulay D, et al: Major pathway of imipramine metabolism is catalyzed by cytochromes P-450 1A2 and P-450 3A4 in human liver. Mol Pharmacol 43:827–832, 1993

Levenson JS: Cardiovascular disease, in Psychiatric Care of the Medical Patient. Edited by Stoudemire A, Fogel BS. New York, Oxford University Press, 1993, pp 539–563

Levy RH, Rettenmeier AW, Anderson GD, et al: Effects of polytherapy with phenytoin, carbamazepine, and stirlpentol on formation of 4-ene-valproate, a hepatotoxic metabolite of valproic acid. Clin Pharmacol Ther 48:225–235, 1990

Li R, Wing LL, Wyatt RJ, et al: Effects of haloperidol, lithium, and valproate on phosphoinositide turnover in rat brain. Pharmacol Biochem Behav 46:323–329, 1993

Lieberman JA, Saltz BL, Johns CA, et al: The effects of clozapine on tardive dyskinesia. Br J Psychiatry 158:503–510, 1991

Livingston MG: Risperidone. Lancet 343:457–460, 1994

Lock JD, Gwirtsman HE, Targ EF: Possible adverse drug interactions between fluoxetine and other psychotropics. J Clin Psychopharmacol 10:383–384, 1990

Loiseau P: Sodium valproate platelet dysfunction and bleeding. Epilepsia 27:55–59, 1981

Lokkegaard H, Andersen NF, Henriksen E, et al: Renal function in 153 manic-depressive patients treated with lithium for more than five years. Acta Psychiatr Scand 71:347–355, 1985

Makkar RR, Fromm BS, Steinman RT, et al: Female gender as a risk factor for torsades de pointes associated with cardiovascular drugs. JAMA 270:2590–2597, 1993

Maoz E, Grossman E, Thaler M, et al: Carbamazepine neurotoxic reaction after administration of diltiazem. Arch Intern Med 152:2503–2504, 1992

Mattson RH, Cramer JA: Valproate interactions with other drugs, in Antiepileptic Drugs, 3rd Edition. Edited by Levy RH, Dreifuss FE, Mattson RH, et al. New York, Raven, 1989, pp 621–632

Maurer PM, Bartkowski RR: Drug interactions of clinical significance with opioid analgesics. Drug Saf 8:30–48, 1993

May RB, Sunder TR: Hematologic manifestations of long-term valproate therapy. Epilepsia 34:1098–1101, 1993

McKee PJ, Blacklaw J, Butler E, et al: Variability and clinical relevance of the interaction between sodium valproate and carbamazepine in epileptic patients. Epilepsy Res 11:193–198, 1992

Mellow AM, Solano-Lopez C, Davis S: Sodium valproate in the treatment of behavioral disturbance in dementia. J Geriatr Psychiatry Neurol 6:205–209, 1993

Mendels J, Johnston R, Mattes J, et al: Efficacy and safety of BID doses of venlafaxine in a dose-response study. Psychopharmacol Bull 29:169–174, 1993

Messiha FS: Fluoxetine: adverse effects and drug-drug interactions. Clin Toxicology 31:603–630, 1993

Metzger E, Friedman R: Prolongation of the corrected QT and torsades de pointes cardiac arrhythmia associated with intravenous haloperidol in the medically ill. J Clin Psychopharmacol 13:128–132, 1993

Meyer MC, Straughn AB: Biopharmaceutical factors in seizure control and drug toxicity. Am J Hosp Pharm 50 (suppl 5):S17–S22, 1993

Miller DD: Effect of phenytoin on plasma clozapine concentrations in two patients. J Clin Psychiatry 52:23–25, 1991

Minthon L, Gustafson L, Dalfelt G, et al: Oral tetrahydroaminoacridine treatment of Alzheimer's disease evaluated clinically and by regional cerebral blood flow and EEG. Dementia 4:322–342, 1993

Morganroth J, Goin JE: Quinidine-related mortality in the short-to-medium-term treatment of ventricular arrhythmias: a meta-analysis. Circulation 84:1977–1983, 1991

Morrison C, Rieder MJ: Practices of epilepsy during pregnancy: a survey of Canadian neurologists. Reprod Toxicol 7:55–59, 1993

Morselli PL: Zolpidem side-effects (letter). Lancet 342(8875):868–869, 1993

Murciano D, Armengaud MH, Cramer PH, et al: Acute effects of zolpidem, triazolam and flunitrazepam on arterial blood gases and control of breathing in severe COPD. Eur Respir J 5:625–629, 1993

Nicholson SD: Extra pyramidal side effects associated with paroxetine. West of England Medical Journal 7:90–91, 1992

Nielsen H: Recombinant human granulocyte colony-stimulating factor (rhG-CSF; filgrastim) treatment of clozapine-induced agranulocytosis. J Intern Med 234:529–531, 1993

Nordenstrom J, Strigard K, Perbeck L, et al: Hyperparathyroidism associated with treatment of manic-depressive disorders by lithium. Eur J Surg 158:207–211, 1992

Nyback H, Hassan M, Junthe T, et al: Clinical experiences and biochemical findings with tacrine (THA). Acta Neurol Scand Suppl 149:36–38, 1993

Ochs HR, Greenblatt DJ, Gugler R, et al: Cimetidine impairs nitrazepam clearance. Clin Pharmacol Ther 34:227–230, 1983

O'Connor CR, Schraeder PL, Kurland AH, et al: Evaluation of the mechanisms of antiepileptic drug-related chronic leukopenia. Epilepsia 35:149–154, 1994

Ohashi T, Fujimoto M, Shimizu H, et al: A case of carbamazepine induced lupus with myositis. Rinsho Shinkeigaku 33:1094–1096, 1993

Ohmori S, Takeda S, Rikihisa T, et al: Studies on cytochrome P450 responsible for oxidative metabolism of imipramine in human liver microsomes. Biological and Pharmacological Bulletin 16:571–575, 1993

Ojemann LM, Wilensky AJ, Temkin NR, et al: Long-term treatment with gabapentin for partial epilepsy. Epilepsy Res 13:159–165, 1992

Okuma T: Effects of carbamazepine and lithium on affective disorders. Neuropsychobiology 27:138–145, 1993

Oles KS, Gal P: Bioequivalency revisited: Epitol versus Tegretol. Neurology 43:2435–2436, 1993

Ozkara C, Dreifuss FE, Apperson-Hansen C: Changes in red blood cells with valproate therapy. Acta Neurol Scand 88:210–212, 1993

Pagliaro LA, Pagliaro AM: Carbamazepine-induced Stevens Johnson syndrome. Hosp Community Psychiatry 44:999–1000, 1993

Patsalos PN, Duncan JS: Antiepileptic drugs. a review of clinically significant drug interactions. Drug Saf 9:156–184, 1993

Patterson BD, Jennings JL: Spiking fever and profuse diarrhea with clozapine treatment (letter). Am J Psychiatry 150:1126, 1993

Pisani F: Influence of co-medication on the metabolism of valproate. Pharm Weekbl [Sci] 14(3A):108–113, 1992

Popper CW: Desipramine deaths may be adrenergic, in New Research Program and Abstracts: American Psychiatric Association Annual Meeting, Philadelphia, PA, May 1994, p 179

Post RM, Ketter TA, Pazzaglia PJ, et al: New developments in the use of anticonvulsants as mood stabilizers. Neuropsychobiology 27:132–137, 1993

Preskorn SH, Alderman J, Chung M, et al: Pharmacokinetics of desipramine coadministered with sertraline or fluoxetine. J Clin Psychopharmacol 14:90–98, 1994

Radulovic LL, Wilder BJ, Leppik IE, et al: Lack of interaction of gabapentin with carbamazepine or valproate. Epilepsia 35:155–161, 1994

Reddig S, Minnema AM, Tandon R: Neuroleptic malignant syndrome and clozapine. Annals of Clinical Psychiatry 5:25–27, 1993

Redington K, Wells C, Petito F: Erythromycin and valproate interaction (letter). Ann Intern Med 116:877–878, 1992

Remington GJ: Clinical considerations in the use of risperidone. Can J Psychiatry 38 (suppl 3):S96–S100, 1993

Rho JM, Donevan SD, Rogawski MA: Mechanism of action of the anticonvulsant felbamate: opposing effects on N-methyl-D-aspartate and gamma-aminobutyric acid A receptors. Ann Neurol 35:229–234, 1994

Roger M, Attali P, Coquelin JP: Multicenter, double-blind, controlled comparison of zolpidem and triazolam in elderly patients with insomnia. Clin Ther 15:127–136, 1993

Rosenqvist M, Bergfeldt L, Aili H, et al: Sinus node dysfunction during long-term lithium treatment. Br Heart J 70:371–375, 1993

Rowe H, Carmichael R, Lemberger L: The effect of fluoxetine on warfarin metabolism in the rat and man. Life Sci 23:807–812, 1978

Safety of terfenadine and astemizole. Medical Letter 34(863):9–10, 1992

Sahakian BJ, Coull JT: Tetrahydroaminoacridine (THA) in Alzheimer's disease: an assessment of attentional and mnemonic function using CANTAB. Acta Neurol Scand Suppl 149:29–35, 1993

Sccrri L, Shall L, Zaki I: Carbamazepine-induced anticonvulsant hypersensitivity syndrome-pathogenic and diagnostic considerations. Clin Exp Dermatol 18:540–542, 1993

Schaff MR, Fawcett J, Zajecka JM: Divalproex sodium in the treatment of refractory affective disorders. J Clin Psychiatry 54:380–384, 1993

Schaffler L, Bourgeois BF, Luders HO: Rapid reversibility of autoinduction of carbamazepine metabolism after temporary discontinuation. Epilepsia 35:195–198, 1994

Schmidt D: Felbamate: successful development of a new compound for the treatment of epilepsy. Epilepsia 34 (suppl 7):S30–S33, 1993

Schneider LS, Olin JT, Pawluczyk S: A double-blind crossover pilot study of l-deprenyl (selegiline) combined with cholinesterase inhibitor in Alzheimers disease. Am J Psychiatry 150:321–323, 1993

Schou M: Effects of long-term lithium treatment on kidney function: an overview. J Psychiatr Res 22:287–296, 1988

Schwartz BJ, Frisolone JA: A case report of clozapine-induced gastric outlet obstruction (letter). Am J Psychiatry 150:1563, 1993

Schweizer E, Feighner J, Mandos LA, et al: Comparison of venlafaxine and imipramine in the acute treatment of major depression in outpatients. J Clin Psychiatry 55:104–108, 1994

Scolnik D, Nulman I, Rovet J, et al: Neurodevelopment of children exposed in utero to phenytoin and carbamazepine monotherapy. JAMA 271:767–770, 1994

Seymour JF: Carbamazepine overdose: features of 33 cases. Drug Saf 8:81–88, 1993

Shaw SH, Curson H, Coquelin JP: A double-blind, comparative study of zolpidem and placebo in the treatment of insomnia in elderly psychiatric in-patients. J Int Med Res 20:150–161, 1992

Shechter Y, Brenner B, Klein E, et al: Carbamazepine (Tegretol)-induced thrombocytopenia. Vox Sang 65:328–330, 1993

Shionoiri H: Pharmacokinetic drug interactions with ACE inhibitors. Clin Pharmacokinet 25:20–58, 1993

Sotalol for cardiac arrhythmias. Medical Letter 35(893):27–28, 1993

Sovner R, Davis JM: A potential drug interaction between fluoxetine and valproic acid (letter). J Clin Psychopharmacol 11:389, 1991

Sperber AD: Toxic interaction between fluvoxamine and sustained release theophylline in an 11-year-old boy. Drug Saf 6:460–462, 1991

Spina E, Pollicino AM, Avenoso A, et al: Fluvoxamine-induced alterations in plasma concentrations of imipramine and desipramine in depressed patients. Int J Clin Pharmacol Res 13:167–171, 1993a

Spina E, Avenoso A, Pollicino AM, et al: Carbamazepine coadministration with fluoxetine or fluvoxamine. Ther Drug Monit 15:247–250, 1993b

Spina E, Pollicino AM, Avenoso A, et al: Effect of fluvoxamine on the pharmacokinetics of imipramine and desipramine in healthy subjects. Ther Drug Monit 15:243–246, 1993c

Stancer HC, Forbath N: Hyperparathyroidism, hypothyroidism, and impaired renal function after 10 to 20 years of lithium treatment. Arch Intern Med 149:1042–1045, 1989

Steens RD, Pouliot Z, Millar TW, et al: Effects of zolpidem and triazolam on sleep and respiration in mild to moderate chronic obstructive pulmonary disease. Sleep 16:318–326, 1993

Stephens JR, Levy RH: Effects of valproate and citrulline on ammonium-induced encephalopathy. Epilepsia 35:164–171, 1994

Steur ENHJ: Increase of Parkinson disability after fluoxetine medication. Neurology 43:211–213, 1993

Stewart DE: High-fiber diet and serum tricyclic antidepressant levels. J Clin Psychopharmacol 12:438–440, 1992

Stoppe G, Muller P, Fuchs T, et al: Life-threatening allergic reaction to clozapine. Br J Psychiatry 161:259–261, 1992

Storey P, Trumble M: Rectal doxepin and carbamazepine therapy in patients with cancer. N Engl J Med 327:1318–1319, 1992

Stoudemire A, Fogel BS (eds): Principles of Medical Psychiatry. Orlando, FL, Grune & Stratton, 1987

Stoudemire A, Fogel BS (eds): Medical-Psychiatric Practice, Vol 1. Washington, DC, American Psychiatric Press, 1991

Stoudemire A, Fogel BS (eds): Psychiatric Care of the Medical Patient. New York, Oxford University Press, 1993a

Stoudemire A, Fogel BS (eds): Medical-Psychiatric Practice, Vol 2. Washington, DC, American Psychiatric Press, 1993b

Stoudemire A, Moran MG, Fogel BS: Psychotropic drug use in the medically ill: part I. Psychosomatics 31:377–391, 1990

Stoudemire A, Moran MG, Fogel BS: Psychotropic drug use in the medically ill: part II. Psychosomatics 32:34–46, 1991a

Stoudemire A, Fogel BS, Gulley LR: Psychopharmacology in the medically ill: an update, in Medical-Psychiatric Practice, Vol 1. Edited by Stoudemire A, Fogel BS. Washington, DC, American Psychiatric Press, 1991b, pp 29–97

Stoudemire A, Brown FW, Cohen-Cole SA: Diagnosis and treatment of psychiatric disorders in the medically ill elderly patient, in Psychiatry, Vol 2. Edited by Michels R. Philadelphia, PA, JB Lippincott, 1993a, pp 1–18

Stoudemire A, Fogel BS, Gulley LR, et al: Psychopharmacology in the medical patient, in Psychiatric Care of the Medical Patient. Edited by Stoudemire A, Fogel BS. New York, Oxford University Press, 1993b, pp 155–206

Stoudemire A, Moran MG, Fogel BS: Psychopharmacology in the medically ill patient, in The American Psychiatric Press Textbook of Psychopharmacology. Edited by Schatzberg AF, Nemeroff CB. Washington, DC, American Psychiatric Press, 1995, pp 783–802

Strouse TB, Skotzko CE, Fawzy FI: Absence of adverse drug interactions between fluoxetine and cyclosporine in organ transplant recipients. Paper presented at the annual meeting of the Academy of Psychosomatic Medicine, New Orleans, LA, November 1993, Abstract 46, p 19

Stuppaeck C, Barnas C, Schwitzer J, et al: The role of carbamazepine in the prophylaxis of unipolar depression. Neuropsychobiology 27:154–157, 1993

Suckow RF, Roose SP, Cooper TB: Effect of fluoxetine on plasma desipramine and 2-hydroxydesipramine. Biol Psychiatry 31:200–204, 1992

Swims MP: Potential terfenadine-fluoxetine interaction (letter). DICP 27:1404–1405, 1993

Szymanski S, Lieberman JA, Picou D, et al: A case report of cimetidine-induced clozapine toxicity. J Clin Psychiatry 52:21–22, 1991

Takahashi N, Aizawa H, Takata S, et al: Acute interstitial pneumonitis induced by carbamazepine. Eur Respir J 6:1409–1411, 1993

Tate JL: Extrapyramidal symptoms in a patient taking haloperidol and fluoxetine. Am J Psychiatry 146:399–400, 1989

Taylor JW, Bell AJ: Lithium-induced parathyroid dysfunction: a case report and review of the literature. DICP 27:1040–1043, 1993

Teo KK, Yusuf S, Furberg CD: Effects of prophylactic antiarrhythmic drug therapy in acute myocardial infarction. JAMA 270:1589–1595, 1993

Thornberg SA, Ereshefsky L: Neuroleptic malignant syndrome associated with clozapine monotherapy. Pharmacotherapy 13:510–514, 1993

Tingelstad JB: The cardiotoxicity of the tricyclics. J Am Acad Child Adolesc Psychiatry 30:845–846, 1991

Troy S, Piergies A, Lucki I, et al: Venlafaxine pharmacokinetics and pharmacodynamics (abstract). Clin Neuropharmacol 15 (suppl 1B):324B, 1992

Update on clozapine. Medical Letter 35(890):16–18, 1993

U.S. Gabapentin Study Group No. 5: Gabapentin as add-on therapy in refractory partial epilepsy: a double-blind, placebo-controlled, parallel-group study. Neurology 43:2292–2298, 1993

Van Amelsvoort T, Bakshi R, Devaux CB, et al: Hyponatremia associated with carbamazepine and oxcarbazepine therapy: a review. Epilepsia 35:181–188, 1994

van Harten J, Holland RL, Wesnes K, et al: Kinetic and dynamic interaction study between fluvoxamine and benzodiazepines. Poster presented at the Second Jerusalem Conference on Pharmaceutical Sciences and Clinical Pharmacology, Jerusalem, May 24–29, 1992a

van Harten J, Stevens LA, Raghoebar M, et al: Fluvoxamine does not interact with alcohol or potentiate alcohol-related impairment of cognitive function. Clin Pharmacol Ther 52:427–435, 1992b

van Harten J, Holland RL, Wesnes K: Influence of multiple-dose administration of fluvoxamine on the pharmacokinetics of the benzodiazepines bromazepam and lorazepam: a randomised, cross-over study (abstract). European Neuropsychopharmacology 2:381, 1992c

van Harten J, Duchier J, Devissaguet J, et al: Pharmacokinetics of fluvoxamine maleate in patients with liver cirrhosis after single-dose oral administration. Clin Pharmacokinet 24:177–182, 1993

Varney NR, Garvey MJ, Cook BL, et al: Identification of treatment-resistant depressives who respond favorably to carbamazepine. Annals of Clinical Psychiatry 5:117–122, 1993

Viner MW, Escobar JI: An apparent neurotoxicity associated with clozapine (letter). J Clin Psychiatry 55:38–39, 1994

von Knorring L, Wahlin A, Nystrom K, et al: Uraemia induced by long-term lithium treatment. Lithium 1:251–253, 1990

von Moltke LL, Greenblatt DJ, Harmatz JS, et al: Cytochromes in psychopharmacology (editorial). J Clin Psychopharmacol 14:1–4, 1994

Wagner ML, Remmel RP, Graves NM, et al: Effect of felbamate on carbamazepine and its major metabolites. Clin Pharmacol Ther 53:536–543, 1993

Waller DG, Edwards JG: Lithium and the kidney: an update. Psychol Med 19:825–831, 1989

Walley T, Pirmohamed M, Proudlove C, et al: Interaction of metoprolol and fluoxetine (letter). Lancet 341:967–968, 1993

Wang JT, Shiu GK, Ong-Chen T, et al: Effects of humidity and temperature on in vitro dissolution of carbamazepine tablets. J Pharm Sci 82:1002–1005, 1993

Warrington SJ: Clinical implications of the pharmacology of sertraline. Int Clin Psychopharmacol 6 (suppl 2):11–21, 1991

Warrington SJ, Lewis Y: Cardiovascular effects of antidepressants: studies of paroxetine in healthy men and depressed patients. Int Clin Psychopharmacol 6 (suppl 4):59–64, 1992

Waters CH, Belai Y, Gott PS, et al: Outcomes of pregnancy associated with antiepileptic drugs. Arch Neurol 51:250–253, 1994

Watkins PB, Zimmerman HJ, Knapp MJ, et al: Hepatotoxic effects of tacrine administration in patients with Alzheimer's disease. JAMA 271:992–998, 1994

Weintraub RG, Gow RM, Wilkinson JL: The congenital long QT syndromes in childhood. J Am Coll Cardiol 16:674–680, 1990

Weller M, Kornhuber J: Clozapine rechallenge after an episode of 'neuroleptic malignant syndrome.' Br J Psychiatry 161:855–856, 1992

Wilens TE, Biederman J, Baldessarini RJ, et al: Electrocardiographic effects of desipramine and 2-hydroxydesipramine in children, adolescents, and adults treated with desipramine. J Am Acad Child Adolesc Psychiatry 32:798–804, 1993

Wilner KD, Lazar JD, Apseloff G, et al: The effects of sertraline on the pharmacodynamics of warfarin in healthy volunteers (abstract). Biol Psychiatry 29:354S–355S, 1991

Wils V: Extrapyramidal symptoms in a patient treated with fluvoxamine (letter). J Neurol Neurosurg Psychiatry 55:330–331, 1992

Wilt JL, Minnema AM, Johnson RF, et al: Torsade de pointes associated with the use of intravenous haloperidol. Ann Intern Med 119:391–394, 1993

Woods DJ, Coulter DM, Pillans P: Interaction of phenytoin and fluoxetine (letter). N Z Med J 107:119, 1994

Woosley RL, Chen Y, Freiman JP, et al: Mechanism of the cardiotoxic actions of terfenadine. JAMA 269:1532–1536, 1993

Wyeth Laboratories: Effexor (venlafaxine) package insert, Philadelphia, PA, December 1993

Yu HY, Shen YZ, Suglyama Y, et al: Drug interaction. Effects of salicylate on pharmacokinetics of valproic acid in rats. Drug Metab Dispos 18:121–126, 1990

Yuksel A, Kartal A, Cenani A, et al: Serum thyroid hormones and pituitary response to thyrotropin-releasing hormone in epileptic children receiving anti-epileptic medication. Acta Paediatr Jpn Overseas Ed 35:108–112, 1993

Zimnitzky B: A fifth case of sudden death in a child taking desipramine, in New Research Program and Abstracts: American Psychiatric Association Annual Meeting, Philadelphia, PA, May 1994, p 181

Zornberg GL, Pope HG Jr: Treatment of depression in bipolar disorder: new directions for research. J Clin Psychopharmacol 13:397–408, 1993

Chapter 3

Treatment of Psychosis in Parkinson's Disease

Stuart S. Rich, M.D.
Joseph H. Friedman, M.D.

When treating psychosis in a patient with Parkinson's disease (PD), the physician faces a dilemma: the dopamine (DA)-receptor–blocking agents (neuroleptics) used to treat psychotic symptoms exacerbate parkinsonism, whereas antiparkinsonian medication essential for mobility may have induced the psychotic symptoms. To manage the symptoms of such a patient properly, it is imperative to consider which symptoms are the primary source of the patient's disability. For example, levodopa may induce a subjectively and functionally benign syndrome of visual hallucinosis, but reducing antiparkinsonian medication may leave the patient unable to walk. In other patients, reducing antiparkinsonian medication may result in an annoying but nondisabling tremor, but leaving the levodopa dosage unchanged would allow frightening and incapacitating hallucinations and paranoia to persist. When no solution is ideal, the physician should discuss with the patient and family how best to strike a balance between control of motor and mental symptoms.

After an overview of PD, we discuss the differential diagnosis, epidemiology, and phenomenology of psychotic syndromes in PD. We examine the current theories of the pathophysiology of psychosis in PD and its treatment. We review the literature on, and our own experience with, the interventions currently available for the treatment of psychosis in PD: typical neuroleptics, clozapine, risperidone, ondansetron, and electroconvulsive therapy (ECT). Finally, we present practical recommendations for treating patients with PD and psychosis.

PARKINSON'S DISEASE: OVERVIEW

Basic Pathophysiology of PD

PD is an idiopathic degenerative disease whose hallmarks are tremor, rigidity, bradykinesia, and postural instability. The principal neuropathological change in PD is degeneration of the pigmented nuclei in the brain stem, particularly the substantia nigra pars compacta (SNpc). The SNpc projects chiefly to the portions of the.striatum related to motor functioning. The degeneration of the SNpc results in a profound deficiency of DA in the striatum, which, in turn, results in the characteristic motoric dysfunction. The aim of pharmacological treatment of PD is to compensate for the lack of dopaminergic input to the striatum.

"Parkinson's Disease" Versus "Parkinsonism"

PD is a disease, whereas parkinsonism refers to the akinetic-rigid syndrome caused by PD and a number of other diseases. PD is by far the most common cause of primary (i.e., not drug-induced) parkinsonism. Treatment of patients with psychosis and parkinsonism is generally the same regardless of the cause of the parkinsonism. However, parkinsonism caused by brain diseases other than PD responds less well to antiparkinsonian treatment than does PD, and patients with PD are the only parkinsonian patients who have been included in systematic studies of the treatment of psychosis.

Treatment of PD

Table 3–1 summarizes the most common pharmacological treatments of PD.

Levodopa.   The mainstay of antiparkinsonian treatment is levodopa, a precursor of DA. For most patients with PD, levodopa is the most effective and best-tolerated therapy. After oral administration (usually in combination with carbidopa, a dopa-decarboxylase inhibitor that does not cross the blood-brain barrier and thus reduces peripheral side effects), levodopa crosses the blood-brain barrier and increases the production of DA by functioning nigral cells. DA at striatal synapses is increased because more DA is produced in the cells of the substriata nigra.

As PD progresses and more nigral cells are lost, patients tend to lose their response to levodopa. Disabling fluctuations in mobility may occur, some of which result from fluctuations in levodopa blood levels, which increasingly affect DA release as more nigral cells are lost. Levodopa/carbidopa is now available in a long-acting preparation (Sinemet CR). The sustained-release formulation smoothes out the fluctuations in blood levels of levodopa, which sometimes helps to smooth out clinical fluctuations.

Although switching to Sinemet CR from regular Sinemet may help to decrease motor fluctuations, it does not alleviate psychotic symptoms. In fact, one study that compared the side effects of Sinemet with Sinemet CR found that Sinemet CR appeared to exacerbate daytime hallucinations (Goetz et al. 1989).

DA agonists.   An alternative approach is to overcome the DA deficiency in the striatum by administration of DA receptor agonists, such as bromocriptine or pergolide. DA agonists are used alone or in combination with levodopa or other antiparkinsonian agents. For most patients, levodopa alone is more effective than a DA agonist alone and results in fewer side effects. There is no evidence that bromocriptine and pergolide differ in terms of psychotogenic properties. However, individual patients may tolerate one of the two better than the other.

Selegiline.   Selegiline, at the doses used in PD, is a selective monoamine oxidase B (MAO-B) inhibitor. Selegiline thus prolongs the presence of DA in the synaptic cleft. It is used as adjunctive therapy to improve the response to other antiparkinsonian regimens and to smooth out fluctuations.

When selegiline was first released, it was thought to have a neuroprotective effect in patients with PD. It was demonstrated that giving selegiline to patients with early PD delayed the need to begin levodopa therapy, raising the possibility that it slows the underlying degenerative process (Shoulson 1992). The concept of neuroprotective treatment is predicated on the idea that the oxidative metabolism of DA accelerates the death of dopaminergic neurons by generating cytotoxic byproducts (Leehey and Boyson 1991). Thus, because selegiline blocks DA oxidation by inhibiting MAO-B, it might retard the degeneration of the remaining dopaminergic nigral cells in patients with PD. Conversely, levodopa might actually accelerate nigral cell death by increasing the flux of DA through oxidative metabolic pathways (Runge and

Table 3–1. Antiparkinsonian medications

Medication	Mechanism of action	Typical prescribing pattern	Side-effect profile
Levodopa/carbidopa	DA precursor; increase in DA production by remaining cells in SNpc/VTA complex	Primary therapy for PD	Classic syndrome of visual hallucinosis in clear sensorium most common; also, delusional or delirious states
Sustained-release levodopa/carbidopa	DA precursor; increase in DA production by remaining cells in SNpc/VTA complex	Substituted for regular Sinemet late in course when fluctuations develop	As above—may improve nighttime side effects at the expense of the daytime effects
Bromocriptine	Postsynaptic DA receptor agonist; stimulation of D_2 receptors	Usually adjunctive therapy	Probably somewhat more likely to cause psychosis than levodopa
Pergolide	Postsynaptic DA receptor agonist; stimulation of D_1 and D_2 receptors	Usually adjunctive therapy	Probably somewhat more likely to cause psychosis than levodopa
Selegiline	MAO-B inhibitor; prolongation of DA in synaptic cleft via inhibition of degradation of DA by MAO-B	Usually early or adjunctive therapy	Often exacerbates or "unmasks" psychotogenic effects of the other anti-PD drugs it is combined with

Amantadine	Increased DA release, DA reuptake blockade, weak anitcholinergic, and weak NMDA receptor blocker	Usually early or adjunctive therapy	High incidence of psychosis in elderly at high doses combined with levodopa; elimination is entirely renal; therefore, side effects are exacerbated with renal impairment (Saint-Cyr et al. 1993)
Anticholinergics (e.g., benztropine or trihexyphenidyl)	Modulation of DA-Ach balance	Usually adjunctive therapy	Especially likely to cause ACS, especially in patients with dementia

Note.   DA = dopamine; SNpc = substantia nigra pars compacta; VTA = ventral tegmental area; PD = Parkinson's disease; MAO-B = monoamine oxidase B; NMDA = *N*-methyl-D-aspartate; ACS = acute confusional state; DA-ACh balance = dopamine-acetylcholine balance.

Horowski 1991). So, as long as it was a putative neuroprotective agent, many neurologists felt obligated to give selegiline to all of their patients with PD. A large multicenter trial, the DATATOP study, was designed to distinguish between a neuroprotective effect of selegiline and a symptomatic effect alone (Anonymous 1993). The most recent analyses of the DATATOP data suggest that selegiline is probably not neuroprotective (LeWitt 1993). In the light of this finding, most neurologists view selegiline as either a symptomatic treatment of early, mild PD or as an adjunct for reducing motor fluctuations in more advanced PD. In either case, its reduced, weak antiparkinsonian action and lack of neuroprotective benefit suggest that it should be discontinued in patients who develop psychosis.

Amantadine.   Amantadine, generally used as an adjunctive treatment in patients with PD, probably acts by increasing release of DA from presynaptic terminals. In addition, it has weak anticholinergic effects and is a noncompetitive N-methyl-D-aspartate (NMDA) receptor blocker at high doses. It can cause psychotic symptoms when used alone for mild PD and can aggravate these symptoms when used as an adjunct in more advanced PD.

Anticholinergics.   Anticholinergic antiparkinsonian drugs are useful in some patients with early disease, especially for tremor. These drugs presumably compensate for DA deficiency by inhibiting cholinergic neurons in the striatum. These agents can cause memory loss, hallucinations, or delirium. There is no evidence that anticholinergic agents differ in their psychotoxicity after allowing for differences in potency.

PSYCHOTIC SYNDROMES IN PARKINSON'S DISEASE

Differential Diagnosis

Psychosis in PD may be caused by antiparkinsonian medication, an acute confusional state, or a comorbid primary mental disorder. It is often a complex combination of these factors.

- *The patient with antiparkinsonian medication–induced psychotic symptoms.* The classic syndrome of psychosis in PD is one of drug-induced hallucinosis in a clear sensorium. Drug-induced psychosis may also be accompanied by delusions, which may be fixed or fluctuating and may be part of a drug-induced acute confusional state.

- *The patient with an acute confusional state.* The syndrome of hallucinosis in a clear sensorium should be distinguished from the acute confusional state (synonymous with *delirium* in U.S. literature and in this chapter). Any of the antiparkinsonian medications—dopaminergic or anticholinergic—can induce a confusional state, but when a patient with treated PD develops an acute confusional state, other causes must be considered. Patients may, for example, develop confusional states because of underlying infection, especially if they have dementia. Parkinsonian patients who have developed dementia are especially likely to become delirious in response to antiparkinsonian medication or to medical illness (Lishman 1987; Saint-Cyr et al. 1993). An underlying medical cause for a psychotic confusional state is especially likely when the onset is acute rather than insidious, when it commences in the context of a stable antiparkinsonian pharmacological regimen, or when it is accompanied by overt symptoms or signs of medical illness. The medical evaluation should be individualized, taking the patient's medical history and risk factors into account. Brain imaging is rarely necessary. Once acute medical illness has been excluded in a confused patient, the delirium is presumed to be drug induced; reducing or eliminating the antiparkinsonian medication is both diagnostic and therapeutic.
- *The patient with a primary mental disorder and parkinsonism.* Whether or not the patient is confused, the psychosis may not be drug induced and may not be caused by an acute confusional state but rather may be caused by a primary mental disorder. Psychotic symptoms are rarely attributable to untreated idiopathic PD alone. The presence of psychotic symptoms in a patient with untreated PD is nearly always a result of a concomitant mental disorder such as bipolar disorder, psychotic depression, or schizophrenia. Primary mental disorders may also be the cause of psychosis in treated PD patients, but psychosis in treated PD more commonly is a side effect of antiparkinsonian treatment.

The patient with a primary mental disorder and PD is more complicated to evaluate than the typical PD patient with drug-induced psychosis (see Case 3: "Premorbid Depression Complicated by PD, Dementia, Delirium, and Psychosis" in the "Case Reports" section later in this chapter). Schizophrenia and PD may coexist (Caligiuri et al. 1993; Crow et al. 1976; J. Friedman et al. 1987). Patients who have been treated with neuroleptics for a preexisting psychotic disorder, such as schizophrenia or a psychotic mood disorder, may develop severe drug-induced parkinsonism. When neuroleptics are withdrawn, the psychosis may recur while the parkinsonism persists, raising the possibility of the exacerbation of preclinical PD or the onset of PD (Rich 1993).

Epidemiology

The median age at onset of PD in the United States is 60 years (Kessler 1978; Martilla 1987; Tanner 1992). The median survival of PD patients is almost equal to that of age-matched control subjects (Martilla et al. 1977; Uitti et al. 1993), and the prevalence of PD in the population aged 65 years or greater is approximately 1%. At age 65 years, Americans have a life expectancy of about 16 years. The likelihood of psychosis in PD increases as the disease advances, so that psychosis in PD is a common problem in the practice of geriatric psychiatry.

Studies of the prevalence of psychosis resulting from pharmacological treatment of PD have resulted in estimates that vary widely, depending on the definition of psychosis used and the selection of the population. For example, drug-induced psychosis has been estimated in different studies to occur in 7% (Greene et al. 1993), 8% (Melamed et al. 1993), and 20% (A. J. Friedman and Sienkiewicz 1991) of patients. Other studies have estimated the prevalence in patients with advanced PD to be as high as 28%–60% (Fischer et al. 1990a). Assuming that only approximately 6%–8% of patients with PD have psychosis (Tanner et al. 1983), at least 15,000 to 30,000 PD patients in the United States are affected by drug-induced psychotic symptoms. The impact is great because psychosis is the best-established predictor of nursing home placement in patients with PD (Goetz and Stebbins 1993).

Advanced age, dementia, treatment with multiple drugs, and treatment with anticholinergics are risk factors for hallucinations in treated patients with PD (Goetz et al. 1982; Tanner et al. 1983).

Phenomenology

The term *psychosis* is variably and imprecisely defined. For the purposes of this discussion, we distinguish between hallucinosis, in which insight is intact and delusions are not present, and psychosis with frank impairment of reality testing. Hallucinations are regarded as "psychotic symptoms," regardless of whether a full syndrome of psychosis is present.

The psychotic symptoms induced by levodopa and the other anti-PD medications include a range of altered perception, thought processes, and emotions (J. H. Friedman 1991). Hallucinations and delusions may occur alone or in combination. An attentional deficit may or may not be present. Hallucinations are mainly visual, and delusions are typically paranoid. Hallucinations are commonly experienced as benign, even when accompanied by unrelated paranoid delusions (Goetz et al. 1982). The psychosis in patients with PD typically lacks the delusions of thought control and the negative symptoms of schizophreniform psychoses.

The phenomenology of levodopa-induced psychosis has been measured with psychiatric rating scales. The Brief Psychiatric Rating Scale (BPRS) (Overall and Gorham 1962) in levodopa-induced psychosis documented in one study that positive psychotic symptoms are the dominant features of the syndrome (M. Parsa, H. Meltzer, personal communication, November 1993). Somatic concern, anxiety, emotional withdrawal, mannerisms and posturing, guilt feelings, tension, grandiosity, depressive mood, hostility, uncooperativeness, blunted affect, and excitement were all rated as absent to mild, whereas conceptual disorganization, suspiciousness, hallucinations, unusual thought content, and disorientation were moderate to marked. In another study, nine parkinsonian patients being treated for psychosis (seven with clozapine) were given the Scale for the Assessment of Positive Symptoms (SAPS; Andreasen 1984) (M. Parsa, H. Y. Meltzer, personal communication, November 1993). Prominent formed, colorful visual hallucinations; paranoid, persecutory delusions; and marked illogical and incoherent thought processes were the most marked abnormalities.

Hallucinations.   Visual hallucinosis is a common complication of all antiparkinsonian medications and can be caused by anticholinergic agents, amantadine, selegiline, levodopa, and DA agonists. In a retrospective study, Goetz and co-workers (1982) examined the phenomenology of hallucinations in PD patients taking dopaminergic and anticholinergic antiparkinsonian medication. They looked at the sensory modality of hallucinations, degree of organization, and emotional impact. They did not specify whether the patients experienced confusional states. Insight into the nature of the hallucinations was not commented on. Interestingly, hallucinations induced by dopaminergic drugs resembled those induced by anticholinergic agents—indeed, two patients who were receiving both types of drugs had identical hallucinatory experiences when the dose of either drug was increased. It is not clear, however, whether their inference that the ensuing hallucinatory phenomena in these two patients were caused by the increased drug dose is valid. The patients were still taking both drugs; their effect may have been additive or synergistic. Most hallucinations were formed visual hallucinations (e.g., of people or animals), often accompanied by auditory hallucinations, especially voices. Patients were about equally likely to experience their hallucinations as threatening or nonthreatening. A minority of patients experienced vague, unformed hallucinations in visual and/or auditory modalities.

Delusions.   Delusions are rare in patients with untreated PD. Such patients probably have a comorbid primary psychotic disorder (see Case 3: "Premorbid Depression Complicated by PD, Dementia, Delirium, and Psychosis"). Delusions in PD usually are a side effect of antiparkinsonian medication. All antiparkinsonian medications, especially anticholinergics, can cause delusions.

Delusions can occur with or without delirium. They are often complex and persecutory. Capgras' syndrome is not rare in delusional PD patients. Patients typically believe that they are targeted for death, that spouses are having sexual affairs, or that their money has been stolen (Jenkins and Groh 1970).

The presence of delusions has little impact on the pharmacological treatment of these patients; it is the same as the pharmacological treatment of patients with hallucinosis. However, delusions may complicate their psychological and behavioral management and may necessitate hospitalization.

Sleep in PD.   Nausieda and co-workers (1982) found sleep complaints in 74% of surveyed PD patients treated with levodopa but found sleep disturbance in 98% of those with psychiatric side effects. It has been suggested that the report of vivid dreams in a parkinsonian patient should be noted as possibly heralding the onset of a psychotic syndrome (Cummings 1992; Nausieda et al. 1982). However, while patients are taking antiparkinsonian medications, vivid dreams are so common that they lack diagnostic specificity.

DIFFERENTIAL PSYCHOTOXICITY OF ANTIPARKINSONIAN MEDICATIONS

It is important to understand the limitations of any proposed hierarchy of the psychotoxicity of antiparkinsonian medications. First, patients vary considerably in their vulnerability to the adverse effects of different antiparkinsonian medications. The distinctive sensitivity of each patient will override general patterns, which should be considered as guidelines for initial interventions to be used until actual reactions of the patient to specific medications are determined. Second, much of what has been written about the differential psychotoxicity of antiparkinsonian drugs necessarily consists of unreferenced assertions and studies of the incidence of side effects of individual agents. Neither of these sources supports firm conclusions. Some studies compared the efficacy and side-effect profile of two different agents in patients who are treated with one or the other as a single agent. Although these studies have a greater degree of validity than the first two sources of information, their use is limited because most patients with advanced PD are treated with multiple medications, and psychosis tends to occur in advanced PD. No large studies have directly examined the issue of differential psychotoxicity of antiparkinsonian agents in patients undergoing treatment under "naturalistic" circumstances. These caveats notwithstanding, we offer the following guidelines.

1. Differential psychotoxicity is best thought of in terms of the risk-benefit ratio of different antiparkinsonian medications.
2. Anticholinergics are the least efficacious and most psychotoxic of the antiparkinsonian agents. They are most useful for treating tremor in patients with early disease whose function is not yet limited by bradykinesia. Anticholinergics sometimes are more effective than levodopa for this indication. The use of anticholinergics early in the disease may allow the physician to delay the institution of levodopa. Because the efficacy of levodopa decreases with time, whereas adverse effects increase, delaying the start of levodopa therapy might prolong the total duration of effective control of the patient's symptoms. It remains controversial whether the loss of efficacy of levodopa with time simply results from disease propensity or whether levodopa actually accelerates the defective process or induces physiological changes that reduce its efficacy.
3. Levodopa/carbidopa is, for the majority of patients, the most effi-

cacious and best-tolerated therapy for PD. It is most likely to be used as monotherapy for most of the patient's disease course.

4. The psychotogenic properties of Sinemet CR do not usually differ noticeably from those of regular Sinemet in clinical practice. However, one comparison study revealed subtle differences in psychotoxicity along with the more expected dramatic differences on motor functioning (Goetz et al. 1989). Sinemet CR may result in increased daytime hallucinations but decreased incidence of sleep disturbances.

5. DA agonists effectively reduce the symptoms of PD and are a close second to levodopa for efficacy. Other medications normally are used as adjuncts in more advanced disease or as primary treatment of mild disease. DA agonists act by stimulating postsynaptic receptors; therefore, they do not increase the DA metabolism in nigral cells. Because increased activity of these cells may increase their vulnerability to degeneration, some neurologists believe that treatment with DA agonists, rather than levodopa, will slow the progression of PD. Indirect evidence and clinical experience suggest that DA agonists cause psychotic syndromes similar to those caused by levodopa but at a significantly higher rate (Saint-Cyr et al. 1993). Consistent with this clinical impression, direct comparison of DA agonist monotherapy (bromocriptine) with levodopa/carbidopa monotherapy has suggested a higher incidence of psychosis with DA agonists (Montastruc et al. 1990).

6. Although selegiline does not appear to be neuroprotective, it certainly potentiates the benefits and the psychotogenic properties of levodopa.

7. Amantadine's risk-benefit ratio and clinical role are similar to that of selegiline.

8. In general, one medication at a higher dose probably is less likely to induce psychosis than two medications at lower doses.

TREATMENT

Adjustment of Antiparkinsonian Medication

Before clozapine was available, the treatment of psychosis in PD included reduction of antiparkinsonian medication, drug holidays, addition of low-potency or mid-range neuroleptics such as thioridazine or molindone, and ECT. However, the usefulness of these approaches is less well documented than that of clozapine, despite having been practiced for a longer period. "Drug holidays" have been used primarily to treat severe motor fluctuations and lack of response to levodopa in previously levodopa-responsive PD patients; little evidence suggests that they ameliorate the problem of levodopa-induced psychosis (Feldman et al. 1986). Interestingly, Mayeux and colleagues (1985) described a patient who became psychotic as a result of levodopa withdrawal. The first intervention should always be an attempt to reduce medication dosage, but if antiparkinsonian treatment has been titrated upward gradually, dosage reduction is likely to result in an unacceptable loss of motor function. In this case, atypical antipsychotics or ECT may be helpful.

Typical Neuroleptics

Although at least one case report describes the efficacy of a neuroleptic (Hale and Bellizzi 1980) in levodopa-induced psychosis, the vast majority report that even low doses of low-potency neuroleptics have major deleterious effects on motor function in patients with PD (J. H. Friedman et al. 1987; Wolk and Douglas 1992). J. Friedman and Lannon (1989), A. J. Friedman and Sienkiewicz (1991), J. H. Friedman (1991), and Cummings (1992) suggest that the psychosis secondary to antiparkinsonian medication be treated by drug withdrawal in the following order: anticholinergic medication, selegiline, and amantadine, followed by reduction of dopaminergic agents if the delusions persist. If drug withdrawal fails, Cummings (1992) has suggested cautious administration of low doses of (typical) neuroleptics as the next step. This has been a common practice because many have argued, especially when clozapine was first released, that even a parkinsonian patient should fail a trial of a typical neuroleptic before taking a drug as potentially toxic as clozapine. One of us (S.S.R.) has taken this route on occasion and discharged patients in satisfactory condition from the hospital on a combination of a typical neuroleptic and levodopa. The co-author (J.H.F.) believes that most such patients eventually decompensate because of drug-induced parkinsonism (Wolk and Douglas 1992), and we now recommend that typical neuroleptics never be administered to patients with PD. The utility of thioridazine and molindone in these patients is certainly greater than that of high-potency neuroleptics, but their advantages probably have been exaggerated. The first step to take after failure of dosage reduction is administration of an atypical neuroleptic. Clozapine is best established for this indication. As other less toxic atypical neuroleptics are tested for treatment of psychosis in PD, they will probably supplant clozapine as the drug of first choice for this indication.

Clozapine

Clozapine is considered the prototypic atypical antipsychotic because it does not cause extrapyramidal side effects and because it relieves both the positive and negative symptoms of schizophrenia more effectively than typical neuroleptics (Kane et al. 1988). Because of its lack of extrapyramidal side effects, it is a useful treatment for psychotic patients with PD.

Pharmacology of clozapine.   Clozapine's affinity is greatest for D_4, 5-HT_{1c}, 5-HT_2 (serotonin), muscarinic, and H_1 histamine receptors (Coward 1992). Clozapine's pharmacological profile both differs from and overlaps with that of typical neuroleptics to a significant degree. The pharmacological basis for the atypical properties of clozapine remains uncertain and controversial despite intensive study.

Clozapine blocks central 5-HT_2 receptors and causes downregulation of these receptors in the frontal cortex and neostriatum in rodents. Its affinity for 5-HT_{1c} receptors is even greater (Canton et al. 1990). The distinctive serotonergic properties of clozapine are strongly suspected to be related to its atypical properties (Meltzer and Gudelsky 1992).

One of the most potent neurotransmitter effects of clozapine is on muscarinic receptors. Clozapine is one to two orders of magnitude more potent as a central anticholinergic agent than other neuroleptic drugs. As with other antimuscarinic agents, clozapine can induce confusion. The only evidence that this may be an anticholinergic effect was its reversal by physostigmine in two cases (Schuster et al. 1977)—the confusion may simply be a nonspecific sedative effect. One of the most difficult to manage side effects of clozapine is drooling (Humpel et al. 1990). This side effect seems paradoxical given clozapine's potent anticholinergic properties. The hypersalivation effect in the presence of anticholinergic blockage is a property that clozapine apparently shares with only one other known drug—substance P. However, clozapine does not appear to affect substance P in the nigrostriatal system. Clonidine, an α_2-agonist, is occasionally helpful in countering clozapine-induced hypersalivation (Grabowski 1992).

Clozapine has antiadrenergic activity both centrally and peripherally. Its affinity for α_1- and α_2-receptors is greater than that for both low- and high-potency antipsychotics. Peripheral blood levels of epinephrine are increased in patients treated with clozapine; this may be caused by end-organ α-receptor blockade.

Clozapine blocks H_1-histamine receptors centrally and causes an increase in γ-aminobutyric acid (GABA) turnover in the neostriatum, in contrast to typical neuroleptics, which reduce GABA turnover (Coward 1992).

Clozapine for schizophrenia.   Clozapine has proven efficacy in the treatment of schizophrenic psychosis (Kane et al. 1988), and the vast majority of the experience with its use is in this population. The safety problem presented by agranulocytosis has been greatly reduced by the institution of an obligatory complete blood count (CBC)-monitoring system. (An update on medical complications of clozapine is found in Chapter 2.)

Clozapine for psychosis in PD.   There have been at least 19 reports on the use of clozapine for treating drug-induced psychosis in PD (Table 3–2). The results from the studies of clozapine are overwhelmingly positive: all studies but one (Wolters et al. 1990) have been open label and reported marked benefit in patients with psychosis, with stable or even improved motor function. Wolters and co-workers (1990) performed the only double-blind trial to date, and it was the one trial with a negative result. However, the doses of clozapine they used are now considered too high both for initiation and for titration. Most investigators recommend initiation with doses of 6.25 to 12.5 mg/day. Wolters and associates used 25 mg as a starting dose. In addition, most physicians now increase doses by 6.25 to 12.5 mg, as tolerated, whereas in the study by Wolters and associates, clozapine was increased by 25 mg/day. In general, the final doses required have been very low (6.25 to 100 mg/day) compared with the doses used in schizophrenia (250 to 450 mg/day), with most patients requiring 50 mg/day or less. It has been noted (Factor and Brown 1992; Factor et al. 1994; Pinter and Helscher 1993) that once psychosis has been controlled with clozapine, the anti-PD drugs sometimes can be increased without recurrence of psychosis; this is consistent with our experience.

In addition to case reports, pilot studies have addressed the effects of clozapine on psychosis in PD with psychiatric rating scales (Factor and Brown 1992; J. H. Friedman et al. 1992; Kang et al. 1991; Parsa et al. 1991). Data from Case-Western Reserve University with the full BPRS showed a pretreatment mean BPRS score of 48 and a posttreatment mean score of 25. One patient treated with less than 20 mg/day of molindone improved from a pretreatment BPRS of 56 to 32 but had worsened parkinsonism (M. Parsa, H. Y. Meltzer, personal communication, November 1993).

At Brown University, the BPRS was completed on five PD patients

Table 3–2. Summary of reports on clozapine for psychosis in PD

Authors	Number of patients	Clozapine dose (mg/day)	Number improved (%)
Scholz and Dichgens (1985)	4	25–100	4 (100)
Ostergaard and Dupont (1988)	16	6.25–100	15 (94)
Roberts et al. (1989)	1	25	1 (100)
Bear et al. (1989)	3	Not specified	3 (100)
Wolters et al. (1990)[a]	6	75–250	0 (0)
Pfeiffer et al. (1990)	5	25–50	3 (60)
Bernardi and Del Zompa (1990)	?	25–37	100%
Kahn et al. (1991)	11	12.5–125	8 (73)
Melamed et al. (1993)	1	100	1 (100)
Lew and Waters (1992)	4	12.5–62.5	2 (50)
Linazasaro and Suarez (1992)	14	35 (mean)	13 (93)
Gershanik et al. (1992)	27	12.5–75	27 (100)
Wolk and Douglas (1992)	5	75–125	3 (60)
Factor and Brown (1992)	8	3.25–75	7 (88)
J. Friedman et al. (1987)	19	6.25–400	15 (79)
Rosenthal et al. (1992)	1	150	1 (100)
Greene et al. (1993)	13	25–125	10 (77)
Parsa et al. (1991)	1	Not specified	1 (100)
Pinter and Helscher (1993)	7	25–125	7 (100)
Total	146		121 (83)

[a]The only double-blind trial.

treated with clozapine for psychosis. The mean BPRS was 45.2 before treatment and 26.8 after 3 months of treatment with clozapine. The Clinical Global Impression Severity (CGIS) changed from a mean of 5 before treatment to 1.6 after treatment (J. Friedman, unpublished observation, October 1987).

Clozapine clearly works best in patients without dementia who have psychosis with a clear sensorium (A. J. Friedman and Sienkiewicz 1991), but it often helps patients with delirium and psychotic features. The risk of adverse effects, particularly worsened confusion, remains highest in this group of patients, who tend to have dementia.

Few patients appear to be unresponsive to the antipsychotic benefits of clozapine. Most treatment failures have been caused by side effects. The intolerable adverse effects have usually been encountered with initial doses of 12.5 to 25 mg. Many of these patients were not given another course of treatment because of the adverse side effects. We believe that the rate of intolerance is lower when clozapine is started at 6.25 mg/day and increased in 6.25- to 12.5-mg/day increments.

Clozapine therapy involves the risk of agranulocytosis and the inconvenience of a weekly blood test and weekly drug pickup. However, the cost of clozapine therapy is modest for most PD patients. Unlike people with schizophrenia, PD patients require very low doses of the drug. If the CBC is done at the office or clinic of the treating physician, or at a low-cost laboratory, blood monitoring is inexpensive as well.

Motoric effects of clozapine in PD. Clozapine has been reported to be helpful for the motor problems of PD and for psychosis. Bennett and colleagues (1993) demonstrated, in six nonpsychotic PD patients, that doses of clozapine of about 300 mg/day produced a marked improvement in "on" time and a reduction in dyskinesias in patients with levodopa-response fluctuations. Baseline parkinsonism scores improved, although sedation, sialorrhea, and orthostatic hypotension were significant. A similar result using 25-mg daily doses of clozapine has been reported (Arevalo and Gershanik 1993).

Four open-label reports describe reduction in tremor in PD patients. Pakkenberg and Pakkenberg (1986) reported reduced tremor in nine of nine PD patients. J. H. Friedman and Lannon (1990) reported reduction in tremor in five of five patients refractory to or intolerant of other PD medications beyond their current dose. All patients had either failed to respond to or to tolerate anticholinergics, leading the investigators to hypothesize that the antitremor effect of clozapine was not simply a result of its anticholinergic potency. Fischer and associates (1990b) reported reduction in tremor in 12 of 12 patients at daily doses of 6.25 to 100 mg. Jansen (1994) reported reduction in tremor in 73% of 22 patients with PD treated with an average dose of 18.2 mg/day of clozapine.

One open-label report describes beneficial effects of clozapine for nocturnal akathisia in PD (Linazasaro et al. 1993).

Agranulocytosis.   The most dangerous side effect of clozapine is agranulocytosis, which has an incidence of approximately 2% in un-monitored patients. Since the institution of the CBC-monitoring system currently in place, only 7 of the first 43,000 patients treated with cloza-pine had fatal reactions related to agranulocytosis (Arellano 1993).

Many clinicians believe that elderly PD patients may be at higher risk for adverse effects of clozapine, and they are reluctant to prescribe it in this population. One of us (J.H.F.) has been involved in a multisite study that tracks data pertinent to the issue of the safety of clozapine in PD. The results of the study of 91 patients over 10 years support the contention that PD patients are not at significantly increased risk for agranulocytosis and that the current monitoring system is adequate for this population, as it is for patients with schizophrenia (J. H. Friedman, unpublished observations, November 1994). Other data suggest that elderly patients may be at somewhat higher risk for agranulocytosis (see Chapter 2). Leukopenia has been rare, and agranulocytosis has been reported in only one PD patient treated with clozapine (Greene et al. 1993).

Other adverse effects of clozapine in PD.   The most troublesome adverse effects of clozapine in PD patients are sedation, hypotension, confusion, and drooling. All these side effects may be dose limiting or responsible for outright intolerance of clozapine. Confusion is espe-cially a problem in patients with dementia. PD patients are at increased risk for orthostatic hypotension relative to the schizophrenic popula-tion because of their older age and the frequent involvement of the au-tonomic nervous system in PD.

Clozapine in atypical parkinsonism.   Successful treatment of psy-chosis with clozapine without exacerbation of parkinsonian symptoms has now been reported in isolated cases of diffuse Lewy bodies disease

(Chacko et al. 1993) and olivopontocerebellar atrophy (Parsa et al. 1993). Clozapine is likely to prove useful in the treatment of any psychosis in a patient with parkinsonism, regardless of whether the course is idiopathic PD.

Beyond Clozapine: Potential New Treatments for Psychosis in PD

Risperidone. Risperidone is the second atypical antipsychotic agent to be approved by the Food and Drug Administration (FDA). At this time (November 1994), it has not been used to treat significant numbers of PD patients. Unlike clozapine, risperidone can cause extrapyramidal effects, although it does so at a rate much lower than that of typical neuroleptics (Chouinard et al. 1993; Lang et al. 1993; van der Linden et al. 1993). We have treated three parkinsonian patients for psychosis with risperidone. One patient suspected of having diffuse Lewy body disease was treated for hallucinations and delusions. He became excessively rigid on 4 mg/day of risperidone, without significant improvement in his psychosis. Another patient with probable PD became hypomanic on carbidopa/levodopa 25/100 mg qid, the lowest dose that would control his PD symptoms. His hypomania resolved on 2 mg/day risperidone without exacerbation of his parkinsonism. The third patient had symptoms diagnosed as idiopathic PD with dementia, levodopa-induced hallucinosis, and intermittent confusion. While in the hospital, 2 mg/day risperidone ameliorated his psychosis without exacerbation of his parkinsonism. One week after discharge, however, his motoric function deteriorated markedly. The literature is in conflict about whether risperidone will become a viable option for the treatment of psychotic parkinsonian patients who cannot tolerate other interventions. Meco and associates (1994) reported benefit, whereas Ford and colleagues (1994) reported worsening parkinsonism. We are not optimistic that risperidone will prove significantly helpful.

Ondansetron. Ondansetron, a 5-HT$_3$ antagonist approved by the FDA as an antiemetic, appears to have antipsychotic properties and is undergoing clinical trials for the treatment of patients with schizophrenia. Ondansetron has been reported to decrease hallucinosis, paranoia, agitation, and confusion in L-dopa–treated PD patients in doses of 12 to 24 mg/day (Melamed et al. 1993; Zoldan et al. 1989).

ECT in PD

The role of ECT in the treatment of psychosis in PD is not yet clearly delineated. This issue is distinct from, but related to, the issues of ECT in mood disorders, in psychotic disorders with and without mood disorder, and in PD without concomitant psychiatric disorder.

ECT in PD without concomitant psychiatric disorder.   It has long been noted that in many patients with PD who are treated with ECT for depression, motoric parkinsonian symptoms also decrease (especially the on-off phenomenon) (Andersen et al. 1987), a response that may be dissociable from the response of the mental symptoms. Similar responses have been seen for neuroleptic-induced parkinsonism (Goswami et al. 1989). Experience with the response of motoric symptoms in the treatment of PD with ECT, which includes a controlled trial with sham ECT in PD patients with severe on-off phenomenon (Andersen et al. 1987), has accumulated to the point that some psychiatrists now recommend that ECT be used to treat advanced PD even in the absence of a psychiatric disorder (Abrams 1989; Fink 1988).

Faber and Trimble (1991) reviewed the use of ECT in PD in detail. The reader is referred to their comprehensive discussion and extensive reference list. We quote from their conclusions: "ECT has antiparkinsonian effects, independent of any effects on mental state. The predictability, magnitude, and duration of such effects cannot be well-specified. . . . We speculate that approximately half of PD patients who receive ECT may be expected to benefit clinically" (pp. 300–301).

Granérus and co-workers (1994) studied 16 patients with advanced PD, all of whom were considered optimally medicated, and administered ECT (four to nine treatments). The patients' pharmacological regimens were not changed. All patients experienced improvement in motor symptoms. Eight had short-lived improvement, 7 patients' improvement lasted 3 to 5 months, and 1 patient's response lasted 18 months. A correlation was found between a lasting response and low levels of monoamine metabolites in the cerebrospinal fluid (CSF) before ECT. Five patients developed confusion during ECT lasting from 1 day to 2 weeks. Development of confusion during ECT was correlated with an abnormal serum-to-CSF albumin ratio before ECT that was considered indicative of disruption of the blood-brain barrier.

The evidence for the efficacy of ECT for the motoric signs of PD is composed largely of case reports and open studies. Examination of these reports raises a number of questions, such as how accurate were the diagnoses? In particular, it is difficult to read reports of parkinsonism that was present only during depressive episodes without wondering whether the patients really had catatonia rather than idiopathic parkinsonism. Still, many of the reports are compelling. The results of the one double-blind trial comparing ECT with sham ECT for the treatment of the on-off phenomenon (Andersen et al. 1987) is certainly positive enough to warrant further research.

Patients who respond well to ECT may be candidates for maintenance ECT (Zervas and Fink 1991). Some evidence suggests that the motoric symptoms of PD most likely respond to ECT in older patients (Douyon et al. 1989) and that the maximal response is usually obtained with relatively few (three to six) treatments (Zervas and Fink 1991). Our own limited experience with maintenance ECT points to a trend toward decreasing efficacy and increasing side effects. Two of three patients refused to continue treatment with maintenance ECT after three or four treatments despite benefit, and the third lost his beneficial response. The two responders could not explain their reluctance but adamantly refused further ECT.

ECT in PD and psychosis.   Clearly, if a patient with PD is psychotic and depressed, ECT is an attractive option if no high-risk factors are present. In the absence of depression, the patient with PD and a dopaminergic-drug-induced psychosis, with or without a confusional state, may or may not be a candidate for ECT, depending on one's view of the evidence.

Only two cases have been reported of successful treatment of levodopa-induced psychosis with ECT (Hurwitz et al. 1988)—although Hurwitz now has treated a total of five such cases (T. A. Hurwitz, personal communication, March 1993). We successfully treated a patient with PD, levodopa-induced psychosis, and minimal evidence of depression using ECT; however, maintenance ECT was unsuccessful because of the short duration of the response. Thus, the role of ECT in the treatment of psychosis in PD awaits clarification by further systematic studies.

We do not concur on the indications for ECT in PD, underscoring the need for further study of this issue. One of us (J.H.F.), a neurologist, believes that ECT is definitely not indicated for (motoric) treatment failures in the absence of psychiatric disorder but is indicated for depression and perhaps for psychosis unresponsive to clozapine. The other (S.S.R.), a psychiatrist, believes that, for patients with PD whose motoric symptoms are inadequately controlled with medication, the current evidence is sufficient to tilt the risk-benefit analysis in favor of an empirical trial of ECT; ECT would also be recommended for levodopa-induced psychoses unresponsive to clozapine.

We agree that ECT is especially useful in the depressed patient with advanced PD whose motoric symptoms are poorly controlled, whose dose of dopaminergic agents is limited by psychotic symptoms, and who is unable to tolerate clozapine. ECT may allow such patients to be managed with lower doses of dopaminergic agents, leading to an improvement in mental status.

Approach to Treatment

As outlined earlier in this chapter, when confronted with a psychotic parkinsonian patient, the first priority is to determine whether the psychotic symptoms are part of an acute confusional state (Figure 3–1). If so, the clinician should identify and treat underlying medical causes for delirium. If these are not found, one should proceed on the assumption that the patient has a drug-induced confusional state. The clinician should attempt to resolve this condition by reducing antiparkinsonian medication. All antiparkinsonian medications can cause delirium; because levodopa has the most favorable risk-benefit ratio, it is best to begin with the reduction or elimination of anticholinergic medication. If this does not accomplish the goal, it is logical to proceed to reduce or eliminate selegiline, amantadine, DA agonists, and eventually levodopa, in that order, if necessary.

Similarly, if the patient has psychotic symptoms without a confusional state, the first step is to reduce antiparkinsonian medications. Again, we suggest that reduction in levodopa preparations should be reserved for last.

If medication-reduction strategies are not efficacious or not tolerated from a motoric point of view, the next step is to institute treatment with clozapine. We recommend a starting dose of 6.25 mg qhs. Some patients' symptoms will resolve on this low dose, but most will require a gradual increase in the dose of clozapine in 6.25-mg increments as tolerated. If the patient requires more than about 50 mg/day, the dose can then usually be increased in greater increments as tolerated. For the parkinsonian patient without a major primary mental disorder, doses of less than 100 mg usually suffice, and it is rare that such a patient

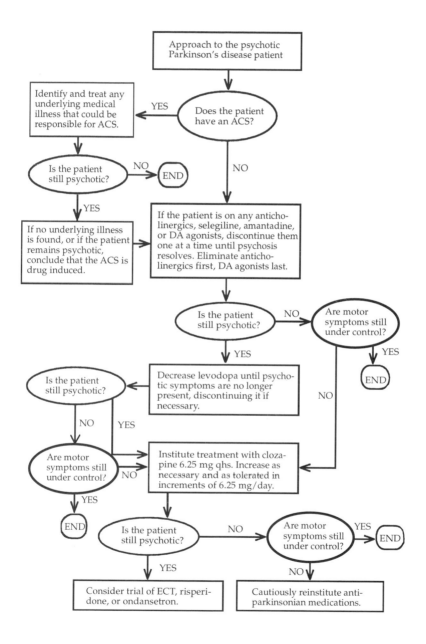

Figure 3–1. Approach to psychotic patients with Parkinson's disease. ACS = acute confusional state; DA = dopamine; ECT = electroconvulsive therapy.

would require as much as 150 mg/day or more. However, patients with primary psychotic disorders tend to require doses in the range used for schizophrenia (i.e., 250 to 450 mg/day). Our experience suggests that the goal should be to increase clozapine until the patient is able to sleep through the night—we have found that this benchmark correlates well with resolution of psychosis. After the psychotic symptoms have been brought under control, if the patient has become more parkinsonian because of previous medication reduction, antiparkinsonian medication can then be cautiously reinstated or increased. This may result in the recurrence of psychotic symptoms; if so, the clozapine may be increased. No data are available to guide the physician on length of patient response. Most patients respond to clozapine within a few days. It is unknown how long the highest tolerated dose should be maintained before it is considered a treatment failure.

If clozapine is not effective at tolerable doses, a trial of ECT may be in order, especially if depression is present and confusion is absent, perhaps followed by maintenance ECT. Initially, ECT in these patients often greatly reduces both mental and motoric disability (one patient nearly sent a wave of cataplexy through an inpatient nursing staff by "kicking up his heels" one day after he could barely walk); nevertheless, ECT is not known to be a successful long-term solution to this problem for the reasons discussed earlier in this chapter.

Other measures to consider, either before attempting ECT or after a patient has an unsuccessful trial of ECT, are a trial of 12 to 24 mg/day ondansetron or of 1 to 3 mg/day risperidone. Our preliminary experience with risperidone in these patients suggests that they should be started at the lowest possible dose (e.g., 0.5 mg qhs) to avoid exacerbation of motoric symptoms. Dosage can be raised by 0.5 mg every 2 to 3 days, using a twice-a-day or three-times-a-day schedule. Some psychotic parkinsonian patients will probably tolerate clozapine best because it has the fewest extrapyramidal side effects, whereas others will respond better on the newer agents if they become sedated, confused, or drool excessively on clozapine.

The vast majority of PD patients with psychosis can be managed as outpatients. Hospitalization may actually worsen the mental state of patients who are confused or who have dementia. It is not necessary to hospitalize every patient who is started on clozapine or given ECT. Patients should be hospitalized for these interventions, however, if concurrent medical conditions place them at high risk for untoward reactions, or if they can neither care for themselves nor permit their usual caregivers to care for them. They are more likely to require hospitalization insofar as they are lacking in insight or are delusional, depressed, suicidal, demented, or confused; all these factors impair patients' abilities to fend safely for themselves in the community.

CASE REPORTS

Following are three case histories that illustrate some issues that arise in the treatment of the psychotic parkinsonian patient, including the heterogeneity of presentation. They are all actual cases from our own clinical practices.

Drug-Induced Visual Hallucinosis in a Clear Sensorium

A 70-year-old woman with a 5-year history of PD came for a routine scheduled visit, reporting that she was doing well on Sinemet 25/100 tid. When asked whether she had had hallucinations, she reported that every night when she got up to go to the bathroom, she saw things that were always in the same location on the floor in the hallway. The first time this occurred she saw "crabs that had the color of lobster." She bent down to touch one, and they all disappeared. She immediately realized it was a hallucination, which she found amusing. Subsequently, she had visual hallucinations every night, always in the same place, when she went to the bathroom. She had no other hallucinations and no other symptoms of mental dysfunction. The nightly visions varied—sometimes she saw bright orange and yellow worms. Although she knew they were not real, she began to wear slippers when she got up at night and would push the worms out of the way with her slippered foot before walking through them so as not to crush any. In describing this she chuckled, pointing out the irrationality of her behavior given the nonexistence of the worms. She found the visions entertaining and did not want her medication reduced simply to resolve the visions.

Drug-Induced Hallucinations and Delusions

A 61-year-old man with a 4-year history of PD and mild dementia developed visual hallucinations of people while taking Sinemet 75/300 daily and selegiline 10 mg daily. He had had no prior psychiatric problems. He intermittently believed that the hallucinations were real, and he worried that they would cause mischief if he did not keep them under observation. He saw them in the leaves of his wife's large houseplant, although they were life-size. He brought in one leaf from the plant and a drawing of the "ringleader of the gang." See Figure 3–2 for his drawings of his hallucinations. He also began writing phrases and letters that were meaningless to others but significant to him and that he could not explain.

The patient developed increased motor disability when we attempted to lower his antiparkinsonian medication. On clozapine 25 mg/day, his psychosis resolved. His motoric function was maintained with the original antiparkinsonian regimen.

Premorbid Depression Complicated by PD, Dementia, Delirium, and Psychosis

A 78-year-old male retired mathematician with PD had a strong family history of depression (both parents committed suicide), a long personal history of severe major depression, and a severe personality disorder. He had no history of psychosis before the onset of PD. He was forced to retire by a gradually progressive dementia. While hospitalized as an inpatient for psychotic depression, it was systematically established that the patient could not tolerate any antiparkinsonian medications without developing a delirium accompanied by florid psychotic features such as Capgras' syndrome. His psychotic depression responded moderately well to ECT; motoric improvement was minimal. He was maintained on the maximum dose of clozapine that he could tolerate (50 mg/day) and 20 mg/day fluoxetine. His incomplete response to ECT deteriorated, despite fluoxetine and a trial of maintenance ECT. He remained chronically depressed and delusional—convinced, for example, that the proof of his most important published theorem was fatally flawed—although he never relapsed into the florid psychotic depression that he presented with. The patient, aside from having a prominent unilateral tremor, was not especially disabled from a motoric point of view. He was fully ambulatory and could perform most of his own activities of daily living. The patient's psychiatrist, neurologist, and family eventually concluded that his quality of life was maximized by not treating his PD, because the psychiatric side effects were not manageable.

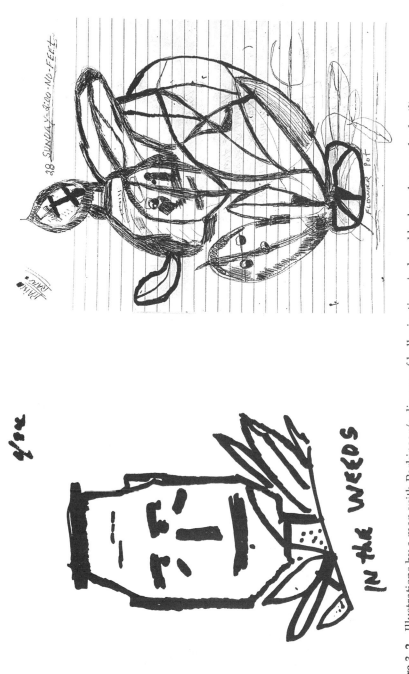

Figure 3–2. Illustrations by a man with Parkinson's disease of hallucinations induced by levodopa and selegiline.

REFERENCES

Abrams R: ECT for Parkinson's disease. Am J Psychiatry 146:1391–1393, 1989

Andersen K, Balldin J, Gottfries C, et al: A double-blind evaluation of electro-convulsive therapy in Parkinson's disease with "on-off" phenomena. Acta Neurol Scand 76:191–199, 1987

Andreasen NC: The scale for the assessment of positive symptoms (SAPS). Iowa City, IA, The University of Iowa, 1984

Anonymous: Effects of tocopherol and deprenyl on the progression of disability in early Parkinson's disease. N Engl J Med 328:176–183, 1993

Arellano F: Agranulocytosis and mortality update, in Standards of Care in Schizophrenia. Washington, DC, Sandoz Pharmaceuticals, 1993

Arevalo GJG, Gershanik OS: Modulatory effect of clozapine on levodopa response in Parkinson's disease: a preliminary study. Mov Disord 8:349–354, 1993

Bear J, Lawson W, Burns S, et al: Clozapine in idiopathic Parkinson's (abstract). Biol Psychiatry 25:163A, 1989

Bennett JP Jr, Landow ER, Schuh LA: Suppression of dyskinesias in advanced Parkinson's disease, II: increasing daily clozapine doses suppresses dyskinesias and improves parkinsonism symptoms. Neurology 43:1551–1555, 1993

Bernardi F, Del Zompa M: Clozapine in the management of psychosis in idiopathic Parkinson's disease (letter). Neurology 40:1151, 1990

Caligiuri MP, Lohr JB, Jeste DV: Parkinsonism in neuroleptic-naive schizophrenic patients. Am J Psychiatry 150:1343–1348, 1993

Canton H, Verrièle L, Colpaert FC: Binding of typical and atypical antipsychotics to $5-HT_{1C}$ and $5-HT_2$ sites: clozapine potently interacts with $5-HT_{1C}$ sites. Eur J Pharmacol 191:93–96, 1990

Chacko RC, Hurley RA, Jankovic J: Clozapine in diffuse Lewy body disease. J Neuropsychiatry Clin Neurosci 5:206–208, 1993

Chouinard G, Jones B, Remington G, et al: A Canadian multicenter placebo controlled study of fixed doses of risperidone and haloperidol in the treatment of chronic schizophrenia. J Clin Psychopharmacol 13:25–40, 1993

Coward DM: General pharmacology of clozapine. Br J Psychiatry 160 (suppl 17):5–11, 1992

Crow TJ, Johnstone EC, McClelland HA: The coincidence of schizophrenia and parkinsonism: some neurochemical implications. Psychol Med 6:227–233, 1976

Cummings JL: Neuropsychiatric complications of drug treatment of Parkinson's disease, in Parkinson's Disease: Neurobehavioral Aspects. Edited by Huber SJ, Cummings JL. New York, Oxford University Press, 1992, pp 313–327

Douyon R, Serby M, Klutchko B, et al: ECT and Parkinson's disease revisited: a "naturalistic" study. Am J Psychiatry 146:1451–1455, 1989

Faber R, Trimble MR: Electroconvulsive therapy in Parkinson's disease and other movement disorders. Mov Disord 6:293–303, 1991

Factor SA, Brown DB: Clozapine prevents recurrence of psychosis in Parkinson's disease. Mov Disord 7:125–131, 1992

Factor SA, Brown D, Molho ES, et al: Clozapine: a two year open trial in Parkinson's disease patients with psychosis. Neurology 44:544–546, 1994

Feldman RG, Kaye JA, Lannon MC: Parkinson's disease: follow-up after "drug holiday." J Clin Pharmacol 26:662–667, 1986

Fink M: ECT for Parkinson's disease? Convulsive Therapy 4:189–191, 1988

Fischer P, Danielczyk W, Simanyi M, et al: Dopaminergic psychosis in advanced Parkinson's disease, in Parkinson's Disease: Anatomy, Pathology, and Therapy. Edited by Streifler MB, Korczyn AD, Melamed E, et al. New York, Raven, 1990a, pp 391–397

Fischer PA, Baas H, Hefner R: Treatment of parkinsonian tremor with clozapine. J Neural Transm Park Dis Dement Sect 2:233–238, 1990b

Ford B, Lynch T, Greene P: Risperidone in Parkinson's disease (letter). Lancet 344:681, 1994

Friedman AJ, Sienkiewicz J: Psychotic complications of levodopa treatment of Parkinson's disease. Acta Neurol Scand 84:111–113, 1991

Friedman J, Lannon M: Clozapine treatment of tremor in Parkinson's disease. Mov Disord 5:225–229, 1990

Friedman J, Max J, Swift R: Idiopathic Parkinson's disease in a chronic schizophrenic patient: long-term treatment with clozapine and L-dopa. Clin Neuropharmacol 10:470–475, 1987

Friedman JH: The management of levodopa psychoses. Clin Neuropharmacol 14:283–295, 1991

Friedman JH, Lannon MC: Clozapine in the treatment of psychosis in Parkinson's disease. Neurology 39:1219–1221, 1989

Friedman JH, Lannon MC, Caley C: Clozapine for movement disorder patients: a retrospective analysis of 38 patients (abstract). Ann Neurol 32:277, 1992

Gershanik O, Garcia S, Papa S, et al: Analysis of the mechanism of action of clozapine in Parkinson's disease (abstract). Mov Disord 7 (suppl 1):101, 1992

Goetz CG, Tanner C, Gilly D, et al: Development and progression of motor fluctuations and side effects in Parkinson's disease: comparison of Sinemet CR vs carbidopa/levodopa. Neurology 39 (suppl 2):63–66, 1989

Goetz CG, Stebbins GT: Risk factors for nursing home placement in Parkinson's disease. Neurology 43:2227–2229, 1993

Goetz CG, Tanner CM, Klawans HL: Pharmacology of hallucinations induced by long term drug therapy. Am J Psychiatry 139:494–497, 1982

Goswami U, Dutta S, Kuruvilla K, et al: Electroconvulsive therapy in neuroleptic-induced parkinsonism. Biol Psychiatry 26:234–238, 1989

Grabowski J: Clonidine treatment of clozapine-induced hypersalivation. J Clin Psychopharmacol 12:69–70, 1992

Granérus A-K, Ekman R, Fall P-A, et al: ECT in Parkinson's disease—predictors to improvement. Presented at the International Parkinson's Disease meeting, Rome, Italy, March 1994

Greene P, Cote L, Fahn S: Treatment of drug-induced psychosis in Parkinson's disease with clozapine. Adv Neurol 60:703–706, 1993

Hale MS, Bellizzi J: Low dose perphenazine and levodopa/carbidopa therapy in a patient with parkinsonism and a psychotic illness. J Nerv Ment Dis 168:312–314, 1980

Humpel C, Knaus GA, Auer B, et al: Effects of haloperidol and clozapine on preprotachykinin-A messenger RNA, tachykinin tissue levels, release and neurokinin-1 receptors in the striato-nigral system. Synapse 6:1–9, 1990

Hurwitz TA, Calne DB, Waterman K: Treatment of dopaminomimetic psychosis in Parkinson's disease with electroconvulsive therapy. Can J Neurol Sci 15:32–34, 1988

Jansen ENH: Clozapine in the treatment of tremor in Parkinson's disease. Acta Neurol Scand 89:262–265, 1994

Jenkins RB, Groh RH: Mental symptoms in Parkinson patients treated with L-DOPA. Lancet 2:177–180, 1970

Kahn N, Freeman A, Juncos JL, et al: Clozapine is beneficial for psychosis in Parkinson's disease. Neurology 41:1699–1700, 1991

Kane J, Honigfeld G, Singer J, et al: Clozapine for the treatment-resistant schizophrenic. Arch Gen Psychiatry 45:789–796, 1988

Kang J, Pfeiffer R, Graber B, et al: Treatment of iatrogenic psychosis in Parkinson's disease with clozapine (abstract). Br J Psychiatry 1991:245S, 1991

Kessler II: Parkinson's disease in epidemiologic perspective. Adv Neurol 19:355–384, 1978

Lang AE, Sandor P, Duff J: Remoxipride in Parkinson's disease: differential response in patients with dyskinesias/fluctuations versus psychosis. Ann Neurol 34:301–302, 1993

Leehey M, Boyson S: The biochemistry of Parkinson's disease, in Current Neurology. Edited by Appel SH. St Louis, MO, Mosby Year Book, 1991, pp 233–286

Lew MF, Waters C: Treatment of parkinsonism with psychosis using clozapine (abstract). Mov Disord 7 (suppl 1):100, 1992

LeWitt PA: Neuroprotection by anti-oxidant strategies in Parkinson's disease. Eur Neurol 1:24–30, 1993

Linazasaro G, Suarez JA: Clozapine in Parkinson's disease: three years experience (abstract). Mov Disord 7 (suppl 1):100, 1992

Linazasaro G, Masso JFM, Suarez JA: Nocturnal akathisia in Parkinson's disease: treatment with clozapine. Mov Disord 8:171–174, 1993

Lishman WA (ed): Organic Psychiatry: The Psychological Consequences of Cerebral Disorder. Oxford, UK, Blackwell Scientific, 1987

Martilla RJ: Epidemiology, in Handbook of Parkinson's Disease. Edited by Koller WC. New York, Marcel Dekker, 1987, pp 35–50

Martilla RJ, Rinne UK, Siirtola T, et al: Mortality of patients with Parkinson's disease treated with levodopa. J Neurol 216:147–153, 1977

Mayeux R, Stern Y, Mulvey K, et al: Reappraisal of temporary levodopa withdrawal ("drug holidays") in Parkinson's disease. N Engl J Med 313:724–728, 1985

Meco G, Alessandria A, Bonifati V, et al: Risperidone for hallucinations in levodopa treated Parkinson disease patients. Lancet 343:1370–1371, 1994

Melamed E, Zoldan J, Friedberg G, et al: Is hallucinosis in Parkinson's disease due to central serotonergic hyperactivity? Mov Disord 8:406–407, 1993

Meltzer HY, Gudelsky GA: Dopaminergic and serotonergic effects of clozapine: implications for a unique clinical profile. Arzneimittelforschung 42:268–272, 1992

Montastruc JL, Rascol O, Rascol A: Comparison of bromocriptine and levodopa as first line treatment of Parkinson's disease: results of a 3-year prospective randomized study. Rev Neurol (Paris) 146:144–147, 1990

Nausieda PA, Weiner WJ, Kaplan LR, et al: Sleep disruption in the course of chronic levodopa therapy: an early feature of the levodopa psychosis. Clin Neuropharmacol 5:183–194, 1982

Ostergaard K, Dupont E: Clozapine treatment of drug induced psychotic symptoms in the late stages of Parkinson's disease. Acta Neurol Scand 78:349–350, 1988

Overall JE, Gorham DR: The Brief Psychiatric Rating Scale. Psychol Rep 10:799–812, 1962

Pakkenberg H, Pakkenberg B: Clozapine in the treatment of tremor. Acta Neurol Scand 73:295–297, 1986

Parsa MA, Ramirez LF, Loula EC, et al: Effect of clozapine on psychotic depression and parkinsonism. J Clin Psychopharmacol 11:330–331, 1991

Parsa MA, Simon M, Dubrow C, et al: Psychiatric manifestations of olivo-ponto-cerebellar atrophy and treatment with clozapine. Int J Psychiatry Med 23:149–156, 1993

Pfeiffer R, Kang J, Graber B, et al: Clozapine for psychosis in Parkinson's disease. Mov Disord 5:239–242, 1990

Pinter MM, Helscher RJ: Therapeutic effect of clozapine in psychotic decompensation in idiopathic Parkinson's disease. J Neural Transm Park Dis Dement Sect 5:135–146, 1993

Rich SS: Drug-induced movement disorders. Rhode Island Medical Journal 76:556–562, 1993

Roberts HE, Dean RC, Stoudemire A: Clozapine treatment of psychosis in Parkinson's disease. J Neuropsychiatry Clin Neurosci 1:190–192, 1989

Rosenthal SH, Fenton ML, Harnett DS: Clozapine for the treatment of levodopa-induced psychosis in Parkinson's disease. Gen Hosp Psychiatry 14:285–286, 1992

Runge I, Horowski R: Can we differentiate symptomatic and neuroprotective effects in parkinsonism? The dopamine agonist lisuride delays the need for levodopa therapy to a similar extent as reported for deprenyl. J Neural Transm Park Dis Dement Sect 3:273–283, 1991

Saint-Cyr J, Taylor AE, Lang AE: Neuropsychological and psychiatric side effects in the treatment of Parkinson's disease. Neurology 43 (suppl 6):S47–S52, 1993

Scholz E, Dichgens J: Treatment of drug induced exogenous psychosis in parkinsonism with clozapine and fluperlapine. Eur Arch Psychiatry Neurol Sci 235:60–64, 1985

Schuster P, Gabriel E, Kufferle B, et al: Reversal by physostigmine of clozapine induced delirium. Clinical Toxicology 10:437–441, 1977

Shoulson I: An interim report of the effect of selegiline (L-deprenyl) on the progression of disability in early Parkinson's disease: the Parkinson Study Group. Eur Neurol 1:46–53, 1992

Tanner CM, Vogel C, Goetz C, et al: Hallucinations in Parkinson's disease: a population study (abstract). Ann Neurol 14:136, 1983

Tanner CM: Epidemiology of Parkinson's disease. Neurol Clin 10:317–329, 1992

Uitti RJ, Ahlskog JE, Maraganore DM, et al: Levodopa therapy and survival in idiopathic Parkinson's disease: Olmstead County Project. Neurology 43:1918–1926, 1993

van der Linden C, Bruggerman R, van Woerkom T: Risperidone in the treatment of Gilles de la Tourette's syndrome. Ann Neurol 34:263–264, 1993

Wolk SI, Douglas CJ: Clozapine treatment of psychosis in Parkinson's disease: a report of five consecutive cases. J Clin Psychiatry 53:373–376, 1992

Wolters EC, Hurwitz RE, Mak E, et al: Clozapine in the treatment of parkinsonian patients with dopaminergic psychosis. Neurology 40:832–834, 1990

Zervas IM, Fink M: ECT for refractory Parkinson's disease. Convulsive Therapy 7:222–223, 1991

Zoldan J, Friedberg G, Goldberg SH, et al: Ondansetron for hallucinosis in advanced Parkinson's disease. Clin Neuropharmacol 12:83–90, 1989

Chapter 4

Neuropsychiatric Aspects of Systemic Lupus Erythematosus

Martin J. Kelly, M.D.
Malcolm P. Rogers, M.D.

Systemic lupus erythematosus (SLE), or lupus, has served as the prototype for the study of modern autoimmune diseases, but the term *lupus* was used for many centuries for most serious skin diseases that gnawed away and destroyed the skin like a wolf (Latin *lupus*, wolf). The disease we now recognize as SLE has been widely written about since the thirteenth century and described at the time of Hippocrates, although it was not until about 1850 that Cazenane specifically separated out *lupus érythèmateau* from the other cutaneous disorders. In the nineteenth century, Kaposi was among the first to note the systemic nature of the disease, noting "various and even dangerous constitutional symptoms may be intimately associated with the process in question," and may have been the earliest to refer to the nearly pathognomonic rash as having a "butterfly" distribution (Talbot 1993).

By the early part of the twentieth century, it was thought that this was a very rare disorder with manifestations throughout the body. By

The authors are grateful to Peter Schur, M.D., Professor of Medicine, Harvard Medical School, and Director, Lupus Center, Brigham and Women's Hospital, Boston, MA, for his review, suggestions, and many helpful tables. The authors also thank Anne Mackin for assistance in the preparation of this manuscript.

the middle of the twentieth century, the term *systemic* lupus erythematosus stressed the fact that almost all body organ systems could be affected by the disorder (Figure 4–1). The "erythematosus" eruptions that occur on the face as well as on oral and nasal mucosa, fingers, hands, and skin surfaces exposed to sunlight are a very frequent, although not an essential, feature of the diagnosis.

Even in recent decades, this condition was thought to be a rare inflammatory autoimmune disorder with a prevalence of only 2 to 3 per 100,000 (Mannik and Gilliland 1974). However, more recent studies suggest that the prevalence may be 15 to 50 per 100,000 (Hahn 1987; Hochberg 1993). This probably reflects the increased clinical awareness of the disorder and the increased sensitivity of the serodiagnostic tests. SLE is much more common in women (nine to one) and more common in blacks than in whites. It is also seen in other racial and ethnic groups. Lupus presents most commonly between ages 20 and 40 years, although it can occur in preadolescence. It is relatively rare after menopause.

DISTINGUISHING SYSTEMIC LUPUS ERYTHEMATOSUS FROM SIMILAR CONDITIONS

Because the implications of the diagnosis are potentially very serious, it is important to distinguish SLE from other conditions that might mimic the syndrome or have somewhat similar symptoms (Table 4–1). These include discoid lupus and the lupuslike syndromes induced by drugs, most commonly medications such as procainamide or hydralazine. No psychotropic medications except for chlorpromazine have been implicated (Table 4–2). Patients with drug-induced lupus syndromes do have positive SLE antibody testing; positive antinuclear antibody (ANA) tests are seen in more than half of the patients taking procainamide and one-third of patients taking hydralazine. The symptoms of drug-induced lupus (polyarthralgias and systemic symptoms) generally resolve fairly promptly on discontinuation of the medication (Table 4–3). Patients with more severe symptoms may benefit from a short course of steroids.

Discoid lupus, which shares the same facial (butterfly) rash, is a much more benign condition, with lesions usually localized to the face and, occasionally, the scalp, ears, and oral mucous membranes. It can be a chronic and distressing disorder, but it does not have the life-

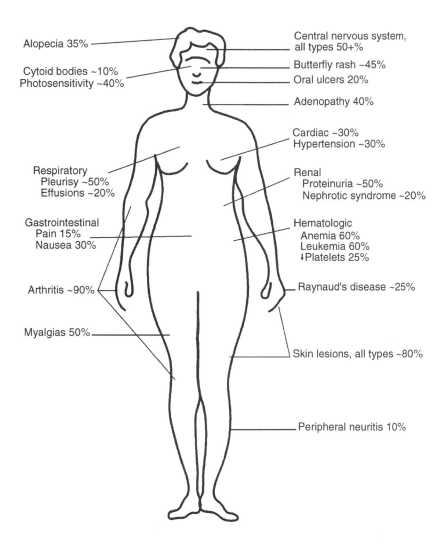

Alopecia 35%

Cytoid bodies ~10%
Photosensitivity ~40%

Central nervous system,
all types 50+%

Butterfly rash ~45%

Oral ulcers 20%

Adenopathy 40%

Cardiac ~30%
Hypertension ~30%

Respiratory
Pleurisy ~50%
Effusions ~20%

Renal
Proteinuria ~50%
Nephrotic syndrome ~20%

Gastrointestinal
Pain 15%
Nausea 30%

Hematologic
Anemia 60%
Leukemia 60%
↓Platelets 25%

Arthritis ~90%

Raynaud's disease ~25%

Myalgias 50%

Skin lesions, all types ~80%

Peripheral neuritis 10%

Figure 4–1.   Clinical presentation of systemic lupus erythematosus.
Source.   Wallace 1993.

Table 4–1. Disorders symptomatically that may resemble systemic lupus
erythematosus

Common	Mixed connective tissue disease
Drug-induced lupus	Fibromyalgia/chronic fatigue
Scleroderma	syndrome
Wegener's granulomatosis	**Less common**
Cutaneous (discoid) lupus	Polymyositis/dermatomyositis
Rheumatoid arthritis	Rheumatic fever
Chronic active hepatitis (lupoid	Sarcoidosis
hepatitis)	Relapsing polychondritis
Vasculitis	Weber-Christian disease
Felty's syndrome	Mixed cryoglobulinemia
Juvenile (rheumatoid) arthritis	Whipple's disease
Sjögren's syndrome	Periodic syndromes

Source. Peter Schur, M.D.

Table 4–2. Lupus-inducing drugs

Definite	Possible	Unlikely
Hydralazine	Phenytoin	Griseofulvin
Procainamide	Penicillamine	Phenylbutazone
	Isoniazid	Oral contraceptives
	Chlorpromazine	Gold salts
	Methyldopa	Penicillins
	Quinidine	Hydrazine
	Sulfonamides	L-Canavanine
	Propylthiouracil	Aminosalicylic acid
	Practolol	Streptomycin
	Acebutolol	Tetracyclines
	Lithium carbonate	Methylthiouracil
	p-Aminosalicylate	Oxyphenisatin
	Nitrofurantoin	Tolazamide
	Tartrazine	Methysergide
	Atenolol	Reserpine
	Metoprolol	Isoquinazepan
	Oxprenolol	
	Mephenytoin	
	Primidone	
	Trimethadione	
	Ethosuximide	
	Methimazole	
	Captopril	
	Chlorthalidone	
	Carbamazepine	
	Phenylethylacetylurea	

Source. Peter Schur, M.D.

threatening implications of systemic lupus. Although the rash has a similar distribution on the face, it usually has some distinguishing clinical features. The rash of systemic lupus is often puffy and erythematous, with telangiectatic characteristics, whereas the rash of discoid lupus is somewhat more scaly and generally lacks puffiness. The skin lesions of discoid lupus are often chronic and eventually show atrophic changes with decreased pigmentation and scarring. Both rashes are exacerbated by exposure to sunlight.

Table 4–3. Clinical and laboratory features of drug-induced lupus

Clinical features	Spontaneous SLE (%)	Drug-induced lupus (%)
Age (yr)	20–40	50
Sex (F:M)	9	1
Race	Blacks > others	All
Acetylation type	Slow-fast	Slow
Onset of symptoms	Gradual	Abrupt
Constitutional symptoms		
(fever, malaise, myalgia)	90	50
Arthritis/arthralgia	95	95
Pleuropericarditis	50	50
Skin rash	74	10–20
Renal disease	50	5
CNS disease	75	0
Hematological disease	Common	Unusual
Immune abnormalities		
ANA	95	95
LE cells	90	90
Anti-dsDNA	80	Rare
Anti-ssDNA	80	Common
Antihistone	25	90
Anti-Sm	20–30	Rare
Anti-RNP	40–50	Rare
Complement	Reduced	Normal
Immune complexes	Elevated	Normal

Note. SLE = systemic lupus erythematosus; CNS = central nervous system; ANA = antinuclear antibody.
Source. Peter Schur, M.D.

DIAGNOSIS OF
SYSTEMIC LUPUS ERYTHEMATOSUS

Criteria have been proposed for the classification of SLE by the American College of Rheumatology (Tan et al. 1982). They recommend that the disorder can be classified as systemic lupus if the patient has at least four of the following symptoms or laboratory findings:

1. Malar (butterfly) rash
2. Discoid rash
3. Photosensitivity
4. Oral ulcers
5. Arthritis
6. Serositis
7   Renal disorder
8. Hematological abnormalities including leukopenia, hemolytic anemia, thrombocytopenia
9. Neurologic disorders including psychosis, seizures, mood disturbance, cognitive changes
10. Positive LE cell or anti-DNA or anti-SM antibody or a false-positive serologic test for syphilis
11. Raised titer of ANAs

It would be relatively easy to diagnose the symptoms in a young woman in her childbearing years presenting with a typical butterfly rash, polyarthralgias, malaise, fever, and weakness. However, the full-blown clinical picture is rarely the initial presentation. More typically, patients will have relatively mild and varying symptoms for months (or years), with occasional bouts of polyarthralgias, fevers, fatigue, or weakness, waxing and waning but often not at a level that comes to clinical attention. Not only do these symptoms mimic many other medical disorders, but they can often imitate psychiatric conditions including somatoform disorders and mood disorders. Mild neuropsychiatric (NP) symptoms, such as decreased concentration, impaired attention, mildly slowed cognition, headaches, emotional lability, and depression, may be easily seen as, or even dismissed as, primary mental disorders before time declares them as lupus.

It may be particularly difficult to diagnose SLE in elderly patients, in whom the presentation may be one of delirium, dementia, or depression. Dennis and co-workers (1992) reported five such cases, all of whom had positive serological tests and all of whom responded well to treatment with steroids. They speculated that the American College of Rheumatology criteria may be inappropriate for the elderly, leading to underrecognition of lupus in patients with subtle mental status changes.

Because a general feeling of malaise and weight loss are common, these very early SLE symptoms may be regarded as a depressive disorder and treated with antidepressants. A reduction in symptoms after receiving antidepressants may reflect the fluctuating nature of the systemic lupus rather than a true response to the medication. The variety and subtlety of early symptoms of the disorder are a diagnostic challenge for the medical community, including psychiatrists.

At times, the delays and frustration in diagnosis, especially the dismissal of early manifestations as psychiatric symptoms, lead to negative attitudes of patients toward the medical profession. Patient groups have helped to educate the public and have advocated effectively for increased support and research. In addition, the specific and sensitive diagnostic tests now available facilitate a definitive diagnosis in the very early stages of the disorder.

The early diagnosis of (milder) cases has led to an apparent increase in 10-year survival, which is probably more than 95% (Hochberg 1993). In general, the clinical picture of SLE can be segregated into two patterns. Most patients have a mild and chronic course, with a gradual decrease in the frequency and intensity of exacerbations as well as a gradual decrease in the probability of major organ system involvement over time. In this group, laboratory abnormalities, including tests for antinuclear antibodies and sedimentation rates, tend to decrease or even normalize.

A smaller number of patients have a more serious and virulent course. They have major organ system involvement, including the cardiac, renal, hematopoietic, and central nervous systems (CNS). The leading cause of death for this population is opportunistic infection, probably followed by renal and CNS complications (Table 4–4).

The natural history of the disorder appears to have been altered in recent decades by treatment with corticosteroids and immunosuppressive drugs (Wallace 1993). Recent moderation in the dosage of these drugs has lessened the drug-induced complications such as steroid-accelerated arteriosclerosis. There is also increased awareness of the significant potential complications of other immunosuppressive drugs, including increased risk of malignancy.

Table 4–4. Clinical features in systemic lupus erythematosus

Manifestations	Approximate frequency (%)	
	At onset	At any time
Nonspecific		
Fatigue		90
Fever	36	80
Weight loss		60
Arthralgia/myalgia	69	95
Specific		
Arthritis		95
Skin		
Butterfly rash	40	50
Discoid lupus	6	20
Photosensitivity	29	58
Mucous ulcers	11	30
Alopecia		71
Raynaud's disease	18	30
Purpura		15
Urticaria		9
Renal	16	50
Nephrosis		18
Gastrointestinal		38
Pulmonary	3	50
Pleurisy		45
Effusions		24
Pneumonia		29
Cardiac		46
Pericarditis		48
Murmurs		23
Electrocardiogram changes		34
Lymphadenopathy	7	50
Splenomegaly		20
Hepatomegaly		25
Central nervous system	12	75
Functional		Most
Psychosis		20
Other psychiatric		50
Seizures		20
Hematologic		90

Source.   Adapted from Peter Schur, M.D.

PSYCHIATRISTS AND
SYSTEMIC LUPUS ERYTHEMATOSUS

Although psychiatrists rarely make the initial diagnosis of SLE, it should be considered in patients who have prominent complaints of physical malaise, weakness, and weight loss disproportionate to their mood symptoms. Early premonitory or mild symptoms of lupus are a challenge to the diagnostic acumen of the psychiatrist but should be considered when the patient does not fit the clinical picture of a primary psychiatric disorder. Demographics (sex, age, and race) and family history of autoimmune disease should influence the degree of suspicion.

Psychiatrists are more frequently challenged by the management of symptoms of patients with an established diagnosis of SLE, typically in the evaluation of new NP symptoms that may or may not be related to SLE. Chronic discouragement and demoralization are not uncommon for patients with a serious chronic disease such as SLE. They need to be distinguished from a primary mood disorder and from a mood disorder secondary to medication, to brain involvement by SLE, or to an opportunistic infection. Similarly, there are risks of an iatrogenic somatoform disorder because of the protean and multifaceted nature of potential lupus symptoms. Some patients must learn that not every somatic symptom they experience is caused by SLE. Supporting the highest level of function and discouraging the patient's formation of an identity as "a lupus patient" are important clinical goals.

The assessment of mood and cognitive symptoms that might be symptoms of SLE, side effects of steroid medication, or caused by a mood disorder can be valuable psychiatric contributions to the overall clinical enterprise. The assessment is especially subtle in patients who have a genetic or developmental vulnerability to mood disorder and also have an established diagnosis of CNS lupus.

PREVALENCE OF NEUROPSYCHIATRIC
SYMPTOMS AND PSYCHOPATHOLOGY IN
SYSTEMIC LUPUS ERYTHEMATOSUS

NP symptoms are one of the widely accepted classification criteria for SLE. NP symptoms include psychosis, seizures, cognitive disturbance, mood disorders, and focal CNS syndromes (Table 4–5). The estimates of the prevalence rates for these conditions have varied from 17% to 71% (Feinglass et al. 1976; Futrell et al. 1992; McCune and Golbus 1988;

Wekking 1993). This wide range probably reflects the difficulty in distinguishing symptoms caused by direct brain involvement from those caused by underlying vascular and immunological problems. In addition, there are a number of methodological difficulties in these studies, including inadequate definitions of NP lupus as well as vagaries of psychiatric nomenclature (Iverson 1993; Iverson and McCracken 1992; Wekking 1993).

Overall, cognitive impairment appears to be the most frequently reported NP symptom, and neuropsychological studies have shown that most patients with lupus have demonstrable cognitive impairment (S. D. Denburg et al. 1993). Depression, psychosis, anxiety, and sleep disturbance are also relatively common. If a patient is to develop psychosis at all, it is likely to occur during the first year of the illness (Ward and Studenski 1991). Some reports estimate the prevalence of general psychiatric symptoms in SLE patients overall as comparable to that for general medical outpatients and below that for psychiatric outpatients (Mitchell and Thompson 1990). However, patients with lupus are more likely to have cognitive impairment or psychotic symptoms than those with other rheumatological disorders such as rheumatoid arthritis (S. D. Denburg et al. 1993; Iverson 1993; Lim et al. 1988; Wekking 1993).

PSYCHIATRIC PRESENTATIONS

The NP manifestations of SLE will precede the diagnosis in more than half of the patients. Case reports document that psychosis and other

Table 4–5.   Incidence of neuropsychiatric systemic lupus erythematosus manifestations

Central nervous system manifestations	Incidence (%)
All types	> 50
Psychosis	≈ 20
Seizures	≈ 15
Peripheral neuropathy	≈ 10
Cognitive disturbance	> 50
Depression	≈ 40
Delirium	≈ 10
Coma	< 5

cognitive impairment disorders, especially delirium, can be the initial presentation (Mavrikakis et al. 1992). In lupus patients with an "organic" or psychotic picture, almost half may have had their mental symptoms before the lupus is diagnosed, according to one estimate (van Dam et al. 1991). However, screening of unselected general psychiatric inpatients for ANAs is not justifiable, because 0.1% or 0.2% of such patients will ultimately show findings specific to SLE (i.e., anti-DNA antibodies) (van Dam et al. 1991). However, testing for ANA would be indicated in a young black woman with psychosis and somatizing features or with a recent onset of depression and a low-grade fever. Principles for determining whether a particular population should be screened routinely are reviewed by Anfinson and Kathol (1993) in their discussion of laboratory testing in medical psychiatry.

There have been many unusual presentations of NP SLE, including catatonia (Mac and Pardo 1983), morbid jealousy (Ravindran et al. 1980), and chorea (Amital-Teplizki and Shoenfeld 1989). It can mimic other NP disorders, including herpes simplex encephalitis, progressive multifocal leukoencephalopathy (Kaye et al. 1992), and vascular dementia.

COGNITIVE IMPAIRMENT IN SYSTEMIC LUPUS ERYTHEMATOSUS

Cognitive problems are common, and they are often missed or minimized. Careful cognitive assessment of SLE patients compared with rheumatoid arthritis patients and with healthy subjects revealed a prevalence of impairment in 68% with SLE versus 17% with rheumatoid arthritis and 14% with healthy matched control subjects at comparable stages of illness. Almost all patients with other active mental symptoms (e.g., psychosis, mood disturbance) also had cognitive disturbances (e.g., memory, concentration problems) (Carbotte et al. 1992). As many as 42% of patients with resolved and inactive NP symptoms had cognitive disturbance (Carbotte et al. 1986, 1992; S. D. Denburg et al. 1987). Interestingly, these studies have not shown a significant association between cognitive disturbance and mood disturbance. The fact that patients whose psychotic or affective symptoms have resolved may be as impaired cognitively as those with active NP symptoms suggests that such patients often have residual and possibly permanent CNS damage. Some patients who have never demonstrated NP symptoms show cognitive disturbances suggestive of sub-clinical CNS involvement.

Three women with SLE and cognitive impairment were studied longitudinally with repeated positron-emission tomography (PET) scans and neuropsychological measures. Areas of diminished glucose metabolism correlated with focal cognitive deficits and waxed and waned in synchrony. For example, one patient with diminished visual-spatial ability showed a right central sulcus PET abnormality; a patient with decreased verbal capacity showed a left superior parietal and pos-terior temporal lesion. The PET scans cleared in association with clini-cal recovery (Carbotte et al. 1992).

In lupus patients not taking steroids, neuropsychological tests often show dysfunction in attention, visuospatial ability, short-term memory, and reaction time. In an individual patient on steroids, how-ever, it may be difficult to distinguish the primary effects of the disease from the consequences of treatment with corticosteroids (Ferstl et al. 1992; Ginsburg et al. 1992; Mulherin et al. 1993). Discrete focal abnor-malities in cognitive tests (e.g., severe visuospatial deficits with normal language) would confirm SLE or a complication rather than steroids as the cause of brain dysfunction.

DIAGNOSTIC ISSUES AND PROBLEMS

Research in this area is complicated by the varying definitions of what should constitute NP disturbance in SLE patients (Wekking 1993). Some clinicians hope to find better correlations with the other manifes-tations of SLE and, perhaps, with antibody titers and imaging studies by splitting patients into relatively homogeneous clinical groups such as "stroke," "suicide attempts," "hallucinations," "confusion," and "sei-zures." However, the splitting approach may lack validity because CNS lupus manifestations are multiple and fluctuating. A better approach is a consensus-derived definition of NP lupus; this includes unmistak-able manifestations such as psychosis, seizure, and stroke and more subtle manifestations of depression and cognitive impairment, which must be accompanied by positive, objective evidence of CNS involve-ment by serologic or brain imaging tests (Singer and Denburg 1990).

After brain involvement is established, the principal differential di-agnostic problem is to distinguish primary CNS lupus (e.g., cerebritis with small vessel vasculitis) from the infectious complications of im-munosuppressive therapy. Another often critical problem is distinguishing large vessel vasculitis or thromboembolism from small vessel disease. These distinctions are important because the specific treatments of these complications are quite different—that is, specific antibiotic therapy for secondary infections, anticoagulant therapy for large vessel thromboembolism or vasculitis, and steroids and/or immunosuppressives for the other problems.

Moreover, an infectious etiology is much more likely if the patient presents with focal neurological deficits, coma, neuropathy, blurring of vision, and myelopathy, whereas "psychiatric" presentations such as depression, psychosis, and decreased cognition are more likely indicative of primary lupus CNS symptoms.

DIAGNOSTIC TESTS IN NEUROPSYCHIATRIC SYSTEMIC LUPUS ERYTHEMATOSUS

Serology and Chemistry

The evaluation for NP SLE includes a general evaluation of the level of lupus disease activity, consisting of a careful history, ANA titers, erythrocyte sedimentation rate, complement studies, complete blood count (CBC), and renal and liver function studies (Table 4–6). The LE cell test ("LE prep") is obsolete. Higher ANA titers increase the probability that a positive ANA is a true positive (i.e., the patient actually has lupus). Other diseases are also associated with a positive ANA (Table 4–7). ANA is negative only in 0.14% of patients with SLE (Griner et al. 1981). Anti-DNA antibodies have about a 95% predictive value for SLE, but they are found in only about 75% of SLE patients. Table 4–8 shows a more detailed profile of autoantibodies seen in patients with SLE.

Table 4–9 summarizes the usefulness of the following diagnostic procedures in identifying the different manifestations of CNS lupus.

Skin Biopsy

When the cause of a patient's rash is uncertain, it is useful to obtain a skin biopsy. Immunofluorescence can be helpful. Typically (in more than 90% of patients with lupus and a rash), it shows many immunoreactive proteins and complement at the dermal-epidermal junction.

Lumbar Puncture

Lumbar puncture is indicated to exclude indolent meningeal infection when the cause of a mental status change in a patient with SLE is not evident from general clinical evaluation and brain imaging. In NP SLE without infection, the cerebrospinal fluid (CSF) may have an increased number of lymphocytes.

Electroencephalogram (EEG)

The EEG is quite important for confirming seizure phenomena, especially in puzzling presentations in which fluctuating or episodic mental symptoms may reflect partial seizure activity. It also may help to distinguish delirium from a primary mental disorder with cognitive dysfunction, such as acute mania. Most patients with delirium have diffuse slowing of the background, unlike most with primary mental disorders (McNamara 1991). Quantitative EEG (QEEG) methods may be more accurate than routine EEG in distinguishing patients with NP SLE from patients with SLE but no NP symptoms. Ritchlin and colleagues (1992) compared topographical QEEG results in 52 patients

Table 4–6. Signs and symptoms suggesting active systemic lupus erythematosus

Malaise	Mouth sores
Poor appetite	Anemia
Weight loss	Leukopenia
Fatigue	Thrombocytopenia
Pallor	Hematuria
Abnormal menses	Pyuria
Fever	Proteinuria
Arthritis	Azotemia
Seizures	Erythrocyte sedimentation rate
Chest pain	elevation
Edema	Complement (C3, C4, CH50)
Hair loss	decreased
Oliguria	Immune complexes
Rashes	Anti-dsDNA

Source.   Peter Schur, M.D.

with SLE, divided into four groups: those with confirmed NP SLE, those with NP symptoms, those without symptoms but with a history of NP SLE, and those with neither symptoms nor history. QEEG was abnormal in 74% of patients with active symptoms and in 28% of those with neither symptoms nor history. The investigators did not evaluate their subjects' response to treatment; therefore, it is unknown whether adding QEEG to clinical evaluation and magnetic resonance imaging

Table 4–7. Diseases and conditions associated with positive antinuclear antibody

Lupus erythematosus	Primary pulmonary fibrosis
Sjögren's syndrome	Vasculitis
Rheumatoid arthritis	Dermatomyositis/polymyositis
Juvenile arthritis	Mixed connective tissue disease
Leprosy	Mixed cryoglobulinemia
Infectious mononucleosis	Aging
Scleroderma	Medications
Liver disease	

Source. Peter Schur, M.D.

Table 4–8. Autoantibodies in patients with systemic lupus erythematosus

Test	Sensitivity (%)	Specificity (%)	Predictive value (%)
Antinuclear antibody	99	80	15–35
dsDNA	70	95	95
ssDNA	80	50	50
Histone	30–80	Moderate	Moderate
Nucleoprotein	58	Moderate	Moderate
Sm	25	99	97
RNP (U1RNP)	50	87–94	46–85
Ro (SS-A)	25–35		
La (SS-B)	15		
PCNA	5	95	95

Source. Adapted from Peter Schur, M.D.

Table 4–9. Usefulness of diagnostic tests in neuropsychiatric evaluation

	Specific serology		Brain imaging					Neuropsychological testing
	Antineuronal, anti-Ribo-P, etc.	Anticardiolipin, diolipin, etc.	CT	MRI	SPECT	LP	EEG	
Psychosis	+++	+	+	+++	+++	++	+	++
Seizures	+	++	++	+++	+++	++	+++	+
Depression	+++	+	+	+	++	+	+	+
Delirium	++	++	+	++	+++	+++	+++	+
Coma	++	++	+	++	+++	+++	+++	+
Cognitive disturbance (memory, concentration)	++	+	+	+	+++	+	++	+++
Fatigue	+	+	+	+	++	+	+	++
Focal CNS (stroke)	+	+++	++	+++	+++	++	++	+

Note. CT = computed tomography; MRI = magnetic resonance imaging; SPECT = single photon-emission computed tomography; LP = lumbar puncture; EEG = electroencephalogram; CNS = central nervous system.

(MRI) would improve the clinician's ability to decide on treatment in patients with SLE and NP symptoms.

Neuropsychological Testing

Neuropsychological testing may be one of the most sensitive indices of subtle or even asymptomatic NP SLE. It also has the advantage of being more directly relevant to the functional and behavioral capacity of the patient. Tests like Bender Gestalt (with immediate and delayed recall), trail making, and verbal fluency usually are easily administered; the Wechsler Adult Intelligence Scale-Revised (WAIS-R) (Wechsler 1987), readily accessible in most clinical settings, is a sensitive screen for nonmemory focal deficits, if the pattern of subtest scores is analyzed and the patient's qualitative approach to the items is carefully observed and recorded.

Brain Imaging

The principal brain imaging tests available are computed tomography (CT) scan, MRI scan, single photon-emission computed tomography (SPECT) scan, and, in some locations, PET scans.

CT scans. When CT scans were introduced in the late 1970s, they represented a major advance. They continue to be a rapid, noninvasive, and relatively inexpensive method for examining brain structures. One of the initial studies reported that long-term steroid users show varying degrees of cerebral atrophy, which, in some cases, improves after a decrease or discontinuation of steroid use; this remains a useful observation (Bentson et al. 1978). There have also been unusual CNS lupus findings, such as calcification in paraventricular areas, for which CT scans may be most useful (Daud and Nuruddin 1988). CT scans continue to have an important role in identifying the presence of hemorrhage or cerebral infarction in an emergent situation (Marstellar et al. 1987). Also, the CT scan is the quickest way to exclude a mass lesion before performing a lumbar puncture in a patient suspected of having meningitis. However, the MRI is the imaging procedure of first choice for the patient with SLE undergoing assessment for brain involvement.

MRIs. With the increased use of MRI in the mid- to late 1980s, the greater sensitivity of MRIs over CT scans in the identification of CNS lupus has clearly emerged (Aisen et al. 1985; Baum et al. 1993; Bell et al. 1991; Miller et al. 1989; Schott et al. 1990; Sibbitt et al. 1989). MRI can demonstrate reversibility of some lesions of CNS lupus. At least three different patterns of disease can be demonstrated by MRI: cerebral infarction, multiple small areas of increased intensity secondary to microinfarctions, and focal areas of increased intensity in the cerebral gray matter.

In one dramatic comparison of MRI versus CT scans (Jacobs et al. 1988), the brains of 13 patients who had experienced signs and symptoms of encephalopathy were examined at autopsy. All patients had had normal CT scans. Four patients with abnormal MRI studies had active CNS disease; however, none of the 9 patients with normal MRI scans did. In another comparison, McCune and co-workers (1988) showed that MRI scans were more likely to show definite focal lesions in patients with clinically localized neurologic deficits or seizures. Overall, focal brain lesions were identified in 53% of 30 well-documented acute NP events, a level of sensitivity replicated in a comparison study (Stimmler et al. 1993) of 51 hospitalized SLE patients. In the latter study, there were 64 separate CNS episodes—two-thirds were attributable to NP SLE and one-third to causes other than SLE. Once again, MRI abnormalities were twice as likely to be found in patients with focal neurologic deficits (73%) than in those without such focal findings (39%). Interestingly, they were also twice as likely to be found in patients with nephritis (79%) than in those without nephritis (38%). MRI abnormalities were equally common in the patients with NP SLE and the patients with other causes for their episodes (e.g., stroke or meningitis). In addition to periventricular increased signal activity, which had been a frequent finding in other MRI studies, enlargement of the prepontine cistern was noted for the first time. Enlargement of this CSF space was previously reported in elderly adults with risk factors for stroke. Both of these findings were associated with the presence of hypertension and lupus nephritis.

Baum and associates (1993) found a 76% prevalence of abnormal MRIs in a consecutive series of 21 outpatients with SLE, unselected for NP symptoms or signs. Twelve patients had focal lesions, mainly in the frontal lobes. More lesions were found in patients with focal signs than in those without them. Ten patients had periventricular hyperintensities. Seven patients with abnormal MRIs had no NP symptoms. Eleven patients had NP symptoms or signs; these were not clearly correlated with MRI findings. Thus, MRI does not in itself confirm or exclude CNS involvement with SLE. It may, however, confirm that a structural abnormality underlies a focal symptom or sign, or exclude some specific complications such as an infarct or abscess.

In conclusion, MRI frequently fails to show abnormalities in diffuse, nonfocal, or subtle CNS lupus, but it is sensitive to focal lesions large enough to produce clear-cut localizing signs on neurologic or cognitive examination.

SPECT scans. Earlier studies of cerebral blood flow (CBF) with oxygen-15 (Pinching et al. 1978) and xenon-133 (Kushner et al. 1987) showed defects in more than three-quarters of patients with known CNS lupus and in many patients who did not have clinically apparent CNS disease. Furthermore, changes during the course of the disease were readily apparent in these scans. CBF seemed least affected in patients with symptoms such as headache or malaise. Those with confusion or psychosis exhibited the greatest reduction in CBF.

Following up on the apparent usefulness of earlier techniques for measuring blood flow, several groups of investigators examined current SPECT scanning technology to evaluate its role in CNS lupus. In the first of these studies, Nossent and colleagues (1991) investigated 20 lupus patients with clinical evidence of cerebral involvement who were also studied with CT scans and serologic tests. Overall, 75% of these patients showed definite regional hypoperfusion. Of the patients who were thought to have active cerebral lupus involvement at the time of the study, 88% had abnormal SPECT scan results. However, the correlation between SPECT findings, CT scan results, overall disease activity, and serologic findings was poor.

Rogers and co-investigators (1992) observed lupus patients showing subtle cognitive and affective changes with SPECT technology using [^{123}I]iodoamphetamine. Eight (44%) of the 18 scans were abnormal, 4 in a diffuse bilateral temporal-parietal pattern previously noted only in Alzheimer's disease. Four had large focal deficits. Neither the existence of the abnormal scan nor the particular pattern of abnormality correlated with the results of other diagnostic tests, however. These preliminary results raised the possibility that SPECT scans might be useful as an additional diagnostic instrument in CNS lupus, particularly in more diffuse and subclinical presentations.

A study by Rubbert and colleagues (1993) reaffirmed the usefulness of SPECT scans but again noted difficulties in correlating the results with the disease activity and serologic findings. They grouped

35 SLE patients into categories—those without NP symptoms, those with definite cognitive deficits or abnormalities on neurological examination, and those with mild symptoms such as headache or memory disturbance. The SPECT scans were classified as either normal, focal, or diffuse. The results showed that SPECT findings were *normal* in 90% of patients *without* CNS symptoms and *abnormal* in 90% of patients *with* overt signs of brain involvement (e.g., with motor or sensory deficits). Seventy-three percent of patients with mild symptoms had abnormal SPECT findings. The majority of the abnormal scans in this group showed focal lesions. These results again suggest that in mild or subtle NP symptoms, without focal NP symptoms or seizures, SPECT scans can be a useful adjunct to MRI.

PET scans.   PET has also been used, in a research context, to demonstrate changes in the CNS of lupus patients. PET scans can assess both CBF and glucose metabolism, both of which have been shown to be abnormal in some patients with NP SLE (Volkow et al. 1988). In one of the four patients in the study by Volkow and others, the PET scan showed improvement after NP recovery, as in the three patients in the report by Carbotte and co-workers (1992) cited earlier in this chapter. Additional studies in the German literature have compared PET scans with other imaging methods (Meyer et al. 1989; Stoppe et al. 1989, 1990). PET scans with fluorodeoxyglucose (FDG) were more sensitive in demonstrating reversible deficits than MRI scans. Meyer and colleagues (1989) concluded that a combination of a PET scan and an MRI constituted the most sensitive diagnostic procedure for NP SLE. However, PET scans are not generally available in the United States. Their high cost and limited availability preclude their routine use in clinical diagnosis of NP SLE.

SEARCH FOR SPECIFIC ANTIBODIES IN NEUROPSYCHIATRIC SYSTEMIC LUPUS ERYTHEMATOSUS

There has been considerable interest in discovering antibodies or other specific immunologic parameters specific to NP lupus. Experience and systematic studies have established that serologic tests are valuable but are not reliable as diagnostic tests for NP SLE. We review some useful serologic tests.

Some patients with lupus erythematosus have antibodies reactive to erythrocytes, lymphocytes, and neurons (Bresnihan et al. 1979). In the study by Bresnihan and colleagues, 11 (92%) of the 12 patients with NP disease had positive antineuronal antibodies, in contrast to 20% of those without evidence of NP involvement.

Bluestein and his group (1981) confirmed these findings. They found increased immunoglobulin G (IgG) antineuronal activity in 20 (74%) of 27 patients with active CNS involvement versus only 2 (11%) of 18 without CNS involvement. Furthermore, they found that patients with more diffuse CNS involvement such as psychosis, encephalopathy, or generalized seizures were far more likely to have increased antineuronal activity than patients with focal lesions such as hemiparesis or chorea (90% versus 25%, respectively).

In 1985, a group from McMaster University performed clinical investigations of a similar nature (How et al. 1985). They used a standardized definition of NP SLE and tested sera from 54 SLE patients and 77 control subjects. The binding of these antibodies was tested against three neuroblastoma and three glioblastoma cell lines. Fifty-five percent of SLE patients with NP SLE had serum binding activity to both the neuroblastoma and glioblastoma cell lines, compared with only 33% of the other SLE patients. The reactivity toward the neuroblastoma cell lines was three times more likely among the NP SLE patient group. Similar to the results of Bluestein and co-workers (1981), NP SLE patients with more diffuse symptomatology had a higher mean titer of neuroblastoma cell line binding than those with focal symptomatology.

Later, others found a significant association between lupus psychosis and another antibody, the antiribosomal P protein (Bonfa et al. 1987). The most interesting aspect of this study was the high degree of correlation between psychosis, but not other CNS manifestations of SLE, and antibody activity against ribosomal P protein. Eighteen (90%) of 20 inpatients with SLE-related psychosis had antiribosomal P protein autoantibodies versus only 3 (15%) of 20 with other nonpsychotic CNS manifestations. Furthermore, levels of these antibodies, also known as anti-P peptide, increased from 5- to 30-fold before and during the active phases of psychosis but not during sepsis or other exacerbations of SLE.

The correlation between IgG antineuronal antibodies and cognitive impairment or nonfocal NP SLE (J. A. Denburg et al. 1987) suggests that there may be specific autoantibody CNS disturbances in specific subtypes of NP SLE. Their investigations suggested that CSF antineuronal antibodies cross a damaged blood-brain barrier (Kelly and Denburg

1987). They found that in patients with SLE, CSF antineuronal antibodies occurred only when serum antineuronal antibodies were present.

A number of studies have identified other specific antibodies in connection with NP SLE: antineurofilament antibody (Robbins et al. 1988), anticardiolipin (ACL) antibodies (Herkes et al. 1988), antiphospholipid antibodies (Asherson and Lubbe 1988), antiganglioside and antigalectocerebroside antibodies (Costallat et al. 1990), anti-CNS antibodies (Klein et al. 1991), and anti-dsDNA/anti-ssDNA antibodies (Senaga and Abdou 1992). So many different specific antibodies have been related to CNS lupus, and so many different assay methods have been proposed, that one author suggested the creation of a library of antigens for testing for the presence of these autoantibodies (Khin and Hoffman 1993).

In certain patients with SLE, ACL antibodies have been associated with thromboembolic phenomena including stroke. One group of investigators (Fields et al. 1990) demonstrated a relationship between MRI evidence of infarctlike lesions and the presence of ACL antibodies. The ACLs are one of a group of antiphospholipid antibodies that include the somewhat misnamed *lupus anticoagulant* (LA). Most of these antibodies occur in SLE but are less commonly detected than in other diseases. A review of the clinical and immunologic features of patients with abnormal ACL antibodies, many without SLE, indicated that stroke and migraine dominated the clinical picture, suggesting the presence of a hypercoagulable state (Chancellor et al. 1991).

Most studies, despite some notable exceptions (Blaser et al. 1993; Hanly et al. 1993; Teh et al. 1992), have supported earlier findings of an association between more diffuse psychiatric symptomatology and antineuronal antibodies (Amital-Teplizki et al. 1992; Chen et al. 1990; Pereira et al. 1992; Schneebaum et al. 1991). Schneebaum's group also noted increased antiribosomal P protein antibodies in SLE patients with NP symptoms. Overall, 19% of 269 patients with SLE had elevated levels of IgG or IgM anti-P antibodies (Schneebaum et al. 1991). Twice as many patients with NP manifestations had elevated antibody ribosomal P antibodies. Furthermore, the frequency of positive test results varied according to the specific nature of CNS involvement. Interestingly, patients with severe depression had the highest association: 88% versus 45% for patients with psychosis. This observation supports the view that depression can be a direct manifestation of brain involvement with SLE.

Unfortunately, there have also been some disappointments and contradictory findings in the efforts to correlate various autoantibodies and NP manifestations of lupus. Hanly and colleagues (1993) studied cognitive abnormalities and a variety of autoantibodies, including antibodies to surface neuronal and lymphocyte antigens, antiribosomal P antibodies, and ACL antibodies. Cognitive impairment was identified in 21% of SLE patients versus 4% of rheumatoid arthritis patients and 4% of healthy subjects. There was no significant difference in the prevalence of antineuronal antibodies, lymphocytotoxic antibodies, anti-P antibodies, or ACL antibodies in the cognitively impaired versus the unimpaired SLE patients. The investigators concluded that the autoantibodies that have been shown to be associated with nervous system manifestations are not likely to be directly involved in the pathogenesis of cognitive dysfunction. This contradicts the results of earlier research (How et al. 1985). Another study failed to demonstrate an association between antiphospholipid antibodies and NP disorders in patients with SLE (Blaser et al. 1993). Antiphospholipid antibodies are currently significant because they are a risk factor for stroke. Aspirin and, in some cases, warfarin are given to mitigate this risk.

Single measurements of anti-P antibody levels in relation to psychosis in SLE are limited (Derkson et al. 1990). The autoantibody levels of two siblings with SLE, both of whom had experienced two episodes of psychosis, were closely followed. In two of three 15-week periods antedating psychosis, anti-P levels rose, then spontaneously dropped. However, in the third period, antibodies to ribosomal protein P were absent. Thus, the presence or absence of anti-P ribosomal antibodies has limited value in predicting the onset of psychosis, and the result of a test for anti-P antibodies may vary according to the precise occasion of testing. This study points out the difference between finding significant correlations and associations in groups of patients and demonstrating diagnostic usefulness of the test for a specific patient in a given clinical situation. The issue is similar to the contrast between the often-replicated finding of ventricular enlargement in schizophrenic patients and the lack of demonstrated clinical utility of ventricular measurement in individual patients with psychosis.

The preponderance of evidence demonstrates some association between a variety of antibodies generally reactive to neural antigens and NP manifestations of SLE. Specific antibodies may correlate with specific subtypes of CNS lupus. Elevations in antiphospholipid or ACL and lupus coagulant antibodies appear to be linked most frequently with cerebral infarctions or stroke (i.e., macrovascular disease), although one report links them to decreased CBF in SLE patients without focal lesions on CT (Maeshima et al. 1993). However, more diffuse manifestations, such as psychosis, diffuse cognitive impairment, and, in at least some reports, depression, have been linked with changes in antineuronal antibodies and antiribosomal P antibodies. It appears that these antibodies do not arise in the CNS; they are systemic (i.e., serum) antibodies that cross a damaged blood-brain barrier.

Although these changes are likely to be of further benefit in research on the underlying pathophysiology of CNS lupus, they are not diagnostically accurate in specific clinical situations. Currently, we do not recommend determination of antineuronal or anti-P antibodies as diagnostic tests for NP SLE. Measurements of serum antiphospholipid antibodies are indicated in the evaluation of stroke in young women, whether or not they are known to have SLE. They should not, however, be used as a test to confirm or exclude NP SLE.

We have attempted to give an overview of the various NP manifestations and the most useful diagnostic tools to help sort them out. Table 4–9 outlines the differential diagnostic usefulness of various serologic and brain imaging tests in the assessment of CNS lupus.

TREATMENT ISSUES

Support groups for patients who have SLE contribute to feelings of empowerment, diminish unnecessary stress, and help patients maintain their quality of life. Such self-help programs lessen patients' depression and anxiety and improve functional capacity (Braden et al. 1993). In our experience, many patients also benefit from individual psychotherapy focused on adjusting their life to the exigencies of the disease and maintaining a sense of hopefulness about the future. Many patients struggle with issues regarding the life-threatening danger of lupus, its impact on their appearance, and its effects on intimate relationships, independence, and pregnancy or plans for pregnancy. All patients with SLE must tolerate considerable uncertainty. Developing the capacity to bear uncertainty frequently is a focus of individual therapy.

NEUROPSYCHIATRIC SYNDROMES

There are a variety of specific treatments for the identified NP problems. Treatment of the underlying SLE is obviously also important (Table 4–10) but generally does not eliminate the need for other specific medications. Seizures require antiepileptic drugs. Psychosis, whatever its etiology, resolves more rapidly with neuroleptics, which should be given in the conservative dosages typically used in "organic" psychoses. Anxiety and insomnia may require benzodiazepines; psychotic patients who are agitated often respond well to a benzodiazepine-neuroleptic combination. Depression of clinical severity may be treated with any of several antidepressants, although bupropion is avoided because of the high incidence of seizures in patients with SLE.

A more controversial issue is whether to use "full-strength" immunosuppressive therapy for suspected CNS lupus associated with cognitive impairment or depression alone. Our general recommendation is to use corticosteroids or other immunosuppressive drugs only for more severe manifestations of CNS lupus, such as psychosis and seizures. Of course, neuroleptics or antiepileptics could be given concurrently. Patients with less severe NP syndromes might also benefit from steroids, but the potential side effects of corticosteroids or immunosuppressive therapy usually outweigh the potential benefits of treat-

Table 4–10. Treatment of specific problems in lupus

Fever: NSAID → Antimalarials → Steroids

Arthralgia/myalgia: NSAID → Acetaminophen → Nortriptyline

Arthritis: NSAID → Antimalarials → Steroids (alternate day) or Methotrexate

Rashes: Sunscreens → Topical steroids → Antimalarials → Steroids

Oral ulcers: Antimalarials

Raynaud's disease: No smoking, caffeine, decongestants → Warm clothing → Biofeedback → (Long-acting) nifedipine → Prazosin

Serositis: Indomethacin → Steroids

Pulmonary: Steroids

Hypertension: Diuretics-ACE inhibitors-Calcium channel blockers-β-blockers-Vasodilators, etc.

Thrombocytopenia/hemolytic anemia: Steroids → Intravenous γ-globulin → Immunosuppressives → Splenectomy

Renal disease: Steroids → Pulse steroids → Immunosuppressives

CNS disease: Organic: Steroids → Antiseizure → Immunosuppressives

---

Note. Arrows refer to initial, or most conservative, treatments and the sequence of progression to more advanced treatment strategies. NSAID = nonsteroidal antiinflammatory drug; ACE = angiotensin-converting enzyme; CNS = central nervous system.
Source. Peter Schur, M.D.

ment. The balance of risks and benefits should, however, be individualized. When cognitive impairment is disabling and the patient has a history of tolerating steroids well, high-dose steroids may be appropriate.

There are no particular restrictions on the choices of psychotropic medications to treat the psychopathology in lupus patients. Severely depressed patients have benefited from antidepressant medications and ECT (Fricchione et al. 1990). A report in the literature stated that fluoxetine was associated with extrapyramidal symptoms in a CNS lupus patient (Fallon and Liebowitz 1991); it is unclear whether lupus causes any unique vulnerability to fluoxetine side effects (see Chapter 2). Sodium valproate has been reported in several cases to have a beneficial effect on NP manifestations of SLE (Kahn et al. 1988).

PSYCHIATRIC EFFECTS OF LUPUS MEDICATIONS

Corticosteroids are the most frequently used immunosuppressant for patients with lupus. In a small percentage of patients given high doses of steroids, a drug-induced psychosis occurs. More commonly, steroids produce modest changes in mood, frequently comprising emotional lability, a low-grade hypomania, anxiety, and insomnia. Steroid-induced psychosis accounts for a very small percentage of psychosis seen in lupus patients. The antimalarial drug hydroxychloroquine, used as an adjunct to steroids or as treatment for mild cases, occasionally has been associated with the development of psychotic symptoms.

Most patients with lupus who present with psychotic symptoms have active CNS involvement and should be treated medically on that basis. While appropriate medical therapy is being rendered, low doses of neuroleptics may be used, keeping in mind that, like other patients with CNS disease, patients with CNS lupus will likely be more sensitive to neuroleptic side effects such as extrapyramidal symptoms and sedation. Neuroleptic medication should be rapidly tapered as the patient's brain disease responds to medical treatment.

SUMMARY

The following "clinical pearls" summarize a number of critical diagnostic and treatment principles garnered from our clinical experience in treating this patient population:

- In lupus patients, sudden mental status changes are presumed to be due to active CNS lupus or other medical causes (such as infections) until proven otherwise.
- In patients with SLE, brain involvement is *far more likely* to be the cause of psychosis than side effects of steroids.
- If a lupus patient has a fever and a mental status change, a lumbar puncture should be done to rule out meningitis. Long-term steroids or other immunosuppressive drugs add to the risk of developing or accelerating a preexisting infection.
- If seizures or specific localizing neurologic signs occur, an MRI is indicated.
- ACL and antiphospholipid antibodies are most likely to be positive in the presence of localizing neurological findings.
- Anticoagulants, either low-dose aspirin or warfarin, are recommended therapies for the antiphospholipid syndrome.
- SPECT scans are of particular value in showing brain change in psychosis and cognitive disturbance and may be abnormal in patients with a normal MRI.
- The more prolonged the psychosis, the higher the likelihood of residual cognitive impairment.
- Cognitive changes associated with CNS lupus often are not reversible.
- If a patient complains of problems with cognitive function, he or she likely has low-grade cerebral involvement even if the initial diagnostic workup shows no abnormality.
- Neuropsychological testing is probably the most sensitive test for CNS lupus but may yield a number of false-positive findings.
- Mood problems in patients with SLE respond better to treatment than cognitive problems, which may persist despite treatment, or improve only slowly.
- Depression can be the first sign of CNS lupus.
- Early diagnosis is better than ongoing denial; early treatment improves the prognosis of the illness.

REFERENCES

Aisen AM, Gabrielsen PO, McCune WJ: MR imaging of systemic lupus erythematosus involving the brain. AJR Am J Roentgenol 144:1027–1031, 1985

Amital-Teplizki H, Shoenfeld Y: Chorea: rare expression of neuropsychiatric manifestation of systemic lupus erythematosus. Isr J Med Sci 25:549–551, 1989

Amital-Teplizki H, Bearman JE, Miele PW Jr, et al: A multidimensional autoantibody analysis specifying systemic lupus erythematosus patients with neuropsychiatric symptomatology. Isr J Med Sci 28:422–427, 1992

Anfinson TJ, Kathol RG: Laboratory and neuroendocrine assessment in medical-psychiatric patients, in Psychiatric Care of the Medical Patient. Edited by Stoudemire A, Fogel BS. New York, Oxford University Press, 1993, pp 105–137

Asherson RA, Lubbe WF: Cerebral and valve lesions in SLE: association with antiphospholipid antibodies. J Rheumatol 15:539–543, 1988

Baum KA, Hopf U, Nehrig C: Systemic lupus erythematosus: neuropsychiatric signs and symptoms related to cerebral MRI findings. Clin Neurol Neurosurg 95:29–34, 1993

Bell CL, Partington C, Robbins M: Magnetic resonance imaging of central nervous system lesions in patients with lupus erythematosus: correlation with clinical remission and antineurofilament and anticardiolipin antibody titers. Arthritis Rheum 34:432–441, 1991

Bentson J, Reza M, Winter J, et al: Steroids and apparent cerebral atrophy on computed tomography scans. J Comput Assist Tomogr 2:16–23, 1978

Blaser KU, Khamashta MA, Herranz MT, et al: Psychiatric disorders in patients with systemic lupus erythematosus: lack of association with antiphospholipid antibodies. Br J Rheumatol 32:646–647, 1993

Bluestein HG, Williams GW, Steinberg AD: Cerebrospinal fluid antibodies to neuronal cells: association with neuropsychiatric manifestations of systemic lupus erythematosus. Am J Med 70:240–246, 1981

Bonfa E, Golombek SJ, Kaufman LD, et al: Association between lupus psychosis and anti-ribosomal P protein antibodies. N Engl J Med 317:265–271, 1987

Braden CJ, McGlone K, Pennington F: Specific psychosocial and behavioral outcomes from the systemic lupus erythematosus self-help course. Health Educ Q 20:29–41, 1993

Bresnihan B, Oliver M, Williams B, et al: An anti-neuronal antibody cross-reacting with erythrocytes and lymphocytes in systemic lupus erythematosus. Arthritis Rheum 22:313–320, 1979

Carbotte RM, Denburg SD, Denburg JA: Prevalence of cognitive impairment in systemic lupus erythematosus. J Nerv Ment Dis 174:357–364, 1986

Carbotte RM, Denburg SD, Denburg JA, et al: Fluctuating cognitive abnormalities and cerebral glucose metabolism in neuropsychiatric systemic lupus erythematosus. J Neurol Neurosurg Psychiatry 55:1054–1059, 1992

Chancellor AM, Cull RE, Kilpatrick DC, et al: Neurological disease associated with anticardiolipin antibodies in patients without systemic lupus erythematosus: clinical and immunological features. J Neurol 238:401–407, 1991

Chen WZ, Zhang NZ, Jiang M: Antineuronal antibodies in neuropsychiatric systemic lupus erythematosus. Chung Hua Nei Ko Tsa Chih 29:161–164, 1990

Costallat LT, de Oliveira RM, Santiago MB, et al: Neuropsychiatric manifestations of systemic lupus erythematosus: the value of anticardiolipin, antigangliosides and antigalactocerebrosides antibodies. Clin Rheumatol 9:489–497, 1990

Daud AB, Nuruddin RN: Solitary paraventricular calcification in cerebral lupus erythematosus: a report of two cases. Neuroradiology 30:84–85, 1988

Denburg JA, Carbotte RM, Denburg SD: Neuronal antibodies and cognitive function in systemic lupus erythematosus. Neurology 37:464–467, 1987

Denburg SD, Carbotte RM, Denburg JA: Cognitive impairment in systemic lupus: a neuropsychological study of individual and group deficits. J Clin Exp Neuropsychol 9:323–339, 1987

Denburg SD, Denburg JA, Carbotte RM, et al: Cognitive deficits in systemic lupus erythematosus. Rheum Dis Clin North Am 19:815–831, 1993

Dennis MS, Byrne EJ, Hopkinson N, et al: Neuropsychiatric systemic lupus erythematosus in elderly people: a case series. J Neurol Neurosurg Psychiatry 55:1157–1161, 1992

Derksen RH, van Dam AP, Gmelig Meyling FH, et al: A prospective study on antiribosomal P proteins in two cases of familial lupus and recurrent psychosis. Ann Rheum Dis 49:779–782, 1990

Fallon BA, Liebowitz MR: Fluoxetine and extrapyramidal symptoms in CNS lupus. J Clin Psychopharmacol 11:147–148, 1991

Feinglass EJ, Arnett FC, Dorsch CA, et al: Neuropsychiatric manifestations of systemic lupus erythematosus: diagnosis, clinical spectrum, and relationship to other features of the disease. Medicine 55:323–339, 1976

Ferstl R, Niemann P, Biehl G, et al: Neuropsychological impairment in autoimmune disease. Eur J Clin Invest 22 (suppl I):16–20, 1992

Fields RA, Sibbitt WL, Toubbeh H, et al: Neuropsychiatric lupus erythematosus, cerebral infarctions, and anticardiolipin antibodies. Ann Rheum Dis 49:114–117, 1990

Fricchione GL, Kaufman LD, Gruber BL, et al: Electroconvulsive therapy and cyclophosphamide in combination for severe neuropsychiatric lupus with catatonia. Am J Med 88:442–443, 1990

Futrell N, Schultz LR, Millikan C: Central nervous system disease in patients with systemic lupus erythematosus. Neurology 42:1649–1657, 1992

Ginsburg KS, Wright EA, Larson MG, et al: A controlled study of the prevalence of cognitive dysfunction in randomly suggested patients with systemic lupus erythematosus. Arthritis Rheum 35:776–782, 1992

Griner PF, Mayewski RJ, Mushlin AI, et al: Selection and interpretation of diagnostic tests and procedures: principles and applications. Ann Intern Med 94:557–592, 1981

Hahn BH: Systemic lupus erythematosus, in Harrison's Principles of Internal Medicine, 11th Edition. Edited by Braunwald E, Isselbacher KJ, Petersdorf RG, et al. New York, McGraw-Hill, 1987, pp 1418–1423

Hanly JG, Walsh NM, Fisk JD, et al: Cognitive impairment and autoantibodies in systemic lupus erythematosus. Br J Rheumatol 32:291–296, 1993

Herkes GK, Cohen MG, Podgorski M, et al: Cerebral systemic lupus erythema-tosus with apnea in a patient with cardiolipin antibodies and oligoclonal bands. J Rheumatol 15:523–524, 1988

Hochberg MC: The epidemiology of systemic lupus erythematosus, in Dubois' Lupus Erythematosus, 4th Edition. Edited by Wallace DJ, Hahn BH. Phila-delphia, PA, Lea & Febiger, 1993, pp 49–53

How A, Dent TB, Liao SK, et al: Antineuronal antibodies in neuropsychiatric systemic lupus erythematosus. Arthritis Rheum 28:789–795, 1985

Iverson GL: Psychopathology associated with systemic lupus erythematosus: a methodological review. Semin Arthritis Rheum 22:242–251, 1993

Iverson GL, McCracken LM: Attributing psychopathology to systemic lupus erythematosus: some methodological considerations. Ann Rheum Dis 51:134–135, 1992

Jacobs L, Kinkel PR, Costello PB, et al: Central nervous system lupus erythema-tosus: the value of magnetic resonance imaging. J Rheumatol 15:601–606, 1988

Kahn D, Stevenson E, Douglas CJ: Effect of sodium valproate in three patients with organic brain syndromes. Am J Psychiatry 145:1010–1011, 1988

Kaye BR, Neuwelt CM, London SS, et al: Central nervous system systemic lupus erythematosus mimicking progressive multi-focal leucoencephalop-athy. Ann Rheum Dis 51:1152–1156, 1992

Kelly MC, Denburg JA: Cerebrospinal fluid immunoglobulins and neuronal antibodies in neuropsychiatric systemic lupus erythematosus and related conditions. J Rheumatol 14:740–744, 1987

Khin NA, Hoffman SA: Brain reactive monoclonal autoantibodies: production and characterization. J Neuroimmunol 44:137–148, 1993

Klein R, Richter C, Berg PA: Antibodies against central nervous system tissue (anti-CNS) detected by ELISA and Western blotting: marker antibodies for neuropsychiatric manifestations in connective tissue diseases. Autoimmu-nity 10:133–144, 1991

Kushner MJ, Chawluk J, Fazekas F, et al: Cerebral blood flow in systemic lupus erythematosus with or without cerebral complications. Neurology 37:1596–1598, 1987

Lim LC, Ron MA, Ormenod IE, et al: Psychiatric and neurological manifesta-tions in systemic lupus erythematosus. Q J Med 249:27–38, 1988

Mac DS, Pardo MP: Systemic lupus erythematosus and catatonia: a case report. J Clin Psychiatry 44:155–156, 1983

Maeshima E, Maeshima S, Yamada Y, et al: Antiphospholipid antibodies and regional cerebral blood flow in systemic lupus erythematosus. Ryumachi 33:125–130, 1993

Mannik M, Gilliland BC: Systemic lupus erythematosus, in Harrison's Princi-ples of Internal Medicine, 7th Edition. Edited by Wintrob MM, Thorn GW, Adams R, et al. New York, McGraw-Hill, 1974, pp 385–390

Marstellar LP, Marstellar HB, Braun A, et al: An unusual CT appearance cere-brates. AJNR 8:737–739, 1987

Mavrikakis ME, Antoniades LG, Germanides JB, et al: Organic brain syndrome with psychosis as an initial manifestation of systemic lupus erythematosus in an elderly woman. Ann Rheum Dis 51:117–119, 1992

McCune WJ, Golbus J: Neuropsychiatric lupus. Rheum Dis Clin North Am 14:149–167, 1988

McCune WJ, MacGuire A, Aisen A, et al: Identification of brain lesions in neuropsychiatric systemic lupus erythematosus by magnetic resonance scanning. Arthritis Rheum 31:159–166, 1988

McNamara ME: Advances in EEG-based diagnostic technologies, in Medical-Psychiatric Practice, Volume 1. Edited by Stoudemire A, Fogel BS. Washington, DC, American Psychiatric Press, 1991, pp 163–192

Meyer GJ, Schober O, Stoppe G, et al: Cerebral involvement in systemic lupus erythematosus (SLE): comparison of positron emission tomography (PET) with other imaging methods. Psychiatry Res 29:367–368, 1989

Miller BH, Johnson G, Tofts PS, et al: Precise relaxation time requirements of normal appearing white matter in inflammatory central nervous system disease. Magn Reson Med 11:331–336, 1989

Mitchell WD, Thompson TL: Psychiatric distress in systemic lupus erythematosus outpatients. Psychosomatics 31:293–300, 1990

Mulherin D, Doherty E, O'Connell A, et al: Assessment of cognitive function in patients with systemic lupus erythematosus. Ir J Med Sci 162:9–12, 1993

Nossent JC, Hovestadt A, Schonfeld DH, et al: Single photon emission computed tomography of the brain in the evaluation of cerebral lupus. Arthritis Rheum 34:1397–1403, 1991

Pereira RM, Yoshinari NH, De Oliveira RM, et al: Antiganglioside antibodies in patients with neuropsychiatric systemic erythematosus. Lupus 1:175–179, 1992

Pinching AJ, Travers RL, Hughes GR, et al: Oxygen-15 brain scanning for detection of cerebral involvement in systemic lupus erythematosus. Lancet 1:898–900, 1978

Ravindran A, Carney MW, Denman AM: Systemic lupus erythematosus presenting as morbid jealousy. Postgrad Med J 56:419–420, 1980

Robbins ML, Kornguth SE, Bell CL, et al: Antineuro filament antibody evaluation in neuropsychiatric systemic lupus erythematosus: combination with anticardiolipin antibody assay and magnetic resonance imaging. Arthritis Rheum 31:623–631, 1988

Rogers MP, Waterhouse E, Nagel JS, et al: I-123 iofetamine SPECT scan in systemic lupus erythematosus patients with cognitive and other minor neuropsychiatric symptoms: a pilot study. Lupus 1:215–219, 1992

Rubbert A, Marienhagen J, Pirner K, et al: Single photon emission computed tomography analysis of cerebral blood flow in the evaluation of central nervous system involvement in patients with systemic lupus erythematosus. Arthritis Rheum 36:1253–1262, 1993

Schneebaum AB, Singleton JD, West SG, et al: Association of psychiatric manifestations of antibodies to ribosomal P proteins in systemic lupus erythematosus. Am J Med 90:54–62, 1991

Schott AM, Colson F, Tebid J, et al: Imagerie en resonance magnetique et neurolupus [Magnetic resonance imaging and (central) nervous system lupus]. Rev Rhum Mal Osteoartic 57:785–790, 1990

Senaga R, Abdou NI: Expression of inactive stage anti-dsDNA idiotypes on anti-ssDNA antibodies in a lupus patient during active stage of lupus cerebritis. J Autoimmun 5:379–392, 1992

Sibbitt WL Jr, Sibbitt RR, Griffey RH, et al: Magnetic resonance and computed tomographic imaging in the evaluation of acute neuropsychiatric disease in systemic lupus erythematosus. Ann Rheum Dis 48:1014–1022, 1989

Singer J, Denburg JA: Diagnostic criteria for neuropsychiatric systemic lupus erythematosus: the results of a consensus meeting. The Ad Hoc Neuropsychiatric Lupus Workshop Group. J Rheumatol 17:1397–1402, 1990

Stimmler MM, Coletti PM, Quismorio FP Jr: Magnetic resonance imaging of the brain in neuropsychiatric systemic lupus erythematosus. Semin Arthritis Rheum 22:335–349, 1993

Stoppe G, Wildhagen K, Meyer GJ, et al: Use of fluoro-deoxyglucose PET in the diagnosis of central nervous system lupus erythematosus and a comparison with CT and MRI. Nuklearmedizin 28:187–192, 1989

Stoppe G, Wildhagen K, Seidel JW, et al: Positron emission tomography in neuropsychiatric lupus erythematosus. Neurology 40:304–308, 1990

Talbot JH: Historical background of discoid and systemic lupus erythematosus, in Dubois' Lupus Erythematosus, 4th Edition. Edited by Wallace DJ, Hahn BH. Philadelphia, PA, Lea & Febiger, 1993, pp 3–6

Tan EM, Cohen AS, Fries JF, et al: The 1982 revised criteria for the classification of SLE. Arthritis Rheum 25:1271, 1982

Teh LS, Bedwell AE, Isenberg DA, et al: Antibodies to protein P in systemic lupus erythematosus. Ann Rheum Dis 51:489–494, 1992

van Dam AP, Wekking EM, Oomen AJ: Psychiatric symptoms as features of systemic lupus erythematosus. Psychother Psychosom 55:132–140, 1991

Volkow ND, Warner N, McIntyre R, et al: Cerebral involvement in systemic lupus erythematosus. Am J Physiol Imaging 3:91–98, 1988

Wallace DJ: The clinical presentation of SLE, in Dubois' Lupus Erythematosus, 4th Edition. Edited by Wallace DJ, Hahn BH. Philadelphia, PA, Lea & Febiger, 1993, pp 318–319

Ward MM, Studenski S: The time course of acute psychiatric episodes in systemic lupus erythematosus. J Rheumatol 18:535–539, 1991

Wechsler D: Wechsler Adult Intelligence Scale—Revised. San Antonio, TX, Psychological Corporation, 1987

Wekking EM: Psychiatric symptoms in systemic lupus erythematosus: an update. Psychosom Med 55:219–228, 1993

Chapter 5

Diagnostic Assessment of Chronic Fatigue Syndrome

Theodore J. Anfinson, M.D.

Fatigue is a common complaint among patients in both primary care and psychiatric settings (Bates et al. 1993; Kroenke et al. 1988). In many patients, this symptom can be attributed to a readily identifiable medical or psychiatric condition; however, a substantial number of chronically fatigued patients present without any clear identifiable etiology. These cases are often very frustrating for both the patient and the clinician. This frustration is fueled in part by the severe degree of disability experienced by patients in the absence of specific physical findings. Clinicians may become skeptical about the nature of the underlying condition responsible for the fatigue. Patients often sense this skepticism, and the physician-patient relationship can become strained as a result.

Patients with this syndrome tend to hold firmly to the notion that their problems are physical in nature (Lane et al. 1991; Powell et al. 1990; Wessely and Powell 1989); epidemiologic data, however, reveal substantial psychiatric comorbidity in these patients (Lane et al. 1991). Attempts by the clinician to address possible psychiatric factors are often perceived by patients as misguided or demeaning paternalistic efforts to dismiss their symptoms. In addition, the popular press and patient advocacy groups have reinforced misconceptions about the disorder by reporting research findings in a fashion that leads the reader to interpret preliminary research results as definitive and final (Stoff and Pellegrino 1992). Patients and clinicians often accept these early reports despite accumulating evidence to the contrary.

Gaining a clear understanding of this disorder has been made difficult by many factors. First, several competing conceptual models of chronic fatigue syndrome (CFS) exist, each reflecting the bias of their respective proponents. These include infectious, immunologic, rheumatologic, myopathic, psychiatric, sociocultural, and anthropologic models. A recent symposium was convened in an attempt to integrate these divergent approaches to this complex topic (Bock and Whelan 1993). Table 5–1 compares the different conceptual models of the syndrome.

Interpretation of the literature surrounding CFS is made more difficult by the fact that several competing sets of diagnostic criteria exist (Holmes et al. 1988; Lloyd et al. 1990; J. C. Sharpe et al. 1991). Furthermore, these criteria are evolving and are inconsistently applied by individual investigators (Schluederberg et al. 1992). The specifics of current diagnostic criteria are controversial (Katon and Russo 1992), and methodologic problems have confounded many avenues of research in this field (Herberman 1991; Katon and Russo 1992; Redmond 1991; Richman et al. 1994). Finally, conflicting data abound regarding issues of etiology, epidemiology, pathophysiology, and treatment (Manu et al. 1992).

It is not easy to determine the most appropriate specialist(s) to treat patients with CFS. Primary care physicians often treat the majority of these patients, whereas specialists in rheumatology, infectious disease, and psychiatry treat others. However, many primary care physicians do not believe that they are prepared to adequately treat the psychological aspects of this disorder. Furthermore, treatment by specialists may result in undue emphasis on one conceptual model of the disorder at the exclusion of others, thus undermining optimal patient care. It has been suggested that physicians with an affinity toward biopsychosocial paradigms of medical care are the ideal candidates to manage the care of patients with CFS (Deale and David 1994).

In this chapter, I first briefly discuss the phenomenology of CFS. Then, I discuss the data surrounding the most prevalent hypotheses on CFS, emphasizing studies concerned with psychiatric comorbidity. In the rest of the chapter, I discuss practical clinical issues involved in the diagnosis and treatment of patients with CFS.

HISTORY OF CHRONIC FATIGUE SYNDROME

Patients with symptoms of severe, chronic, debilitating fatigue have been described for centuries. Numerous diagnostic terms have been used to describe these patients, including febricula, neurasthenia, epidemic neuromyasthenia, benign myalgic encephalitis, chronic brucellosis, and the more contemporary terms of hypoglycemia, environmental sensitivity, chronic candidiasis, chronic Epstein-Barr virus (EBV) infection, fibromyalgia, and, finally, CFS (Goldenberg 1988; Greenberg 1990; Shorter 1993; Straus 1991).

The earliest accounts of chronically fatigued patients appeared in the writings of Hippocrates and his predecessors, noting a high prevalence among women in wealthy families. In 1750, Sir Richard Manningham published a description of a condition he termed *febricula*, emphasizing its features of low-grade fever, lassitude, and subtle cognitive dysfunction (Straus 1991). In the late nineteenth century, George Beard introduced the term *neurasthenia*, noting the imprecision of the earlier phrase *nervous exhaustion*, advocated by Austin Flint (Straus 1991). The concept of neurasthenia had a tremendous influence on the field of psychiatry, notably in the work of Janet and Freud (Greenberg 1990). It remained a part of psychiatric nosology until the publication of DSM-III (American Psychiatric Association 1980).

Earlier in the twentieth century, several clusters of cases occurred resembling what we now call CFS. Many of them occurred in the setting of other epidemics or were believed to be precipitated by an acute respiratory illness (Goldenberg 1988). Table 5–2 summarizes these reports. The modern infectious hypothesis of CFS was probably born out of these clusters of cases.

In more recent years, other controversial entities have emerged that superficially resemble CFS, including hypoglycemia, environmental sensitivity, and chronic candidiasis. It is striking to note the resistance among these patients to alternative explanations for their symptoms. Patients with these syndromes are often desperately ill and appear to require external explanations for their symptoms. Apart from their similar clinical manifestations, these disorders resemble each other in the fact that few direct data support the involvement of the purported etiologic explanations for any of these conditions (Straus 1991). Misinterpretation of normal variations of laboratory data has often played a role in the belief that a known physiologic or environmental variable is responsible (Meador 1965; Straus 1991; Yager and Young 1974).

The initial finding of abnormal antibodies to EBV in patients with chronic fatigue was seized by clinicians and patient advocacy groups as an explanation for the chronic fatigue and disability experienced by these patients (Jones et al. 1985; Straus 1988; Straus et al. 1985). Subse-

Table 5–1. Conceptual models for the chronic fatigue syndrome

Model	Evidence for model	Evidence against model	Comments
Infectious disease	Clustering of cases; frequent history of antecedent febrile illness; nonspecific immune abnormalities similar to those seen after viral illness	Koch's postulates never fulfilled; seroepidemiology unable to distinguish patients from control subjects; predominance of white, middle-aged women	Patients accept serologic findings as evidence of their disease; research continues regarding other potential relationships with infectious etiologies
Immune disorder	Abnormal distribution of immunoglobulin G subtypes; impaired natural killer cell cytotoxicity, mitogen-induced T-cell proliferation, delayed-type hypersensitivity	Considerable disagreement between studies regarding specifics of immune abnormalities; immune abnormalities overlap with those seen in affective illness	Immune abnormalities may represent nonspecific response to illness regardless of etiology
Sleep disorder	Impaired onset of sleep, α intrusion into non-REM sleep	High prevalence of primary obstructive sleep apnea in some series	Shortened REM latency seen in depression is not a feature of CFS
Muscle disorder	Abnormal histochemistry, distribution of muscle fiber types in CFS patients	Microscopic findings nonspecific; functional muscle testing reveals central origin of fatigue	Functional testing is most consistent with deconditioning

| Psychiatric disorder | High prevalence of affective, anxiety, somatization disorders in CFS patients | Phenomenology of illness somewhat different from primary psychiatric samples; no family, outcome data to support hypothesis | Primary/secondary distinction not resolved; affective and anxiety states may share common etiology with symptom of fatigue |
| Sociocultural phenomenon | CFS primarily a Western phenomenon; attribution of illness onset to social sources | | Potential iatrogenic role for producing disability in patients; media may influence choice of CFS label |

Note.   REM = rapid eye movement; CFS = chronic fatigue syndrome.

Table 5–2. Clusters of benign myalgic encephalomyelitis

Location	Year	Female:male	No. of cases	Most prominent chronic symptoms at follow-up
Los Angeles County Hospital	1934	5:1	210	Myalgias, fatigue at 7 years
Iceland (Akureyi)	1948	2:1	465	Myalgias, muscle tenderness, fatigue, nervousness at 6 years in 80%
Royal Free Hospital	1955	10:1	292	Myalgias, fatigue common at 1 year
Florida (Punta Gorda)	1956	2:1	62	Fatigue, myalgias, depression common at 6 months
Alaska	1951	3:1	175	Fatigue, myalgias, paresthesias in 110 of 175 at 2 years
Australia (Adelaide)	1949	1:1	800	Myalgias, emotional stability common at 2 years

Note. Follow-up was incomplete except in Florida cases (all evaluated at 6 months) and Alaska cases (all examined at 2 years).
Source. Adapted from Goldenberg 1988.

quent research, however, revealed this association to be quite weak and led to the development of the more descriptive term *chronic fatigue syndrome*, removing from the name any assumption regarding etiology (Holmes et al. 1988; Koo 1989; Straus 1991). The search for an infectious etiology continues, but research efforts are proceeding along other avenues toward a more comprehensive view of this complex syndrome.

SIGNS AND SYMPTOMS OF CHRONIC FATIGUE SYNDROME

In 1988, the Centers for Disease Control (CDC) in Atlanta published a preliminary set of working criteria for the newly renamed chronic fatigue syndrome (Holmes et al. 1988). The result of a consensus panel, these criteria were intended to reflect the clinical phenomenology as it was then understood (Table 5–3). In 1992, a subsequent panel published modifications and clarifications of the CDC criteria to address issues that had become apparent after the initial publication (Table 5–4) (Schluederberg et al. 1992). Shortly after the CDC criteria were published, Australian and British investigators published separate definitions of the disorder (Lloyd et al. 1990; J. C. Sharpe et al. 1991). Table 5–5 compares the three definitions of CFS.

The main feature of the disorder is chronic debilitating fatigue of unknown etiology. Other symptoms may include fever, postexertional malaise, sore throat, painful lymph nodes, weakness, arthralgias, headaches, confusion, memory deficits, and sleep disturbance. Physical findings may include nonexudative pharyngitis, cervical and/or axillary adenopathy, alterations in body temperature, and impaired tests of balance. Tables 5–6 and 5–7 summarize the relative frequency of these findings in one sample of CFS patients (Komaroff 1993).

There is some dispute about the reliability of some of the physical findings reported in CFS. For example, the finding of pharyngeal erythema is quite subjective and has less reliability than other more objective findings. Even the data concerning objective findings are inconsistent— for example, abnormalities in body temperature, revealing 20%–30% of patients with a low body temperature, 50%–70% with normal body temperature, and 10%–20% with fever. This pattern is different from healthy people, but it approaches a normal distribution, making it difficult to interpret body temperature findings in individual patients. Furthermore, patients often vehemently report physical abnormalities that cannot be confirmed by physical examination (Komaroff 1993).

Table 5–3. Centers for Disease Control case definition of chronic fatigue
syndrome

Must fulfill both major criteria and the following minor criteria: 6 or more of
the 11 symptom criteria and 2 or more of the 3 physical criteria; or 8 or more
of the 11 symptom criteria.

Major criteria

1. New onset of persistent or relapsing debilitating fatigue or easy
   fatigability in a person who has no previous history of similar symptoms,
   which does not resolve with bed rest and is severe enough to reduce or
   impair average daily activity below 50% of the patient's premorbid
   activity level for a period of at least 6 months.
2. Other clinical conditions that may produce similar symptoms must be
   excluded by thorough evaluation, based on history, physical examination,
   and appropriate laboratory findings. See Table 5–4 for list of exclusionary
   disorders.

Minor criteria

Symptom criteria

To fulfill a symptom criterion, a symptom must have begun at or after the
time of onset of increased fatigability and must have persisted or recurred
over a period of at least 6 months (individual symptoms may or may not
have occurred simultaneously). Symptoms include

1. Mild fever—oral temperatures between 37.5°C and 38.6°C, if measured
   by the patient, or chills. (Note: oral temperatures of > 38.6°C are less
   compatible with chronic fatigue syndrome and should prompt studies for
   other causes of illness.)
2. Sore throat.
3. Painful lymph nodes in the anterior or posterior cervical or axillary
   distribution.
4. Unexplained generalized muscle weakness.
5. Muscle discomfort or myalgia.
6. Prolonged (24 hours or greater) generalized fatigue after levels of exercise
   that would have been easily tolerated in the patient's premorbid state.
7. Generalized headaches (of a type, severity, or pattern that is different
   from headaches the patient may have had in the premorbid state).
8. Migratory arthralgia without joint swelling or redness.
9. Neuropsychologic complaints (one or more of the following: photophobia,
   transient visual scotomata, forgetfulness, excessive irritability, confusion,
   difficulty thinking, inability to concentrate, depression).
10. Sleep disturbance (hypersomnia or insomnia).
11. Description of the main symptom complex as initially developing over a
    few hours to a few days (this is not a true symptom but may be

(continued)

Table 5–3. Centers for Disease Control case definition of chronic fatigue
syndrome *(continued)*

considered as equivalent to the above symptoms in meeting the
requirements of the case definition).

Physical criteria

Physical criteria must be documented by a physician on at least two
occasions, at least 1 month apart. Symptoms include

1. Low-grade fever—oral temperature between 37.6°C and 38.6°C or rectal
   temperature between 37.8°C and 38.8°C. (See note under Symptom
   criterion 1.)
2. Nonexudative pharyngitis.
3. Palpable or tender anterior or posterior cervical or axillary lymph nodes.
   (Note: lymph nodes > 2 cm in diameter suggest other causes. Further
   evaluation is warranted.)

Source. Adapted from Holmes et al. 1988.

EPIDEMIOLOGY OF FATIGUE AND
CHRONIC FATIGUE SYNDROME

The prevalence of fatigue is obviously highly dependent on the nature
of the sampled population. Community studies, followed by studies in
primary care and tertiary care centers, reveal increasing prevalence
rates of fatigue and CFS; furthermore, associated psychiatric comorbidity increases with progression from community to tertiary populations (Katon and Walker 1993).

Community Studies

In a comprehensive review of community and primary care studies,
Lewis and Wessely (1992) noted a wide range—from 7% to 45%—of
prevalence rates of fatigue among community samples. Fatigue was
almost always more prevalent in females, and the duration of fatigue
was greater among females as well.

A retrospective analysis of data collected during the Epidemiologic
Catchment Area (ECA) study revealed subjective complaints of chronic
fatigue in 23% of patients (Price et al. 1992). Again, females were nearly
twice as likely to report fatigue as males. Only 1 of 13,528 patients met
an approximation of the CDC case definition for CFS. This study has
been criticized by CFS advocates for its retrospective design, the absence of certain CFS symptoms in the Diagnostic Interview Schedule

Table 5–4. Clarifications of Centers for Disease Control case definition criteria for chronic fatigue syndrome

Illness category	Exclusions	Inclusions[a]	Recommended tests[b]
Chronic medical conditions	Major conditions to be considered in differential diagnoses include malignancy, autoimmune disease, inflammatory disease, endocrine disease, neurologic disease, and chronic organic disease		*Standard:* urinalysis, complete blood count with differential, serum electrolytes, blood urea nitrogen, glucose, creatinine, calcium, thyroid function tests, erythrocyte sedimentation rate, and antinuclear antibodies
		Fibromyalgia[c]	Tender point examination[c] *Optional or as clinically indicated:* serum cortisol, rheumatoid factor, and immunoglobulin levels
Postinfectious disease	Chronic active hepatitis B or C; Lyme borreliosis, inadequately treated; human immunodeficiency virus (HIV) infection, tuberculosis	Infectious mononucleosis, adequately treated infection that is not typically associated with chronicity: toxoplasmosis, brucellosis, Lyme borreliosis[d]	Tuberculin skin test, Lyme serology in endemic area, HIV serology when indicated

| Psychiatric and behavioral disorders | Psychoses: psychotic depression, bipolar disorder, schizophrenia | Major depression: recurrent, or nonrecurrent; somatoform disorders; anxiety disorders: generalized or panic disorder | *Screen:* General Health Questionnaire (Goldberg and Hillier 1979) or combination of self-report instrument[e] |
| | Substance abuse | | For patients with positive screening results: *Structured interview:* Diagnostic Interview Schedule version IIIA (Robins et al. 1981) or Structured Clinical Interview for the *Diagnostic and Statistical Manual of Mental Disorders, Third Edition Revised* (DSM-III-R) |

[a]Stratified by individual category in analysis of data.
[b]Tests are to be used in conjunction with completed detailed medical history and comprehensive physical examination.
[c]See Wolfe F, Smythe HA, Yunus MB, et al: "Criteria for Fibromyalgia (abstract)." *Arthritis and Rheumatism* 32 (suppl):S47, 1989.
[d]Recognized recrudesence and chronicity of active *Borrelia* infection was considered an exception.
[e]Zung Self-Rating Anxiety Scale (Zung 1971), Symptom Checklist-90 (Derogatis 1977), Beck Depression Inventory (Beck 1978).
Source. Adapted from Schluederberg et al. 1992.

Table 5–5. Comparison of chronic fatigue syndrome case definitions

	CDC	United Kingdom	Australian
Fatigue duration	At least 6 months	At least 6 months	At least 6 months
Fatigue severity	50% decrease in activities	Severe and disabling	Causing disruption of daily activities
Other characteristics of fatigue	New onset required	Definite onset required	Not required
Cognitive dysfunction	No requirement (may be present)	Must "affect mental functioning"	Required
Other diagnoses	Medical conditions associated with fatigue excluded	Medical conditions associated with fatigue excluded	Medical conditions associated with fatigue excluded
Minor criteria, both symptoms and clinical	Required	Not required	Not required

Note.   CDC = Centers for Disease Control.
Source.   Adapted from Bates et al. 1993.

(Robins et al. 1981) employed in the ECA study, and the absence of physical examination and laboratory data (Robin et al. 1993).

Preliminary data from the multicenter CDC CFS surveillance study have resulted in minimum CFS prevalence estimates of 2.0 to 7.3 per 100,000, with prevalence rates based on prorated data of 4.6 to 11.3 per 100,000. These represent an underestimation of the true prevalence, as

Table 5–6. Frequency of symptoms reported in chronic fatigue syndrome

Symptom	Frequency (%)
Fatigue	100
Impaired cognition	50–85
Depression	50–85
Pharyngitis	50–75
Anxiety	50–70
Postexertional malaise	50–60
Premenstrual worsening	50–60
Stiffness/"gelling"	50–60
Visual blurring	50–60
Nausea	50–60
Muscle weakness	40–70
Arthralgias	40–50
Tachycardia	40–50
Headaches	35–85
Dizziness	30–50
Paresthesias	30–50
Dry eyes	30–40
Dry mouth	30–40
Diarrhea	30–40
Anorexia	30–40
Cough	30–40
Finger swelling	30–40
Night sweats	30–40
Painful lymph nodes	30–40
Rash	30–40
Low-grade fever	20–95
Myalgias	20–95
Sleep disorder	15–90

Source. Estimated from work by Komaroff and Buchwald; adapted from Komaroff 1993.

a result of the relatively low participation of eligible referring physicians (45%) and the fact that all cases meeting screening criteria were not referred. Demographically, more than 80% of CFS patients were women, and most were white, with a mean age at onset of 30 years (Gunn et al. 1993).

Primary Care Studies

Cathebras and colleagues (1992) evaluated the prevalence of fatigue in 686 patients attending two family medicine clinics. They noted that 93 patients (13.6%) presented with a chief complaint of fatigue, and it was the major reason for presentation in 46 patients (6.7%). Fatigued patients were more likely than nonfatigued control subjects to have symptoms currently diagnosed as major depressive disorder (17.2% versus 8.8%) or lifetime symptoms diagnosed as major depression or anxiety disorders (45.2% versus 28.2%).

In a sample of 1,159 consecutive patients in two primary care clinics, 276 (24%) presented with complaints indicating that fatigue was a major problem contributing to their visit (Kroenke et al. 1988). One hundred two of these patients were extensively evaluated, and 26 fatigued patients were demographically matched and compared with 26 nonfatigued control subjects. Only 29 fatigued patients (28%) had improved at 1-year follow-up. Kroenke and co-workers noted that labo-

Table 5–7. Physical examination findings in chronic fatigue syndrome

Finding	Frequency (%)
Inflamed pharynx	40–60
Posterior cervical adenopathy	20–40
Abnormal Romberg test (for balance)	10–20
Impaired tandem gait (test of balance)	15–25
Macular rash	10–20
Fever (T > 99.6°F; 37.56°C) at a single office visit	10–20
Low body temperature (T < 97.0°F; 36.4°C)	20–30
Hepatomegaly	5–20
Splenomegaly	5–20
Axillary adenopathy	5–15

Source. Estimated from work by Komaroff and Buchwald; adapted from Komaroff 1993.

ratory testing was not useful in detecting unsuspected medical illnesses or in determining the cause of the patients' fatigue. They also noted that 56% of *all* fatigued patients had Beck Depression Inventory (BDI) (Beck 1978) scores of ≥ 10; of *matched* fatigued patients, 46% had BDI scores of ≥ 10 compared with 0 of 26 nonfatigued control subjects. (In primary care samples, a cutoff score of 10 on the BDI is a more sensitive indicator of the presence of depression; a BDI score of 13 is a more specific indicator of depression [Nielsen and Williams 1980].) In the above-noted sample, 34 (33%) of fatigued patients had a BDI score of 13.

In a more recent prospective study of 1,000 consecutive patients in a primary care clinic, 271 (27%) reported at least 6 months of severe fatigue that interfered with their daily functioning (Bates et al. 1993). Of these chronically fatigued patients, 186 (69%) had either a medical or psychiatric condition potentially accountable for the fatigue. Eighty-five patients (8.5%) had chronic fatigue without an apparent cause. Table 5–8 illustrates the relative frequencies of the various medical and psychiatric disorders associated with fatigue in this sample.

Tertiary Care Studies

Manu and colleagues (1988a) investigated the prevalence of CFS in a consecutive sample of 135 patients presenting to a referral clinic with fatigue of more than 6 months' duration. They noted that only 6 patients (4%) met the CDC criteria for CFS. Four patients (3%) had medical disorders considered to be a major cause of the fatigue. In contrast, 91 patients (67%) met the criteria for a clinically active psychiatric disorder, including major depressive disorder (50%), somatization disorder (14%), panic disorder (8%), and dysthymia (6%). Thirty-four patients (25%) met an insufficient number of criteria for CFS. Results from a continuation study involving 405 patients confirmed the high rate of psychiatric disorder among these patients. Table 5–9 illustrates the relative frequencies of medical and psychiatric diagnoses in patients attending a tertiary chronic fatigue clinic (Manu et al. 1993).

Prevalence rates may vary based on population and methodologic differences between studies; however, other findings relevant to CFS have been replicated. The majority of cases are white, middle-aged, well-educated women. CFS patients have a high lifetime prevalence of major depression and somatization disorder and tend to adhere to the belief that their fatigue has a physical rather than a psychological cause (Manu et al. 1992).

CHRONIC FATIGUE SYNDROME AS INFECTIOUS DISEASE

An infectious etiology is the most prevalent hypothesis regarding CFS. Its origins are in the observation of epidemic-like clustering of cases (Table 5–2). Initial reports of abnormal EBV serologies supported the clinical viewpoint that CFS was a form of chronic viral infection (Jones

Table 5–8. Medical and psychiatric disorders associated with chronic fatigue in a prospective sample of 1,000 primary care patients

	Self-report ($n = 121$)	Additional diseases found by chart review ($n = 65$)	All ($n = 186$)
Medical disorders			
Diabetes	45	2	47
Heart disease	27	4	31
Lung disease	15	3	18
Rheumatoid arthritis	13	3	16
Anemia (hematocrit < 0.34)	0	9	9
Cancer	7	1	8
Chronic pain	0	8	8
HIV infection	0	7	7
Kidney disease	4	1	5
Liver disease	2	1	3
Hypothyroidism, without therapy	0	3	3
Sarcoidosis	2	0	2
Multiple sclerosis	2	0	2
Tuberculosis	1	0	1
Systemic lupus	1	0	1
Other organic illness	2	8	10
Psychiatric and substance abuse disorders			
Substance abuse	0	6	6
Recent or current major depression	0	5	5
Schizophrenia, other major psychosis (not depression)	0	4	4

Note. HIV = human immunodeficiency virus.
Source. Adapted from Bates et al. 1993.

et al. 1985; Straus 1988; Straus et al. 1985). Other studies failed to replicate these initial findings and noted that EBV serologic patterns in these patients were quite variable, did not distinguish between patients and control subjects, and did not correlate with clinical symptoms (Buchwald et al. 1987; Gold et al. 1990; Hellinger et al. 1988; Holmes et al. 1987; Hotchin et al. 1989; Koo 1989).

Other herpesviruses have been implicated in the pathophysiology of CFS, including cytomegalovirus (CMV) and human herpesvirus 6 (HHV6). Acute CMV may trigger a fatigue response, but there is little

Table 5–9. Medical and psychiatric disorders associated with chronic fatigue in a prospective sample of 405 patients attending a tertiary care chronic fatigue clinic

	Number of patients
Medical disorders	
Obstructive sleep apnea	5
Periodic hypersomnia	2
Periodic nocturnal limb movements	2
Temporal lobe epilepsy	2
Lyme disease	2
Epstein-Barr infection	2
Cytomegalovirus infection	1
Hepatitis B infection	1
Hepatitis C infection	1
Hypothyroidism	2
Hypopituitarism	1
Polymyalgia rheumatica	2
Systemic lupus	1
Asthmatic bronchitis	2
Pulmonary sarcoidosis	1
Anemia	1
Psychiatric diagnoses	
Major depression	236
Dysthymia	32
Bipolar disorder, depressed	4
Anxiety disorders	82
Somatization disorder	39
Hypochondriasis	2

Source. Adapted from Manu et al. 1993.

evidence of active CMV infection in CFS patients (Straus 1993). HHV6 is a ubiquitous virus, acquired in childhood. The study methodology and serologic data for HHV6 follow similar patterns to those concerning EBV; initial reports suggested an association between HHV6 and CFS but were followed by the accumulation of less convincing evidence (Straus 1993).

Enterovirus involvement in CFS is limited to unreplicated data suggesting a higher prevalence of enterovirus DNA sequences in CFS patients than in control subjects (Behan et al. 1993). Furthermore, a retrovirus does not appear to play a significant role in the pathophysiology of CFS (Folks et al. 1993).

CHRONIC FATIGUE SYNDROME AS DISORDER OF IMMUNE REGULATION

Several abnormalities of immune system functioning have been reported in patients with CFS, involving both the humoral and the cellular arms of the immune system.

Humoral Immunity

Although total serum levels are within the reference range for immunoglobulins (Ig) A, G, and M (Behan et al. 1985; Lloyd et al. 1989), some investigators have noted differences in IgG subclasses in CFS patients. In a controlled study of 78 CFS patients and 71 control subjects, the CFS patients had statistically significant reductions in total IgG, IgG1, IgG2, and IgG3. It should be noted, however, that none of the patients had values of these Ig levels more than two standard deviations from the control population mean (Wakefield et al. 1990). The investigators emphasized that 1) normal ranges of IgG subclasses have yet to be clearly defined, and 2) the degree of reduction in IgG subclasses was not consistent with that noted in clinically significant humoral immunodeficiency states (Lloyd et al. 1993b). Other investigators have noted evidence of humoral activation in CFS patients as manifested by nonsignificant trends toward increases in IgG2 levels (Lane et al. 1992). Increases in specific IgG levels directed at viral antigens (EBV, CMV, Coxsackie, enteroviruses) have not been shown to distinguish CFS patients from control subjects and thus have little diagnostic utility (Holmes et al. 1987; Miller et al. 1991).

Eighty-three percent of highly selected patients with CFS had histories of atopy (inhalant, food, or drug allergy), whereas 50% of these patients had histories of skin-test reactivity to food and inhalant antigens (Straus et al. 1988b). Olson and colleagues (1986a, 1986b) noted increased IgE levels in patients with chronic fatigue symptoms and evidence of EBV exposure compared with EBV-exposed patients without chronic fatigue symptoms.

Cellular Immunity

The most consistent findings relevant to altered cellular immunity in CFS patients involve impaired cytotoxicity of natural killer (NK) cells to the K562 erythroleukemia cell line and impaired mitogen-induced T-cell proliferation (Caliguri et al. 1987). Quantitative evaluations of both T cells and NK cells reveal marked inconsistencies between studies (Lloyd et al. 1993b). Impaired delayed-type hypersensitivity is more common among CFS patients than control subjects, with CFS patients exhibiting rates of cutaneous anergy ranging from 21%–54%, compared with 0%–15% among control subjects (Lloyd et al. 1989, 1990, 1992; Murdoch 1988). These alterations in cellular immunity are similar to those observed to occur in patients with viral infections (Griffen 1991).

Several nonspecific abnormalities of the immune system have been observed in CFS; however, the measurement of immune parameters should be regarded as a research tool designed to facilitate our understanding of this disorder. It is premature to regard the measurement of immune parameters as a clinically useful tool until more progress has been made in more clearly defining the clinical sample to be tested, establishing normal values for the parameters in question, and improving standardization of assay performance.

CHRONIC FATIGUE SYNDROME AS SLEEP DISORDER

Sleep impairment is a common complaint among patients with CFS, fibromyalgia, and mood disorders. Furthermore, patients with primary sleep disorders, such as sleep apnea and periodic limb movements of sleep, often complain of fatigue, myalgia, and vague cognitive dysfunction. Studies comparing chronic fatigue patients with control patients have revealed that CFS patients have more difficulty falling asleep, spend less time sleeping, have reduced rapid eye

HIGH ROYDS HOSPITAL
MEDICAL LIBRARY

movement (REM) sleep, and have greater α-electroencephalogram (EEG) activity during non-REM sleep (Whelton et al. 1992). These results are similar to those in patients with fibromyalgia (Moldofsky 1993; Moldofsky et al. 1988). Of interest is the finding that the shortened REM latency that has been observed in some patients with major depression is less commonly seen in patients with chronic fatigue–like syndromes (Moldofsky 1993).

CHRONIC FATIGUE SYNDROME AS MUSCLE DISORDER

Because fatigue and myalgias are common symptoms of primary muscle disorders, the role of primary muscle pathology in CFS was evaluated. The most common morphologic changes included abnormalities of muscle fiber size, fiber type prevalence, and degenerative and regenerative changes. The data between studies are inconsistent, and most of the morphologic changes can be explained on the basis of deconditioning (Behan et al. 1985; Edwards et al. 1993). Studies of muscle contractile properties revealed no abnormalities, however, and patients with CFS had higher perceived exertion scores in relation to heart rate (Edwards et al. 1993). The data suggest that the fatigue experienced by patients with CFS is not of peripheral origin but results from an abnormal central drive (Edwards et al. 1993; Wood et al. 1991).

CHRONIC FATIGUE SYNDROME AND ITS RELATIONSHIP TO FIBROMYALGIA

Although overwhelming fatigue is a requirement for the diagnosis of CFS, pain symptoms are also common in this population. Myalgias are present in 20%–95% of CFS patients (Komaroff 1993). Furthermore, patients with the fibromyalgia syndrome often complain of debilitating fatigue. Table 5–10 compares the criteria for CFS and fibromyalgia. Goldenberg and colleagues (1990) noted that the majority of patients complaining of chronic fatigue or those meeting CDC criteria for CFS also met criteria for fibromyalgia. A review of demographic characteristics reveals striking similarities between these groups (Goldenberg 1988, 1989; Goldenberg et al. 1990). Based on these findings, the CDC has suggested that fibromyalgia be considered a subset of CFS (Table 5–4) (Schluederberg et al. 1992).

CHRONIC FATIGUE SYNDROME AS PSYCHIATRIC DISORDER

Significant psychiatric comorbidity is undisputed among patients with chronic fatigue. Such patients are known to have high prevalence rates of depression, somatization disorder, and personality disturbances. Controversy surrounds the interpretation of these data. Are the psychiatric symptoms merely a reaction to the stress of chronic illness, or are the psychiatric disorders responsible for the fatigue?

In a sample of 405 patients attending a tertiary chronic fatigue clinic, Manu and colleagues (1993) noted that 74% of patients met criteria for psychiatric disorders, whereas 4.2% had both medical and psychiatric diagnoses, and only 2.7% had medical diagnoses to explain their fatigue.

In a comprehensive review of the topic, Katon and Walker (1993) noted that a high association existed between anxiety and mood disorders and the symptom of fatigue in community, primary, and tertiary care samples. Furthermore, they noted that the prevalence of affective illness increased linearly with progression from community to tertiary populations.

Issues of the validity of CFS as a psychiatric illness have yet to be evaluated with family history methods and treatment outcome data.

Phenomenological differences between major depression and CFS are often cited as evidence against CFS as a primary psychiatric illness. Data revealing the absence of shortened REM latency in CFS patients and conflicting data regarding immune abnormalities when comparing CFS and depressed patients suggest that, at least, intriguing differences exist between patients with major depression and CFS, as currently defined (Lloyd et al. 1993b).

APPROACH TO THE PATIENT WITH CHRONIC FATIGUE

The Dilemma

The very nature of CFS, with its cluster of nonspecific symptoms and the absence of pathognomonic findings, makes the physician's evaluation very difficult. CFS is, by definition, a diagnosis of exclusion, with unlimited potential diagnostic possibilities. The difficulty is in determining how far to proceed with the diagnostic evaluation before sum-

Table 5–10. Comparison of diagnostic criteria for chronic fatigue syndrome and fibromyalgia

Chronic fatigue syndrome[a]	Fibromyalgia[b]
Major (mandatory) criteria	Major (mandatory) criteria
1. Exclusion of any systemic condition that may cause similar symptoms	1. Exclusion of any systemic condition that may cause similar symptoms
2. New onset of persistent or relapsing severe fatigue	2. Generalized aches or stiffness involving three or more anatomic sites for at least 3 months
	3. At least six typical and reproducible tender points
Symptom criteria	Minor criteria
1. Debilitating fatigue for at least 6 months	1. Generalized fatigue
2. Chronic headaches	2. Chronic headaches
3. Sleep disturbances	3. Sleep disturbances
4. Neuropsychiatric symptoms	4. Neuropsychiatric symptoms
5. Migratory joint pains	5. Subjective joint swelling but no objective swelling
6. Unexplained muscle weakness	6. Numbness, tingling sensation
7. Myalgias	7. Irritable bowel syndrome
8. Sore throat	8. Modulation of symptoms by activity, weather, or stress
9. Painful lymph nodes	
10. Fatigue prevents usual activity	
11. Symptoms began abruptly	
12. Fever	
Physical criteria	
1. Low-grade fever	
2. Nonexudative, inflamed pharynx	
3. Palpable or tender cervical or axillary lymph nodes	

[a]Must fulfill major criteria and either six or more of the symptom criteria and two or more of the physical criteria or eight or more of the symptom criteria (Holmes et al. 1988).
[b]Must fulfill major criteria and at least four of the minor criteria (Goldenberg 1987).
Source. Adapted from Goldenberg et al. 1990.

marizing the results and initiating treatment. The approach to the diagnosis of nonspecific complaints is influenced by a number of factors, including societal and patient expectations, the bias of the examiner, the relative availability of diagnostic tests, reimbursement systems, the presence of incentives to perform laboratory testing, and the overvaluation of a particular diagnostic test's ability to distinguish disease from nondisease (Mechanic 1993). The physician must consider these factors at initiation of the diagnostic process.

In its clarification of the CFS criteria, the CDC recommended an initial laboratory evaluation battery (Table 5–4). It should be stressed that the intent of this initial battery was to obtain as homogeneous a sample as possible in research settings (Schluederberg et al. 1992). Such laboratory testing, however, has not been shown to increase the diagnostic yield in clinical samples (Kroenke et al. 1988; Lane et al. 1990). It is important to note that, in any screening laboratory evaluation, the number of false-positive results increases as an exponential function of the number of tests in the battery: $(1-P)^n$, where P is the probability that a positive test result reflects true disease, and n is the number of tests obtained. Thus, although the initial cost of a screening battery may seem reasonable, the diagnostic testing seldom concludes with the initial battery. A cascade effect ensues, wherein one false-positive test stimulates a series of subsequent evaluations, which inevitably contain ambiguous or false-positive results, stimulating more diagnostic testing, and so on.

A common style of clinical logic also contributes to the potential for excessive diagnostic testing in patients with CFS. When confronted with nonspecific syndromes with potential physical or psychiatric etiologies, many physicians elect to use a linear logic model, wherein all potential physical illness is excluded first, followed sequentially by a consideration of psychiatric possibilities (Engel 1980). This approach may be appropriate for illnesses that have limited numbers of medical diagnostic possibilities; however, in CFS, this approach is inefficient and expensive and yields little useful information. Not only does this strategy fail to identify unrecognized disease, but it also increases the cost of medical care, increases the risk of iatrogenic disease, and reinforces the illness behavior of the patient (Mechanic 1993). A history-based strategy consisting of simultaneous consideration of psychiatric and medical possibilities is more cost-effective and diagnostically efficient, given the high psychiatric morbidity in this population.

The Evaluation

The initial evaluation of the chronically fatigued patient must include a complete history of the present illness, assessing both physical and psychological symptoms, a review of current medications, past medical and psychiatric history, family medical and psychiatric history, review of systems, and a complete physical examination. The patient's prior records should be reviewed whenever possible.

After the historical information is obtained, judicious use of the clinical laboratory should follow. Inexpensive screening tests for common illnesses are most appropriate, including urinalysis, blood glucose, renal function, and thyroid function (Anfinson and Kathol 1992). The examiner must consider the expense and diagnostic utility of further testing.

Tests that are *not recommended* in the routine evaluation of chronic fatigue patients include viral serologies (including those for EBV), lymphocyte subset analysis, Ig levels, serum cortisol, rheumatoid factor, porphyrin levels, and expensive and invasive tests such as magnetic resonance imaging and lumbar puncture.

Selection of further diagnostic testing must be based on the results of the initial database. Because of the ubiquitous nature of fatigue, the dictation of an algorithmic approach to further laboratory studies in the chronically fatigued patient is beyond the scope of this chapter. Note that diabetes, cardiopulmonary disorders, rheumatoid arthritis, and anemia accounted for 65% of the cases of chronic fatigue in a primary care sample, whereas medical disorders of all types accounted for only 7% of fatigue in a tertiary care sample (Bates et al. 1993; Manu et al. 1993). The reader is referred elsewhere for a general discussion of a directed approach to the use of the clinical laboratory in psychiatric patients (Anfinson and Kathol 1993).

Viral Serologies

Frequently, a patient presents with a history of symptoms that were diagnosed as CFS based on abnormal EBV serology results. As noted previously, EBV titers contribute little to the diagnosis of CFS. For the patient, however, these results represent tangible evidence of their illness and validate their suffering. Therefore, it is important in this situation not to summarily dismiss these findings as irrelevant or to question the competence of the clinician who obtained these results. A posture of objective data collection and patient education is more appropriate, explaining to the patient that indeed it appears that exposure to EBV has taken place in the past. It is also appropriate at this point to explain to the patient that the role of EBV in the perpetuation of symptoms is poorly understood and that, until more research is done, the appropriate treatment strategy is to alleviate symptoms and improve the level of functioning, independent of the viral serology profile. Table 5–11 illustrates the interpretation of EBV serologic patterns to assist the clinician in this situation.

General Approach to Treatment

The approach to treatment of the CFS patient is similar to the approach applied to other chronic illnesses such as chronic pain, fibromyalgia, somatization disorder, and even disorders with established pathophysiology such as multiple sclerosis and systemic lupus erythematosus. The most important factor involves a supportive physician-patient relationship.

Supportive treatment of patients with chronic illnesses such as CFS involves the following basic principles of providing supportive psychotherapy modified for the presence of somatic symptoms: elicit a detailed history of the patient's complaint(s); attempt to understand the possible affective meaning of symptoms for the patient; validate the patient's suffering; openly acknowledge any prior difficulty the patient may have experienced with the medical system in a supportive, noncritical fashion; examine the patient; and initiate consultation or laboratory investigation only in the presence of objective evidence of a change in the patient's status. It is important to direct attention away from discovering a definitive cause for the patient's symptoms and toward a program directed at alleviation of symptoms and long-term supportive care with the overall goal of maximizing the patient's potential functioning (Sapira 1977; Wessely et al. 1989).

Pharmacological Strategies

No treatment of CFS has shown efficacy in replicated controlled trials. Negative results have been shown for acyclovir, liver extract–folic acid–cyanocobalamin (LEFAC), and dialyzable leukocyte extract. Conflicting data exist for intravenous Ig therapy. Positive, but unreplicated, studies have been published for essential fatty acid and

Table 5–11. Serologic tests for Epstein-Barr virus

Antibody	Relationship with infectious mononucleosis (or inapparent acute infection)	Diagnostic use
VCA-IgM	Peaks early and usually disappears by 3–4 months	Presence indicates recent infection
VCA-IgG	Peaks early, persists indefinitely	Present in 90%–98% of adults; higher titers in acute infection and chronic illness
EA-D or EA-R	Found in 75%–95% of acute infections; titers decline and generally not present by 9 months	Found in low titers in 10%–40% of adults; titers higher in chronic illness and with aging
EBNA	Negative during first month; peaks at 1–4 months after infection and persists indefinitely	If low or absent in a seropositive patient, indicates abnormal immune response

Note. VCA-IgM = immunoglobulin M antibody to Epstein-Barr virus (EBV) viral capsid antigen; VCA-IgG = immunoglobulin G antibody to EBV viral capsid antigen; EA-D = diffuse pattern of immunofluorescence of early antigen; EA-R = pattern of immunofluorescence of early antigen restricted to cytoplasmic or perinuclear staining; EBNA = antibody to EBV nuclear antigen.
Source. Adapted from Goldenberg 1988.

intramuscular magnesium therapies. Uncontrolled data reveal a potential response to bupropion, little response to interferon-α, and conflicting results for cognitive-behavior psychotherapy. These studies are summarized in Table 5–12.

It is interesting that despite the overwhelming data on the high prevalence of psychiatric comorbidity in this population, not a single controlled trial of antidepressant therapy in CFS patients has been published. Clinicians and reviewers have been forced to rely on the case literature and to extrapolate from data on other populations (Blondel-Hill and Shafran 1993; Goodnick and Sandoval 1993; Gracious and Wisner 1991).

Lessons From Fibromyalgia Literature

Although no controlled studies exist for use of antidepressants in CFS patients, data support their use in patients with fibromyalgia. Given the above-noted similarity between these syndromes, it is worthwhile to review this literature. Table 5–13 summarizes these studies. Thus, until controlled data in CFS patients become available, it is reasonable to consider using antidepressants to treat patients with CFS. If a patient meets criteria for a current major depressive episode in the context of their complaints of chronic fatigue, the patient should be considered for an empirical trial of antidepressants. Currently, it is not clear which antidepressant would be preferable to use in this patient population. Studies of the use of antidepressants in fibromyalgia patients have been performed primarily with tricyclics, with generally positive results (symptom reduction) in a substantial number of patients (Moran and Dubester 1993).

Cognitive-Behavior Strategies

The data are mixed concerning the efficacy of cognitive-behavior therapy in the treatment of CFS, but favorable results were observed with a combined approach of antidepressant and cognitive-behavior treatment (Butler et al. 1991; Lloyd et al. 1993a).

It is not difficult to discover distorted cognitions in patients with CFS (Deale and David 1994). Such distortions may take the form of polarized thinking regarding issues of prognosis or the ability to perform exercise; e.g., "I will *never* get better," or "exercise makes me worse; I can't do *anything*." Selective abstraction is manifest by atten-

Table 5–12. Controlled and uncontrolled trials in the treatment of chronic fatigue syndrome

Treatment	N at entry/ N completing study	Population characteristics	Design	Results	Comments	Reference
Acyclovir	27/24	CDC criteria	Double blind, placebo controlled, crossover	No significant difference between acyclovir and control	Association noted between psychological test results and patients' sense of well-being	Straus et al. 1988a
Liver extract–folic acid–cyanocobalamin (LEFAC)	15/14	CDC criteria	Double blind, placebo controlled, crossover	No significant difference between LEFAC and placebo	High placebo response rate noted	Kaslow et al. 1989
Essential fatty acids	63/32	Antecedent viral illness (diagnosed on clinical grounds) requirement for entry into study; symptom criteria similar to British criteria	Double blind, placebo controlled	Fatty acid–treated group: 77% improved at 1 month, 85% at 3 months; placebo group: 23% improved at 1 month, 17% at 3 months	High drop-out rate; four-point scale used to measure depression; comprehensive assessment of affective morbidity not performed	Behan et al. 1990

Treatment	N	Criteria	Design	Results	Comments	Reference
Intravenous immunoglobulin (IgG) therapy	49/49	Australian criteria	Double blind, placebo controlled	43% response rate in IgG group versus 12% placebo response rate	Several factors may have undermined blinding of study	Lloyd et al. 1990
Intravenous IgG therapy	30/28	CDC criteria	Double blind, placebo controlled	No significant change from baseline in either placebo or IgG group; no significant difference between placebo and IgG groups	Lower doses of IgG used than in Lloyd study	Peterson et al. 1990
Intramuscular magnesium	32/31	CDC criteria	Double blind, placebo controlled	12/15 treated patients reported benefit versus 3/17 placebo patients; energy, pain, and emotional reactions subsets of Nottingham Health Profile Score (Hunt et al. 1985) significantly improved	Small statistical difference in red blood cell magnesium content between chronic fatigue syndrome patients and control subjects not replicated by another group (Deulofeu et al. 1991)	Cox et al. 1991

(continued)

Table 5–12. Controlled and uncontrolled trials in the treatment of chronic fatigue syndrome *(continued)*

Treatment	N at entry/ N completing study	Population characteristics	Design	Results	Comments	Reference
Cognitive-behavior psychotherapy (CBT)	50/32	British criteria	Open trial	Significant response in several functional domains	High drop-out rate; no control group; 20 patients meeting Research Diagnostic Criteria (Spitzer et al. 1978) for major depression were also treated with dothiepin (a tricyclic)	Butler et al. 1991
Bupropion	9/9	CDC criteria; patients either fluoxetine non-responders (n = 6) or intolerant of side effects (n = 3)	Open trial	6/9 (67%) had 40% reduction in HRSD and BDI scores; fall in plasma homovanillic acid correlated with improvement	1 patient met DSM-III-R criteria for major depressive episode; 4 met criteria for dysthymia; response of other CFS symptoms to bupropion not assessed	Goodnick et al. 1992

Dialyzable leukocyte extract (DLE) and CBT	90/88	Australian criteria	Randomized; DLE versus placebo portion double blinded	DLE no better than CBT; CBT no better than regular clinic attendance	74% met DSM-III-R criteria for major depression; trend for all patients to improve, regardless of treatment	Lloyd et al. 1993a
Interferon-α	20/20	CDC criteria	Open trial; randomized to immediate treatment versus treatment at 3 months	3 (15%) recovered; 2 (10%) improved; 15 (75%) not improved	No control group	Brook et al. 1993

Note. CDC = Centers for Disease Control; CFS = chronic fatigue syndrome; HRSD = Hamilton Rating Scale for Depression (Hamilton 1960); BDI = Beck Depression Inventory (Beck 1978); DSM-III-R = *Diagnostic and Statistical Manual of Mental Disorders,* 3rd Edition, Revised.

Table 5–13. Controlled and uncontrolled antidepressant trials in the treatment of fibromyalgia

Treatment	N at entry/ N completing study	Population characteristics	Design	Results	Comments	Reference
Amitrip-tyline 25 mg tid	20/1	Smythe and Moldofsky fi-brositis criteria (Smythe 1972); patients re-fractory to heat, massage, and NSAIDs	Open trial	Two patients im-proved; 12 pa-tients discontin-ued therapy within 4 weeks, 19 patients within 3 months; 70% because of a lack of efficacy, 35% because of side effects	High drop-out rate; no formal psychia-tric assessment	Wysenbeek et al. 1985
Amitrip-tyline 50 mg/day	70/59	Smythe and Moldofsky fibrositis criteria	Double blind, placebo con-trolled	Amitriptyline associated with improvements in sleep, patient and physician global assess-ments, morning stiffness, and pain analog scores; point tenderness not improved with amitriptyline	Anticholinergic side effects un-dermined blind-ing of study; 50% of placebo group had meaningful improvement in symptoms	Carette et al. 1986

Amitriptyline, 25 mg/day and naproxen 500 mg bid	62/58	Yunus criteria for fibromyalgia (Wolfe et al. 1989)	Double blind, placebo controlled; treatment groups: amitriptyline versus naproxen versus both versus placebo	Amitriptyline associated with improvement in many symptoms; naproxen not associated with significant response	Sample size too small to determine whether naproxen had additive effect with amitriptyline	Goldenberg et al. 1986
Maprotiline 75 mg/day or clomipramine 75 mg/day	37/18	Smythe and Moldofsky fibrositis criteria	Triple crossover design: maprotiline versus clomipramine versus placebo	Maprotiline associated with improvement in HRSD scores; clomipramine associated with improvement in trigger points	High drop-out rate	Bibolotti et al. 1986
Dothiepin 75 mg/day	60/52	Campbell fibrositis criteria (Campbell et al. 1983)	Double blind, placebo controlled	Trigger point scores, subjective pain experience improved with dothiepin	60% side-effect rate in treated group versus 20% in placebo group	Caruso et al. 1987

(continued)

Table 5–13. Controlled and uncontrolled antidepressant trials in the treatment of fibromyalgia *(continued)*

Treatment	*N* at entry/ *N* completing study	Population characteristics	Design	Results	Comments	Reference
Amitriptyline 50 mg/day	39/36	Smythe and Moldofsky fibrositis criteria	Double blind, placebo controlled, crossover	55% of treatment group moderately or markedly improved versus 22% of placebo group; point tenderness not improved with amitriptyline		Scudds et al. 1989

Note. NSAID = nonsteroidal antiinflammatory drugs; HRSD = Hamilton Rating Scale for Depression (Hamilton 1960).

tion given to certain aspects of the illness (abnormal laboratory values) at the exclusion of others; e.g., "but I have Epstein-Barr disease, therefore, I can't hope to return to functioning."

Helpful paradigms to use with patients may be the stress and deconditioning hypotheses (Wessely et al. 1989). For those patients reluctant to focus on psychiatric aspects of their illness, the stress model is a nonthreatening way to explain to the patient that their psychological distress is a common accompaniment to chronic illness. Likewise, the exercise physiology data support the major role that deconditioning plays in the perpetuation of chronic fatigue states (Edwards et al. 1993). Explaining to the patient the nature of the inactivity–pain with activity "vicious cycle" may prove to be a helpful approach to overcome the patient's initial reluctance to begin an exercise regimen. Table 5–14 summarizes a basic cognitive approach to CFS patients.

CONCLUSION

Until better data become available, the most appropriate management of CFS patients' symptoms involves a supportive relationship, attentive to the psychosocial and psychological needs of the patient, with judicious use of laboratory evaluation and psychotropic and/or nonsteroidal antiinflammatory agents when it seems appropriate. Chronic fatigue appears to be a heterogenous syndrome with no known specific

Table 5–14. Behavioral strategies in the treatment of chronic fatigue syndrome

- Regular exercise, with which the patient feels comfortable.
- A graded increase in exercise, involving walking, swimming, and so on.
- Encouragement of exercises such as yoga and calisthenics.
- Gradual exposure to all avoided activity.
- Cognitive work to break the association between increase in symptoms and stopping or avoiding the activity.
- Further cognitive strategies involving alternative explanations for symptoms. For example, if the patient admitted to thinking "I feel tired, I must have done too much," one might ask the patient to look for alternative explanations, such as "I may be tired because I haven't been doing much lately."
- No further visits to specialists or hospitals unless agreed with therapist.
- Involvement of a cotherapist.

Source.   Adapted from Wessely et al. 1989.

etiology. Some patients appear to have a diagnosable psychiatric illness, such as major depressive disorder, although the effectiveness of antidepressants in this population has not been determined in controlled clinical trials. Until more definitive data are available regarding specific etiologies for this syndrome, clinicians should keep an open mind but, nevertheless, remain skeptical of both explanatory models of the disorder and claims of purported treatment unless they are based on sound scientific research.

REFERENCES

American Psychiatric Association: Diagnostic and Statistical Manual of Mental Disorders, 3rd Edition. Washington, DC, American Psychiatric Association, 1980

Anfinson TJ, Kathol RG: Screening laboratory evaluation in psychiatric patients—a review. Gen Hosp Psychiatry 14:248–257, 1992

Anfinson TJ, Kathol RG: Laboratory and neuroendocrine assessment in medical-psychiatric patients, in Psychiatric Care of the Medical Patient. Edited by Stoudemire A, Fogel BS. New York, Oxford University Press, 1993, pp 105–137

Bates DW, Schmitt W, Buchwald D, et al: Prevalence of fatigue and chronic fatigue syndrome in a primary care practice. Arch Intern Med 153:2759–2765, 1993

Beck AT: Depression Inventory. Philadelphia, PA, Philadelphia Center for Cognitive Therapy, 1978

Behan PO, Behan WM, Bell EJ: The postviral fatigue syndrome—an analysis of the findings in 50 cases. J Infect 10:211–222, 1985

Behan PO, Behan WMH, Horrobin D: Effect of high doses of essential fatty acids on the postviral fatigue syndrome. Acta Neurol Scand 82:209–216, 1990

Behan PO, Behan WMH, Gow JW, et al: Enteroviruses and postviral fatigue syndrome. Ciba Found Symp 173:146–159, 1993

Bibolotti E, Borghi C, Paculli E, et al: The management of fibrositis: a double-blind comparison of maprotiline, chlorimipramine and placebo. Clinical Trials Journal 23:269–280, 1986

Blondell-Hill E, Shafran SD: Treatment of chronic fatigue syndrome—a review and practical guide. Drugs 46:639–651, 1993

Bock GR, Whelan J: Chronic fatigue syndrome. Ciba Found Symp 173:1–345, 1993

Brook MG, Bannister BA, Weir WRC: Interferon-α therapy for patients with chronic fatigue syndrome. J Infect Dis 168:791–792, 1993

Buchwald D, Sullivan JL, Komaroff AL: Frequency of 'chronic active Epstein-Barr virus infection' in a general medical practice. JAMA 257:2303–2307, 1987

Butler S, Chalder T, Ron M, et al: Cognitive behaviour therapy in chronic fatigue syndrome. J Neurol Neurosurg Psychiatry 54:153–158, 1991

Caliguri M, Murray C, Buchwald D, et al: Phenotypic and functional deficiency of natural killer cells in patients with chronic fatigue syndrome. J Immunol 139:3306–3313, 1987

Campbell SM, Clark S, Tindall EA, et al: Clinical characteristics of fibrositis, I: a "blinded" controlled study of symptoms and tender points. Arthritis Rheum 26:817–824, 1983

Carette S, McCain GA, Bell DA, et al: Evaluation of amitriptyline in primary fibrositis—a double blind, placebo controlled study. Arthritis Rheum 29:655–659, 1986

Caruso I, Sarzi Puttini PC, Boccassini L, et al: Double-blind study of dothiepin versus placebo in the treatment of primary fibromyalgia syndrome. International Journal of Medical Research 15:154–159, 1987

Cathebras PJ, Robbins JM, Kirmayer LJ, et al: Fatigue in primary care: prevalence, psychiatric comorbidity, illness behavior, and outcome. J Gen Intern Med 7:276–286, 1992

Cox IM, Campbell MJ, Dowson D: Red blood cell magnesium and chronic fatigue syndrome. Lancet 337:757–760, 1991

Deale A, David AS: Chronic fatigue syndrome: evaluation and management. J Neuropsychiatry 6:189–194, 1994

Derogatis LR: The SCL-90. Baltimore, MD, Clinical Psychometric Research, 1977

Deulofeu R, Gascon J, Gimeniz, N, et al: Magnesium and chronic fatigue syndrome (letter). Lancet 338:641, 1991

Edwards RHT, Gibson H, Clague JE, et al: Muscle histopathology and physiology in chronic fatigue syndrome. Ciba Found Symp 173:102–131, 1993

Engel GL: The clinical application of the biopsychosocial model. Am J Psychiatry 137:535–544, 1980

Folks TM, Heneine W, Khan A, et al: Investigation of retroviral involvement in chronic fatigue syndrome. Ciba Found Symp 173:160–175, 1993

Gold D, Bowden R, Sixbey J, et al: Chronic fatigue—a prospective clinical and virologic study. JAMA 264:48–53, 1990

Goldberg DP, Hillier VF: A scaled version of the General Health Questionnaire. Psychol Med 90:139–145, 1979

Goldenberg DL: Fibromyalgia syndrome. JAMA 257:2782–2787, 1987

Goldenberg DL: Fibromyalgia and other chronic fatigue syndromes: is there evidence for chronic viral disease? Semin Arthritis Rheum 18:111–120, 1988

Goldenberg DL: Fibromyalgia and its relationship to chronic fatigue syndrome, viral illness and immune abnormalities. J Rheumatol 16 (suppl 19):91–93, 1989

Goldenberg DL, Felson DT, Dinerman H: A randomized, controlled trial of amitriptyline and naproxen in the treatment of patients with fibromyalgia. Arthritis Rheum 29:1371–1377, 1986

Goldenberg DL, Simms RW, Geiger A, et al: High frequency of fibromyalgia in patients with chronic fatigue seen in a primary care practice. Arthritis Rheum 33:381–387, 1990

Goodnick PJ, Sandoval R: Psychotropic treatment of chronic fatigue syndrome and related disorders. J Clin Psychiatry 54:13–20, 1993

Goodnick PJ, Sandoval R, Brickman A, et al: Bupropion treatment of fluoxetine-resistant chronic fatigue syndrome. Biol Psychiatry 32:834–838, 1992

Gracious B, Wisner KL: Nortriptyline in chronic fatigue syndrome: a double blind, placebo-controlled single case study. Biol Psychiatry 30:405–408, 1991

Greenberg DB: Neurasthenia in the 1980s: chronic mononucleosis, chronic fatigue syndrome, and anxiety and depressive disorders. Psychosomatics 31:129–137, 1990

Griffen DE: Immunologic abnormalities accompanying acute and chronic viral infections. Rev Infect Dis 13 (suppl 1):S129–S133, 1991

Gunn WJ, Connell DB, Randall B: Epidemiology of chronic fatigue syndrome: the Centers for Disease Control study. Ciba Found Symp 173:83–101, 1993

Hamilton M: A rating scale for depression. J Neurol Neurosurg Psychiatry 23:56–62, 1960

Hellinger WC, Smith TF, Van Scoy RE, et al: Chronic fatigue syndrome and the diagnostic utility of antibody to Epstein-Barr early antigen. JAMA 260:971–973, 1988

Herberman RB: Sources of confounding in immunologic data. Rev Infect Dis 13 (suppl 1):S84–S86, 1991

Holmes GP, Kaplan JE, Stewart JA, et al: A cluster of patients with a chronic mononucleosis–like syndrome. is Epstein-Barr virus the cause? JAMA 257:2297–2303, 1987

Holmes GP, Kaplan JE, Gantz NM, et al: Chronic fatigue syndrome: a working case definition. Ann Intern Med 108:387–389, 1988

Hotchin NA, Read R, Smith DG, et al: Active Epstein-Barr virus infection in post-viral fatigue syndrome. J Infect 18:143–150, 1989

Hunt SM, McEwen J, McKenna SP: Measuring health status: a new tool for clinicians and epidemiologists. J R Coll Gen Pract 35:185–188, 1985

Jones JF, Ray CG, Minnich LL, et al: Evidence for active Epstein-Barr virus infection in patients with persistent, unexplained illnesses: elevated anti-early antigen antibodies. Ann Intern Med 102:1–7, 1985

Kaslow JE, Rucker L, Onishi R: Liver extract–folic acid–cyanocobalamin vs placebo for chronic fatigue syndrome. Arch Intern Med 149:2501–2503, 1989

Katon W, Russo J: Chronic fatigue syndrome criteria—a critique of the requirement for multiple physical complaints. Arch Intern Med 152:1604–1609, 1992

Katon WJ, Walker EA: The relationship of chronic fatigue to psychiatric illness in community, primary care and tertiary care samples. Ciba Found Symp 173:193–211, 1993

Komaroff AL: Clinical presentation of chronic fatigue syndrome. Ciba Found Symp 173:43–61, 1993

Koo D: Chronic fatigue syndrome—a critical appraisal of the role of Epstein-Barr virus. West J Med 150:590–596, 1989

Kroenke K, Wood DR, Mangelsdorff AD, et al: Chronic fatigue in primary care—prevalence, patient characteristics, and outcome. JAMA 260:929–934, 1988

Lane TJ, Matthews DA, Manu P: The low yield of physical examination and laboratory investigations of patients with chronic fatigue. Am J Med Sci 299:313–318, 1990

Lane TJ, Manu P, Matthews DA: Depression and somatization in the chronic fatigue syndrome. Am J Med 91:335–344, 1991

Lane TJ, Manu P, Matthews DA: Immunologic abnormalities in patients with chronic fatigue and the chronic fatigue syndrome. Clin Res 40:559A, 1992

Lewis G, Wessely S: The epidemiology of fatigue: more questions than answers. J Epidemiol Community Health 46:92–97, 1992

Lloyd A, Wakefield D, Dwyer J, et al: Immunological abnormalities in the chronic fatigue syndrome. Med J Aust 151:122–124, 1989

Lloyd A, Hickie I, Wakefield D, et al: A double-blind, placebo-controlled trial of intravenous immunoglobulin therapy in patients with chronic fatigue syndrome. Am J Med 89:561–568, 1990

Lloyd A, Hickie I, Hickie C, et al: Cell-mediated immunity in patients with chronic fatigue syndrome, healthy control subjects, and patients with major depression. Clin Exp Immunol 87:76–79, 1992

Lloyd AR, Hickie I, Boughton CR, et al: The prevalence of chronic fatigue syndrome in an Australian population. Med J Aust 153:522–588, 1990

Lloyd AR, Hickie I, Brockman A, et al: Immunologic and psychologic therapy for patients with chronic fatigue syndrome: a double-blind, placebo-controlled trial. Am J Med 94:197–203, 1993a

Lloyd AR, Wakefield D, Hickie I: Immunity and the pathophysiology of chronic fatigue syndrome. Ciba Found Symp 173:176–192, 1993b

Manu P, Lane TJ, Matthews DA: The frequency of chronic fatigue syndrome in patients with symptoms of persistent fatigue. Ann Intern Med 109:554–556, 1988a

Manu P, Matthews DA, Lane TJ: The mental health of patients with a chief complaint of chronic fatigue—a prospective evaluation and follow-up. Arch Intern Med 148:2213–2217, 1988b

Manu P, Lane TJ, Matthews DA: The pathophysiology of chronic fatigue syndrome: confirmations, contradictions, and conjectures. Int J Psychiatry Med 22:397–408, 1992

Manu P, Lane TJ, Matthews DA: Chronic fatigue and chronic fatigue syndrome: clinical epidemiology and aetiological classification. Ciba Found Symp 173:23–42, 1993

Meador CK: The art and science of nondisease. N Engl J Med 272:92–95, 1965

Mechanic D: Chronic fatigue syndrome and the treatment process. Ciba Found Symp 173:318–341, 1993

Miller NA, Carmichael HA, Calder BD, et al: Antibody to Coxsackie B virus in diagnosing postviral fatigue syndrome. BMJ 302:140–143, 1991

Moldofsky H: Fibromyalgia, sleep disorder and chronic fatigue syndrome. Ciba Found Symp 173:262–279, 1993

Moldofsky H, Saskin P, Lue FA: Sleep and symptoms in fibrositis syndrome after a febrile illness. J Rheumatol 15:1701–1704, 1988

Moran MG, Dubester SN: Connective tissue diseases, in Psychiatric Care of the Medical Patient. Edited by Stoudemire A, Fogel BS. New York, Oxford University Press, 1993, pp 739–756

Murdoch JC: Cell-mediated immunity in patients with myalgic encephalitis syndrome. N Z Med J 101:511–512, 1988

Nielsen AC, Williams TA: Depression in ambulatory medical patients: prevalence by self-report questionnaire and recognition by nonpsychiatric physicians. Arch Gen Psychiatry 37:999–1004, 1980

Olson GB, Kanaan MN, Gersuk GM, et al: Correlation between allergy and persistent Epstein-Barr virus infections in chronic active Epstein-Barr virus infected patients. J Allergy Clin Immunol 78:308–314, 1986a

Olson GB, Kanaan MN, Kelley LM, et al: Specific allergen-induced Epstein-Barr nuclear antigen-positive B cells from patients with chronic active Epstein-Barr virus infections. J Allergy Clin Immunol 78:315–320, 1986b

Peterson PK, Shepard J, Macres M, et al: A controlled trial of intravenous immunoglobulin G in chronic fatigue syndrome. Am J Med 89:554–560, 1990

Powell R, Dolan R, Wessely S: Attribution and self-esteem in depression and chronic fatigue syndromes. J Psychosom Res 34:665–673, 1990

Price RK, North CS, Wessely S, et al: Estimating the prevalence of chronic fatigue syndrome and associated symptoms in the community. Public Health Rep 107:514–522, 1992

Redmond CK: Analysis of clinical, epidemiologic, and laboratory data on chronic fatigue syndrome. Rev Infect Dis 13 (suppl 1):S90–S93, 1991

Richman JA, Flaherty JA, Rospenda KM: Chronic fatigue syndrome: have flawed assumptions been derived from treatment-based studies? Am J Public Health 84:282–284, 1994

Robin R, Lipkin DM, Hume DW: Taking exception to chronic fatigue prevalence findings by Price, et al. Public Health Rep 108:135–137, 1993

Robins LN, Helzer JE, Croughan J, et al: National Institute of Mental Health Diagnostic Interview Schedule: its history, characteristics, and validity. Arch Gen Psychiatry 38:381–389, 1981

Sapira JD: Reassurance therapy: what to say to symptomatic patients with benign diseases. Ann Intern Med 77:603–604, 1977

Schluederberg A, Straus SE, Peterson P, et al: Chronic fatigue syndrome research—definition and medical outcome assessment. Ann Intern Med 117:325–331, 1992

Scudds RA, McCain GA, Rollman GB, et al: Improvements in pain responsiveness in patients with fibrositis after successful treatment with amitriptyline. J Rheumatol 16 (suppl 19):98–103, 1989

Sharpe JC, Archard LC, Banatavala JE, et al: A report—chronic fatigue syndrome: guidelines for research. J R Soc Med 84:118–121, 1991

Shorter E: Chronic fatigue in historical perspective. Ciba Found Symp 173:6–22, 1993

Smythe HA: Non-articluar rheumatism and the fibrositis syndrome, in Arthritis and Allied Conditions, 8th Edition. Edited by Hollander JL, McCarty DJ. Philadelphia, PA, Lea & Febiger, 1972, pp 874–884

Spitzer RL, Endicott J, Robins E: Research Diagnostic Criteria: rationale and reliability. Arch Gen Psychiatry 35:773–782, 1978

Stoff JA, Pellegrino CR (eds): Chronic Fatigue Syndrome—The Hidden Epidemic, 2nd Edition. New York, Harper Collins, 1992

Straus SE: The chronic mononucleosis syndrome. J Infect Dis 157:405–412, 1988

Straus SE: Intravenous immunoglobulin treatment for the chronic fatigue syndrome. Am J Med 89:551–553, 1990

Straus SE: History of chronic fatigue syndrome. Rev Infect Dis 13 (suppl 1):S2–S7, 1991

Straus SE: Studies of herpesvirus infection in chronic fatigue syndrome. Ciba Found Symp 173:132–145, 1993

Straus SE, Tosato G, Armstrong G, et al: Persisting illness and fatigue in adults with evidence of Epstein-Barr virus infection. Ann Intern Med 102:7–16, 1985

Straus SE, Dale JK, Tobi M, et al: Acyclovir treatment of the chronic fatigue syndrome: lack of efficacy in a placebo-controlled trial. N Engl J Med 319:1692–1698, 1988a

Straus SE, Dale JK, Wright R, et al: Allergy and the chronic fatigue syndrome. J Allergy Clin Immunol 81:791–795, 1988b

Wakefield D, Lloyd A, Brockman A: Immunoglobulin subclass abnormalities in patients with chronic fatigue syndrome. Pediatr Infect Dis J 9:S50–S53, 1990

Wessely S, Powell R: Fatigue syndromes: a comparison of chronic "postviral" fatigue with neuromuscular and affective disorders. J Neurol Neurosurg Psychiatry 52:940–948, 1989

Wessely S, David A, Butler S, et al: The management of the chronic "post-viral" fatigue syndrome. J R Coll Gen Pract 39:26–29, 1989

Whelton CL, Salit I, Moldofsky H: Sleep, Epstein-Barr virus infection, musculoskeletal pain, and depressive symptoms in chronic fatigue syndrome. J Rheumatol 19:939–943, 1992

Wolfe F, Smythe HA, Yunus MB, et al: Criteria for fibromyalgia (abstract). Arthritis Rheum 32 (suppl):S47, 1989

Wood GC, Bentall RP, Gopfert M, et al: A comparative psychiatric assessment of patients with chronic fatigue and muscle disease. Psychol Med 21:619–628, 1991

Wysenbeek J, Mor F, Lurie Y, et al: Imipramine for the treatment of fibrositis: a therapeutic trial. Ann Rheum Dis 44:752–753, 1985

Yager J, Young RT: Non-hypoglycemia is an epidemic condition. N Engl J Med 291:907–908, 1974

Zung WW: A rating instrument for anxiety disorders. Psychosomatics 12:371–379, 1971

Chapter 6

Psychiatric Aspects of HIV Infection and AIDS: An Overview and Update

Joel J. Wallack, M.D.
Philip A. Bialer, M.D.
Steven L. Prenzlauer, M.D.

The acquired immunodeficiency syndrome (AIDS) pandemic is now well into its second decade, and, despite a well-organized effort by the global medical community, the numbers of persons infected with the human immunodeficiency virus (HIV) continue to rise while a definitive cure remains elusive. To date, more than a quarter of a million people in the United States have AIDS, and more than 1 million are estimated to be infected with HIV. The World Health Organization (WHO) estimates that 13 million men, women, and children worldwide are HIV infected, and each day the number increases by 5,000. By the year 2000, as many as 40 million people could be infected (CDC 1993e).

The role of the psychiatrist in the fight against AIDS is clearly indispensable; however, it is also increasingly complex. In fact, the psychiatric AIDS literature has become so extensive that selected bibliographies have been published to assist the psychiatrist in sorting through this information (Bialer et al. 1993; Wallack et al. 1991). HIV spectrum disease is associated with frequent neuropsychiatric sequelae, as well as functional psychiatric disorders. The emotional and psychiatric trauma of this disease extends beyond the patient to his or her family and partners and to those at risk ("the worried well"). Furthermore, until effective treatments that will eradicate AIDS are available, mental health specialists will be called on to develop and provide psychoeducational and behavioral interventions designed to reduce high-risk behaviors, thereby helping to control the spread of HIV infection. Toward this effort, in 1986, the American Psychiatric Association, with support from the National Institute of Mental Health, established an AIDS Education Project to provide training courses and materials to assist psychiatrists and other mental health professionals in meeting the challenges of this epidemic (American Psychiatric Association 1990a).

SHIFTING DEMOGRAPHICS OF THE AIDS EPIDEMIC

During 1992, the Centers for Disease Control (CDC 1993c) received reports of 47,095 cases of AIDS, with the majority (50.8%) attributable to transmission among homosexual and bisexual men. Also during 1992, HIV infection became the number one cause of death among men aged 25 to 44 years and the fourth leading cause of death among women in this age group. A higher incidence of mortality was noted among blacks and Hispanics than among other racial and ethnic groups (CDC 1993d). However, the number of reported cases among homosexual and bisexual men decreased in both 1991 and 1992 as the number of cases attributable to injecting drug use (IDU) increased, approaching one-fourth of all reported cases. Clearly, heterosexual contact accounted for the largest proportionate increase (17.1%); 59.4% of this group were women. In fact, in 1992, for the first time, the number of AIDS cases among women infected through heterosexual contact exceeded those infected through IDU. Nearly two-thirds of these women (56.8%) were exposed through heterosexual sex with an injecting drug user. The significant increase in the number of women with AIDS is primarily accounted for by a large increase in infection among non-Hispanic black women. Overall, however, injecting drug users and men who have sex with men continue to account for 80.3% of the AIDS cases (CDC 1993c). Most tragically, the increasing number of women infected during childbearing age has led to a concurrent increase in the number of cases of AIDS among children and infants aged 0 to 4 years, almost all of whom (95.8%) were infected perinatally (CDC 1993c, 1993d).

The future incidence of AIDS cases reported in the United States will be significantly affected by revisions in the CDC classification system for HIV infection. To emphasize the clinical importance of the CD4+ T-lymphocyte count in the categorization of HIV infection, the CDC replaced its 1986 classification system (CDC 1986) and, effective January 1, 1993, expanded its AIDS case surveillance definition to include all HIV-infected persons who have less than 200 CD4+ T lymphocytes/mm^3 or a CD4+ T-lymphocyte percentage of total lymphocytes less than 14%. Three clinical conditions were also added: pulmonary tuberculosis, recurrent pneumonia, and invasive cervical cancer (CDC 1992a). The previous 23 clinical conditions in the case definition published in 1987 (CDC 1987) were retained. Although it is estimated that 120,000 to 190,000 of the more than 1 million Americans who are HIV infected would be found to have CD4+ T-lymphocyte counts below 200 cells/mm^3, many are unaware that they are HIV infected or are unaware of their immunologic status. Nonetheless, the CDC anticipated that the number of cases reported in 1993 under the new expanded definition would increase by approximately 75% (CDC 1992a) before leveling off in subsequent years. In fact, the number of AIDS cases reported to the CDC in 1993 was 106,949, more than double the 1992 total (CDC 1994). At least one study has demonstrated that the new case definition will result in a significant increase in the median patient survival time when compared with survival time of those previously diagnosed under the 1987 definition (Vella et al. 1994). Therefore, those providing care to AIDS patients will need to understand the greater variability in prognoses that will result from the new classification system to provide appropriate information and counseling.

EARLY HISTORY OF THE AIDS EPIDEMIC

AIDS was first recognized as a new clinical entity in 1981 with the appearance of uncommon diseases among young homosexual men in San Francisco, Los Angeles, and New York City, which included *Pneumocystis carinii* pneumonia (PCP) and Kaposi's sarcoma (Gottlieb et al. 1981; Masur et al. 1981). At first, researchers assumed the cause of this syndrome was related to homosexual lifestyle; however, AIDS cases were soon reported among intravenous drug users, transfusion recipients, adults from Central Africa and Haiti, and infants of mothers who were either injecting drug users or had AIDS. This progression of risk groups eventually led to the conclusion that AIDS was caused by a common infectious agent (Francis et al. 1983; Ward and Drotman

1992). Before we continue the history of the AIDS epidemic, we briefly review basic information regarding cellular immunity.

ASSESSING IMMUNOLOGIC STATUS: SURFACE GLYCOPROTEINS AND THE CD4+ CELL COUNT

All human lymphocytes have a variety of surface glycoproteins that are essential to the cell's proper functioning. These glycoproteins are particularly important to the understanding of immunologic activity. The CD3 (T3) cell marker is found on all adult lymphocytes. Those lymphocytes with the CD4 (T4) cell surface marker, known as helper cells, induce immunologic reactions, in contrast to the cells with CD8 (T8) surface markers, suppressor cells, which control or suppress immunologic responses. Over the course of HIV infection, CD4+ T lymphocytes are destroyed, leading to the opportunistic infections and malignancies characteristic of AIDS. Under the new AIDS classification system (CDC 1992a), CD4+ cell counts are used to define clinical AIDS. Monitoring of the CD4+ cell count allows for the clinical staging of the disease status of the HIV-infected patient (Saag 1992). Although variation exists among laboratories, total CD4+ cell counts are usually 500 to 1,600 cells/mm^3 in adults. Patients can also be followed clinically by use of the CD4:CD8 ratio (normal 0.5 to 2.0) or by the CD4 percentage, which measures the number of CD4+ cells as a percentage of all lymphocytes (normal 40% to 70%).

Abnormal CD4+ T-lymphocyte cell counts are by themselves not diagnostic of HIV infection; confirmatory HIV testing is still required.

SEARCH FOR THE CAUSATIVE AGENT OF AIDS

Asymptomatic patients with hemophilia and intravenous drug users were often noted to have inverted CD4+ T-lymphocyte helper to CD8+ T-lymphocyte suppressor cell ratios; this was also the finding among AIDS patients and some asymptomatic homosexual men. However, unlike those noninfected patients whose abnormal T-cell ratios were caused by an increase in the number of suppressor T cells as a result of antigen stimulation, the AIDS patients and asymptomatic infected patients actually had a decrease in T-helper cells. Because the human T-lymphotropic virus (HTLV) was, at that time, the only virus known to infect T-helper lymphocytes and that could be transmitted by blood, by sexual contact, and from mothers to newborns, researchers began to search for an HTLV-related causative organism for AIDS (Essex 1992).

Eventually, it was demonstrated that AIDS was indeed linked to a T-lymphotropic retrovirus (Gallo et al. 1984), which was eventually termed *human immunodeficiency virus type 1* (HIV-1) (Coffin et al. 1986). The origin of HIV-1 has been subject to much speculation. One theory is that HIV-1 originated in central Africa and traveled to the large cities that now comprise the "AIDS belt" of Africa. Possibilities include a subhuman primate transmission to humans as early as the mid-1950s (Nahmias et al. 1986) or migration of a few resistant human carriers from previously isolated tribes. However, no groups of Africans have, yet, shown greater resistance to AIDS or disease progression. Therefore, a primate origin seems more likely (Essex 1992). In fact, all types of HIV-1 appear to be avirulent when injected into chimpanzees, and interestingly, a virus that could be a progenitor of HIV-1 has been isolated from a central African chimpanzee (Huet et al. 1990).

A second human immunodeficiency virus (HIV-2) was discovered among Africans in Mozambique and Angola. This virus is clearly much less virulent than HIV-1, but there have been some case reports of HIV-2–associated AIDS (Paulsen et al. 1989). For the remainder of this chapter, when we use the term *HIV*, we are referring specifically to HIV-1.

MECHANISMS OF INFECTION AND VIROLOGY

HIV is a member of the lentivirus subfamily of retroviruses. Human lentiviruses encode an enzyme, RNA-dependent DNA polymerase or reverse transcriptase, which allows viral RNA to be transcribed into DNA. This new proviral DNA integrates into the host cellular genome and can then continue to replicate within the host. Therefore, a person with evidence of HIV infection should be considered permanently infected (Mitsuyasu 1989). However, the infected cells can remain in a "latent" state during which little or no viral RNA or proteins are produced. The virus can therefore elude the host's immune system, and, even after antibody production, severe immunodeficiency may not be seen for months or even years.

HIV infection leads to progressive destruction of infected cells, including CD4 (helper) T lymphocytes. This eventually leads to the gross cellular immune dysfunction characteristic of AIDS. Other cells targeted by HIV include T and B lymphocytes, monocyte-macrophages, and the cellular components of the central nervous system (CNS), among other sites. HIV has been found in a number of body fluids—most frequently, in blood or cerebrospinal fluid (CSF) and, less frequently or in lower concentration, in saliva, tears, urine, and breast milk. HIV is also found in stool, semen, and vaginal secretions; the concentration of HIV is directly related to the number of infected cells. Therefore, the presence of inflammation or venereal infection may lead to a greater number of HIV-infected cells being present (Mitsuyasu 1989). HIV attaches to specific surface molecules on the target cells, among them, the CD4 antigen. Cells with the CD4 surface antigen, such as the T4-lymphocyte helper cells, are therefore readily attacked.

The outcome of HIV infection depends on the host's immune reaction to the virus, which includes both suppression of HIV replication and direct killing of the infected cells. Some patients with active immune systems have been able to delay the onset of the active disease for more than 10 years (J. A. Levy 1992).

Maternal-to-Infant Transmission

There is a 15%–40% chance of an HIV-infected mother giving birth to an HIV-infected infant. It is believed that most infections occur during the third trimester of pregnancy. Infants can also become infected from the breast milk of an HIV-infected mother. Therefore, it is recommended that these women do not breast-feed (American Psychiatric Association 1993a).

Zidovudine (AZT) has been shown to significantly reduce the rate of transmission of HIV from mothers to their infants. In a recent multisite study by the Pediatric AIDS Clinical Trials Group (Connor et al. 1994), a regimen of AZT was administered to HIV-infected pregnant women beginning between 14 and 34 weeks of gestation, continued throughout pregnancy, and then given to their infants for the first 6 weeks of life. The risk of maternal-to-infant transmission of HIV was reduced from 25.5% in the placebo-treated group to 8.3% in the AZT-treated mothers and infants. These early results are very encouraging, but long-term follow-up is essential to rule out any late effects of AZT on these infants. The study did not address AZT use in the first trimester.

HIV TESTING

It is important to understand that AIDS is a clinical syndrome with an evolving and expanding case definition. We do not test for a syndrome. "AIDS testing," rather, is an effort to identify evidence of HIV infection, the causative agent of AIDS.

The first tests included expensive and time-consuming methods to isolate the virus via tissue cultures. However, once the causative agent of AIDS was discovered, more specific tests were soon developed that identified host antibodies to HIV. The two most common tests currently in use are the enzyme-linked immunosorbent assay (ELISA) and the Western blot. The reliability of these tests depends on the production of antibodies by the host and the absence of cross-reacting antibodies (Saag 1992). The overall reliability of these tests, when used properly and in combination, is quite high.

The presence of antibodies indicates that a host response to the virus has occurred. However, this does not in any way indicate a resolution of the infection. Retroviruses, such as HIV, integrate within the viral genome (DNA) of the host cell. Once an adult has produced HIV antibodies (i.e., becomes seropositive), virus can usually be isolated from the patient. The presence of HIV antibodies, therefore, is generally considered evidence of persistent infection. One exception to this rule is found with infants less than age 18 months, born to HIV-seropositive mothers. Immunoglobulin G (IgG) antibodies may cross the placenta and then gradually decrease until undetectable. Thus, HIV serologic testing of umbilical cord blood is not a reliable indicator of newborn HIV infection (Weiss 1992).

Antibody Responses

The majority of HIV-infected individuals will achieve a detectable antibody response shortly after exposure to HIV. Approximately 90% will have evidence of antibodies within 6 months of infection (Summergrad and Glassman 1991). However, some reports indicate significant lag times in some individuals from the time of infection until measurable antibody response (Imagawa et al. 1989). Generally, 4 to 8 weeks after infection, at the time of seroconversion, the patient may experience a brief flulike illness, characterized by fever, rash, myalgia, and fatigue; some may also have neurologic symptoms. This time-limited illness, usually lasting a few days to a few weeks, is associated with active replication of the virus within the host, followed by increasing serum levels of virus-specific antibodies (Davey et al. 1992).

Enzyme-Linked Immunosorbent Assay (ELISA) Test

The ELISA is generally used as a screening test; therefore, it is highly sensitive at the expense of specificity. Thus, the predictive value of the ELISA will vary with the population being tested. When the probability of infection is high, the positive predictive value of a reactive ELISA is quite high. Similarly, when testing an asymptomatic person at low risk for HIV infection, the reliability of a nonreactive ELISA is also high. If such a low-risk person has a positive test, a false-positive result must be considered. As many as 1% of healthy blood donors may test positive, and as many as 90% of these will prove to be false positives (Levine and Bayer 1985).

Often, the interval between exposure and testing is unknown, and a negative result could reflect testing during the latency period, before the onset of circulating antibodies. In this case, a repeat test in a few months will help to confirm seronegativity. Therefore, it is important for the clinician to keep in mind that a single negative HIV test in an individual at high risk for exposure does not rule out the possibility of infection.

A positive ELISA can be caused by several factors, in addition to HIV infection. Therefore, all positive results must be verified by repeat testing and subsequent confirmation, usually with the Western blot, which has very low false-positive and false-negative rates.

In 1991, publicly funded counseling and testing programs provided more than 2 million HIV tests (CDC 1992b). Testing rates of people at risk for HIV infection are lower among blacks, Hispanics, and those with less than a high school education. A 1991–1992 assessment of high-risk populations in southern Los Angeles County revealed that 37% had either not been tested or failed to obtain their test results. Of particular concern is the finding that only 55% of female sexual partners of male injecting drug users, who otherwise have no risk factors for infection, were themselves tested (CDC 1993a).

Impact of Widespread Testing

Because of the potential benefits of early identification and treatment of asymptomatic seropositive individuals as well as the essential importance of modifying high-risk behaviors among this growing group, widespread HIV testing has been encouraged. Concerns have been expressed, however, regarding the potential physical and emotional impact of undergoing testing and the distress of receiving test results. This distress related to testing might lead to an increase in high-risk behaviors (e.g., unprotected sex, alcohol and drug use) and suicidal potential or to a negative impact on disease progression by adversely affecting immune processes (Marzuk 1991; Perry et al. 1991; Solomon 1989). Perry and co-workers (1990b) found that after testing, anxiety and depression were actually reduced, even among those testing positive for HIV. Similarly, these investigators found that suicidal ideations decreased over the 2 months after testing, regardless of the patient's serostatus (Perry et al. 1990c).

To help patients to better understand and cope with the process of HIV testing, both pre- and posttest counseling are now standard.

HIV TEST COUNSELING

Individual counseling is generally considered preferable, and, if possible, the same clinician should see the patient both pre- and posttest. The goals of pretest counseling include educating patients regarding the accuracy and meaning of HIV testing, informing them of reporting requirements and confidentiality issues, evaluating their coping abilities and the potential emotional impact of the test results, and helping patients to decide whether testing is both indicated and advisable. Patients must understand the meaning of both positive and negative test results and the possibilities of false-positive or false-negative results. High-risk behaviors must be identified, with a clear goal of reducing future risks of additional exposure or possible transmission of infection. Practical information such as safe sex techniques or proper cleansing of syringes and needles should be frankly discussed. Appropriate literature for patients to take home is often helpful and can reinforce proper behaviors.

Posttest counseling begins with notification of the test results and an interpretation of the meaning of the results. The patient's emotional reaction must be assessed, and appropriate follow-up must be provided as needed. Those who test HIV positive must be made aware that they are considered infected and infectious for life. In HIV-positive women of childbearing age, the risk of mother-to-infant HIV transmission during or after pregnancy must be discussed. For patients who test seropositive, as well as those who test seronegative but are still considered at risk for infection, the counselor must thoroughly review high-risk practices and risk-reduction strategies. The HIV-positive patient should be referred for appropriate medical follow-up and should be given information regarding community support and crisis intervention services. If possible, the patient should not be left alone during the first few days after notification because of the potential for severe emotional reactions, including impulsive self-destructive behaviors (American Psychiatric Association 1993c; Perry and Markowitz 1988).

A variety of psychoeducational counseling interventions have been studied. Perry and his colleagues (1991) demonstrated significant decreases in distress among seronegative subjects who received standard pre- and posttest counseling, counseling plus an interactive video program, or counseling plus individual stress prevention training. Among those who tested seropositive, the brief stress prevention training program significantly decreased emotional distress, whereas the other two interventions showed no significant increase in distress measures. These findings are important and may help to reduce the frequently expressed concerns regarding potential adverse effects of voluntary testing.

PSYCHIATRIC DIAGNOSIS

Prevalence of Psychiatric Morbidity in HIV

Although there have been no studies of psychiatric morbidity among those with HIV-related illness on the scale of the Epidemiologic Catchment Area Program (Regier et al. 1984, 1988), the psychological and neuropsychiatric manifestations of HIV infection are now well documented. However, it is difficult to provide a simple overview of the research regarding psychiatric diagnoses in HIV illness because of the various methodologies used, cohorts studied, and the complexities of the science of HIV.

Early reports of the psychiatric manifestations of AIDS were often based on clinical experience rather than on actual data. Nonetheless, they provided a sound basis for understanding the problems facing this population. The patients' emotional reactions and phases of situational distress were well described (Morin et al. 1984; Nichols 1983, 1985), and the relative frequencies of specific psychiatric diagnoses, particularly adjustment disorders, major depression, and cognitive impairment, were also reported (Holland and Tross 1985). Retrospective chart reviews of patients hospitalized for the treatment of HIV-related illnesses also confirmed that adjustment disorders, mood disturbances, and "organic" mental syndromes (as defined in DSM-III [American Psychiatric Association 1980]) were the most frequently diagnosed psychiatric disorders (Dilley et al. 1985; Perry and Tross 1984). In addition, several case reports described AIDS patients with CNS syndromes that sometimes mimicked functional psychiatric disorders (Hoffman 1984; Lowenstein and Sharfstein 1984; Nurnberg et al. 1984).

More recently, structured scales and interviews have been used to study psychiatric morbidity among HIV patients. At least two studies have shown a relatively high lifetime prevalence of depressive, anxiety, and nonopiate substance use disorders in cohorts of homosexual men, regardless of HIV serostatus (Atkinson et al. 1988; Williams et al. 1991). A group of men and women at risk for HIV infection who were interviewed before serologic testing also had a high lifetime prevalence of mood disorder (Perry et al. 1990a). Perry and colleagues (1993) also discovered that an abnormal score indicative of psychopathology on a series of anxiety and depression scales administered at the time of HIV testing was the most reliable predictor of the presence of psychopathology 1 year later. Some studies have shown increased distress in HIV-seropositive men compared with those with full-blown AIDS (Chuang et al. 1989; Tross and Hirsch 1988). Other studies have shown distress and depression to be associated with HIV-related symptoms (Ostrow et al. 1989). Although these reports imply that patients with AIDS may be at high risk for developing psychiatric disorders during the course of their illnesses, it is important to note that the majority of these subjects who were in the early stage of HIV disease had no significant psychiatric morbidity.

Some reports have focused on the psychiatric diagnoses among HIV patients who required admission to general inpatient psychiatric units. Of 60 patients admitted to San Francisco General Hospital, the most common diagnoses were dementia (30%), adjustment disorder with depressed mood (22%), major depression (12%), and schizophrenia (10%) (Baer 1989). A similar study of 91 patients admitted to St. Vincent's Hospital in New York City revealed that many received more than one diagnosis—49 (54%) had symptoms diagnosed as a cognitive impairment syndrome, of which 30 (33%) were more specifically diagnosed with dementia, 43 (47%) had substance use/dependence, and 22 (24%) had an adjustment disorder (Wiener et al. 1994). At both hospitals, the patients with dementia had the longest lengths of stay.

Women represent a rapidly increasing segment of the AIDS population, but, for the most part, they have not been adequately included in AIDS psychosocial research. Using structured interviews, Brown and Rundell (1993) conducted a prospective study of psychiatric morbidity among military women infected with HIV. Interestingly, 31% of the subjects had hypoactive sexual desire disorder at initial contact, with a significant increase to 41% of the sample at follow-up interviews. Excluding hypoactive sexual desire disorder, phobias, and DSM-III-R (American Psychiatric Association 1987) "V" code diagnoses, only 24% of the women had symptoms diagnosed as an Axis I disorder by the time of their second assessment. Few of these women revealed clinically significant anxiety or depression on the Hamilton Anxiety Scale (Hamilton 1959) and Hamilton Rating Scale for Depression (Hamilton 1960). Only one woman reported suicidal ideation, and none reported suicidal gestures or attempts during the course of the study. The investigators compared these findings with similar studies of HIV-infected men in the military; the men experienced higher frequencies of suicidal ideation and behavior and had more psychiatric hospitalizations. The results of the military studies also differed from those of a study of 62 women with psychiatric diagnoses who attended an urban AIDS clinic, the majority of whom had a history of IDU and were socioeconomically deprived. Psychological distress, as measured by depression and anxiety on self-report scales, was found in 40%–45% of this sample (Bialer et al. 1992). Although some authors have reported higher levels of depressive symptoms among HIV-infected women (Fleishman and Fogel 1994), it is not yet clear if there is a gender difference in overall psychiatric morbidity among the HIV population. Further studies exploring the psychosocial circumstances, coping styles, and psychiatric phenomenology in male and female cohorts are needed.

Tables 6–1 and 6–2 summarize the frequencies of psychiatric diagnoses among 819 HIV-infected patients seen for psychiatric consultation over a 3-year period at a major New York City teaching hospital.

AIDS Dementia Complex

AIDS dementia complex (ADC), a syndrome first described and defined in 1986 by Navia and his group (Navia et al. 1986a), was added to the surveillance case definition of AIDS in 1987 (CDC 1987). *Subacute encephalitis* (Snider et al. 1983) and *HIV encephalopathy* (Levy et al. 1985) are terms that have also been used for this syndrome. In 1991, a working group of the American Academy of Neurology AIDS Task Force proposed the term *HIV-1–associated cognitive/motor complex,* along with a set of diagnostic criteria (Working Group 1991) (Table 6–3). This name may more accurately describe the phenomenologic manifestations of HIV brain disease, but for the purposes of this discussion, we will continue to use *AIDS dementia complex.*

Clinically, patients with ADC present with cognitive deficits that include impairment in attention and concentration, mental slowing, and forgetfulness. Motor symptoms such as unsteady gait, tremor, and impaired fine rapid finger or hand movements may also be present. In addition, there may be behavioral changes typically manifested by ap-

Table 6–1. Psychiatric diagnoses (DSM-III-R) among HIV-infected patients seen for inpatient consultation from 1989–1993[a]

Diagnosis	AIDS/ARC (*n* = 529)	HIV+ (*n* = 140)
Dementia[b]	122	25
Organic mood disorder[c]	81	27
Delirium[d]	68	7
Organic mental syndrome not otherwise specified[e]	64	24
Substance use/dependence	197	122
Adjustment disorder	83	24
Schizophrenia	16	7
Major depression	10	2
Anxiety disorder	4	1
Schizoaffective disorder	3	3
Personality disorder	102	61

Note. AIDS = acquired immunodeficiency syndrome; ARC = AIDS-related complex; HIV+ = human immunodeficiency virus positive.
[a]From the Consultation-Liaison Psychiatry Service, Beth Israel Medical Center, New York City.
[b]DSM-IV: dementia due to HIV disease.
[c]DSM-IV: mood disorder due to a general medical condition or substance-induced mood disorder.
[d]DSM-IV: delirium due to a general medical condition or substance-induced delirium.
[e]DSM-IV: mental disorder not otherwise specified due to a general medical condition or cognitive disorder not otherwise specified.

athy, decreased emotional responsiveness, and lethargy. Because these symptoms have a wide range of severity, a system to classify patients, from stage 0 (no ADC) to stage 4 (severe ADC), has been proposed (Price and Brew 1988; Sidtis and Price 1990) (Table 6–4). The clinical course of ADC is variable, however, and placing a patient at stage 0.5 or 1 should not imply that he or she will necessarily progress to more severe stages.

Prevalence and incidence.   The actual prevalence and yearly incidence of ADC are unknown. Various authors have estimated that 66% (Price et al. 1988) to 90% (Brew 1993) of HIV-infected patients will develop ADC by the late stages of their illness. In contrast, recent epidemiologic studies have reported that frequencies of ADC range from 7%–28% (Day et al. 1992; Janssen et al. 1992; McArthur et al. 1993), although methodologic problems of the studies may have influenced

Table 6–2.   Psychiatric diagnoses (DSM-III-R) among HIV-infected patients seen for outpatient consultation from 1989–1993[a]

Diagnosis	AIDS/ARC (n = 94)	HIV+ (n = 56)
Adjustment disorder	24	23
Major depression	15	5
Organic mood disorder[b]	12	7
Dementia[c]	10	0
Organic mental syndrome not otherwise specified[d]	8	4
Substance use/dependence	37	32
Schizophrenia	1	3
Anxiety disorder	8	3
Personality disorder	30	27

Note.   AIDS = acquired immunodeficiency syndrome; ARC = AIDS-related complex; HIV+ = human immunodeficiency virus positive.
[a]From the Consultation-Liaison Psychiatry Service, Beth Israel Medical Center, New York City.
[b]DSM-IV: mood disorder due to a general medical condition or substance-induced mood disorder.
[c]DSM-IV: dementia due to HIV disease.
[d]DSM-IV: mental disorder not otherwise specified due to a general medical condition or cognitive disorder not otherwise specified.

Table 6–3.   Criteria for clinical diagnosis of central nervous system disorders in adults and adolescents

---

HIV-1–associated cognitive/motor complex

All of the following diagnoses require laboratory evidence for systemic HIV-1 infection (enzyme-linked immunosorbent assay test confirmed by Western blot, polymerase chain reaction, or culture)

I. Sufficient for diagnosis of AIDS

   A. HIV-1–associated dementia complex[a]

   Probable (must have *each* of the following):

   1. Acquired abnormality in at least *two* of the following cognitive abilities (present for at least 1 month): attention/concentration, speed of processing of information, abstraction/reasoning, visuospatial skills, memory/ learning, and speech/ language. The decline should be verified by reliable history and mental status examination. In all cases, when possible, history should be obtained from an informant, and examination should be supplemented by neuropsychological testing.

   Cognitive dysfunction causing impairment of work or activities of daily living[b] (objectively verifiable or by report of a key informant). This impairment should not be attributable solely to severe systemic illness.

   2. At least *one* of the following:

   a. Acquired abnormality in motor function or performance verified by clinical examination (e.g., slowed rapid movements, abnormal gait, limb incoordination, hyperreflexia, hypertonia, or weakness), neuropsychological tests (e.g., fine motor speed, manual dexterity, perceptual motor skills), or both.

   b. Decline in motivation or emotional control or change in social behavior. This

---

Note. HIV-1 = human immunodeficiency virus type 1; AIDS = acquired immunodeficiency syndrome; HTLV-I = human T-lymphotropic virus type I.

[a]For research purposes, HIV-1–associated dementia complex can be coded to describe the major features:

   HIV-1–associated dementia complex requires criteria 1, 2a, 2b, 3, and 4.

   HIV-1–associated dementia complex (motor) requires criteria 1, 2a, 3, and 4.

   HIV-1–associated dementia complex (behavior) requires criteria 1, 2b, 3, and 4.

[b]The level of impairment due to cognitive dysfunction should be assessed as follows:

Mild: Decline in performance at work, including work in the home, that is conspicuous to others. Unable to work at usual job, although may be able to work at a much less demanding job. Activities of daily living or social activities are impaired but not to a degree making the person completely dependent on others. More complicated daily tasks or recreational activities cannot be undertaken. Capable of basic self-care such as feeding, dressing, and maintaining personal hygiene, but activities such as handling money, shopping, using public transportation, driving a car, or keeping track of appointments or medications is impaired.

Moderate: Unable to work, including work in the home. Unable to function without some assistance of another in daily living, including dressing, maintaining personal hygiene, eating, shopping, handling money, and walking, but able to communicate basic needs.

Severe: Unable to perform any activities of daily living without assistance. Requires continual supervision. Unable to maintain personal hygiene, nearly or absolutely mute.

(continued)

Table 6–3. Criteria for clinical diagnosis of central nervous system disorders in adults and adolescents *(continued)*

---

may be characterized by any of the following: change in personality with apathy, inertia, irritability, emotional lability, or new onset of impaired judgment characterized by socially inappropriate behavior or disinhibition.

3. Absence of clouding of consciousness during a period long enough to establish the presence of #1.
4. Evidence of another etiology, including active central nervous system opportunistic infection or malignancy, psychiatric disorders (e.g., depressive disorder), active alcohol substance use, or acute or chronic substance withdrawal, must be sought from history, physical and psychiatric examination, and appropriate laboratory and radiologic investigation (e.g., lumbar puncture, neuroimaging). If another potential etiology (e.g., major depression) is present, it is *not* the cause of the above cognitive, motor, or behavioral symptoms and signs.

Possible (must have *one* of the following):
1. Other potential etiology present (must have *each* of the following):
   a. As above (see *Probable*) #1, 2, and 3.
   b. Other potential etiology is present, but the cause of #1 above is uncertain.
2. Incomplete clinical evaluation (must have *each* of the following):
   a. As above (see *Probable*) #1, 2, and 3.
   b. Etiology cannot be determined (appropriate laboratory or radiologic investigations not performed).

B. HIV-1–associated myelopathy
Probable (must have *each* of the following):
1. Acquired abnormality in lower-extremity neurologic function disproportionate to upper-extremity abnormality verified by reliable history (lower-extremity weakness, incoordination, and/or urinary incontinence) and neurologic examination (paraparesis, lower-extremity spasticity, hyperreflexia, or the presence of Babinski signs, with or without sensory loss).
2. Myelopathic disturbance (see #1) is severe enough[c] to require constant unilateral support for walking.
3. Although mild cognitive impairment may be present, criteria for HIV-1–associated dementia complex are not fulfilled.
4. Evidence of another etiology, including neoplasm, compressive lesion, or multiple sclerosis must be sought from history, physical examination, and appropriate laboratory and radiologic investigations (e.g., lumbar puncture, neuroimaging, myelography). If another potential etiology is present, it is *not* the cause of the myelopathy. This diagnosis cannot be made in a patient infected with both HIV-1 and HTLV-I; such a patient should be classified as having possible HIV-1–associated myelopathy.

---

[c]The severity of HIV-1–associated myelopathy should be graded as follows:
Mild: Ambulatory but requires constant unilateral support (e.g., cane) for walking.
Moderate: Requires constant bilateral support (e.g., walker) for walking.
Severe: Unable to walk even with assistance; confined to bed or wheelchair.

(continued)

Table 6–3. Criteria for clinical diagnosis of central nervous system disorders in adults and adolescents *(continued)*

Possible (must have *one* of the following):

  1. Other potential etiology present (must have *each* of the following):

   a. As above (see *Probable*) #1, 2, and 3.

   b. Other potential etiology is present, but the cause of the myelopathy is uncertain.

  2. Incomplete clinical evaluation (must have *each* of the following):

   a. As above (see *Probable*) #1, 2, and 3.

   b. Etiology cannot be determined (appropriate laboratory or radiologic investigations not performed).

 II. Not sufficient for diagnosis of AIDS

 HIV-1–associated minor cognitive/motor disorder

 Probable (must have *each* of the following):

  1. Cognitive/motor/behavioral abnormalities (must have *each* of the following):

   a. At least *two* of the following acquired cognitive, motor, or behavioral symptoms (present for at least 1 month) verified by reliable history (when possible, from an informant):

    1) Impaired attention or concentration

    2) Mental slowing

    3) Impaired memory

    4) Slowed movements

    5) Incoordination

    6) Personality change, or irritability or emotional lability

   b. Acquired cognitive/motor abnormality verified by clinical neurologic examination or neuropsychological testing (e.g., fine motor speed, manual dexterity, perceptual motor skills, attention/concentration, speed of processing of information, abstraction/reasoning, visuospatial skills, memory/learning, or speech/language).

  2. Disturbance from cognitive/motor/behavioral abnormalities (see #1) causes mild impairment of work or activities of daily living[d] (objectively verifiable or by report of a key informant).

  3. Does not meet criteria for HIV-1–associated dementia complex or HIV-1–associated myelopathy.

  4. *No* evidence of another etiology, including active central nervous system opportunistic infection or malignancy, or severe systemic illness determined by appropriate history, physical examination, and laboratory and radiologic investigation (e.g., lumbar puncture, neuroimaging). The above features should not be attributable solely to the effects of active alcohol or substance

---

[d]Able to perform all but the most demanding aspects of work or activities of daily living. Performance at work is mildly impaired but able to maintain usual job; social activities may be mildly impaired, but person is not dependent on others. Can feed self, dress, and maintain personal hygiene, handle money, shop, use public transportation, or drive a car, but complex daily tasks such as keeping track of appointments or medications may be occasionally impaired.

(continued)

Table 6–3. Criteria for clinical diagnosis of central nervous system disorders in adults and adolescents *(continued)*

use, acute or chronic substance withdrawal, adjustment disorder, or other psychiatric disorders.

Possible (must have *one* of the following):

1. Other potential etiology present (must have *each* of the following):
   a. As above (see *Probable*) #1, 2, and 3.
   b. Other potential etiology is present and the cause of the cognitive/motor/behavioral abnormalities is uncertain.
2. Incomplete clinical evaluation (must have *each* of the following):
   a. As above (see *Probable*) #1, 2, and 3.
   b. Etiology cannot be determined (appropriate laboratory or radiologic investigations not performed).

Source. Reprinted from Working Group of the American Academy of Neurology AIDS Task Force: "Nomenclature and Research Case Definitions for Neurologic Manifestations of Human Immunodeficiency Virus-Type 1 (HIV-1) Infection." *Neurology* 41:778–785, 1991. Used with permission.

these lower percentages. Portegies and associates (1993) speculated that the introduction of AZT has lowered the incidence of ADC, but this has not yet been proven. We suspect the current prevalence and incidence of ADC are somewhere between the above extremes.

It is not clear why only a certain percentage of HIV-infected patients develop ADC. Each strain of HIV may have a different neurovirulence, or certain cofactors, as yet undetermined, may play a role in the etiology of ADC.

Pathogenesis.   The pathogenesis of ADC is unknown, but several theories have been offered. Autopsy studies have demonstrated direct infection by HIV of the CNS. Pathologic findings include multinucleated giant cells and diffuse white matter pallor (Navia et al. 1986b; Sharer 1992). Although these pathologic changes may be associated with the presence and severity of ADC, one study found them in only 50% of their sample (Glass et al. 1993). Indirect mechanisms, such as the production of neurotoxic cytokines by infected macrophages or other activated cells, are now largely thought to be crucial to the development of ADC. Quinolinic acid (Freese et al. 1990; Heyes et al. 1989; Martin et al. 1992) and tumor necrosis factor-α (Glass et al. 1993; Merrill 1992) have been implicated. Alternatively, the gp120 envelope coat protein of HIV has been shown to be neurotoxic by increasing intracellular calcium (Dreyer et al. 1990). Current research efforts are exploring the CNS excitatory *N*-methyl-D-aspartate (NMDA) receptors, which are thought to be involved in the pathogenesis of a range of acute and chronic neurologic disorders (Lipton and Rosenberg 1994). Activation of NMDA receptors can also result in an influx of intracellular calcium, which may lead to neuronal injury or death. Theoretically, NMDA receptor antagonists such as dextromethorphan or calcium channel blockers such as nimodipine could have a beneficial effect in patients

Table 6–4. Staging scheme for the AIDS dementia complex (ADC)

ADC stage	Characteristics
Stage 0 (normal)	Normal mental and motor function
Stage 0.5 (equivocal/subclinical)	Either minimal or equivocal *symptoms* of cognitive or motor dysfunction characteristic of ADC or mild signs (snout response, slowed extremity movements) but *without impairment of work or capacity to perform activities of daily living* (ADL); gait and strength are normal
Stage 1 (mild)	Unequivocal evidence (symptoms, signs, neuropsychological test performance) of functional intellectual or motor impairment characteristic of ADC but able to perform *all but the more demanding aspects of work or ADL;* can walk without assistance
Stage 2 (moderate)	Cannot work or maintain the more demanding aspects of daily life but able to perform *basic activities of self-care;* ambulatory but may require a single prop
Stage 3 (severe)	*Major intellectual incapacity* (cannot follow news or personal events, cannot sustain complex conversation, considerable slowing of all output), *or motor disability* (cannot walk unassisted, requiring walker or personal support, usually with slowing and clumsiness of arms as well)
Stage 4 (end stage)	*Nearly vegetative;* intellectual and social comprehension and responses are at a rudimentary level, nearly or absolutely mute; paraparetic or paraplegic with double incontinence

Source. Reprinted from Sidtis JJ, Price RW: "Early HIV-1 Infection and the AIDS Dementia Complex." *Neurology* 40:323–326, 1990. Used with permission.

with ADC (M. Teitelman, personal communication, April 1994). However, the clinical usefulness of these agents has not yet been demonstrated. Regardless of the mechanism, ADC generally occurs late in the course of HIV disease and is most commonly associated with immunologic decline (Brew 1993; Sidtis and Price 1990).

Diagnosis.   The diagnosis of ADC is clinical, and all HIV-infected patients with acute or chronic mental status changes should have a complete neurologic evaluation. The workup should include a cognitive history (especially from others who know the patient), a thorough neurologic examination to evaluate motor changes, a neuroradiologic evaluation to exclude opportunistic infections and neoplasms, CSF examination to rule out infectious or inflammatory processes, and selective neuropsychological testing if clinically indicated.

ADC can only be diagnosed after other potential causes of cognitive, motor, and behavioral symptoms have been ruled out. Efforts to identify diagnostic tests that are specific for ADC have had mixed success. Magnetic resonance imaging (MRI) may be more sensitive than computed tomography (CT) in the detection of subcortical white matter abnormalities, but no significant difference in the presence of these lesions has been found between patients with and without dementia (Broderick et al. 1993) or between HIV-seropositive men and seronegative control subjects (Bornstein et al. 1992). Some studies have suggested that certain patterns of regional cerebral dysfunction, as demonstrated by positron-emission tomography (PET) or single photon-emission computed tomography (SPECT), may be specific for patients with ADC (LaFrance et al. 1988; Pohl et al. 1988; van Gorp et al. 1992), but further research is needed in this area. Routine CSF analysis in patients with ADC is usually nonspecific; however, elevated concentrations of surrogate markers in the CSF, namely β_2-microglobulin (McArthur et al. 1992), neopterin (Brew et al. 1990), and quinolinic acid (Heyes et al. 1991b), have been shown to be associated with dementia in HIV patients. McArthur and co-workers (1992) reported that levels of CSF β_2-microglobulin greater than 3.8 mg/L have a high positive predictive value for the diagnosis of ADC; however, longitudinal studies are needed to determine the sensitivity, specificity, and clinical usefulness of these markers.

Neuropsychology.   Neuropsychological testing is a helpful adjunct in the evaluation of patients for ADC, but abnormal test scores alone do not provide a diagnosis of dementia. The American Academy of Neurology recommends testing these domains: attention/concentration, speed of processing information, motor functioning, abstraction/reasoning, visuospatial skills, memory/learning, and speech/language (Working Group 1991). The Mini-Mental State Exam (Folstein et al. 1975) is not recommended as a clinically useful test for the deficits seen in ADC, but certain bedside screening tests may be helpful. These include Trailmaking Tests A and B, Finger Tapping Tests, Rey Auditory Verbal Learning Test, and Verbal Fluency Tests. Some have advocated the use of computer software packages that measure reaction times as a simple way of covering several of the domains of cognition (Martin et al. 1992; Worth et al. 1993).

Perhaps no area in the field of AIDS psychiatry has generated more controversy than the question of neuropsychological deficits in asymptomatic HIV-positive individuals. This area has been difficult to study adequately, because many patients infected with HIV have histories confounded by psychoactive substance use, head injuries, or preexisting psychiatric disorders. For more detailed critical evaluations of the numerous studies on this topic and their differing results, the reader is referred to other reviews (Grant and Heaton 1990; Ingraham et al. 1990; Perry 1990; Sidtis and Price 1990).

Discussions of the potential impact of subtle neuropsychological deficits in asymptomatic HIV-seropositive individuals involved in high-risk occupations or responsible for public safety (e.g., police officers, airline pilots, physicians) are complicated by many factors, including confidentiality of HIV status, individual versus public rights, and the perception of discrimination. Although a multisite study conducted by WIIO did find abnormalities on neuropsychological testing in asymptomatic HIV-positive individuals, there was no association of these findings with the ability to perform all but the most demanding tasks of daily living (Maj 1990; Maj et al. 1994). Studies to date have not demonstrated a clear indication for routine HIV testing of people in high-risk occupations. More research is needed to ascertain whether HIV seropositivity could affect the functioning of individuals involved in high-risk or hazardous occupations.

Depression: Relationship to Disease Progression

The Medical Outcomes Study (Wells et al. 1989) showed the effect of depression on medical patients in the community. Depressed patients had worse physical and social functioning and more bodily pain than nondepressed subjects. Clinical practice indicates that these findings are also true for patients with chronic illnesses such as AIDS. Although research in psychoneuroimmunology has not yet precisely elucidated the relationship between depression and immune function in HIV-infected patients, some investigators speculate that psychological distress may play an important role in disease progression and outcome (Antoni et al. 1990; Gorman and Kertzner 1990; Kiecolt-Glaser and Glaser 1988; Temoshok 1988). At least one study has shown a more rapid rate of decline in CD4+ lymphocyte counts in depressed versus nondepressed HIV-infected patients, although depression was not significantly associated with earlier AIDS diagnosis or mortality (Burack et al. 1993). However, the difference in actual numbers of CD4+ lymphocytes between the two groups in this study was very small, and other studies have not been able to demonstrate a significant relationship between depression and CD4+ cell count, stage of illness, progression of disease, or mortality (Lyketsos et al. 1993a; Perry et al 1992; Rabkin et al. 1991). In fact, in all of the above studies as well as others (Hays et al. 1992; Ostrow et al. 1989; Perry et al. 1993), the most significant factor associated with depression and distress was the report of HIV-related physical symptoms such as fever, night sweats, lymphadenopathy, diarrhea, herpetic pain, oral thrush, and fatigue. Although the exact relationship of psychological distress with immune function, physical symptoms, and disease progression in the HIV population is unclear, the clinician must continue to carefully assess and treat depression in these patients.

When an HIV-infected patient presents with symptoms of psychomotor slowing, withdrawal, and apathy, the clinician has the difficult task of differentiating between depression and ADC. Scales such as the Center for Epidemiologic Studies—Depression Scale (CES-D) (Radloff 1977) or Hamilton Rating Scale for Depression have been useful research tools, but their clinical applications may be limited in patients with medical symptoms that may contribute to higher scores. Melancholic symptoms such as frequent crying, loss of self-esteem, hopelessness, and suicidal ideation are probably more indicative of a depressive syndrome than of ADC. Also, as stated earlier in this chapter, ADC is less likely to occur in HIV patients until they become physically symptomatic and/or have signs of immunologic decline. Finally, the clinician must be aware that patients with ADC can also be depressed, and both diagnoses must then be addressed.

Suicidality

An often-cited study showed the rate of suicide in men with AIDS in New York City in 1985 to be 35 times higher than in age-matched men without AIDS (Marzuk et al. 1988). A national study of suicide in men with AIDS, using the same methods as Marzuk et al., reported a rate 7.4 times higher than demographically matched men in the general population (Cote et al. 1992). Interestingly, the suicide rate significantly declined from 1987 to 1989, and Cote and others speculated that an improvement in medical therapies and quality of life for patients with AIDS had contributed to this phenomenon. In addition, rates of suicide attempts (Rundell et al. 1992) and suicidal ideation (Perry et al. 1990c) have been reported to be high compared with the general population. Some have found suicidal ideation to be significantly higher in HIV-positive patients without full-blown AIDS (McKegney and O'Dowd 1992; O'Dowd et al. 1993). The presence of pain has also been shown to be associated with suicidality in this population (Breitbart 1993).

Certain predisposing factors may indicate a high risk for suicidality among HIV patients. These include previous suicide attempts, substance use, sexual identity difficulties, recent loss of significant others, and cognitive dysfunction. Depression is a known risk factor for suicide in the general population, and one study has shown that depressed AIDS patients are less likely to consent to some medical interventions that could prolong life (Fogel and Mor 1993). Further studies are needed to determine which factors have the highest predictive value for suicide in HIV patients. However, because of the increased rate of suicide in this population, this issue must be evaluated on an individual basis.

Manic Syndromes

Manic episodes occurring in patients with AIDS as a result of medication side effects (O'Dowd and McKegney 1988) or opportunistic infection (Johannessen and Wilson 1988) have been reported. However, evidence is emerging of a growing number of patients presenting with manic symptoms as a manifestation of HIV illness itself (El-Mallakh 1991). In selected series of HIV patients, investigators have reported prevalence rates of manic syndromes of 2.4% (Halman et al. 1993), 8% (Lyketsos et al. 1993c), and 30% (Boccellari et al. 1988). Although some subjects may have had preexisting bipolar disorder, neurodiagnostic evaluations, including neuropsychological testing in these and other studies (Kieburtz et al. 1991), indicate that manic symptoms represent a mood disorder secondary to HIV infection of the CNS in most patients. Except for the difference in the behavioral presentation, the neurodiagnostic findings also suggest that a manic syndrome in an AIDS patient may represent a clinical variation of ADC.

PSYCHOPHARMACOLOGIC AND SOMATIC THERAPIES

Psychopharmacologic management of symptoms of HIV-infected patients requires an understanding of HIV illness and the various associated neuropsychiatric symptoms and syndromes. The specific psychotropic medication used depends on the patient's symptomatology and concurrent medical status. In addition, the clinician must be acutely aware of the increased likelihood of side effects from psychotropic medications as a result of the neurotropism of HIV and its direct effects on the CNS. One must also consider the frequent interactions and side effects of the numerous medications used to treat AIDS and its associated neoplasms and infections. For a further discussion of the neuropsychiatric side effects of AIDS treatments, see Appendix 6–1 at the end of this chapter.

Antidepressants

Antidepressant medications can be used safely and effectively in HIV-infected patients. Differences exist in medication-specific side effects but not in clinical efficacy. Some have reported response rates to antidepressant treatment as high as 85%–89% in selected samples of HIV-infected patients (Rabkin and Harrison 1990; Treisman et al. 1993). Because of their low side-effect profile and low lethality in overdose, the selective serotonin reuptake inhibitors (SSRIs) should be considered first-line medications in this population (Bhugra et al. 1990; Fernandez 1990; Hintz et al. 1990). Fluoxetine, sertraline, and paroxetine are well tolerated and effective in HIV-infected patients with depression (Batki et al. 1993; Levine et al. 1990; Perkins and Evans 1991). Paroxetine would be more likely to inhibit the cytochrome P_{450}-2D6 isoenzyme than either fluoxetine or sertraline, thereby increasing levels of medications metabolized by this enzyme (see Chapters 1 and 2).

The initial choice of an SSRI also may be theoretically warranted. Tryptophan is the precursor of the neurotransmitter serotonin and of the excitatory neurotoxin quinolinic acid. Recent evidence suggests that there is a disproportionate shift in the metabolism of tryptophan in HIV-infected individuals, resulting in increased serum and CSF concentrations of quinolinic acid; this may also lead to a hyposerotonergic state (Heyes et al. 1991a, 1992a, 1992b; Javitt and Zukin 1990; Larsson et al. 1989; Launay et al. 1989; Werner et al. 1988).

In this population, doses of psychotropic drugs should be carefully selected (e.g., 5 to 10 mg of fluoxetine) to minimize side effects. Additional caution should be taken to monitor for activation, gastrointestinal, extrapyramidal, and hyperserotonergic effects (Sternbach 1991). The newer serotonin and norepinephrine reuptake inhibitors such as venlafaxine may also prove useful in these patients. Although nausea is a relatively common side effect with venlafaxine, its lower affinity for muscarinic, histaminergic, and α-adrenergic receptors results in an overall favorable side-effect profile.

Tricyclic antidepressants (TCAs) have also been demonstrated to be effective medications for HIV-infected individuals (Hintz et al. 1990; Rabkin and Harrison 1990). The secondary amines (e.g., nortriptyline, desipramine) are recommended because of their lower side-effect profile, but as HIV disease progresses, deleterious side effects may still occur. Sometimes, lower dosages than those usually required for the non-HIV-infected population are both tolerated and effective. Often medication-specific properties can be helpful in given clinical situations. For example, when agitation is a significant component of the depression, one of the more sedating antidepressants (e.g., doxepin) may be used. Depression with a significant component of psychomotor retardation can be targeted by using a more activating agent such as desipramine or protriptyline. Parenteral forms of some of the TCAs are available (Fernandez 1990); however, because of pain at the injection site and risk of infection, they should only be used when oral administration is not possible and for a very limited time (Fernandez 1990). Depression associated with concomitant pain syndromes, such as neuropathic pain, may also benefit from TCA therapy. Treatment with TCAs should be initiated with low dosages. The patient must be carefully monitored for hypotension, cardiac, and anticholinergic side effects including dry mouth (which may predispose the patient to oral candidiasis) or urinary retention. TCAs may cause a deterioration in cognitive functioning or may even precipitate an overt delirium (Storch 1991).

Other agents available to treat depression include trazodone, maprotiline, and buproprion. However, because HIV-infected patients are at increased risk for seizures (Wong et al. 1990) and the safety of bupropion for these patients has not been established, we would only use buproprion in asymptomatic patients and not as a first-choice drug. The monoamine oxidase inhibitors (MAOIs) can be used in HIV-infected patients; however, based on the need for dietary restrictions and the potential for dangerous drug interactions, this drug class should be avoided if possible. Sleep difficulties are common in this population, and trazodone, 25 to 50 mg at bedtime, is quite effective and safe.

Augmentation strategies for depression may be useful in patients who have a partial response or who are refractory to standard treatment with an SSRI. Low-dose TCAs (25 to 50 mg of desipramine or 10 mg of nortriptyline), lithium carbonate (300 to 600 mg), triiodothyronine (T_3) (25 to 50 µg), or buspirone (5 to 10 mg tid) (Joffe and Schuller 1993; Sussman 1994) are effective adjuvants when added to the SSRIs. If lithium is used, neurotoxicity can develop at relatively low or therapeutic serum levels. When TCAs are added, SSRI serum levels can significantly increase. However, the safety and efficacy of these strategies has not been systematically evaluated in patients who are HIV positive or who have AIDS. It is also highly likely that patients who are HIV positive or who have AIDS are more sensitive to side effects from combinations of psychotropics.

Psychostimulants

Psychostimulants have been demonstrated to be effective in the treatment of depression in severely medically ill patients and in patients with ADC, especially when the patients have symptoms of apathy, amotivation, or mild to moderate cognitive deficits (Fernandez et al. 1988a; Holmes et al. 1989). Methylphenidate, in a dosage range of 5 to 60 mg/day, is well tolerated. Treatment should be initiated with doses of 5 to 10 mg twice daily—at 8:00 A.M. and noon—and carefully titrated upward every 1 or 2 days until a good clinical response is observed. Dextroamphetamine may be used in patients who do not respond to methylphenidate. Pemoline can be given sublingually; it is usually started at 18.75 mg in the morning and can be used in patients who have difficulty swallowing or tolerating oral medications. The clinician should monitor the patient for signs of extreme activation, tremor, increase in blood pressure or heart rate, or the emergence of psychotic symptoms. Some clinicians might be concerned with using methylphenidate or dextroamphetamine in a group at high risk for drug dependence and abuse. However, in our clinical experience, this has not been a problem, and we have found these agents to be very effective.

Electroconvulsive Therapy

In selected individuals, such as those with psychotic depression, electroconvulsive therapy (ECT) should be considered. Little, however, has been published regarding the use of ECT in HIV-infected patients (Schaerf et al. 1989). Before initiating ECT, the HIV-infected patient must be evaluated for significant cognitive deficits and/or CNS lesions, such as toxoplasmosis or lymphoma, as these complications may preclude its use.

Antimanic Medications

Mania in the HIV patient may be a manifestation of preexisting psychiatric illness, CNS effects of HIV-related conditions, or side effects of medications such as AZT (Dauncey 1988; Gabel et al. 1986; Johannessen and Wilson 1988; Kieburtz et al. 1991; Lyketsos et al. 1993b; Maxwell et al. 1988; O'Dowd and McKegney 1988; Schmidt and Miller 1988). The clinician must aggressively treat the acutely manic patient because of the risk for impaired judgment, the potential for hyperactive sexual behavior, and poor impulse control. Those with a premorbid history of bipolar disorder may be given standard lithium treatment; however, patients with advanced HIV disease may be at increased risk for lithium-induced side effects, including neurotoxicity, diarrhea, polyuria, and polydipsia (Tanquary 1993). Therefore, anticonvulsants (e.g., valproic acid) may be better choices to treat patients with AIDS-related mania (Halman et al. 1993). Because of the greater risk of myelosuppression by carbamazepine, sodium valproate may be preferred. However, in HIV-infected patients with mania, clinicians must closely monitor hepatic enzymes, coagulation factors, and complete blood count (including platelets). Note that both HIV and AZT may independently cause myelosuppression.

Neuroleptics in mania.   High-potency neuroleptics (e.g., haloperidol, fluphenazine) are also quite useful in the management of mania in HIV-infected patients. However, increased sensitivity to extrapyramidal side effects of the neuroleptics has been well documented (Breitbart et al. 1988; Hriso et al. 1991). Risperidone, with its relatively low propensity for extrapyramidal side effects, may prove to be a first-line drug for these patients, because patients with AIDS are believed by most clinicians to be more susceptible to neuroleptic-induced neurologic side effects (see below and Chapter 2). Lorazepam (often in combination with a neuroleptic) or clonazepam have also been shown to be effective in the treatment of acutely manic HIV patients (Budman and Vandersall 1990).

Anxiolytics

Anxiety, when present, can range from mild agitation to severe panic states. Benzodiazepines are the drugs of choice for the acute or chronic treatment of anxiety. Benzodiazepines themselves differ in their therapeutic potency and elimination half-lives (American Psychiatric Association 1990b). It is extremely important to keep this in mind when treating patients with HIV disease. Benzodiazepines with short or intermediate half-lives (e.g., alprazolam, lorazepam, oxazepam) accumulate less extensively and are cleared more rapidly. The clinician should be aware of the potential for abuse, tolerance, and disinhibition. Patients who are cognitively impaired or who have dementia may become confused or delirious when they are given benzodiazepines and should therefore be frequently monitored. Despite its long half-life, clonazepam is often well tolerated and effective (see Chapter 2). Because of the risk of hypotension, the β-blocker propranolol should be used cautiously (Fernandez 1990) in acutely ill patients. Traditional antihistamines have anticholinergic side effects with risk of cognitive impairment and should be avoided. On first glance, buspirone, a nonbenzodiazepine agent with virtually no sedation or abuse potential, seems promising and has been reported to be effective (Batki 1990). However, it usually takes between 2 and 4 weeks to achieve therapeutic response; therefore, it cannot be used in acute situations. A case of buspirone-induced psychosis has also been reported (Trachman 1992).

Neuroleptics

Psychotic symptoms may be seen in HIV-infected patients with schizophrenia, delusional disorders, and mood disorders with psychotic features. Patients with substance use disorder (both intoxication and withdrawal states) may also present with psychotic symptoms. The treatment approach is always dictated by the clinical situation. By and large, the approach to the psychotic patient with HIV is similar to the treatment of the non-HIV-infected patient (Ostrow et al. 1988; Perry and Markowitz 1986; Wolcott et al. 1989). For severe anxiety or in situations in which benzodiazepines are not indicated, low-dose neuroleptics are quite useful. Often, low oral divided doses of haloperidol (0.25 to 1 mg) or chlorpromazine (10 to 50 mg) are well tolerated. However, HIV-infected individuals can be extremely sensitive to the extrapyramidal side effects of neuroleptics. Medication-induced extrapyramidal side effects and neuroleptic malignant syndrome have been reported in patients with HIV illness (Burch and Montoya 1989; Hriso et al 1991; Lazarus 1990; Rapoport 1989; Swenson et al. 1989). Neuroleptics can and should be used in this population when indicated. The increased risk of the extrapyramidal side effects of antiemetics when used in HIV patients has also been observed (Edelstein and Knight 1987; Hollander et al. 1985; Manger and Warner 1990; Rodgers 1992). Molindone has been reported to be effective in the treatment of HIV-infected patients with delirium who had severe reactions to other neuroleptics (Fernandez and Levy 1993). At the time of this writing, there have been no studies of risperidone in this population. However, as mentioned earlier, with its lower incidence of extrapyramidal side effects at usual therapeutic doses (6 mg/day or less), risperidone may become a first choice in the HIV-infected individual with psychosis.

Treatment of Delirium

Delirium is a very common diagnosis among HIV-infected patients (Baer 1989; Fernandez et al. 1989a; O'Dowd and McKegney 1990), and the potential etiologies are extraordinarily varied (Bialer et al. 1991). The distress caused to the patient, family members, and staff as well as the potential for brain damage and death necessitate quick and aggressive treatment of delirium. In addition, the acutely agitated patient poses a risk for self-injury and exposure of HIV to others.

Because of the low incidence of significant sedation, hypotension, hypothermia, or anticholinergic side effects, we have primarily used haloperidol for the treatment of delirium, usually at low doses. Despite its high side-effect profile, low-dose chlorpromazine is also often well tolerated and effective. For extremely agitated patients, a combination of environmental and behavioral interventions, along with aggressive chemotherapeutic management, is warranted. In the hospital setting, intravenous haloperidol with or without intravenous lorazepam can be used for the acute management of severe agitation (Adams 1988; Adams et al. 1986; Fernandez et al. 1988b, 1989b; Tesar et al. 1985). However, Fernandez and colleagues (1989b) reported notable extrapyramidal side effects in 17 of 38 patients receiving this regimen. Cardiac arrhythmias and lengthening of the Q-T interval on electrocardiogram leading to torsades de pointes have also been reported with the use of intravenous haloperidol (Metzger and Friedman 1993) (see also Chapter 2). Risk factors for this potentially lethal arrhythmia during intravenous haloperidol treatment include dilated cardiomyopathy and history of alcohol abuse. Under these conditions, cardiac monitoring is indicated if intravenous haloperidol is used.

Treatment of Dementia

Dementia during the course of AIDS is a common finding. However, treatment of ADC is so far quite limited, and current attention is focused on the use of antiretroviral medications. AZT may reduce the progression of ADC or may cause improvement in cognitive functioning. Although debate still exists as to whether AZT will prevent asymptomatic patients or patients with mild neuropsychiatric symptoms from developing ADC, the findings of some recent studies appear promising (Portegies et al. 1993; Sidtis et al. 1993; Tozzi et al. 1993). AZT appears to be most helpful in slowing disease progression in the early stages of HIV infection, but the benefit appears to be time limited, and progressive disease appears to be inevitable (Bartlett 1993).

Psychotherapeutic Interventions

Psychotherapeutic treatment continues to be an integral part of the management of symptoms in many patients with HIV illness. A complete discussion of the topic is beyond the scope of this chapter. However, psychiatrists working with the HIV population must have an adequate knowledge of the psychological aspects of medical illness and patient-coping behaviors. In addition, therapists must be sensitive to sociocultural issues for each patient (Bing et al. 1990). Psychotherapeutic interventions and the role of the therapist can take many different forms as a reflection of the variable course of the illness (Fawzy et al. 1991; Perry and Markowitz 1986; Perry et al. 1991; Schaffner 1990). These include therapy with "the worried well," pre- and post-HIV serologic test counseling, crisis intervention, and individual psychotherapy that is adaptable to the specific and changing needs of the patient (Markowitz et al. 1992). These various therapies include psychoeducation and supportive, interpersonal, cognitive-behavioral, and psychodynamic psychotherapy (Adler and Beckett 1989; Baker and Heather 1993; Kelly and St. Lawrence 1989; Markowitz et al. 1992). Before undertaking any psychotherapeutic intervention, the clinician must conduct a complete biopsychosocial evaluation (Cohen 1990). Particular attention should be paid to the assessment of the patient's cognitive state, past and current sexual activity, substance use history, support systems, and personality traits and defenses. The evaluation must include an understanding of the patient's coping strategies used throughout his or her life.

Ongoing attention to the issues of suicide and suicidal ideation and risk must be appreciated. Suicidal ideation can be the manifestation of a specific psychiatric syndrome, secondary to side effects of medications, or a response to a specific crisis or stressor. Suicidal ideation often occurs in response to feelings of loss of control (e.g., bodily functions, ambulation, pain) or secondary to overwhelming despair from having experienced the loss of others. These patients often raise the issue of "rational" suicide. They must be carefully assessed to identify treatable psychiatric symptoms and syndromes, including acute and progressive organic states, side effects of some medications (e.g., interferon-induced depression and suicidal ideation), and uncontrolled pain (Breitbart 1993). Suicidal ideations may be transiently intensified as a result of psychotherapeutic explorations of underlying guilt, rage, shame, and loss. Such interventions must therefore carefully consider the patient's available support systems and previous patterns of adaptation and coping.

Group psychotherapy is an important treatment modality for many individuals with HIV disease (Beckett and Rutan 1990; Chung and Magraw 1992; Fawzy et al. 1989; Levine et al. 1991; Tunnell 1991). Health outcome studies of individuals with serious illness who were treated with supportive group therapy reported encouraging qualitative and quantitative potential benefits. These included a decrease in emotional distress, better health status, and even a potential increase in survival time (Fawzy et al. 1990a, 1990b; Spiegel et al. 1989). For patients with chronic severe illnesses such as AIDS, groups that utilize a supportive-expressive approach are most helpful (Spira and Spiegel 1993). With this approach, the emphasis is on emotional expression of thoughts and feelings to oneself and to others in the group, fostering group support, and learning ongoing coping strategies. These groups focus on the patient's current life and near future (as opposed to the past). Spira and Spiegel (1993) also recommend that these groups meet regularly and be ongoing (not time limited). Homogeneity of the group's members is recommended. However, homogeneity is less important for shorter-term focused groups.

For the HIV population, groups are often composed of patients at various stages of HIV illness. Although some difficulties may arise, such as sicker patients feeling isolated, in general, these groups can allow for role modeling. Less ill members of the group can benefit from observing how those with more advanced illness cope. The clinician facilitating the group helps to foster open expression of emotion, group interaction, and support. Issues of death and dying, loss, disability, and family are always addressed. Specific coping skills, such as relaxation, meditation, stress and pain reduction exercises, and self-hypnosis can be taught. Outside social interaction among group members is encouraged. Resources for groups or other psychosocial support services include local hospitals, AIDS clinics, and AIDS-related community-based organizations such as New York's Gay Men's Health Crisis (GMHC) or the San Francisco Shanti Project.

AIDS AND SEVERELY MENTALLY ILL PATIENTS

HIV seroprevalence rates between 4.0% and 16.3% have been reported among psychiatric inpatients in New York City (Cournos et al. 1991; Empfield et al. 1993; Lee et al. 1992; Meyer et al. 1993; Sacks et al. 1992; Volavka et al. 1991). A study of 183 patients with severe mental illness revealed that 52% had been sexually active in the previous 6 months, and, despite exclusion of patients with a primary diagnosis of substance use disorder, 18% had injected drugs since 1978. Only 10% of the sexually active patients reported consistent condom use despite good performance on AIDS knowledge testing (Satriano et al. 1993). Unprotected heterosexual intercourse was the most frequent HIV risk activity among severely mentally ill patients. Past homosexual activity and the use of injectable drugs certainly remained as serious risk factors (Cournos et al. 1993).

AIDS AND INJECTING DRUG USERS

During 1992, intravenous drug use accounted for 29.5% of all reported AIDS cases (CDC 1993c). The majority, heterosexual men, pose an enormous risk to their female sexual partners (now the fastest growing at-risk group among women) and subsequently to their children through perinatal infection. Seroprevalence rates among intravenous drug users have been reported to be as high as 50%–60% in the New York City metropolitan area and in Puerto Rico. More than 70% of the AIDS patients who use intravenous drugs are either black or Hispanic.

Drug use is associated with behavioral disinhibition leading to unsafe sexual and needle-use practices; direct immunosuppressive effects of the opiates, cocaine, and alcohol; and increased morbidity secondary to drug injecting. In high-prevalence areas, numerous education and prevention programs were created to decrease needle use and needle sharing, offer easier access to treatment, and teach safe needle use and cleansing. Needle exchange and distribution programs do not appear to increase drug use as initially feared and may actually lead to decreased IDU (American Psychiatric Association 1993b; Des Jarlais et al. 1994; Watters et al. 1994). AIDS educational outreach programs have proven successful with inner city intravenous drug users in decreasing injecting drug use and injection-related risk behaviors including needle sharing (Des Jarlais 1989; Des Jarlais et al. 1990). It is clear that altering drug use behaviors is inseparable from efforts to control the spread of HIV infection.

AIDS AND TUBERCULOSIS

The AIDS epidemic has resulted in a major second epidemic of tuberculosis (TB). Geographic areas with high HIV prevalence rates have seen the greatest increases in TB case reporting; New York City has the highest prevalence of TB in the United States. In 1992, the CDC received reports of 26,673 cases of TB throughout the United States (CDC 1993b). Individuals coinfected with HIV and TB have a much greater risk of developing active TB than people who are not HIV infected. Such coinfected individuals require longer courses of anti-TB drugs for both prophylaxis and active treatment (CDC 1992a). Pulmonary TB is the most common site for presentation among HIV-infected individuals, but extrapulmonary disease with or without coexisting pulmonary TB may appear in 40%–75% of patients with HIV and TB. As HIV disease progresses, the proportion of patients with extrapulmonary TB increases (Friedland and Klein 1992). Because of the frequent association of TB with HIV infection, the CDC (1989) recommends that all persons with TB receive HIV testing with counseling.

All patients with HIV infection should be screened for latent TB infection. If the patient's tuberculin skin test status is unknown, or if it is known to be previously negative and he or she has not been tested in the last 12 months, the patient should be tested with a Mantoux test using five test units (intermediate strength) of tuberculin purified protein derivative (PPD). For HIV-infected patients, a 5-mm or greater induration, measured 48 to 72 hours after the test, is considered positive and warrants further investigation. HIV-infected patients may have suppressed reactions to PPD skin tests because of anergy, particularly if their CD4+ cell counts decline. People with anergy will have a negative PPD test regardless of infection with *Mycobacterium tuberculosis*. Some experts have recommended, therefore, that HIV-infected individuals should be evaluated for anergy in conjunction with the PPD by testing with at least two companion antigens (e.g., candida and tetanus toxoid). People with ≥ 3-mm induration to any of the antigens (including PPD) are not considered anergic. All HIV-infected patients with signs or symptoms suggestive or TB (e.g., cough, hemoptysis, weight loss) should receive chest X rays and, if indicated, sputa smears to rule out active TB, regardless of PPD results.

Staff working with these patients must also be tested at least yearly and, possibly, every 6 months if exposed regularly to high-risk patients. If a patient with active or suspected TB requires inpatient psychiatric care, an appropriate isolation room equipped with ultraviolet air disinfection and negative pressure air exchange must be available. Staff must be trained and familiar with appropriate infection control equipment and procedures, and other patients on the ward must be protected from exposure (American Thoracic Society 1992).

It is beyond the scope of this chapter to describe the various chemotherapies for TB infection, but one drug interaction is significant in treating injecting drug users who have TB. Rifampin, a commonly used anti-TB drug, induces hepatic enzymes and will rapidly metabolize methadone. When rifampin is prescribed to a patient on methadone, the methadone dosage often must be increased by 25%–50%. Many antimycobacterial drugs used to treat TB are associated with neuropsychiatric side effects. See Appendix 6–1 for a detailed description.

REFERENCES

Adams F: Emergency intravenous sedation of the delirious medically ill patient. J Clin Psychiatry 49 (suppl):22–26, 1988

Adams F, Fernandez F, Andersson BS: Emergency pharmacotherapy and delirium in the critically ill cancer patient: intravenous combination drug approach. Psychosomatics 27 (suppl 1):33–37, 1986

Adler G, Beckett A: Psychotherapy of the patient with an HIV infection; some ethical and therapeutic dilemmas. Psychosomatics 30:203–208, 1989

American Psychiatric Association: Diagnostic and Statistical Manual of Mental Disorders, 3rd Edition. Washington, DC, American Psychiatric Association, 1980

American Psychiatric Association: Diagnostic and Statistical Manual of Mental Disorders, 3rd Edition, Revised. Washington, DC, American Psychiatric Association, 1987

American Psychiatric Association: A Psychiatrist's Guide to AIDS and HIV Disease: AIDS Primer. Washington, DC, American Psychiatric Association AIDS Education Project, 1990a

American Psychiatric Association: Benzodiazepine Dependence: Toxicity and Abuse. Task Force on Benzodiazepine Dependency. Washington, DC, American Psychiatric Press, 1990b

American Psychiatric Association: Children and AIDS, in AIDS and HIV Disease: A Mental Health Perspective. Washington, DC, American Psychiatric Association AIDS Education Project, 1993a, pp 117–136

American Psychiatric Association: HIV and substance abuse, in AIDS and HIV Disease: A Mental Health Perspective. Washington, DC, American Psychiatric Association AIDS Education Project, 1993b, pp 88–101

American Psychiatric Association: HIV testing and counseling, in AIDS and HIV Disease: A Mental Health Perspective. Washington DC, American Psychiatric Association AIDS Education Project, 1993c, pp 169–176

American Thoracic Society: Control of tuberculosis in the United States. Am Rev Respir Dis 146:1623–1633, 1992

Antoni MH, Schneiderman N, Fletcher MA, et al: Psychoneuroimmunology and HIV-1. J Consult Clin Psychol 58:38–49, 1990

Atkinson JH, Grant I, Kennedy CJ, et al: Prevalence of psychiatric disorders among men infected with human immunodeficiency virus. Arch Gen Psychiatry 45:859–864, 1988

Baer JW: Study of 60 patients with AIDS or AIDS-related complex requiring psychiatric hospitalization. Am J Psychiatry 146:1285–1288, 1989

Baker A, Heather N: Evaluation of a cognitive-behavioral intervention for HIV prevention among injecting drug users. AIDS 7:247–256, 1993

Bartlett JG: Zidovudine now or later? N Engl J Med 329:351–352, 1993

Batki SL: Buspirone in drug users with AIDS or AIDS-related complex. J Clin Psychopharmacol 10 (suppl 3):111S–115S, 1990

Batki SL, Manfredi LB, Murphy JM, et al: Treatment of cocaine abuse and depression in HIV-infected injection drug users. Paper presented at the IXth International Conference on AIDS, Berlin, Germany, June 1993

Beckett A, Rutan JS: Treating persons with ARC and AIDS in group psychotherapy. Int J Group Psychother 40:19–29, 1990

Bhugra D, Moorey S, Minnie C: Antidepressant and cognitive behavior therapy for an AIDS patient. Am J Psychiatry 147:256–260, 1990

Bialer PA, Wallack JJ, Snyder SL: Psychiatric diagnosis in HIV-spectrum disorders. Psychiatr Med 9:361–375, 1991

Bialer PA, Prenzlauer SL, Getter EV, et al: Psychological distress in HIV-infected women, in Abstracts of the VIII International Conference on AIDS. Amsterdam, The Netherlands, July 1992, Abstract PoB 3764, p 218

Bialer PA, Wallack JJ, King M, et al: C/L database: AIDS, 1993 update. Gen Hosp Psychiatry 15:20S–22S, 1993

Bing EG, Nichols SE, Goldfinger SM, et al: The many faces of AIDS: opportunities for intervention. New Dir Ment Health Serv 48:69–92, 1990

Boccellari A, Dilley JW, Shore MD: Neuropsychiatric aspects of AIDS dementia complex: a report on a clinical series. Neurotoxicology 9:381–390, 1988

Bornstein RA, Chakeres D, Brogan M, et al: Magnetic resonance imaging of white matter lesions in HIV infection. J Neuropsychiatry Clin Neurosci 4:174–178, 1992

Breitbart W: Suicide risk and pain in cancer and AIDS patients, in Emerging Issues in Cancer Pain: Research and Practice. Edited by Foley CR. New York, Raven, 1993, pp 49–65

Breitbart W, Marrotta RF, Call P: AIDS and neuroleptic malignant syndrome. Lancet 2:1488–1489, 1988

Brew BJ: HIV-1-related neurological disease. J Acquir Immune Defic Syndr 6 (suppl 1):S10–S15, 1993

Brew BJ, Bhalla RV, Paul M, et al: CSF neopterin in HIV-1 infection. Ann Neurol 28:556–560, 1990

Broderick DF, Wippold FJ, Clifford DB, et al: White matter lesions and cerebral atrophy on MR images in patients with and without AIDS dementia complex. AJR Am J Roentgenol 161:177–181, 1993

Brown GR, Rundell JR: A prospective study of psychiatric aspects of early HIV disease in women. Gen Hosp Psychiatry 15:139–147, 1993

Budman CL, Vandersall TA: Clonazepam treatment of acute mania in an AIDS patient (letter). J Clin Psychiatry 51:212, 1990

Burack JH, Barrett DC, Stall RD, et al: Depressive symptoms and CD4 lymphocyte decline among HIV-infected men. JAMA 270:2568–2573, 1993

Burch EA, Montoya J: Neuroleptic malignant syndrome in an AIDS patient. J Clin Psychopharmacol 9:228–229, 1989

Centers for Disease Control: Classification system for human T-lymphotropic virus type III/lymphadenopathy-associated virus infections. MMWR 35:334–339, 1986

Centers for Disease Control: Revision of the CDC surveillance case definition for acquired immunodeficiency syndrome. MMWR 36 (suppl):1S–15S, 1987

Centers for Disease Control: Tuberculosis and human immunodeficiency virus infection: recommendations of the Advisory Committee for the Elimination of Tuberculosis. MMWR 38:236, 1989

Centers for Disease Control: 1993 revised classification system for HIV infection and expanded surveillance case definition for AIDS among adolescents and adults. MMWR 41:1–19, 1992a

Centers for Disease Control: Publicly funded HIV counseling and testing—United States, 1991. MMWR 41:613–617, 1992b

Centers for Disease Control and Prevention: Self-reported HIV antibody testing among persons with selected risk behaviors—Southern Los Angeles County, 1991–1992. MMWR 42:786–789, 1993a

Centers for Disease Control and Prevention: Tuberculosis morbidity—United States, 1992. MMWR 42:363, 1993b

Centers for Disease Control and Prevention: Update: acquired immunodeficiency syndrome—United States 1992. MMWR 42:547–557, 1993c

Centers for Disease Control and Prevention: Update: mortality attributable to HIV infection among persons aged 25–44 years—United States, 1991 and 1992. MMWR 42:869–872, 1993d

Centers for Disease Control and Prevention: Worlds AIDS day—December 1, 1993. MMWR 42:869, 1993e

Centers for Disease Control and Prevention: HIV/AIDS Surveillance Report 5(4):1–33, 1994

Chuang HT, Devins GM, IIunsley J, et al: Psychosocial distress and well-being among gay and bisexual men with human immunodeficiency virus infection. Am J Psychiatry 146:876–880, 1989

Chung JY, Magraw MM: A group approach to psychosocial issues faced by HIV-positive women. Hosp Community Psychiatry 43:891–894, 1992

Coffin J, Haase A, Levy JA, et al: Human immunodeficiency viruses (letter). Science 232:697, 1986

Cohen MAA: Biopsychosocial approach to the human immunodeficiency virus epidemic: a clinicians primer. Gen Hosp Psychiatry 12:98–123, 1990

Connor EM, Sperling RS, Gelber R, et al: Reduction of maternal-infant transmission of human immunodeficiency virus type 1 with zidovudine treatment. N Engl J Med 331:1173–1180, 1994

Cote TR, Biggar RJ, Dannenberg AL: Risk of suicide among persons with AIDS. a national assessment. JAMA 268:2066–2068, 1992

Cournos F, Empfield M, Horvath E, et al: HIV seroprevalence among patients admitted to two psychiatric hospitals. Am J Psychiatry 148:1225–1230, 1991

Cournos F, McKinnon K, Meyer-Bahlburg H, et al: HIV risk among persons with severe mental illness: preliminary findings. Hosp Community Psychiatry 44:1104–1106, 1993

Dauncey K: Mania in the early stages of AIDS (letter). Br J Psychiatry 152:716–717, 1988

Davey RT, Vasudevachari MB, Lane HC: Serologic tests for human immunodeficiency virus infection, in AIDS—Etiology, Diagnosis, Treatment and Prevention, 3rd Edition. Edited by Devita VT, Hellman S, Rosenberg SA. Philadelphia, PA, JB Lippincott, 1992, pp 141–155

Day JJ, Grant I, Atkinson JH, et al: Incidence of AIDS dementia in a two-year follow-up of AIDS and ARC patients on an initial phase II AZT placebo-controlled study: San Diego cohort. J Neuropsychiatry Clin Neurosci 4:15–20, 1992

Des Jarlais DC: AIDS prevention program for intravenous drug users: diversity and evaluation. International Review of Psychiatry 1:101–108, 1989

Des Jarlais DC, Friedman SR, Woods JS: Intravenous drug use and AIDS, in Behavioral Aspects of AIDS. Edited by Ostrow DG. New York, Plenum, 1990, pp 139–155

Des Jarlais DC, Friedman SR, Sotheran JL, et al: Continuity and change within an HIV epidemic: injecting drug users in New York City, 1984 through 1992. JAMA 271:121–127, 1994

Dilley JW, Ochitill HN, Perl M, et al: Findings in psychiatric consultations with patients with acquired immune deficiency syndrome. Am J Psychiatry 142:82–85, 1985

Dreyer EB, Kaiser PK, Offermann JT, et al: HIV-1 coat protein neurotoxicity prevented by calcium channel antagonists. Science 248:364–367, 1990

Edelstein H, Knight RT: Severe parkinsonism in two AIDS patients taking prochlorperazine. Lancet 2(8554):341–342, 1987

El-Mallakh RS: Mania in AIDS: clinical significance and theoretical considerations. Int J Psychiatry Med 21:383–391, 1991

Empfield M, Cournos F, Meyer I, et al: HIV seroprevalence among homeless patients admitted to a psychiatric inpatient unit. Am J Psychiatry 150:47–52, 1993

Essex M: Origin of AIDS, in AIDS—Etiology, Diagnosis, Treatment, and Prevention, 3rd Edition. Edited by DeVita VT, Hellman S, Rosenberg SA. Philadelphia, PA, JB Lippincott, 1992, pp 3–11

Fawzy FI, Namir S, Wolcott DL: Structured group intervention model for AIDS patients. Psychiatr Med 7:35–45, 1989

Fawzy FI, Cousins N, Fawzy NW, et al: A structured psychiatric intervention for cancer patients, I: changes over time in methods of coping and affective disturbance. Arch Gen Psychiatry 47:720–725, 1990a

Fawzy FI, Kemeny M, Fawzy NW, et al: A structured psychiatric intervention for cancer patients, II: changes over time in immunological measures. Arch Gen Psychiatry 47:729–735, 1990b

Fawzy FI, Fawzy NW, Pasnau RO: A model of a psychiatric intervention for AIDS patients. Psychiatr Med 9:409–422, 1991

Fernandez F: Psychiatric complications in HIV-related illnesses, in American Psychiatric Association AIDS Primer. Washington, DC, American Psychiatric Association, 1990, pp 21–34

Fernandez F, Levy JK: The use of molindone in the treatment of psychotic and delirious patients infected with the human immunodeficiency virus: case reports. Gen Hosp Psychiatry 15:31–35, 1993

Fernandez F, Levy JK, Galizzi H: Response of HIV-related depression to psychostimulants: case reports. Hosp Community Psychiatry 39:628–631, 1988a

Fernandez F, Holmes VF, Adams F, et al: Treatment of severe refractory agitation with haloperidol drip. J Clin Psychiatry 49:239–241, 1988b

Fernandez F, Holmes VF, Levy JK, et al: Consultation-liaison psychiatry and HIV-related disorders. Hosp Community Psychiatry 40:146–153, 1989a

Fernandez F, Levy JK, Mansell PW: Management of delirium in terminally ill AIDS patients. Int J Psychiatry Med 19:165–172, 1989b

Fleishman JA, Fogel B: Coping and depressive symptoms among people with AIDS. Health Psychol 13:156–169, 1994

Fogel BS, Mor V: Depressed mood and care preferences in patients with AIDS. Gen Hosp Psychiatry 15:203–207, 1993

Folstein MF, Folstein SE, McHugh PR: Mini-Mental State: a practical method for grading the cognitive state of patients for the clinician. J Psychiatr Res 12:189–198, 1975

Francis DP, Curran JW, Essex M: Epidemic acquired immune deficiency syndrome (AIDS): epidemiologic evidence for a transmitted agent (editorial). J Natl Cancer Inst 71:1–4, 1983

Freese A, Swartz KJ, During MJ, et al: Kynurenine metabolites of tryptophan: implications for neurologic diseases. Neurology 40:691–695, 1990

Friedland G, Klein R: Tuberculosis and other bacterial infections in AIDS, in AIDS—Etiology, Diagnosis, Treatment, and Prevention, 3rd Edition. Edited by DeVita VT, Hellman S, Rosenberg SA. Philadelphia, PA, JB Lippincott, 1992, pp 180–193

Gabel RH, Barnard N, Norko M, et al: AIDS presenting as mania. Compr Psychiatry 27:252–254, 1986

Gallo RC, Sahahuddin SZ, Popovic M, et al: Frequent detection and isolation of cytopathic retroviruses (HTLV III) from patients with AIDS and at risk for AIDS. Science 224:500–503, 1984

Glass JD, Wesselingh SL, Selnes OA, et al: Clinical-neuropathological correlation in HIV-associated dementia. Neurology 43:2230–2237, 1993

Gorman JM, Kertzner R: Psychoneuroimmunology and HIV-1 infection. J Neuropsychiatry Clin Neurosci 2:241–252, 1990

Gottlieb MS, Schroff R, Schanker HM, et al: Pneumocystis carinii pneumonia and mucosal candidiasis in previously healthy homosexual men: evidence of a new acquired cellular immunodeficiency. N Engl J Med 305:1425–1431, 1981

Grant I, Heaton RK: Human immunodeficiency virus-type 1 (HIV-1) and the brain. J Consult Clin Psychol 58:22–30, 1990

Halman MH, Worth JL, Sanders KM, et al: Anticonvulsant use in the treatment of manic syndromes in patients with HIV-1 infection. J Neuropsychiatry Clin Neurosci 5:430–434, 1993

Hamilton M: The assessment of anxiety states by rating. Br J Med Psychol 32:50–55, 1959

Hamilton M: A rating scale for depression. J Neurol Neurosurg Psychiatry 23:56–62, 1960

Hays RB, Turner H, Coates TJ: Social support, AIDS-related symptoms, and depression among gay men. J Consult Clin Psychol 3:463–469, 1992

Heyes MP, Rubinow D, Lane C, et al: Cerebrospinal fluid quinolinic acid concentrations are increased in acquired immune deficiency syndrome. Ann Neurol 26:275–277, 1989

Heyes MP, Brew BJ, Martin A, et al: Cerebrospinal fluid quinolinic acid concentrations are increased in acquired immune deficiency syndrome. Adv Exp Med Biol 294:687–690, 1991a

Heyes MP, Brew BJ, Martin A, et al: Quinolinic acid in cerebrospinal fluid and serum in HIV-1 infection; relationship to clinical and neurological status. Ann Neurol 29:202–209, 1991b

Heyes MP, Saito K, Markey SP: Human macrophages convert L-tryptophan to the neurotoxin quinolinic acid. Brain Res 570:237–250, 1992a

Heyes MP, Saito K, Crowley JS, et al: Quinolinic acid and kynurenine pathway metabolism in inflammatory and non-inflammatory neurological disease. Brain 115 (pt 5):1249–1273, 1992b

Hintz A, Kuck J, Peterkin JJ, et al: Depression in the context of human immunodeficiency virus infection: implications for treatment. J Clin Psychiatry 51:497–501, 1990

Hoffman RS: Neuropsychiatric complications of AIDS. Psychosomatics 25:393–400, 1984

Holland JC, Tross S: The psychosocial and neuropsychiatric sequelae of the acquired immunodeficiency syndrome and related disorders. Ann Intern Med 103:760–764, 1985

Hollander H, Golden J, Mendelson T, et al: Extrapyramidal symptoms in AIDS patients given low-dose metoclopramide or chlorpromazine (letter). Lancet 2(8465):1186, 1985

Holmes VF, Fernandez F, Levy JK: Psychostimulant response in AIDS-related complex patients. J Clin Psychiatry 50:5–8, 1989

Hriso W, Kuhn T, Masdeu JC, et al: Extrapyramidal symptoms due to dopamine blocking agents in patients with AIDS encephalopathy. Am J Psychiatry 148:1558–1561, 1991

Huet T, Cheynier R, Meyerhaus A, et al: Genetic organization of a chimpanzee lentivirus related to HIV-1 (letter). Nature 345:356–359, 1990

Imagawa DT, Lee MH, Wolinsky SM, et al: Human immunodeficiency virus type 1 infection in homosexual men who remain seronegative for prolonged periods. N Engl J Med 320:1458–1462, 1989

Ingraham LJ, Bridge TP, Janssen R, et al: Neuropsychological effects of early HIV-1 infection: assessment and methodology. J Neuropsychiatry Clin Neurosci 2:174–182, 1990

Janssen RS, Nwanyanwu OC, Selik RM, et al: Epidemiology of human immunodeficiency virus encephalopathy in the United States. Neurology 42:1472–1476, 1992

Javitt DC, Zukin SR: The role of excitatory amino acids in neuropsychiatric illness. J Neuropsychiatry Clin Neurosci 2:44–52, 1990

Joffe RT, Schuller DR: An open study of buspirone augmentation of serotonin reuptake inhibitors in refractory depression. J Clin Psychiatry 54:269–271, 1993

Johannessen DJ, Wilson LG: Mania with cryptococcal meningitis in two AIDS patients. J Clin Psychiatry 49:200–201, 1988

Kelly ST, St. Lawrence JS: Behavioral intervention to reduce AIDS risk activities. J Consult Clin Psychol 57:60–67, 1989

Kieburtz K, Zettelmaier AE, Ketonen L, et al: Manic syndromes in AIDS. Am J Psychiatry 148:1068–1070, 1991

Kiecolt-Glaser JK, Glaser R: Psychological influences on immunity: implications for AIDS. Am Psychol 4:892–898, 1988

LaFrance ND, Pearlson GD, Schaerf FW, et al: I-123 IMP-SPECT in HIV-related dementia. Advances in Functional Neuroimaging 1:9–15, 1988

Larsson M, Hagberg L, Norkrans G, et al: Indole-amine deficiency in blood and cerebrospinal fluid from patients with human immunodeficiency virus infection. J Neurosci Res 23:441–446, 1989

Launay JM, Copel L, Callebert J, et al: Serotonin and human immunodeficiency viruses. Nouv Rev Fr Hematol 31:159–161, 1989

Lazarus A: EPS, NMS, and AIDS. Biol Psychiatry 28:551–552, 1990

Lee H, Travin S, Bluestone H: HIV-1 in inpatients. Hosp Community Psychiatry 43:181–182, 1992

Levine C, Bayer R: Screening blood, public health and medical uncertainty. Hastings Cent Rep Special Supplement, August, 1985, pp 8–11

Levine S, Anderson D, Bystritsky A, et al: A report of eight HIV-seropositive patients with major depression responding to fluoxetine. J AIDS 3:1074–1077, 1990

Levine SH, Bystritsky A, Baron D, et al: Group psychotherapy for HIV-seropositive patients with major depression. Am J Psychother 45:413–424, 1991

Levy JA: Viral and immunologic factors in HIV infection, in The Medical Management of AIDS, 3rd Edition. Edited by Sande MA, Volberding PA. Philadelphia, PA, WB Saunders, 1992, pp 18–32

Levy RM, Bredesen DE, Rosenblum ML: Neurologic manifestations of the acquired immunodeficiency syndrome (AIDS): experience at UCSF and review of the literature. J Neurosurg 62:475–495, 1985

Lipton SA, Rosenberg PA: Excitatory amino acids as a final common pathway for neurologic disorders. N Engl J Med 330:613–623, 1994

Lowenstein RJ, Sharfstein SS: Neuropsychiatric aspects of the acquired immune deficiency syndrome. Int J Psychiatry Med 13:255–260, 1984

Lyketsos CG, Hoover DR, Guccione M, et al: Depressive symptoms as predictors of medical outcomes in HIV infection. JAMA 270:2563–2567, 1993a

Lyketsos CG, Hanson AL, Fishman M, et al: Mania early and late in the course of HIV infection. Am J Psychiatry 150:326–327, 1993b

Lyketsos CG, Hanson AL, Fishman M, et al: Manic syndrome early and late in the course of HIV. Am J Psychiatry 150:326–327, 1993c

Maj M: Organic mental disorders in HIV-1 infection. AIDS 4:831–840, 1990

Maj M, Satz P, Janssen R, et al: WHO neuropsychiatric AIDS study, cross sectional phase II: neuropsychological and neurological findings. Arch Gen Psychiatry 51:51–61, 1994

Manger TJ, Warner JF: Neuroleptic malignant syndrome associated with prochlorperazine. South Med J 83:73–74, 1990

Markowitz JC, Klerman GL, Perry SW: Interpersonal psychotherapy of depressed HIV-positive outpatients. Hosp Community Psychiatry 43:885–890, 1992

Martin A, Heyes MP, Salazar AM, et al: Progressive slowing of reaction time and increasing cerebrospinal fluid concentrations of quinolinic acid in HIV-infected individuals. J Neuropsychiatry Clin Neurosci 4:270–279, 1992

Marzuk PM: Suicidal behavior and HIV illnesses. International Review of Psychiatry 3:365–371, 1991

Marzuk PM, Tierney H, Tardiff K, et al: Increased risk of suicide in persons with AIDS. JAMA 259:1333–1337, 1988

Masur H, Michelis MA, Greene JB, et al: An outbreak of community-acquired *Pneumocystis carinii* pneumonia: initial manifestations of cellular immune dysfunction. N Engl J Med 305:1431–1438, 1981

Maxwell S, Scheftner WA, Kessler HA, et al: Manic syndrome associated with zidovudine treatment (letter). JAMA 259:3406–3407, 1988

McArthur JC, Nance-Sproson TE, Griffin DE, et al: The diagnostic utility of elevation in cerebrospinal fluid β2-microglobulin in HIV-1 dementia. Neurology 42:1707–1712, 1992

McArthur JC, Hoover DR, Bacellar H, et al: Dementia in AIDS patients: incidence and risk factors. Neurology 43:2245–2252, 1993

McKegney FP, O'Dowd MA: Suicidality and HIV status. Am J Psychiatry 149:396–398, 1992

Merrill JE: Cytokines and retroviruses. Clin Immunol Immunopathol 64:23–27, 1992

Metzger E, Friedman R: Prolongation of the corrected QT and torsades de pointes cardiac arrhythmia associated with intravenous haloperidol in the medically ill. J Clin Psychopharmacol 13:128–132, 1993

Meyer I, McKinna K, Cournos F, et al: HIV seroprevalence among long-stay patients in a state psychiatric hospital. Hosp Community Psychiatry 44:282–284, 1993

Mitsuyasu RT: Medical aspects of HIV spectrum disease. Psychiatr Med 7:5–22, 1989

Morin SF, Charles KA, Malyon AK: The psychologic impact of AIDS on gay men. Am Psychol 39:1288–1293, 1984

Nahmias AJ, Weiss J, Yao X, et al: Evidence for human infection with an HTLV-III/LAV-like virus in Central Africa, 1959 (letter). Lancet 1:1279–1280, 1986

Navia BA, Jordan BD, Price RW: The AIDS dementia complex, I: clinical features. Ann Neurol 19:517–524, 1986a

Navia BA, Cho ES, Petito CK: The AIDS dementia complex, II: neuropathology. Ann Neurol 19:525–535, 1986b

Nichols SE: Psychiatric aspects of AIDS. Psychosomatics 24:1083–1089, 1983

Nichols SE: Psychosocial reactions of persons with the acquired immunodeficiency syndrome. Ann Intern Med 103:765–767, 1985

Nurnberg HG, Prudic J, Fiori M, et al: Psychopathology complicating acquired immune deficiency syndrome (AIDS). Am J Psychiatry 141:95–96, 1984

O'Dowd MA, McKegney FP: Manic syndrome associated with zidovudine (letter). JAMA 260:3587, 1988

O'Dowd MA, McKegney FP: AIDS patients compared with others seen in psychiatric consultation. Gen Hosp Psychiatry 12:50–55, 1990

O'Dowd MA, Biderman DJ, McKegney FP: Incidence of suicidality in AIDS and HIV-positive patients attending a psychiatry outpatient program. Psychosomatics 34:33–40, 1993

Ostrow D, Grant I, Atkinson H: Assessment and management of the AIDS patient with neuropsychiatric disturbances. J Clin Psychiatry 49:14–22, 1988

Ostrow DG, Monjan A, Joseph J, et al: HIV-related symptoms and psychological functioning in a cohort of homosexual men. Am J Psychiatry 146:737–742, 1989

Perkins DO, Evans DL: Fluoxetine treatment of depression in patients with HIV infection. Am J Psychiatry 148:807–808, 1991

Perry S, Fishman B, Jacobsberg L, et al: Effectiveness of psychoeducational interventions in reducing emotional distress after human immunodeficiency virus antibody testing. Arch Gen Psychiatry 48:143–147, 1991

Perry S, Fishman B, Jacobsberg L, et al: Relationships over 1 year between lymphocyte subsets and psychosocial variables among adults with infection by human immunodeficiency virus. Arch Gen Psychiatry 49:396–401, 1992

Perry S, Jacobsberg L, Card CAL, et al: Severity of psychiatric symptoms after HIV testing. Am J Psychiatry 150:775–779, 1993

Perry SW: Organic mental disorders caused by HIV: update on early diagnosis and treatment. Am J Psychiatry 147:696–710, 1990

Perry SW, Markowitz JC: Psychiatric interventions for AIDS spectrum disorders. Hosp Community Psychiatry 37:1001–1006, 1986

Perry SW, Markowitz JC: Counseling for HIV testing. Hosp Community Psychiatry 39:731–739, 1988

Perry SW, Tross S: Psychiatric problems of AIDS inpatients at the New York Hospital: a preliminary report. Public Health Rep 99:200–205, 1984

Perry SW, Jacobsberg LB, Fishman B, et al: Psychiatric diagnosis before serologic testing for the human immunodeficiency virus. Am J Psychiatry 147:89–93, 1990a

Perry SW, Jacobsberg LB, Fishman B, et al: Psychological response to serological testing for HIV. AIDS 4:145–152, 1990b

Perry SW, Jacobsberg L, Fishman B: Suicidal ideation and HIV testing. JAMA 263:679–682, 1990c

Pohl P, Vogl G, Fill H, et al: Single photon emission computed tomography in AIDS dementia complex. J Nucl Med 29:1382–1386, 1988

Portegies P, Entig RH, de Gans J, et al: Presentation and course of AIDS dementia complex: 10 years of follow-up in Amsterdam, the Netherlands. AIDS 7:669–675, 1993

Poulsen AG, Aaby P, Fredericksen K, et al: Prevalence of and mortality from human immunodeficiency virus type 2 in Bissau, West Africa. Lancet 1:827–830, 1989

Price RW, Brew BJ: The AIDS dementia complex. J Infect Dis 158:1079–1083, 1988

Price RW, Brew BJ, Sidtis J, et al: The brain in AIDS: central nervous system HIV-1 infection and AIDS dementia complex. Science 239:586–592, 1988

Rabkin JG, Harrison WM: Effect of imipramine on depression and immune status in a sample of men with HIV infection. Am J Psychiatry 147:495–497, 1990

Rabkin JG, Williams JBW, Remien RH, et al: Depression, distress, lymphocyte subsets, and human immunodeficiency virus symptoms on two occasions in HIV-positive homosexual men. Arch Gen Psychiatry 48:111–119, 1991

Radloff LS: The CES-D scale: a self-report depression scale for research in the general population. Applied Psychological Measurement 1:385–401, 1977

Rapoport A: Unilateral akathesia (letter). Neurology 39:1648, 1989

Regier DA, Myers JK, Kramer M, et al: The NIMH Epidemiologic Catchment Area (ECA) Program: historical context, major objectives, and study population characteristics. Arch Gen Psychiatry 41:934–941, 1984

Regier DA, Boyd JH, Burke JD, et al: One-month prevalence of mental disorders in the United States. Arch Gen Psychiatry 45:977–986, 1988

Rodgers C: Extrapyramidal side effects of antiemetics presenting as psychiatric illness. Gen Hosp Psychiatry 14:192–195, 1992

Rundell JR, Kyle KM, Brown GR, et al: Risk factors for suicide attempts in a human immunodeficiency virus screening program. Psychosomatics 33:24–27, 1992

Saag MS: AIDS testing now and in the future, in The Medical Management of AIDS, 3rd Edition. Edited by Sande MA, Volberding PA. Philadelphia, WB Saunders, 1992, pp 33–53

Sacks M, Dermatis H, Looser-Ott S, et al: Seroprevalence of HIV and risk factors for AIDS in psychiatric inpatients. Hosp Community Psychiatry 43:736–737, 1992

Satriano J, Herman R, Koplan M, et al: HIV risk reduction groups for people with serious mental illness. Paper presented at the NIMH Conference Mental Health Issues in HIV/AIDS Research: Clinical Challenges and Research Directions, Bethesda, MD, November 8–9, 1993

Schaerf FW, Miller RR, Lipsey JR, et al: ECT for major depression in four patients infected with human immunodeficiency virus. Am J Psychiatry 146:782–784, 1989

Schaffner B: Psychotherapy with HIV-infected persons. New Dir Ment Health Serv 48:5–6, 1990

Schmidt U, Miller D: Two cases of hypomania in AIDS. Br J Psychiatry 152:839–842, 1988

Sharer LR: Pathology of HIV-1 infection of the central nervous system: a review. J Neuropathol Exp Neurol 51:3–11, 1992

Sidtis JJ, Price RW: Early HIV-1 infection and the AIDS dementia complex. Neurology 40:323–326, 1990

Sidtis JJ, Gatsonis C, Price RW, et al: Zidovudine treatment of the AIDS dementia complex; results of a placebo-controlled trial. Ann Neurol 33:343–349, 1993

Snider W, Simpson D, Nielson S, et al: Neurological complications of acquired immune deficiency syndrome: analysis of 50 patients. Ann Neurol 14:403–418, 1983

Solomon GF: Psychoneuroimmunology and human immunodeficiency virus infection. Psychiatr Med 7:47–57, 1989

Spiegel D, Bloom J, Kraemer HC, et al: The beneficial effect of psychosocial treatment on survival of metastatic breast cancer patients: a randomized prospective outcome study. Lancet 12:888–891, 1989

Spira JL, Spiegel D: Group psychotherapy of the medically ill, in Psychiatric Care of the Medical Patient. Edited by Stoudemire A, Fogel BS. New York, Oxford University Press, 1993, pp 31–50

Sternbach H: The serotonin syndrome. Am J Psychiatry 148:705–713, 1991

Storch DD: Caution with use of tricyclics in patients with AIDS (letter). Am J Psychiatry 148:1750, 1991

Summergrad P, Glassman RS: Human immunodeficiency virus and other infectious disorders affecting the central nervous system, in Medical-Psychiatric Practice, Vol 1. Edited by Stoudemire A, Fogel B. Washington, DC, American Psychiatric Press, 1991, pp 243–284

Sussman N: The potential benefits of serotonin receptor-specific agents. J Clin Psychiatry 55 (suppl 2):45–51, 1994

Swenson JR, Erman M, Labelle J, et al: Extrapyramidal reactions: neuropsychiatric mimics in patients with AIDS. Gen Hosp Psychiatry 11:248–253, 1989

Tanquary J: Lithium neurotoxicity at therapeutic levels in AIDS patients. J Nerv Ment Dis 181:518–519, 1993

Temoshok L: Psychoimmunology and AIDS, in Psychological Neuropsychiatric and Substance Abuse Aspects of AIDS. Edited by Bridge PT. New York, Raven, 1988, pp 187–197

Tesar GE, Murray GB, Cassem NH: Use of high-dose intravenous haloperidol in the treatment of agitated cardiac patients. J Clin Psychopharmacol 5:344–347, 1985

Tozzi V, Narciso P, Galgani S, et al: Effects of zidovudine in 30 patients with mild to end-stage AIDS dementia complex. AIDS 7:683–692, 1993

Trachman SB: Buspirone induced psychosis in a human immunodeficiency virus infected man. Psychosomatics 33:332–335, 1992

Treisman GJ, Lyketsos CG, Fishman M, et al: Psychiatric care for patients with HIV infection; the varying perspectives. Psychosomatics 34:432–439, 1993

Tross S, Hirsch DA: Psychological distress and neuropsychological complications of HIV infection and AIDS. Am Psychol 43:929–934, 1988

Tunnell G: Complications in group psychotherapy with AIDS patients. Int J Group Psychother 41:481–498, 1991

van Gorp WG, Mandelkern MA, Gee M, et al: Cerebral metabolic dysfunction in AIDS: findings in a sample with and without dementia. J Neuropsychiatry Clin Neurosci 4:280–287, 1992

Vella S, Chiesi A, Volpi A, et al: Differential survival of patients with AIDS according to the 1987 and 1993 CDC case definitions. JAMA 271:1197–1199, 1994

Volavka J, Convit A, Czobar P, et al: HIV seroprevalence and risk behaviors in psychiatric inpatients. Psychiatry Res 39:109–114, 1991

Wallack JJ, Snyder S, Bialer PA, et al: An AIDS bibliography for the general psychiatrist. Psychosomatics 32:243–254, 1991

Ward JW, Drotman DP: Epidemiology of HIV and AIDS, in AIDS and Other Manifestations of HIV Infection, 2nd Edition. Edited by Wormser GP. New York, Raven, 1992, pp 1–15

Watters JK, Estilo MJ, Clark GL, et al: Syringe and needle exchange as HIV/AIDS prevention for injection drug users. JAMA 271:115–120, 1994

Weiss SH: Laboratory detection of human retroviral infection, in AIDS and Other Manifestations of HIV Infection, 2nd Edition. Edited by Wormser GP. New York, Raven, 1992, pp 95–106

Wells KB, Stewart A, Hays RD, et al: The functioning and well-being of depressed patients. JAMA 262:914–919, 1989

Werner ER, Fuchs D, Hausen A, et al: Tryptophan degradation in patients infected by human immunodeficiency virus. Biol Chem 369:337–340, 1988

Wiener PK, Schwartz MA, O'Connell RA: Characteristics of HIV-infected patients in an inpatient psychiatric setting. Psychosomatics 35:59–65, 1994

Williams JBW, Rabkin JG, Remien RH, et al: Multidisciplinary baseline assessment of homosexual men with and without human immunodeficiency virus infection, II: standardized clinical assessment of current and lifetime psychopathology. Arch Gen Psychiatry 48:124–130, 1991

Wolcott DL, Fawzy FI, Namir S: Clinical management of psychiatric disorders in HIV spectrum disease. Psychiatr Med 7:107–127, 1989

Wong MC, Suite ND, Labar DR: Seizures in human immunodeficiency virus infection. Arch Neurol 47:640–642, 1990

Working Group of the American Academy of Neurology AIDS Task Force: Nomenclature and research case definitions for neurologic manifestations of human immunodeficiency virus-type 1 (HIV-1) infection. Neurology 41:778–785, 1991

Worth JL, Savage CR, Baer L, et al: Computer-based neuropsychological screening for AIDS dementia complex. AIDS 7:677–681, 1993

Appendix 6–1

NEUROPSYCHIATRIC SIDE EFFECTS OF MEDICATIONS COMMONLY USED IN AIDS PATIENTS

Antiretrovirals

Didanosine (ddI, Videx)	Agitation, amnesia, ataxia, depression, dizziness, neuropathy
Zalcitabine (ddC, Hivid)	Headaches, dizziness, fatigue, neuropathy
Zidovudine (AZT, Retrovir)	Agitation, arthralgia, depression, headaches, insomnia, mania, myopathy, pain, restlessness; AZT-induced anemia may lead to fatigue and mimic depression; may have role in delaying onset or palliating AIDS dementia syndrome; AZT together with acyclovir can cause severe drowsiness and lethargy

Pneumocystis carinii pneumonia (PCP) prophylaxis and treatment

Atovaquone (Mepron)	Anorexia, anxiety, dizziness, insomnia
Dapsone (USP)	Agitation, depression, headaches, insomnia, mania, neuropathy, psychosis; rifampin may lower dapsone level
Pentamidine (Pentam)	Anxiety, ataxia, confusion, decreased appetite, depression, dizziness, drowsiness, emotional lability, fatigue, hallucinations, insomnia, memory loss, neuropathy, paranoia, paresthesias, seizures, tremors
Sulfadoxine/ pyrimethamine (Fansidar)	Anxiety, apathy, ataxia, depression, fatigue, hallucinations, insomnia, muscle weakness, peripheral neuropathy, seizures, tinnitus, vertigo
Trimethoprim/sulfame-thoxazole (Bactrim)	Anorexia, apathy, ataxia, decreased appetite, depression, hallucinations, headaches, insomnia, mutism, nervousness, psychosis, vertigo

Opportunistic infections (antivirals)

Acyclovir (Zovirax)	Confusion, depression, dizziness, hallucinations, headaches, insomnia, myalgia, paresthesias, pain, paranoia, somnolence, visual difficulties; used with AZT can cause severe lethargy and drowsiness; neuropsychiatric side effects are more frequent with concomitant renal failure and also with intravenous administration
Foscarnet (Foscavir)	Agitation, anxiety, body pain, confusion, muscle contractions, depressions, dizziness, fatigue, hallucinations, headaches, insomnia, paresthesias, neuropathy, pain, seizures, somnolence; may cause renal impairment
Ganciclovir (Cytovene, DHPG)	Agitation, ataxia, coma, confusion, delirium, dizziness, dreaming increased, hallucinations, headaches, insomnia, malaise, nervousness, paresthesias, psychosis, retinal detachment, tremors; 5% of patients have neurological side effects

Opportunistic infections (antifungals)

Amphotericin B (Fungizone IV)	Anorexia, body pain, delirium, headaches, hearing loss, malaise, tinnitus, vertigo, vision problems, weight loss
Fluconazole (Diflucan)	Headaches, seizures; rifampin lowers fluconazole level
Ketoconazole (Nizoral)/ itraconazole (Sporanox)	Depression, dizziness, hallucinations, headaches, somnolence, suicidality; decreased serum testosterone level, can lead to impotence

Opportunistic infections (antibacterials)

Amikacin (Amikin)	Anxiety, auditory and vestibular toxicities, body pain, depression, dizziness, hall, headaches, insomnia, neuromuscular blockade/paralysis, paresthesias, tremors, vertigo
Azithromycin (Zithromax)	Dizziness, fatigue, headaches, somnolence, vertigo
Capreomycin (Capastat)	Auditory and vestibular toxicities, paralysis
Ciprofloxacin (Cipro)	Agitation, anorexia, ataxia, catatonia, delirium, depersonalization, depression, dizziness, hallucinations, headaches, insomnia, irritability, lethargy, mania, photosensitivity, tremors

Clarithromycin (Biaxin)	Headaches
Clofazimine (Lamprene)	Depression, dizziness, fatigue, headaches, orange-brown skin discoloration, visual disturbances
Cycloserine (Seromycin)	Depression, headaches, neuropathy, psychosis, seizures; monitoring levels can help to facilitate management; severe psychotic episodes are common
Ethambutol (Myambutol)	Confusion, decreased red-green color discrimination, decreased visual acuity, disorientation, dizziness, hallucinations, headaches, neuropathy, optic neuritis
Isoniazid (INH)	Agitation, ataxia, depression, euphoria, hallucinations, mania, memory disturbance, muscle twitching, neuropathy, optic neuritis, paranoia, paresthesias, psychosis, seizures
Pyrazinamide (PZA)	Arthralgia, myalgia
Rifampin (Rifadin, Rimactane)	Anorexia, ataxia, confusion, decreased concentration, drowsiness, dizziness, fatigue, headaches, muscle weakness, neuropathy; may decrease methadone level and thus can precipitate opiate withdrawal

Miscellaneous

Dronabinol (Marinol)	Anxiety, confusion, psychosis
Epoetin alfa (Procrit)	Headaches, seizures
Interferon alfa-2a (Roferon-A)	Anxiety, depression, dizziness, impotence, insomnia, lethargy, numbness, paresthesia, paranoia, suicidal ideation
Sargramostim (Prokine, GM-CSF)	Arthalgias, headaches, myalgias

Chapter 7

Neuropsychiatric Sequelae of Mild Traumatic Brain Injury

John G. Tierney, M.D.
Barry S. Fogel, M.D.

This chapter is a practical guide for the general psychiatrist treating patients with neuropsychiatric sequelae of mild traumatic brain injury (TBI). The 1989 Interagency Head Injury Task Force Report identified TBI as the leading killer and cause of disability among children and young adults and estimated that 2 million head injuries occur each year, with 75,000 to 100,000 deaths and economic costs that approached $25 billion per year (Department of Health and Human Services 1989). Transport-related events are the single largest cause of new brain injury.

Of the 2 million injuries that occur each year, approximately 80%–90% are classified as mild (Kraus 1987). These "mild" injuries are associated with significant lifetime costs, because of their effects on occupational performance and their potential for causing or aggravating psychotic disorders (Max et al. 1991).

The TBI literature is difficult to review and summarize because of inconsistent definitions for various syndromes and conditions. Consequently, we begin this chapter with a definition of terms and subsequently limit the discussion to mild TBI caused by closed head injury (CHI). We focus on the neuropsychiatric sequelae of mild TBI, especially problems of accurate diagnostic assessment, and the treatment of common manifestations of mild CHI such as postconcussional syndromes, mood disorders, cognitive deficits, and impaired impulse control. This is not a comprehensive review, but, wherever possible, we have cited seminal papers and review articles for the reader interested in more detailed information. Very little systematic research on CHI diagnosis and treatment is available; therefore, most of the recommendations made here are based on extrapolations from other neuropsychiatric populations by experts who specialize in the treatment of severe TBI (Szymanski and Linn 1992).

DEFINITIONS AND DIAGNOSTIC CRITERIA

Definitions and diagnostic criteria are important in the approach to any psychiatric intervention; however, they are particularly important in TBI because the condition lacks definitive systematic research on treatment, and such research requires relatively homogeneous study populations. Unfortunately, there is no generally accepted classification of post-TBI neuropsychiatric syndromes. Neurologists, neurosurgeons, psychiatrists, and physical therapists each have nomenclature unique to their perspectives on the condition, and even within these groups, there are disagreements on the definition of terms. For example, in a series of studies of "mild" TBI, the maximum duration of loss of consciousness (LOC) varied from 0 to 60 minutes (Kraus and Sorenson 1994).

TBI may be characterized by the type and severity of the injury. The three broad types of injury are 1) penetrating brain injury (PBI), 2) open head injury (i.e., involving a break in the integrity of the dura) (OHI), and 3) CHI (Gualtieri 1988). The severity of the TBI is typically described as severe, moderate, or mild, based on the duration of LOC, the duration of posttraumatic amnesia, and the severity of neurologic deficit on presentation for treatment. General psychiatrists will most likely encounter mild TBI caused by CHI because it is the most common type and because the clinical features of the posttraumatic period often overlap with features of primary mental disorders (Kraus 1987; Jane et al. 1985). The criteria listed below are generally accepted classifications for severity of TBI (Rimel et al. 1981, 1982; Szymanski and Linn 1992):

Severe TBI: LOC > 2 weeks **OR**
Posttraumatic amnesia > 2 weeks **OR**
Glasgow coma score (GCS) (Teasdale and Jennett 1974) < 8

Moderate TBI: Neither mild nor severe
Mild TBI: LOC < 30 minutes **AND**
        Posttraumatic amnesia of 1–24 hours **AND**
        Initial GCS 13–15

Table 7–1 lists DSM-IV (American Psychiatric Association 1994) diagnoses commonly used in patients with behavioral complications of TBI. Precise diagnosis of psychiatric syndromes after TBI, however, at times requires departure from the DSM-IV system. In the DSM-IV, the diagnosis of major depression implies the absence of a causative medical condition. Strictly following the DSM-IV, one could only identify a major depression syndrome after TBI as a *mood disorder due to a general medical condition.* DSM-IV describes *general medical condition* as a convenient shorthand to refer to conditions outside the "Mental Disorder" section of the *International Classification of Diseases* (ICD). This is particularly problematic when using DSM-IV nomenclature to describe TBI patients because, in most cases, the diagnostic criteria for a "pure" psychiatric condition are much more specific and descriptive than those for a mental disorder due to a general medical condition. For example, the diagnosis of a major depressive episode requires at least five of nine depressive symptoms during the same 2-week period. Specifically, one

Table 7–1. DSM-IV diagnoses potentially applicable to patients with traumatic brain injury (TBI)[a]

Diagnosis	
Delirium	Personality change (due to TBI)
Amnestic disorder (due to TBI)	(specify type)
Dementia due to head trauma	Disinhibited
Mood disorder (due to TBI)	Aggressive
With manic features	Labile
With depressive features	Apathetic
With mixed features	Paranoid
Anxiety disorder (due to TBI)	Other
Psychotic disorder (due to TBI)	Combined
With delusions	Unspecified
With hallucinations	Postconcussional disorder (not official in DSM-IV)
	Sleep disorder (due to TBI)

[a]Also code 854.00 head injury on Axis III.
Source. American Psychiatric Association 1994.

of the symptoms must be either 1) depressed mood or 2) loss of interest or pleasure. On the other hand, to diagnose a depression in a TBI patient as a mood disorder due to a general medical condition, the only necessary feature is a depressed mood or loss of interest or pleasure in most activities. Consequently, in describing behavioral complications of TBI, the available DSM-IV criteria tend to be more vague and less rigorous than those for primary mental disorders. Table 7–2 contrasts DSM-IV criteria for a major depressive episode with criteria for a mood disorder due to a general medical condition.

A practical expedient taken by many clinicians is to clinically designate the patient's symptoms as a *major depressive syndrome due to TBI* but to code a diagnosis for administrative purposes as mood disorder due to a general medical condition.

Although difficulties exist with the use of DSM-IV nomenclature in TBI, DSM-IV introduced two new diagnostic categories that should help improve diagnostic clarity. The new categories are dementia due to head trauma and postconcussional disorder. The DSM-IV task force believed that insufficient evidence existed to warrant official validation of the postconcussional disorder in DSM-IV; however, unofficial criteria have been published to facilitate systematic clinical research. This is an important change for clinicians working with TBI patients, and we discuss the proposed disorder in greater detail later in this chapter. Along with these changes, the DSM-IV modified the definition of organic personality syndrome, and the category became *personality change due to a general medical condition.* As with mood disorders, the criteria for personality change due to a general medical condition are broad and rather nonspecific. Nevertheless, this is an important diagnostic category for psychiatrists working with TBI patients because of the high frequency of personality changes seen after TBI. We discuss these changes in greater detail in the "Clinical Features" section later in this chapter. Table 7–3 lists the criteria for personality change.

ETIOLOGY

Important insights into the behavioral manifestations of CHI are found even in the limited research currently available on the mechanisms and pathogenesis of damage in these types of injury. Brain damage in TBI may result from contusions, lacerations, hematomas, diffuse axonal injury, and neurotoxicity of substances released from brain cells as a consequence of trauma (Silver et al. 1992). Both hematomas and diffuse axonal injury can be either immediate or delayed consequences of the initial injury.

Direct or primary damage occurs when brain tissue comes into contact with bony protuberances of the skull and typically causes a contusion or laceration. In addition to this direct, or coup, injury there is commonly a contrecoup injury at a point on the brain opposite the impact site (Graham et al. 1987). *Contusion* is not a clinical term but rather a pathological condition to describe superficial damage or "brain bruise" to the cortical convolutions (Strub and Black 1988). Many, but not all, contusions can be diagnosed in the living patient by

Table 7–2. Modified DSM-IV criteria for major depressive episode versus mood disorder due to a general medical condition

Major depressive episode	Mood disorder due to a general medical condition
A. At least five of the following have been present during the same 2-week period . . . at least one of the symptoms is either 1) depressed mood or 2) loss of interest or pleasure	A. A prominent and persistent disturbance in mood characterized by either (or both): 1. Depressed mood or loss of interest or pleasure in most activities
1. Depressed mood	2. Elevated, expansive, or irritable mood
2. Diminished interest or pleasure	
3. Weight loss or gain	B. Evidence from history, physical examination, or laboratory findings of a general medical condition judged to be etiologically related to the disturbance
4. Insomnia or hypersomnia	
5. Psychomotor agitation or retardation	
6. Fatigue or loss of energy	
7. Feelings of worthlessness or excessive or inappropriate guilt	C. Disturbance does not occur exclusively during the course of delirium or dementia
8. Diminished ability to think or concentrate	
9. Recurrent thoughts of death	D. Disturbance is not better accounted for by another mental disorder
B. The symptoms cause clinically significant distress or impairment in social, occupational, or other important areas of functioning	
	E. Symptoms cause significant distress or impairment in social, occupational, or other functioning
C. Not due to the direct effects of a substance (e.g., drugs of abuse, medication) or a general medical condition (e.g., hypothyroidism)	

Source. American Psychiatric Association 1994.

brain imaging. The frontal and temporal poles and the inferior surfaces of these lobes are characteristic sites of this damage (Graham et al. 1987). Damage to these areas commonly results in syndromes named for their location—that is, frontal, orbitofrontal, and temporal lobe syndromes. These syndromes are characterized by well-known constellations of symptoms. Decreased executive cognitive function is a characteristic feature of frontal lobe change, disinhibition is associated with orbitofrontal damage, and memory loss is typical of temporal lobe damage. Personality changes occur with damage to any of the three sites (Levin 1987).

Indirect damage is typically the result of rotational or angular acceleration injuries, common to CHI and to secondary neurotoxicity. Even in the absence of direct skull impact and mechanical injury, rotational acceleration can cause profound damage (Adams et al. 1982). In the literature, definitions of the microscopic pathophysiology of acceleration forces and the brain damage they cause are emerging (White and Krause 1993). This mechanism of injury is associated with shear

Table 7–3. Traumatic brain injury and modified DSM-IV criteria for personality change due to a general medical condition

---

A. A persistent personality disturbance that represents a change from the individual's previous characteristic personality pattern
B. There is evidence from the history, physical examination, or laboratory findings of a general medical condition judged to be etiologically related to the personality change
C. The disturbance is not better accounted for by another mental disorder (including other mental disorders due to a general medical condition)
D. The disturbance causes clinically significant distress or impairment in social, occupational, or other important areas of functioning
E. The disturbance does not occur exclusively during delirium and does not meet criteria for dementia

Specify type:
• Disinhibited
• Aggressive
• Labile
• Apathetic
• Paranoid
• Other
• Combined
• Unspecified

Source.   American Psychiatric Association 1994.

damage to capillaries and blood vessels (e.g., hematomas), the mid-brain, and to long tracts, including monoaminergic projections to the cerebral cortex from brain stem nuclei. Currently, it is widely accepted that the acceleration-deceleration common to TBI (especially in motor vehicle accidents) often causes diffuse axonal injury (Adams et al. 1982; Blumberg et al. 1989; Jane et al. 1985). In diffuse axonal injury, axons may be torn mechanically by shear forces at the time of injury, or the internal cytoskeleton of the axon may be disrupted, leading to delayed disruption of the axon's function. The damage induced by blunt head trauma may be multifactorial; transient shear forces mechanically de-form tissue, while extensive depolarization of neurons triggers a cas-cade of excitatory neurotransmitter release, excitotoxicity, hypoxia, free radical formation, acidosis, and subsequent cellular injury or death (Faden et al. 1989; Siesjo 1993). Povlishock and co-workers (1993) em-phasized that trauma damages the axonal cytoskeleton, leading to focal impairment of anterograde axoplasmic transport, progressive axonal swelling, and ultimately disconnection of the axon. The continuum of axonal injury suggested by Povlishock and co-workers (1993) helps to explain the delayed onset of conditions such as amnesia, dementia, and seizures and, perhaps most significantly for clinicians, suggests a mechanism for significant neuropsychiatric symptoms to develop after an apparently mild injury. Regardless of the exact mechanism finally described, diffuse injury is consistently observed in this type of injury, and the long tracts of the central nervous system (CNS), particularly the long-fiber tracts of the brain stem, are physically most susceptible to this type of damage (Jane et al. 1985). By definition, diffuse axonal injury lesions are located diffusely throughout the brain. As Gualtieri (1993) describes, "The combination of cortical, subcortical, and brain-stem injury is characteristic of CHI" (p. 518).

Even severe diffuse axonal injury may be difficult to identify by computed tomography (CT) or magnetic resonance imaging (MRI), al-though MRI is more sensitive than CT, and serial CT scans are more sensitive than single scans. Currently, these imaging techniques cannot definitively exclude the diagnosis of axonal injury. LOC at the time of injury implies some degree of diffuse axonal injury. According to Strub and Black (1988), "The midbrain is one of the points of maximum rota-tion in CHI and the ascending activating system at this level suffers an initial injury, with a prolonged coma when damage is significant" (p. 342). The authors go on to explain that dysfunction of these ascend-ing fibers may be responsible for the attention and concentration problems experienced by victims of minor injuries even when consciousness is quickly regained. In addition, long-fiber tracts projecting from brain stem nuclei transmit neurotransmitters norepinephrine and serotonin to the entire cerebral cortex, so relatively small axonal injuries in the midbrain may have effects on mood that are similar to those seen in stroke (Morrison et al. 1979; Robinson and Szetela 1981).

The clinical significance of this pathophysiology for the clinician is threefold.

1. Frontal, orbitofrontal, and temporal lobe symptoms and syndromes are common after TBI and should be considered in the differential diagnosis of postinjury mental changes.
2. Diffuse axonal injury in the brain stem most likely accounts for damage to the reticular activating system, resulting in stupor, coma, delirium, or inattention in the acute postinjury period and subsequent problems with attention and arousal as the patient recovers from moderate and severe injury.
3. Damage to the long-fiber tracts such as projections from the locus coeruleus and raphe nuclei may interrupt monoamine pathways and partially explain the mood and anxiety disorders that frequently occur after TBI.

CLINICAL FEATURES

The clinical features of TBI are as diverse as the brain is complicated. Almost any clinical feature is possible after TBI, ranging from deficit behaviors and negative symptoms to disinhibited behaviors and positive symptoms. Among the most common neuropsychiatric sequelae of mild TBI are cognitive deficits, mood disorders, personality changes, and impulse control problems. Some patients meet criteria for primary psychiatric disorders such as delirium, dementia due to head trauma, or mood disorder with depressive features due to a general medical condition. However, some people have a recognized constellation of symptoms after TBI that is not typical of any of the primary psychiatric disorders, whereas their cognitive impairment is not severe enough to warrant the diagnosis of delirium or dementia, and their vegetative symptoms are not severe enough to meet criteria for DSM-IV depressive disorders. In this section, we examine the clinical features common to mild TBI and their relationship to primary mental disorders and to the new DSM-IV diagnostic category postconcussional disorder.

As mentioned earlier in this chapter, mild TBI may represent 80%–90% of all TBIs (Kraus 1987), and, although diagnostic ambiguity limits the quality of epidemiological studies to date, carefully conducted studies increasingly indicate that many patients with mild TBI develop symptom clusters consistent with postconcussional disorder (Kraus 1987; Levin 1987). Despite these studies, *postconcussional syndrome* borders on being a pejorative term for those clinicians who still associate postconcussion symptoms with *compensation neurosis* (Lishman 1988). Brown and associates (1994) attribute this "perpetuating myth of compensation neurosis" to the lack of a specific diagnostic framework specifically for sequelae of milder head injuries. In an excellent review of mild head injury, McAllister (1994) points to flaws in early studies that supported the theory of compensation neurosis and to increasing numbers of studies that demonstrate that patients elaborating symptoms for secondary gain represent only a small fraction of patients with postconcussional symptoms (Binder 1986; Bornstein et al. 1988; Dikmen et al. 1986; Keshavan et al. 1981; Rimel et al. 1981).

Terminology and definitions are as problematic with postconcussional disorder as with other aspects of TBI. However, McAllister (1994) clarifies that, whereas postconcussional disorder is described as a constellation of symptoms commonly associated with mild TBI, many of its symptoms can be seen as late consequences of more severe injuries. Therefore, for this chapter, and in keeping with our interpretation of the intent of the DSM-IV diagnostic category, mild TBI describes the severity of the injury, and postconcussional disorder is a syndrome that follows TBI that is often, but not necessarily, mild. Table 7–4 shows research criteria for the DSM-IV diagnostic category postconcussional disorder.

These criteria can be broken into three clusters of postconcussional symptoms: 1) a somatic cluster (e.g., headache, fatigue, and dizziness); 2) a cognitive cluster (e.g., attention, concentration, and memory); and 3) an affective cluster (e.g., irritability, anxiety, and depression) (Brown et al. 1994). In a commonly quoted multicenter study, Levin and others (1987a) compared neurobehavioral function of 57 patients with mild TBI at 1 week, 1 month, and 3 months after injury with 56 selected control subjects. Almost all the patients with TBI (82%–93%) in the Levin study reported postconcussion symptoms at the initial evaluation. Headache, decreased energy, and dizziness were the most frequently reported symptoms, occurring at rates of 71%, 60%, and 53%, respectively. These symptoms were still prominent at the 3-month follow-up, but the rates dropped to 47%, 22%, and 22%, respectively. In a similar study of 424 patients with TBI, Rimel and colleagues (1981) reported 78% of patients complained of headache and 60% complained of decreased memory at 3-month follow-up.

How long the postconcussional symptoms persist is a controversial

Table 7–4. Traumatic brain injury and DSM-IV research criteria for postconcussional disorder

A. A history of head trauma that has caused significant cerebral concussion.

B. Evidence from neuropsychological testing or quantified cognitive assessment of difficulty in attention (concentrating, shifting focus of attention, performing simultaneous cognitive tasks) or memory (learning or recalling information).

C. Three (or more) of the following occur shortly after the trauma and last at least 3 months:

   (1) becoming fatigued easily
   (2) disordered sleep
   (3) headache
   (4) vertigo or dizziness
   (5) irritability or aggression on little or no provocation
   (6) anxiety, depression, or affective lability
   (7) changes in personality (e.g., social or sexual inappropriateness)
   (8) apathy or lack of spontaneity

D. The symptoms in Criteria B and C have their onset following head trauma or else represent a substantial worsening of preexisting symptoms.

E. The disturbance causes significant impairment in social or occupational functioning and represents a significant decline from a previous level of functioning. In school-age children, the impairment may be manifested by a significant worsening in school or academic performance dating from the trauma.

F. The symptoms do not meet criteria for dementia due to head trauma and are not better accounted for by another mental disorder (e.g., amnestic disorder due to head trauma, personality change due to head trauma).

Source. American Psychiatric Association 1994. Used with permission.

subject. According to one prospective study of 54 patients' relatives at 1, 6, and 12 months post-TBI, the level of family stress did not appear to depend on how long the patient was in the hospital, the degree of physical disability, or even the severity of injury but rather on personality change and the relative's perception of the symptoms arising from the head injury (Oddy et al. 1978). Levin (1987) points out that the patient's premorbid personality and the postinjury environment also contribute to the longer-term psychosocial outcome. McAllister (1994) concludes that most patients show progressive resolution of symptoms in the first 1 to 3 months after injury; however, some will have persistent sequelae at 6 and 12 months or even longer. With the introduction of the new diagnostic category (albeit unofficial), another problem arises: the potential overlap of this proposed syndrome with existing categories of mood disorder due to a general medical condition, dementia, and delirium. Especially when, as we discussed in the "Definitions" section, the criteria for disorders due to a general medical condition are less precise than those for primary mental disorders. The extent of this overlap remains unanswered; it may be resolved by further experience with the provisional category in DSM-IV.

POSTTRAUMATIC STRESS DISORDER AND PATIENTS WITH TRAUMATIC BRAIN INJURY

TBIs often occur during a psychologically traumatic event. For example, a concussion may be sustained in an automobile accident in which a person is killed or maimed. Mild TBI may occur in connection with a mugging or in the context of domestic violence. In these situations, the patient may develop a posttraumatic stress disorder (PTSD), with symptoms that greatly confound the assessment of the neurologic lesions.

Difficulty concentrating is a symptom of PTSD, but its presence is not required for the diagnosis. However, recent neuropsychological studies of patients with PTSD suggest that many patients with PTSD not related to cerebral trauma have demonstrable cognitive deficits. For example, Uddo and co-investigators (1993) compared 16 Vietnam combat veterans with PTSD with 15 control subjects; the PTSD subjects had worse verbal learning with more perseverative errors and greater sensitivity to proactive interference. They also had decreased verbal fluency and impaired visual tracking. Bremner and associates (1993), in a similarly designed study, found that Vietnam combat veterans with

PTSD performed worse than control subjects on two widely used memory tests: the Wechsler Memory Scale (Wechsler 1987) and the Selective Reminding Test (Buschke and Fuld 1974). Intelligence quotient (IQ) did not differ between patients and control subjects. Gurvits and associates (1993) used somewhat different measures in a similar study but did not find a difference between combat veterans with PTSD and control subjects on neuropsychological measures. They did find more neurologic soft signs in the PTSD patients. When only general intelligence tests such as the Wechsler Adult Intelligence Scale—Revised (Wechsler 1981) are given, differences between PTSD patients and control subjects are minimal (Dalton et al. 1989).

When a patient with a history of TBI has active symptoms of PTSD, the interpretation of neuropsychological test results must take into account the potential cognitive effects of PTSD, just as major depression must be considered as an influence on test performance. Impairments in attention and memory can be attributed to PTSD, but highly localizing findings such as constructional apraxia or nominal aphasia cannot. It is unknown whether frontal lobe damage can be reliably diagnosed in a patient with an active PTSD. As in the case of depression, assessment of primary neurologic deficits is most valid if the patient can be retested after successful psychiatric treatment of the PTSD. Prognoses for both clinical and legal purposes should be qualified until a serious attempt is made to treat the PTSD.

ASSESSMENT

The neuropsychiatric assessment of patients with recent TBI requires systematic observation to 1) document the constellation of symptoms, 2) grade the nature and severity of injury, 3) diagnose the individual syndrome or disorder, 4) track the course of recovery, and 5) gauge the effectiveness of interventions. Because many interventions in this patient population are empirical trials, the assessment of the individual should clearly delineate the syndrome, target symptoms, treatment goals, and measures of successful intervention. To grade the injury, information about the presence or absence and duration of features such as coma, LOC, initial GCS, and posttraumatic amnesia or delirium is of particular importance. The key elements of the assessment are 1) the premorbid and current history from the patient *and* a corroborating source, 2) the clinical interview, 3) the neuropsychiatric mental status examination, 4) neuropsychological testing, and 5) laboratory testing.

HISTORY

In patients with TBI, a systematic history is an important cornerstone of the assessment, and it is essential to successful diagnosis, treatment planning, and prediction of outcome and prognosis. The TBI history should focus on three periods surrounding the injury: 1) the premorbid or pretraumatic period, 2) the peritraumatic period, and 3) the current or posttraumatic period (Lishman 1988). Patient presentations can vary markedly after TBI. Some patients present with mild TBI symptoms and are unaware that they were ever injured, whereas others present with severe deficits (Silver et al. 1992). Therefore, the most effective history and assessment should be flexible enough to elicit and characterize a spectrum of conditions ranging from the subtle cognitive deficits of a mild postconcussional disorder to the potentially severe behavioral disinhibition of a frontal lobe syndrome. A sample approach to the assessment of patients with TBI is outlined in Table 7–5.

Pretraumatic or Premorbid History

The premorbid history is always important in a psychiatric evaluation; however, it is especially important in patients with TBI, because certain premorbid conditions 1) overlap with potential behavioral consequences of TBI (e.g., preexisting attention-deficit hyperactivity disorder [ADHD] or poor impulse control); 2) are associated with a worse prognosis (e.g., alcohol abuse predisposes to dementia and repeated head injuries); and 3) can be used to establish targets for recovery (e.g., a person with premorbid dementia cannot be expected to improve beyond baseline level of cognitive or behavioral function after a head injury). A combination of factors such as age, social involvement, social support, and employment and education level affect prognosis. For example, a high premorbid education and occupation level is associated with a better prognosis for return to work after head injury (Levin 1987; Rimel et al. 1981). Advanced age implies a worse prognosis for any given level of injury severity.

Peritraumatic History

The peritraumatic history is necessary to grade the injury, and corroborating sources are particularly important for supplying information about the presence or absence and duration of features such as coma,

Table 7–5.   Neuropsychiatric evaluation of patients with traumatic brain injury

Chief complaint	Elicit symptoms from mild to severe
History of present illness	
Peritrauma history	
Recollection of injury?	Date
Loss of consciousness? (LOC)	Severity and duration of LOC
Coma?	Severity and duration of coma
	• Glasgow Coma Score (GCS) (Teasdale and Jennett 1974): initial and subsequent
	• Galveston Orientation and Amnesia Test (GOAT) scores (Levin et al. 1979): initial and subsequent
Last memory before injury?	i.e., retrograde amnesia
First memory after injury?	i.e., duration of posttraumatic amnesia or anterograde amnesia
Oculovestibular problems	i.e., eye findings are indicative of severe brain stem injuries
Focal hemispheric lesions	i.e., hematomas, contusions
Posttrauma history	
Current symptoms?	For example, in mild injury:
	• Confusion
	• Headache
	• Dizziness
	• Irritability
	• Decreased concentration
	• Sensitivity to noise or light
Premorbid history	Ideally obtained from family or close friend (e.g., for frontal lobe syndromes)
Age	
Psychiatric	Especially:
	• Attention-deficit hyperactivity disorder
	• Axis II (e.g., antisocial)
	• Depression
	• Alcoholism
	• Drug abuse
	• Cognitive problems
	• Behavioral problems
Education level	School performance, records

(continued)

Table 7–5.   Neuropsychiatric evaluation of patients with traumatic brain injury *(continued)*

Employment	Work records
Social	Relationships, social support, personality
Legal	Antisocial behavior, pending litigation
Psychiatric review of symptoms	Delirium, dementia, psychosis, mood, anxiety, etc.
Past medical history	Emphasis on previous head injuries
Past surgical history	
Neuropsychiatric mental status examination	Clinical examination of diverse cognitive functions
	Mini-Mental State Exam (Folstein et al. 1975)
	Mental Status Examination in Neurology (Strub and Black 1993)
	Neuropsychological testing from focused to comprehensive (based on indications)
Symptom screens/checklists	GCS
	GOAT
	Neurobehavioral Rating Scale (NBRS) (Levin et al. 1987b)
	Organic Aggression Scale (OAS) (Silver and Yudofsky 1991)
Laboratory	Computed tomography (CT) (limited usefulness, especially around bony surfaces)
	Magnetic resonance imaging (MRI) (preferable to CT but will not always detect diffuse axonal injury and may be within normal limits in mild injuries)
	Electroencephalogram (limited usefulness)
	Single photon-emission computed tomography (SPECT)

LOC, initial GCS, and retrograde and anterograde amnesia. These factors are used to categorize the injury as mild, moderate, or severe, and they are essential to treatment planning for each stage of recovery from TBI and to anticipate the behavioral problems associated with each stage. Peritraumatic history is also key to establishing a prognosis; for example, "Daily administration of the Galveston Orientation and Amnesia Test (GOAT) (Levin et al. 1979) to consecutive admissions for TBI has disclosed that patients with mild head injury (initial GCS of 13–15, normal neurological findings, and no extracranial injuries requiring surgery or hospitalization longer than 48 hours) typically improve to the normal range with 48 hours" (Levin 1987, p. 449).

CLINICAL INTERVIEW AND NEUROPSYCHIATRIC MENTAL STATUS EXAMINATION

The clinical interview and neuropsychiatric mental status examination should be tailored to the particular stage of recovery and severity of injury. Ideally, the examination should probe functions governed by various lobes of the brain and their integration, with particular emphasis on frontal, orbitofrontal, and temporal lobe functions, because these areas are those most commonly damaged by TBI caused by CHI. Tests such as the GCS, GOAT, and Mini-Mental State Exam (MMSE) (Folstein et al. 1975) are used to characterize gross deficits, particularly during early stages of recovery from moderate to severe injury. As recovery progresses, or when injuries are less severe and patients have more functional and cognitive capacity, systematic and bedside clinical neuropsychological testing such as the collection of tests outlined by Strub and Black (1993) progressively assess the range from basic functions to higher cortical functions. More specifically, the examination should test attention; fluency; set shifting; language function; memory (immediate, recent, remote, verbal, and visual); higher cognitive functions such as calculation, abstraction, and construction; and executive function. Executive function has increasingly been appreciated as relevant to disability in other psychiatric disorders such as ADHD, schizophrenia, and dementia, and scales are available that appear to show sensitivity, reliability, validity, and clinical utility (Fogel 1994; Royal et al. 1993). Corroborative history remains important for evaluation of mental status, and scales given by caregivers such as the Organic Aggression Scale (OAS) (Silver and Yudofsky 1987, 1991) and the Neurobehavioral Rating Scale (NBRS) (Levin et al. 1987b) are invaluable for characterizing current behaviors and their response to intervention.

Mild TBI often requires particularly meticulous evaluation because, even though the injury is mild, functional disability may be significant. However, more comprehensive and sophisticated testing may be necessary to quantify and objectify the neurological basis of the disability following mild TBI than that following severe TBI. Patients should be carefully evaluated for personality changes, mood changes, and anxiety symptoms. Structured interviews and inventories such as the Structured Clinical Interview for DSM-III-R (SCID) (Spitzer et al. 1992), Minnesota Multiphasic Personality Inventory (MMPI) (Hathaway and McKinley 1943), and Hamilton Depression Scale (Ham-D) (Hamilton 1960) may identify discrete psychiatric disorders and comorbid Axis II problems, but they may also suggest multiple mental disorders, none of which captures the relationship of the symptoms to the brain injury. Formal neuropsychological testing may not be necessary if the history and a detailed bedside examination are consistent with a diagnosis that explains the patient's symptoms and disability.

NEUROPSYCHOLOGICAL TESTING

There are essentially two primary reasons—clinical and forensic—to conduct formal neuropsychological testing in patients with mild TBI. Clinically, "The principal roles of formal neuropsychological testing in TBI patients are to delineate specific and sometime subtle functional weakness, to help in planning specific treatment strategies, and to assess patients' course and response to treatment" (Gualtieri 1993, p. 525). Neuropsychological testing for legal purposes often relates to questions of malingering, degree of disability, and estimation of appropriate compensation. The adversarial nature of the American legal system often requires a comprehensive neuropsychological evaluation even if it is not directly relevant. Regardless of the express purpose of the testing, the neuropsychologist must examine five domains: 1) attention, 2) language, 3) memory, 4) cognition, and 5) executive function. In the following section, we briefly review these three aspects of neuropsychological testing.

Clinically Driven Neuropsychological Testing

From a clinical standpoint, as with all other areas of medicine, random, or "shotgun," testing is expensive and, if not hypothesis driven, often produces confusing and even misleading results. In addition, patients with TBI are notoriously fatigable, and long, arduous testing may compromise test validity. Therefore, clinically, it is always best to formulate hypotheses to subsequently accept or reject based on the results of tests that specifically measure or evaluate those hypotheses (Fogel and Faust 1993). Such hypotheses often concentrate on delineation of functionally important cognitive deficits, along with areas of preserved function that might be useful in compensatory strategies. Once the clinical decision is made to conduct formal neuropsychological testing, the clinician must find someone with experience and training in assessment of TBI patients because, just as not all psychiatrists are experienced in the assessment of TBI, not all psychologists or psychometricians are experienced in the formal neuropsychological testing of this population. Finally, the clinician should work closely with the neuropsychologist to formulate the hypotheses to be tested and to design the most appropriate battery of tests to assess the questions raised. "In general, the clinical evaluation of TBI does not require expensive neurodiagnostic procedures of comprehensive neuropsychologic testing . . . however, if the issue is litigation, one may be urged to spare no expense to identify an objective neuropathic finding" (Gualtieri 1993, p. 525).

Forensically Driven Neuropsychological Testing

A discussion of forensic psychiatry is beyond the scope of this chapter; however, the following generalizations intend to help clinicians involved in litigation of a TBI case. A major advantage of formal neuropsychological testing for forensic work is the test reliability and validity achieved by expert neuropsychologists that typically cannot be attained with informal, bedside, or clinical testing. This reliability and validity are valued in the courtroom. However, the reliability of various test instruments may be known only for certain test populations, and validity estimates do not extend to subjective inferences from test data. Thus, if the patient is a minority, is not a native speaker of English, or has a comorbid psychiatric illness, conclusions must be qualified. Also, if the patient has an active mental syndrome, whether primary or caused by the TBI, the psychiatrist should point out that a definitive prognosis cannot be made until psychiatric treatment has been attempted and the response to treatment has been assessed.

Neuropsychological Test Domains

As noted earlier in this chapter, neuropsychological testing comprises five domains: 1) attention, 2) language, 3) memory, 4) cognition, and 5) executive function. Each domain contains more or less challenging tasks. The more difficult tasks within each domain depend to some extent on the interaction of other domains. For example, making lists of words of a given category is a language task but draws on attention, memory, and executive function. Patients with impairments after TBI often show intact brain function in all domains, with impaired speed and/or accuracy in more complex functions. According to Levin (1987), "Memory deficit, reduced speed of information processing, inflexibility in problem solving, and socially inappropriate behavior impose the major constraints on quality of life . . . even in cases with seemingly adequate intelligence on conventional tests" (p. 461). Thus, key elements of neuropsychological testing of the patient with mild TBI include *timed tests* and demonstrations that a patient may fail a complex task but accurately perform its component subtasks. Table 7–6 outlines basic tests of the five domains as they might be used with various degrees of TBI and/or stages of recovery.

NEURODIAGNOSTIC EVALUATION OF PATIENTS WITH LATE EFFECTS OF MILD TRAUMATIC BRAIN INJURY

A common problem facing the psychiatrist is the diagnostic assessment of the patient with persistent neuropsychiatric symptoms after a TBI with minimal or no LOC. In such patients, a CT scan may have been normal shortly after the injury, and the severity of injury would not have warranted an intensive neurodiagnostic workup. When postconcussional symptoms fail to resolve and the patient experiences functional disability, diagnostic testing must be reconsidered. The precise timing of the decision for further workup depends on the severity of the symptoms and whether they are steadily improving. However, any patient experiencing impaired occupational function more than 3 months after an apparently minor brain injury requires further neurodiagnostic assessment.

In this situation, MRI is the procedure of choice; it is generally more sensitive than CT, and it is specifically more sensitive to damage to cerebral white matter caused by axonal injury from shearing forces (Honda et al. 1992; Ichise et al. 1994; Levin et al. 1993; Yokota et al. 1992). MRI also images the behaviorally crucial orbital frontal and anterior temporal regions more clearly than CT. Anatomic damage to the frontal or temporal lobes or to central cerebral white matter strongly supports a primarily neurologic component to the patient's complaints.

It has become increasingly clear, however, that many patients with neuropsychiatric symptoms and/or cognitive deficits not explained by

Table 7–6.   Neuropsychological testing of patients with traumatic brain injury

---

Moderate to severe traumatic brain injury

Acute	Orientation and amnesia
	• Glasgow Coma Score (GCS) (Teasdale and Jennett 1974)
	• Galveston Orientation and Amnesia Test (GOAT) (Levin et al. 1979)
	• Mini-Mental State Exam (MMSE) (Folstein et al. 1975)
Subacute to chronic	Acute tests plus:
	Clinical/bedside neuropsychology testing (e.g., Mental Status Examination in Neurology [Strub and Black 1993])
	Attention
	• Attention: Digit Span
	• Vigilance: Signaling to a target letter in a sequence of letters
	Language
	• Basic: Aphasia screen
	• Comprehensive:
	Word finding with time limits
	Naming
	Comprehension
	Complex language
	Memory testing
	• Immediate (e.g., digits forward)
	• Recent/remote (e.g., verbal and visual memory testing)
	Cognitive testing
	• Wechsler Adult Intelligence Scale—Revised (Wechsler 1981)
	• Cognitive stress testing (e.g., Paced Auditory Serial Addition Test) (Gronwall 1977)
	Executive functions/frontal lobes
	• Go/no go tests
	• Primitive reflexes
	• Distraction tasks
	• Set shifting
	• Wisconsin Card Sort (Berg 1948)
	• Word lists
	• Trail Making (Reitan 1958)

(continued)

Table 7-6. Neuropsychological testing of patients with traumatic brain injury *(continued)*

Neurobehavioral scales
- Organic Aggression Scale (OAS) (Silver and Yudofsky 1991)
- Neurobehavioral Rating Scale (NBRS) (Levin et al. 1987b)

Mild traumatic brain injury

All the above plus:

Careful screening for psychiatric comorbidity:
- Structured Clinical Interview for DSM-III-R (SCID) (Spitzer et al. 1992)
- Minnesota Multiphasic Personality Inventory (MMPI) (Hathaway and McKinley 1943)
- Hamilton Depression Screen (Ham-D) (Hamilton 1960)

---

anatomic lesions will have abnormal regional cerebral perfusion that does correlate with the observed symptoms and deficits. The perfusion abnormalities are identified by single photon-emission computed tomography (SPECT), using the radionuclide Tc-99m-HMPAO. The following recent reports support the role of SPECT with HMPAO in establishing a neurologic basis for persistent symptoms after mild TBI:

- Ichise and colleagues (1994) studied the correlation of CT, MRI, SPECT, and neuropsychological testing in 29 patients with TBI and 17 control patients; 15 of the TBI patients had minor injuries. SPECT demonstrated more abnormalities than CT or MRI in the TBI subgroup with minor injuries, and SPECT abnormalities were correlated more strongly with poor performance on neuropsychologic tests than were MRI abnormalities.
- Nedd and associates (1993) compared SPECT findings with CT scans in 16 patients with mild to moderate TBI. SPECT was abnormal in 87.5% of the patients, whereas CT scans were abnormal in 37.5%. When both scans were abnormal, SPECT usually showed a larger area of abnormality. SPECT, but not CT, showed contrecoup abnormalities in five cases.
- Gray and co-workers (1992) compared CT scans with SPECT results in 53 patients with a history of remote TBI, of whom 20 had minor

head injury. Of those 20, 12 (60%) had SPECT abnormalities and 5 (25%) had CT abnormalities.

- Newton and others (1992) evaluated CT, MRI, and SPECT in 19 patients with a history of CHI. SPECT showed more focal abnormalities than CT or MRI, alone or in combination. The number of SPECT lesions was positively correlated with increased functional disability and worse outcome on the Glasgow Outcome Scale; the overall estimate of cerebral blood flow was inversely correlated with disability.

Formal neuropsychological testing is indicated when the patient's principal complaints or disabilities are cognitive. Correlation of the extent and severity of cognitive test findings with functional brain imaging helps to distinguish the unequivocally "organic" cases from those in which issues of mood, coping style, beliefs, and environmental factors may be more relevant in causing or perpetuating symptoms and disability.

The results of the diagnostic evaluation are used to place the patient on a continuum of treatment approaches that range from purely rehabilitative to mainly psychotherapeutic. Although it is virtually always helpful to acknowledge that both primary brain changes and the patient's individual circumstances will influence the outcome, patients seem to respond to a clear and thoughtful delineation of their brain damage.

PSYCHOTROPIC MEDICATIONS AND MILD TRAUMATIC BRAIN INJURY

In this section, we briefly discuss several classes of psychotropic medications and their relative advantages and disadvantages for patients with mild TBI. (For a more complete review of this material, interested readers are referred to Gualtieri [1988] and Silver and Yudofsky [1994].) As mentioned earlier in this chapter, there are very few reports of systematic studies of the use of psychotropic medications in patients with sequelae of TBI. Medications are selected by extrapolating from their known effects in other medical populations and the clinician's risk-benefit analysis of particular psychotropic side-effect profiles and possible drug interactions. The constraints of prescribing medications in the TBI population are very similar to those of the geriatric population. Therefore, as in elderly patients who tend to be more sensitive to the intended and the unintended effects of medication, the clinician treating a patient with TBI should begin medication at lower doses, prolong titration, and extend clinical trials before switching medications (Table 7–7).

Dopamine Antagonists

Neuroleptics are indicated in patients with TBI for psychosis or severe agitation, with or without the full syndrome of delirium. These conditions are uncommon in patients with mild TBI. Consideration should be given to the increased vulnerability of brain-injured patients to extrapyramidal side effects, including neuroleptic malignant syndrome. Appropriate precautions are 1) to minimize dosage and use adjunctive benzodiazepines for general sedation, 2) to monitor carefully for extrapyramidal side effects and treat symptoms promptly with amantadine, and 3) to give neuroleptics for an explicitly limited time—then reevaluate the patient. On theoretical grounds, atypical neuroleptics, with their much lower rates of extrapyramidal side effects, would be the drugs of choice for psychosis or severe agitation after TBI. However, orthostatic hypotension and sedation are associated with these medications and can be problematic in patients with TBI, as is the tendency to produce seizures with clozapine. Risperidone, with its lower propensity to cause seizures, may prove to be a more suitable choice.

The use of neuroleptics in brain-injured patients is somewhat controversial, based on the study by Feeney and colleagues (1982) in which rats were experimentally brain injured and then treated with placebo, amphetamines, amphetamines followed by haloperidol, or haloperidol alone. The amphetamine group recovered motor function more quickly than the placebo, amphetamine/haloperidol, or haloperidol groups. The investigators then postulated that recovery of function in humans with TBI may be slowed by haloperidol. This is a major extrapolation from limited animal data that has not, to our knowledge, been confirmed by human studies.

Dopamine Agonists

In contrast to neuroleptics, there are several reports in the case literature of positive effects of dopamine agonists such as amantadine and L-dopa on the level of arousal of obtunded or comatose patients with TBI and of calming effects of dopamine agonists in agitated patients (Chandler et al. 1988; Gualtieri et al. 1989; Horiguchi et al. 1990; Ross and Stewart 1981). All were cases of severe brain injury; any benefit of

Table 7–7. Psychotropic medications and mild traumatic brain injury

Medications	Indications	Advantages	Disadvantages	Starting dosage (range)
Psychostimulants				
Methylphenidate	Attention deficits, memory, learning, apathy, anergia, frontal lobe symptoms	Short half-life	May be too activating for some patients	5 mg bid (up to 60 mg/day in 2–4 divided doses)
Dextroamphetamine				5 mg bid (up to 45 mg/day in 2–4 divided doses) (controlled-release preparations available for qd dosage)
Dopamine agonists				
Amantadine	Same as stimulants		Confusion	50 mg bid (up to 200 mg bid)
Dopamine antagonists				
Haloperidol	Delirium, dyscontrol, severe agitation, psychosis	Less anticholinergic	Extrapyramidal effects Tardive dyskinesia risk Possible slowing of TBI recovery Risk of lowering seizure threshold	0.5 mg bid
Fluphenazine	Same as haloperidol	Less likely to affect seizure threshold	Same as above	0.5 mg bid (up to 2 mg tid)

Molindone	Same as above	Low antidopaminergic effects No weight gain	Low sedation Weight loss possible	5 mg bid (up to 10 mg tid)
Risperidone	Same as above	Less extrapyramidal effects	Sedation[a] Orthostatic hypotension	0.5 mg bid (up to 2 mg tid)
Antidepressants *Tricyclics*				
Amitriptyline	Depression, anxiety, mood lability, chronic pain	Best established for migraine therapy	Most sedating and anticholinergic Affects cardiac conduction	10 mg qhs (up to 300 mg/day depending on tolerance and serum levels)
Nortriptyline	Same as above	Less orthostatic hypotension	Too sedating for some patients Affects cardiac conduction	10 mg qhs (up to serum level of 50–150 ng/ml)
Desipramine	Same as above	Less anticholinergic	Too activating for some patients Affects cardiac conduction Associated with sudden cardiac death in children	10 mg qhs (up to 300 mg/day, depending on tolerance and serum levels)

(continued)

Table 7–7. Psychotropic medications and mild traumatic brain injury (continued)

Medications	Indications	Advantages	Disadvantages	Starting dosage (range)
MAOIs Tranylcypromine	Same as above	Not anticholinergic No cardiotoxicity Broad spectrum of antidepressant action	Orthostatic hypotension Diet restrictions and risk of hypertensive crisis and drug interactions Sedating for some/activating for others Sexual dysfunction	10 mg qam (up to 60 mg/day in 2–4 divided doses)
Phenelzine	Same as above	No cardiotoxicity, documented antimigraine action, and antiphobic action	Orthostatic hypotension Diet restrictions and risk of hypertensive crisis and drug interactions Weight gain Sexual dysfunction	15 mg bid (up to 90 mg/day in 2–4 doses)
SSRIs Fluoxetine	Same as above	Few medically serious side effects	Long half-life Too activating for some patients Slows P_{450} system	5 mg qam (up to 60 mg/day)
Sertraline	Same as above	Same as above	Slows P_{450} system	25 mg qam (up to 200 mg/day)

Paroxetine	Same as above		Slows P$_{450}$ system	10 mg qam (up to 60 mg/day)
Other antidepressants				
Bupropion	Same as above	Few side effects	Seizure risk,[b] agitation, psychosis	75 mg bid (up to 150 mg tid) with antiepileptic drug
Trazodone	Same as above	Sedation Not anticholinergic No quinidine-like effects	Orthostatic hypotension Rare priapism	25 mg qhs (up to 400 mg qd)
Lithium	Mania, aggression, antidepressant adjunct		Sedation, cognitive slowing, tremor, ataxia	300 mg bid (up to serum level of 1.0 mEq/L)
Antiepileptic drugs				
Carbamazepine	Chronic aggression, mania, mood lability, seizures		Blood dyscrasias, hepatotoxicity, hyponatremia, drug interactions	100 mg bid (up to serum level of 12 µg/ml)
Valproic acid	Same as above		Bleeding disorders, hepatotoxicity, pancreatitis, drug interactions	250 mg bid (up to serum level of 100 µg/ml)

(continued)

Table 7–7. Psychotropic medications and mild traumatic brain injury (*continued*)

Medications	Indications	Advantages	Disadvantages	Starting dosage (range)
β-Blockers				
Propranolol	Chronic aggression, anxiety	Antimigraine effect	Sedation, hypotension, bradycardia, sexual dysfunction; can aggravate asthma	20 mg bid (up to threshold of bradycardia)
Benzodiazepines				
Lorazepam	Insomnia, agitation, anxiety	Conjugative metabolism and few, if any, active metabolites	Sedation, disinhibition, delirium, dependence	0.5 mg lorazepam (up to 1 mg tid)
Oxazepam	Same as above	Same as above	Same as above	10 mg bid (up to 15 mg tid)
Temazepam	Same as above	Same as above	Same as above	15–30 mg qhs
Buspirone	Same as above	Infrequent sedation Does not cause dependence	Dizziness, nausea, insomnia	5 mg bid (up to 30 mg tid)

Note.   TBI = traumatic brain injury; MAOIs = monoamine oxidase inhibitors; SSRIs = selective serotonin reuptake inhibitors.
[a] A stimulant may be coadministered with risperidone if the drug is of marked benefit apart from sedation.
[b] In patients with TBI, this drug should be given together with an antiepileptic drug.

dopamine agonists for mildly injured patients remains to be demonstrated. Gualtieri and colleagues (1989) emphasize that amantadine, their dopamine agonist of choice, either helps rapidly and decisively or does not help at all. Regardless of whether amantadine is indicated for agitation after TBI, it is a drug of choice for patients with TBI who develop extrapyramidal side effects when given neuroleptics.

Psychostimulants

The distinction between psychostimulants and dopamine agonists is somewhat artificial, because most of the so-called psychostimulants are presumed to work via dopamine mechanisms. Methylphenidate, dextroamphetamine, and pemoline have long been used in children with ADHD. Lipper and Tuchman (1976) claim the first case of an adult TBI patient treated with dextroamphetamine. They targeted confusion, paranoia, and memory deficits. Interestingly, the investigators also reported a potentiation of the dextroamphetamine effect by concomitant use of amitriptyline. Since that time, animal studies (Feeney et al. 1982), case reports (Crisostomo et al. 1988), and at least one controlled study (Gualtieri and Evans 1988) have reported positive effects of stimulants, particularly for problems of arousal, attention deficit, and anergia. Wroblewski and co-workers (1992) conducted a retrospective study of 30 TBI cases treated with methylphenidate and concluded that no increased seizure incidence was attributable to methylphenidate treatment. The patients studied had mainly moderate to severe brain injuries.

Antidepressants

Currently available antidepressants can be divided into four main categories—tricyclic antidepressants (TCAs), selective serotonin reuptake inhibitors (SSRIs), monoamine oxidase inhibitors (MAOIs), and others (e.g., bupropion, trazodone, and venlafaxine). To date, no class has been shown to have greater antidepressant efficacy than another. TBI-related mood disorders and affective symptoms may be more resistant to drug treatment than primary major depression or dysthymia (Saran 1985; Varney et al. 1987). Because there are no known differences in efficacy between the classes, antidepressant selection is based on the side-effect profile most tolerable for each patient and their likely effect on target symptoms causing the most distress or disability.

TCAs. TCAs are efficacious for severe vegetative symptoms and provide readily available blood level determinants to guide dosage and detect pharmacokinetic interactions. Their primary drawbacks include orthostatic hypotension, sedation, agitation, anticholinergic effects, and effects on intraventricular cardiac conduction. Patients with TBI may be at increased risk for sedation, agitation, or confusion, and those who spent much time in bed during their recovery may be especially prone to orthostatic hypotension. Secondary amines such as nortriptyline and desipramine tend to be better tolerated than the tertiary amines. Starting with daily doses of 10 mg of desipramine or nortriptyline, or equivalent, as recommended for elderly patients (Salzman 1982), is advisable for patients with TBI.

SSRIs. The SSRIs, generally lacking anticholinergic, hypotensive, and cardiac conduction effects, have become increasingly used as first-line antidepressants. Nevertheless, side effects including nervousness, anxiety, insomnia, and nausea are common and can exacerbate underlying problems for patients with TBI. Many patients complain of sedation, especially during the mid-to-late afternoon. Also, diminished libido or sexual dysfunction attributable to the SSRI may aggravate sexual problems caused by the brain injury. The SSRIs inhibit hepatic cytochrome P_{450} and thus may cause pharmacokinetic interactions with hepatically metabolized drugs such as carbamazepine (DeVane 1992; Somni et al. 1987). Among the SSRIs, fluoxetine has the longest effective half-life (1 to 3 days for the drug and 7 to 15 days for its active metabolite). This may facilitate maintaining therapeutic serum levels in patients prone to miss taking medication, but it can also prolong the duration of side effects if problems develop. Consequently, many physicians prefer the relative advantage of SSRIs with shorter half-lives such as sertraline.

When prescribing SSRIs to patients with TBI, conservative starting doses are 5 mg/day for fluoxetine, 5 mg/day for paroxetine, and 25 mg/day for sertraline.

MAOIs. MAOIs are excellent antidepressants, especially for the treatment of patients with atypical depression and anxiety disorders such as social phobia and agoraphobia. This class lacks anticholinergic effects and direct cardiotoxic effects and has indirect dopamine agonist effects that may alleviate apathy. Apart from the inconvenience of dietary restrictions, other potential disadvantages include orthostatic hypotension and effects on sleep—either daytime sedation, insomnia, or both. (Details on MAOIs and their drug interactions are provided other texts [Stoudemire et al. 1993].)

Others (bupropion, trazodone, and venlafaxine). Trazodone is relatively free of cardiac effects, especially anticholinergic effects, and it is an excellent sedative commonly used as an adjunct for insomnia. However, it has significant orthostatic effects and can cause priapism, especially in young men, and trazodone is usually too sedating to patients in doses that are adequate to treat major depression. A reasonable initial dosage in a patient with TBI who has insomnia would be 25 mg qhs; this would be increased if tolerated until the patient slept through the night without a significant morning sedation.

Bupropion has minimal anticholinergic effects and does not cause orthostatic hypotension. However, it is associated with a relatively higher seizure rate than the TCAs or SSRIs (0.4% for bupropion versus 0.1%–1.0% for TCAs) (Johnston et al. 1991). Also, agitation or insomnia may be early side effects of the medication. Because patients with TBI are at increased risk for seizures, bupropion is not recommended for this population, unless given together with an antiepileptic drug.

Venlafaxine, a recently approved antidepressant with combined serotonin and norepinephrine reuptake inhibition, has side effects similar to those of the SSRIs but may be more effective for severe or melancholic depression. Experience with patients with TBI is limited.

Lithium

Lithium is a mood-stabilizing agent with neurologic side effects, especially tremor, in patients without gross brain disease. Patients with TBI are more vulnerable to tremor, ataxia, and sedation and may be intolerant of nonneurologic side effects such as polyuria (Schiff et al. 1982). However, lithium is important for treatment of mania, aggression, and emotional lability and as an antidepressant adjunct. Because of the lower therapeutic index of lithium in patients with TBI, Silver and Yudofsky (1994) recommend limiting its use to those TBI patients with mania or with irritability associated with cyclic mood fluctuations.

Antiepileptic Drugs

Antiepileptic drugs are used in patients with TBI 1) to treat seizures, 2) to stabilize mood or control impulsive behavior, and 3) to treat paroxysmal posttraumatic symptoms that are not clearly epileptic, such as sudden-onset headaches, dizzy spells, or anxiety attacks. Carbamazepine and valproate, because of their increasing use in the treatment of bipolar disorder, are the agents most often prescribed by psychiatrists. Some nonpsychiatrists continue to initiate antiepileptic drug therapy with phenobarbital and/or phenytoin; these agents usually do not improve mood and behavior and may, at times, aggravate them.

The mood-stabilizing antiepileptic drugs carbamazepine and valproate should be considered as treatment for mood instability, impulsivity, and episodic neurologic symptoms, particularly those that have a sudden onset. Their efficacy as symptomatic therapies in patients with TBI has much anecdotal support but essentially no confirmation by placebo-controlled clinical trials. However, it is clear that they can help patients whose symptoms do not warrant a diagnosis of epilepsy as well as people with normal or abnormal, but nonepileptiform, electroencephalograms.

In many cases, much time and money are spent in pursuit of a electroencephalographic abnormality, when the more important question of whether antiepileptic drugs will help would be better answered by a planned clinical trial with systematic assessment of target symptoms. A 4-week trial, in which patients' blood levels reach the therapeutic range for epilepsy, will determine whether an antiepileptic drug will be useful. If there is no benefit or only partial benefit, and the drug is tolerated, the dose should be increased, up to the top end of the therapeutic range for epilepsy. If there is no benefit or partial benefit at a level at which side effects limit further dosage increase, an alternative antiepileptic drug should be tried.

The important consideration in selecting an initial drug is the differing side-effect profile of the two drugs. Carbamazepine has cardiac conduction effects resembling those of the TCAs. It also can cause or aggravate ataxia, impaired coordination, or diplopia. Valproate often causes gastrointestinal upset. Both drugs rarely cause hepatitis or suppress blood counts, so significant preexisting hepatic or hematologic disease is a relative, but not absolute, contraindication to both (see Stoudemire et al. 1991).

A reasonable starting dose of carbamazepine is 100 mg bid. Doses should be increased by 100 mg/day, with 2 or 3 days between increases unless more rapid loading is required by the patient's clinical condition (e.g., mania, frequent seizures). For valproate, a reasonable starting dose is 250 mg bid. Doses should be increased by 250 mg/day, with at least 2 days between increases unless the clinical condition warrants rapid loading. Usual maximum trough serum levels are 12 µg/ml for carbamazepine and 100 µg/ml for valproate.

Patients with unstable but mainly depressed mood, and those with paroxysmal symptoms of epilepsy and depression, often respond to a combination of an antidepressant with a mood-stabilizing antiepileptic drug. When undertaking such therapies, note the following considerations regarding drug interactions:

- SSRIs raise carbamazepine levels by inhibiting their hepatic metabolism. Carbamazepine blood levels should be rechecked after starting an SSRI, and dosage should be reduced if necessary.
- Valproate competes with antidepressants for protein binding and may increase the clinical effect of antidepressants without raising their blood levels.
- Carbamazepine induces the hepatic metabolism of antidepressants and may lower their blood levels for a given oral dose.

(These drug interactions are discussed in some detail in Chapter 2.)

Benzodiazepines

In the literature on TBI, the use of benzodiazepines is generally discouraged because of the risk of exacerbating delirium, confusion, sedation, cognitive impairment, psychomotor coordination, and/or falls. If benzodiazepines are used in patients with TBI, we suggest relatively short-acting, low-potency preparations without active metabolites, such as lorazepam, oxazepam, or temazepam.

Buspirone

There is an emerging case literature that buspirone is especially useful for the treatment of disinhibition and aggression in patients with TBI (Gualtieri 1991a, 1991b; Levine 1988; Tiller et al. 1988). However, other investigators report that, in their clinical experience, buspirone is periodically associated with an increase in aggression and disinhibition (Silver and Yudofsky 1994). The inconsistent literature is partially explained by the highly variable bioavailability of buspirone because of its extensive but variable first-pass metabolism. Any standard fixed dose of buspirone will be too high for some patients and too low for other patients.

A reasonable starting dose is from 2.5 to 5.0 mg bid; if tolerated but ineffective, the dose is increased gradually to obtain therapeutic benefit until the patient develops side effects of dizziness, tinnitus, or increased irritability or until a limiting dose of 60 mg/day (20 mg tid) is reached. If there are no side effects on 60 mg/day, some clinicians will raise the dose to 90 to 100 mg/day to achieve a therapeutic effect.

CONCLUSION

In summary, until recently, the terminology of TBI literature has been unclear and variable from study to study. For example, *delirium*, although presumed to be a common post-TBI syndrome, is a term rarely seen in TBI research (Trzepacz 1994), and even the fundamental descriptions and definitions of TBI itself vary. This lack of clarity limits the value of epidemiologic, phenomenologic, and treatment studies conducted to date. Therefore, we began this chapter by narrowing the focus on a most common subtype of TBI, the mild CHI, and not coincidentally, it is the type of injury most likely to be seen by psychiatrists. In addition, we examined current DSM-IV diagnostic criteria and their application to TBI patients, with the hope that improved diagnostic rigor will benefit the individual patient now and improve the quality of research for the benefit of the entire TBI population in the future.

REFERENCES

Adams JH, Graham DL, Murray LS, et al: Diffuse axonal injury due to nonmissile head injury: an analysis of 45 cases. Ann Neurol 12:557–563, 1982

American Psychiatric Association: Diagnostic and Statistical Manual of Mental Disorders, 4th Edition. Washington, DC, American Psychiatric Association, 1994

Berg GE: A simple objective test for measuring flexibility in thinking. J Gen Psychol 39:15–22, 1948

Binder LM: Persisting symptoms after mild head injury: a review of the postconcussive syndrome. J Clin Exp Neuropsychol 8:323–346, 1986

Blumberg PC, Jones NR, North JB: Diffuse axonal injury in head trauma. J Neurol Neurosurg Psychiatry 52:838–841, 1989

Bornstein RA, Miller HB, van Schoor T: Emotional adjustment in compensated head injury patients. Neurosurgery 23:622–627, 1988

Bremner J, Douglas S, Tammy M, et al: Deficits in short-term memory in posttraumatic stress disorder. Am J Psychiatry 150:1015–1019, 1993

Brown SJ, Fann JR, Grant I: Postconcussional disorder: time to acknowledge a common source of neurobehavioral morbidity. J Neuropsychiatry Clin Neurosci 6:15–22, 1994

Buschke H, Fuld PA: Evaluating storage, retention and retrieval in disordered memory and learning. Neurology 14:1019–1025, 1974

Chandler MC, Barnhill JB, Gualtieri CT: Amantadine for the agitated head-injury patient. Brain Inj 2:309–311, 1988

Crisostomo EA, Duncan PW, Propst M, et al: Evidence that amphetamine with physical therapy promotes recovery of motor function in stroke patients. Ann Neurol 23:94–97, 1988

Dalton J, Pederson S, Ryan J: Effects of post traumatic stress disorder on neuropsychological test performance. International Journal of Clinical Neuropsychology 11:121–124, 1989

Department of Health and Human Services: Interagency Head Injury Task Force report. Washington, DC, U.S. Government Printing Office, 1989

DeVane CL: Pharmacokinetics of selective serotonin re-uptake inhibitors. J Clin Psychiatry 53 (suppl 2):13–20, 1992

Dikmen S, McLean A, Temkin N: Neuropsychological and psychosocial consequences of minor head injury. J Neurol Neurosurg Psychiatry 49:1227–1232, 1986

Faden AI, Demediuk P, Panter S, et al: The role of excitatory amino acids and NMDA receptors in traumatic brain injury. Science 244:798–800, 1989

Feeney DM, Gonzalez A, Law WA: Amphetamine, haloperidol and experience interact to affect rate of recovery after motor cortex surgery. Science 217:855–857, 1982

Fogel BS: The significance of frontal system disorders for medical practice and health policy. J Neuropsychiatry Clin Neurosci 6:343–347, 1994

Fogel BS, Faust D: Neurologic assessment, neurodiagnostic test, and neuropsychology in medical psychiatry, in Psychiatric Care of the Medical Patient. Edited by Stoudemire A, Fogel BS. New York, Oxford University Press, 1993, pp 367–413

Folstein MF, Folstein SE, McHugh PR: Mini-Mental State: a practical method for grading the cognitive state of patients for the clinician. J Psychiatr Res 12:189–198, 1975

Graham DI, Adams JH, Gennarelli TA: Pathology of brain damage in head injury, in Head Injury, 2nd Edition. Edited by Cooper PR. Baltimore, MD, Williams & Wilkins, 1987, pp 72–88

Gray BG, Ichise M, Chung DG, et al: Technetium-99m-HMPAO SPECT in the evaluation of patients with a remote history of traumatic brain injury: a comparison with x-ray computed tomography. J Nucl Med 33:52–58, 1992

Gronwall D: Paced Auditory Serial Addition Test: a measure of recovery from concussion. Percept Mot Skills 44:367–373, 1977

Gualtieri CT: Pharmacotherapy and the neurobehavioral sequelae of closed head injury. Brain Inj 2:101–129, 1988

Gualtieri CT: Buspirone for the behavior problem patients with organic brain disorders. J Clin Psychopharmacol 11:280–281, 1991a

Gualtieri CT: Buspirone: neuropsychiatric effects. Journal of Head Trauma Rehabilitation 6:90–92, 1991b

Gualtieri CT: Traumatic brain injury, in Psychiatric Care of the Medical Patient. Edited by Stoudemire A, Fogel BS. New York, Oxford University Press, 1993, pp 517–535

Gualtieri CT, Evans RW: Stimulant treatment for the neurobehavioral sequelae of traumatic brain injury. Brain Inj 2:273–290, 1988

Gualtieri CT, Chandler M, Coons TB, et al: Amantadine: a new clinical profile for traumatic brain injury. Clin Neuropharmacol 12:258–270, 1989

Gurvits T, Lasko N, Schachter S, et al: Neurological status of Vietnam veterans with chronic posttraumatic stress disorder. J Neuropsychiatry Clin Neurosci 5:183–188, 1993

Hamilton M: A rating scale for depression. J Neurol Neurosurg Psychiatry 23:56–62, 1960

Hathaway SR, McKinley JC: Minnesota Multiphasic Personality Inventory. Minneapolis, MN, University of Minnesota, 1943

Honda E, Tokunaga T, Oshima Y, et al: MRI findings of closed head injury in children with special reference to the effect of central shearing force. No Shinkei Geka 20:235–242, 1992

Horiguchi J, Inami Y, Shoda T: Effects of long-term amantadine treatment on clinical symptoms and EEG of a patient in a vegetative state. Clin Neuropharmacol 13:84–88, 1990

Ichise M, Chung DG, Wang P, et al: Technetium-99m-HMPAO SPECT, CT and MRI in the evaluation of patients with chronic traumatic brain injury: a correlation with neuropsychological performance. J Nucl Med 35: 217–226, 1994

Jane JA, Steward O, Gennarelli T: Axonal degeneration induced by experimental noninvasive minor injury. J Neurosurg 62:96–100, 1985

Johnston JA, Lineberry CG, Ascher JA, et al: A 102-center prospective study of seizure in association with bupropion. J Clin Psychiatry 52:450–456, 1991

Keshavan MS, Channabasavanna SM, Reddy GNN: Post-traumatic psychiatric disturbances: patterns and predictors of outcome. Br J Psychiatry 138:157–160, 1981

Kraus JF: Epidemiology of head injury, in Head Injury. Edited by Cooper PR. Baltimore, MD, William & Wilkins, 1987, pp 1–19

Kraus JF, Sorenson SB: Epidemiology, in Neuropsychiatry of Traumatic Brain Injury. Edited by Silver JM, Yudofsky SC, Hales RE. Washington, DC, American Psychiatric Press, 1994, pp 3–41

Levin HS: Neurobehavioral sequelae of head injury, in Head Injury, 2nd Edition. Edited by Cooper PR. Baltimore, MD, Williams & Wilkins, 1987, pp 442–463

Levin HS, O'Donnell VM, Grossman RG: The Galveston Orientation and Amnesia Test: a practical scale to assess cognition after head injury. J Nerv Ment Dis 167:675–684, 1979

Levin HS, Mattis S, Ruff RM, et al: Neurobehavioral outcome following minor head injury: a three-center study. J Neurosurg 66:234–243, 1987a

Levin HS, High WM, Goethe KE, et al: The Neurobehavioral Rating Scale: assessment of the behavioral sequelae of head injury by the clinician. J Neurol Neurosurg Psychiatry 50:183–193, 1987b

Levin HS, Culhane KA, Mendelsohn D, et al: Cognition in relation to magnetic resonance imaging in head-injured children and adolescents. Arch Neurol 50:897–905, 1993

Levine AM: Buspirone and agitation in head injury. Brain Inj 2:165–167, 1988

Lipper S, Tuchman MM: Treatment of chronic post-traumatic organic brain syndrome with dextroamphetamine: first reported case. J Nerv Ment Dis 162:366–371, 1976

Lishman WA: Physiogenesis and psychogenesis in the "post-concussional syndrome." Br J Psychiatry 153:460–469, 1988

Max W, MacKenzie E, Rice D: Head injuries: costs and consequences. Journal of Head Trauma Rehabilitation 6:76–91, 1991

McAllister TM: Mild traumatic brain injury and the postconcussive syndrome, in Neuropsychiatry of Traumatic Brain Injury. Edited by Silver JM, Hales RE, Yudofsky SC. Washington, DC, American Psychiatric Press, 1994, pp 357–392

Morrison JH, Molliver ME, Grzanna R: Noradrenergic innervation of cerebral cortex: widespread effects of local cortical lesions. Science 205:313–316, 1979

Nedd K, Sfakianakis G, Ganz W, et al: 99mTc-HMPAO SPECT of the brain in mild to moderate traumatic brain injury patients: compared with CT—a prospective study. Brain Inj 7:469–479, 1993

Newton MR, Greenwood RJ, Britton KE, et al: A study comparing SPECT with CT and MRI after closed head injury. J Neurol Neurosurg Psychiatry 55:92–94, 1992

Oddy M, Humphrey M, Uttley D: Stresses upon the relatives of head-injured patients. Br J Psychiatry 133:507–513, 1978

Povlishock J-T: Pathophysiology of traumatically induced axonal injury in animals and man. Ann Emerg Med 22:980–986, 1993

Reitan RM: Validity of the Trail Making Test as an indicator of organic brain damage. Percept Mot Skills 8:271–276, 1958

Rimel RW, Giordani B, Barth JT, et al: Moderate head injury: completing the clinical spectrum of brain trauma. Neurosurgery 11:344–351, 1981

Rimel RW, Giordani B, Barth JT, et al: Disability caused by minor head injury. Neurosurgery 9:221–228, 1982

Robinson RG, Szetela B: Mood change following left-hemispheric brain injury. Ann Neurol 9:447–453, 1981

Ross ED, Stewart RM: Akinetic mutism from hypothalamic damage: successful treatment with dopamine agonists. Neurology 31:1435–1439, 1981

Royal DR, Roderick KM, True JE, et al: Executive impairment among the functionally dependent: comparisons between schizophrenic and elderly subjects. Am J Psychiatry 150:1813–1819, 1993

Salzman C: A primer on geriatric psychopharmacology. Am J Psychiatry 139:67–74, 1982

Saran AS: Depression after minor closed head injury: role of dexamethasone suppression test and antidepressants. J Clin Psychiatry 46:335–338, 1985

Schiff HB, Sabin TD, Geller A, et al: Lithium in aggressive behavior. Am J Psychiatry 139:1346–1348, 1982

Siesjo BK: Basic mechanisms of traumatic brain damage. Ann Emerg Med 22:959–969, 1993

Silver JM, Yudofsky SC: Documentation of aggression in the assessment of the violent patient. Psychiatric Annals 17:375–384, 1987

Silver JM, Yudofsky SC: The Overt Aggression Scale: overview and clinical guidelines. J Neuropsychiatry Clin Neurosci 3:522–529, 1991

Silver JM, Yudofsky SC: Psychopharmacology, in Neuropsychiatry of Traumatic Brain Injury. Edited by Silver JM, Yudofsky SC, Hales RE. Washington, DC, American Psychiatric Press, 1994, pp 631–670

Silver JM, Hales RE, Yudofsky SC: Neuropsychiatric aspects of traumatic brain injury, in The American Psychiatric Press Textbook of Neuropsychiatry. Edited by Hales RE, Yudofsky SC. Washington, DC, American Psychiatric Press, 1992, pp 363–395

Somni RW, Crimson ML, Bowden CL: Fluoxetine: a serotonin-specific, second generation antidepressant. Pharmacotherapy 7:1–15, 1987

Spitzer RL, Williams JB, Gibon M, et al: Structured Clinical Interview for DSM-III-R. Arch Gen Psychiatry 49:624–636, 1992

Stoudemire A, Fogel BS, Gulley LR: Psychopharmacology in the medically ill: an update, in Medical-Psychiatric Practice, Vol 1. Edited by Stoudemire A, Fogel BS. Washington, DC, American Psychiatric Press, 1991, pp 29–98

Stoudemire A, Fogel BS, Gulley LR, et al: Psychopharmacology in the medical patient, in Psychiatric Care of the Medical Patient. Edited by Stoudemire A, Fogel BS. New York, Oxford University Press, 1993, pp 155–206

Strub RL, Black FW: Closed head trauma, in Neurobehavioral Disorders: A Clinical Approach, 2nd Edition. Philadelphia, PA, FA Davis, 1988, pp 313–348

Strub RL, Black FW (eds): The Mental Status Examination in Neurology. Philadelphia, PA, FA Davis, 1993

Szymanski H-V, Linn R: A review of the postconcussion syndrome. Int J Psychiatry Med 22:357–375, 1992

Teasdale G, Jennett B: Assessment of coma and impaired consciousness: a practice scale. Lancet 2:81–84, 1974

Tiller JWG, Dakis JA, Shaw JM: Short-term buspirone treatment in disinhibition with dementia (letter). Lancet 2:510, 1988

Trzepacz PT: Delirium, in Neuropsychiatry of Traumatic Brain Injury. Edited by Silver JM, Yudofsky SC, Hales RE. Washington, DC, American Psychiatric Press, 1994, pp 189–218

Uddo M, Vasterling J, Brailey K, et al: Memory and attention in combat-related post-traumatic stress disorder (PTSD). Journal of Psychopathology and Behavioral Assessment 15:43–52, 1993

Varney NR, Martzke JS, Roberts RJ: Major depression in patients with closed head injury. Neuropsychology 1:7–9, 1987

Wechsler D: Wechsler Adult Intelligence Scale—Revised. San Antonio, TX, Psychological Corporation, 1981

Wechsler D: Wechsler Memory Scale—Revised. San Antonio, TX, Psychological Corporation, 1987

White BC, Krause GS: Brain injury and repair mechanisms: the potential for pharmacologic therapy in closed-head trauma. Ann Emerg Med 22:970–979, 1993

Wroblewski BA, Leary JM, Phelan AM, et al: Methylphenidate and seizure frequency in brain injured patients with seizure disorders. J Clin Psychiatry 53:86–89, 1992

Yokota H, Yasuda K, Mashiko K, et al: Magnetic resonance imaging in diffuse brain injury. No Shinkei Geka 20:15–20, 1992

Chapter 8

Psychiatric Aspects of "Chemical Sensitivity" Syndromes

Donald W. Black, M.D.
Patricia J. Sparks, M.D., M.P.H.

Every so often a new medical subculture emerges that grows in "fits and starts." *Clinical ecology* is one such example. Its advocates claim that a new diagnosis has evolved, partially as a result of the growing complexity of modern life (Crook 1992; Cullen 1987; Levin and Byers 1987; McLellan 1987; Rea et al. 1992). Characterized by an exquisite sensitivity to common foods, chemicals, and microorganisms (e.g., *Candida albicans*), the condition has been described as causing a variety of ill-defined symptoms affecting nearly every organ system. Most frequently called *environmental illness* (EI), this term recognizes the clinical ecologists' belief that agents in our environment cause this mysterious condition. Other terms that have become popular recognize its different features. *Multiple chemical sensitivity* recognizes the sensitivity to different chemical agents that is often considered a defining feature of the disorder. The terms *allergic to everything* and *total environmental allergy* reflect the focus on allergic mechanisms as an etiologic factor. An abnormal immune system has been implicated, and several terms reflect this belief (e.g., *immune dysregulation syndrome, chemical acquired immunodeficiency syndrome [chemical AIDS]*). Other terms have focused on the seemingly new aspect of the illness (e.g., *twentieth century disease, ecologic illness*). Some patients are believed to be primarily sensitive to *C. albicans* and are reported to have *candidiasis* or *yeast disease*. The common ground among these terms is that a patient's symptoms or complaints are considered to stem from abnormal reactions to common substances present in the air or ingested in foods and liquids.

THE CLINICAL ECOLOGIST AND ENVIRONMENTAL ILLNESS

The history of EI is reminiscent of other medical conditions that emerged, were embraced by a group of practitioners, and were later abandoned, such as neurasthenia in the late nineteenth century and chronic brucellosis in the 1950s (Abbey and Garfinkle 1991; Imboden et al. 1959). Nontraditional practitioners proclaiming to have explanations and treatments for conditions that other physicians explain as primarily functional, subjective, or psychological see themselves as on the "cutting edge." These practitioners' beliefs are reinforced by their ready acceptance from patients, many of whom feel abandoned by the mainstream medical community; their insurance companies; and, often, their families and friends. Although clinical ecologists feel misunderstood and rejected by their colleagues, they believe they are filling an important void in the health care system.

Clinical ecologists believe that EI is common. They estimate prevalence rates to be as high as 2%–10% of the general population (Mooser 1987), based on the assumption that the condition is either frequently unrecognized or masked by the label of a traditional medical diagnosis (e.g., fibromyalgia). An estimated 500 clinical ecologists (or "environmental physicians") practice in the United States (American College of Physicians 1989). However, no estimates are available for the even larger number of physicians and other health care practitioners who may be sympathetic to clinical ecology's beliefs and practices. Because, for all practical purposes, they are excluded from participation in traditional medical forums, clinical ecologists have developed their own professional organizations, literature, and educational programs. They practice according to their beliefs and provide care for their patients in special hospitals and clinics.

Clinical ecologists have become increasingly influential, partially because of the large number of patients they diagnose with EI and treat. Their patients have developed a network of support groups, have pursued worker's compensation benefits, and have sought to influence legislation and gain official recognition through the courts. Multiple chemical sensitivity is currently recognized as a disease by the Social Security Administration and the Department of Housing and Urban Development (Hileman 1991). Many patients have claimed that EI merits recognition under the recently enacted American Disabilities Act. If recognized, this law would mandate that employers accommodate people who claim to have unusual sensitivities to chemicals in the workplace.

Despite the growing popularity and acceptance of clinical ecology's beliefs and practices, EI has not been embraced by the mainstream medical community (American Academy of Allergy and Immunology 1981, 1986; American College of Physicians 1989; American Medical Association 1992; Black 1993; California Medical Association 1986; Salvaggio 1991; Terr 1992). In perhaps the strongest criticism to date, the American Medical Association ([AMA] 1992) recently concluded that "Until such accurate, reproducible, and well-controlled studies are available, the AMA Council on Scientific Affairs believes that multiple chemical sensitivity should not be considered a recognizable syndrome" (p. 3467). The California Medical Association (1986), the American Academy of Allergy and Immunology (1981, 1986), and the American College of Physicians (1989) have all issued position papers critical of clinical ecology and its recommended testing procedures and therapies. Criticisms have included the lack of acceptable case definitions for EI (Black 1993), the lack of reproducible laboratory or physical abnormalities (American Academy of Allergy and Immunology 1981, 1986; American College of Physicians 1989; American Medical Association 1992; California Medical Association 1986; Salvaggio 1991), the use of unorthodox testing procedures (American Academy of Immunology 1991; American College of Physicians 1989; American Medical Association 1992; California Medical Association 1986; Jewett et al. 1990), and unproven treatments (American Academy of Allergy and Immunology 1981, 1986; American College of Physicians 1989; American Medical Association 1992; California Medical Society 1986; Salvaggio 1991). Currently, no scientifically acceptable methods exist to definitively establish or exclude the existence of EI, a fact that has helped to undermine its credibility in the medical community.

Distinguishing EI From Other Conditions

EI must be differentiated from the chronic fatigue syndrome (CFS) (see Chapter 5) and the sick-building syndrome, both controversial, media-popularized conditions. CFS, characterized by disabling exhaustion and weakness, has received considerable attention (Schluederberg et al. 1992). The Centers for Disease Control and Prevention has established diagnostic criteria, and both infectious and immunologic mechanisms have been investigated. Many clinical ecologists link CFS with EI, and patients who have EI may also have their symptoms diagnosed as CFS (Crook 1992). The sick-building syndrome has also been linked to EI, because many people are thought to have developed EI from very-low-level chemical exposures in the workplace (Gots 1993). The term is used to describe work-related irritations of the skin and mucous membranes as well as various subjective symptoms (e.g., headache, fatigue, difficulty concentrating), reported by workers in modern buildings, that hypothetically occur when the supply of outside air is minimized. Sick-building syndrome is actually a misnomer, because no specific syndrome has been described, and it covers a heterogeneous mix of complaints and illnesses ranging from the deadly Legionnaire's disease caused by bacteria residing in an air conditioning system to subjective complaints caused by the irritant effects of formaldehyde "off-gassing" from particle board. Building-related complaints are typically investigated by industrial hygienists who can assign causes in about 25% of cases. A recent study found that increasing the supply of outside air did not appear to affect workers' perceptions of their office environment or their reporting of symptoms attributed to the sick-building syndrome (Menzies et al. 1993). Many cases are thought to be of functional or psychological origin.

EI should also be distinguished from objectively defined physical illnesses attributed to allergic mechanisms, for example, contact dermatitis, allergic alveolitis, or occupational exposures to well-recognized toxins such as organophosphate insecticides or carbon monoxide. In these conditions, in contrast to EI, active disease and the causal relationships of the findings to environmental exposure are more readily established. Furthermore, in cases of toxic exposure, effects occur through specific and dose-related mechanisms. In practice, occupational disease and EI may be confused; many people whose symptoms are diagnosed as EI may also have a bonafide occupation-related condition (Sparks et al. 1994). Readers who are interested in additional information on occupational diseases are referred to *Occupational Medicine: Principles and Practical Applications* (Zenz 1988).

DEFINITION AND DIAGNOSIS OF ENVIRONMENTAL ILLNESS ACCORDING TO CLINICAL ECOLOGISTS

Multiple chemical sensitivity syndrome (a form of EI) has been defined as "an acquired disorder characterized by recurrent symptoms, referable to multiple organ systems, occurring in response to demonstrable exposure to many chemically unrelated compounds at doses far below those established in the general population to cause harmful effects. No single widely accepted test of physiologic function can be shown to correlate with the symptoms" (Cullen 1987, p. 657). Other definitions for EI have been offered and all are unified by their attribution of a polysymptomatic disorder to environmental agents. (Agents are also referred to as allergens, antigens, incitants, or offenders.) Symptoms referable to every organ system have been implicated, as indicated in a popular pamphlet issued by the Human Ecology Action League (HEAL), a support group for people with EI: "It [Environmental illness] includes reactions to today's increasingly chemical environment, which can produce headaches, fatigue, abdominal distention, roving pains as well as a host of mental problems that range from fuzzy thinking or falling asleep to hyperactivity, sudden anger, irritability or depression or even schizophrenia" (p. 3).

The array of symptoms attributed to EI is virtually unlimited, as are its putative causes, which include both natural and synthetic chemicals (although an emphasis is generally on synthetic products), natural gas, electromagnetic radiation, viruses, fungi, yeast, wood dust, and common foods (Crook 1992; Rea et al. 1992). Specific chemicals frequently cited as a cause of EI include formaldehyde, phenol, ethanol, ammonia, hydrocarbons, and petrochemicals. In certain cases, endogenous hormones (e.g., progesterone) have been identified as a causative factor. More typically, patients with EI attribute their illness to a combination of agents.

The clinical ecologist makes the diagnosis based on the patient's personal history of exposure to presumed environmental contaminants and the subsequent development of physical or emotional symptoms of illness (Levin and Byers 1987; Rea et al. 1992). An inventory is taken of the patient's diet to check for foods that may have led to allergies or sensitivities. Antibiotic use is assessed, because broad-spectrum antibiotics are thought by clinical ecologists to predispose to bacterial overgrowth, thereby releasing toxins into the bowel or allowing *C. albicans* to proliferate.

Elimination diets and oral food challenges (to test for the effects of certain foods that may have been implicated) have been used in the diagnostic process (Levin and Byers 1987; McLellan 1987). Testing may begin with a 1-week washout (or fast) followed by single food challenges; positive results are indicated by the appearance of subjective symptoms of illness. Provocation-neutralization testing is also thought to be useful. In this procedure, small amounts of dilute chemicals are injected intradermally or administered sublingually or by inhalation in a specially constructed aluminum and glass booth. Tests are rarely performed in a blinded fashion or with the use of placebo controls. Sensitivities are diagnosed by the appearance or disappearance of subjective symptoms. These tests are important because they later play a role in treatment provided by the clinical ecologist.

Other laboratory tests have become important, particularly as the immune system has been implicated in many current etiologic theories of EI. Clinical ecologists may assess levels of serum immunoglobulins, complement, and circulating antibodies or quantitative counts of lymphocyte subsets (Levin and Byers 1987). Various chemicals, including organic solvents, hydrocarbons, pesticides and insecticides, and heavy metals, are sought after, even at very low levels, in samples of blood, urine, fat, hair, or other tissues (Rea et al. 1992).

THEORIES BEHIND CHEMICAL SENSITIVITY

Initial explanations focused on allergies to foods and chemicals (Randolph 1952; Randolph and Moss 1980; Rowe 1930). Eventually, more sophisticated explanations developed, involving the formation of circulating immune complexes or autoantibodies or the release of inflammatory mediators from cell membranes caused by toxic free radicals (Levine and Reinhardt 1983). Damage to T cells, resulting in an inversion of the normal helper/suppressor T-cell ratio, has been implicated (Levin and Byers 1987). More recently, an olfactory-limbic system model has been proposed (Bell 1992). In this model, chemicals are thought to stimulate firing of olfactory pathways, leading to behavioral, autonomic, and endocrine system dysfunction. This theory is based on a concept of *kindling,* in which progressively smaller amounts of chemical agents cause progressively greater reactions. Some also believe that electromagnetic phenomena have a role in producing symptoms (Rea et al. 1992). None of these intriguing theories has been supported by credible research.

Several concepts are thought to be crucial in the development of EI (Rea et al. 1992). *Total body load* is the concept that the immune system can handle a limited quantity of antigens, and symptoms result from an overload or excess burden of an agent. Once a sensitivity has developed, the patient is thought to be predisposed to develop sensitivities to other agents; this is called the *spreading phenomenon*. A *switch phenomenon* has been described in which symptoms' patterns change over time; for example, a person who predominantly complains of fatigue and lassitude might begin to complain of joint pain and discomfort. A *bipolarity phenomenon* has also been described in which stimulation by a chemical agent is followed by a period of depression and exhaustion.

TREATMENT OF CHEMICAL SENSITIVITY BY CLINICAL ECOLOGISTS

Treatment offered by clinical ecologists is determined in part by the patient's personal history and the results of challenge testing; it aims to reduce the total body burden of chemicals. Avoidance of offending substances is the main pillar of treatment, because it is thought to decrease total body load, allowing for recovery of overworked "detoxification systems" (Levin and Byers 1987; McLellan 1987; Rea et al. 1992). Patients may be instructed to create a "safe" room or to construct homes that are as free of offending materials as possible. Patients are advised to eliminate drapery, carpeting, formaldehyde-containing insulation, or other products thought to produce dangerous fumes (by "off-gassing"). The goal is to create an oasis free of harmful materials. Randolph and Moss (1980) describe an "ecology unit" for sensitive patients at their hospital that incorporates these beliefs, which creates an "old-fashioned appearance." "The couch in the lounge, for instance, is made of well-worn leather and the chairs are fashioned from wood and metal, upholstered with cotton or felt and covered with natural fabrics. All of the bedding is made of simple, untreated cotton, and such things as sponge rubber pillows or mattresses, draw sheets, upholstered furniture, rug pads or even tubing made with rubber are forbidden" (pp. 203–204). Plastics and other synthetic materials are forbidden. Some patients are advised to use oxygen or charcoal filter masks to prevent chemical exposures, particularly when the patient must leave the home. Others are advised to move to different locations to escape polluted environments. Several communities have been established for chemically sensitive persons—for example, Wimberly,

Texas, which is located in a rural area far from heavy industry (Hall 1993). Local businesses have evolved to cater to their unique clientele.

Special diets are frequently prescribed, usually based on challenge test results (Levin and Byers 1987; McLellan 1987; Rea et al. 1992). These diets may include avoidance of particular foods, additives, and dyes; the use of bottled spring water is advised. Rotation diets have been developed for patients sensitive to many foods. In theory, when patients follow the diet, no one food is allowed to build up in the system because the patient does not eat the same food twice in the 4 to 5 days estimated for the complete digestion of food and passage of residue. In rare cases, intravenous hyperalimentation is prescribed.

Immunotherapy is commonly recommended (McLellan 1987). After the challenge testing has identified specific sensitivities, small doses of a chemical are used to relieve symptoms. Doses are self-administered either subcutaneously or sublingually after subjective symptoms appear or before anticipated exposure to the offending agent. Neutralizing substances include various organic chemicals, hormones, food extracts, and natural substances (e.g., histamine, serotonin).

Detoxification is a relatively recent addition to the treatment arsenal. It usually takes place at a special hospital or clinic (McLellan 1987). Through a number of steps, including physical exercise followed by forced sweating and cooling showers, it is believed that undesirable chemicals can be washed from the body. This routine may be repeated daily over several weeks.

Other treatments are based, in part, on symptoms reported, the patient's history, and the clinical ecologist's own experiences and preferences. Treatment may include oral nystatin or ketoconazole, antifungal agents that fight chronic yeast infections and prevent systemic toxin release caused by yeast overgrowth in the bowel. Yogurt douches have been prescribed to women to help fight yeast infections (Crook 1992; McLellan 1987). Enemas using spring water or coffee are believed to rid the digestive tract of toxins (Trowbridge and Walker 1986). Vitamin supplements, antioxidants, essential fatty acids, and supplements (e.g., garlic) may be prescribed (McLellan 1987). The variety of treatments is limited only by the imagination and resourcefulness of the clinical ecologist. All of these treatments have been widely prescribed to treat patients with EI; however, none has been supported by controlled clinical trials. One controlled study of nystatin therapy for "candidiasis hypersensitivity" syndrome was negative (Dismukes et al. 1990).

CLINICAL DESCRIPTION OF PERSONS REPORTED TO HAVE ENVIRONMENTAL ILLNESS

Several controlled (Black et al. 1990, 1993; Pearson et al. 1983; Simon et al. 1990, 1993) and uncontrolled (Brodsky 1983; Fiedler et al. 1992; Stewart and Raskin 1985; Terr 1986, 1989) studies in the literature describe people whose symptoms have been diagnosed as EI or multiple chemical sensitivity. The studies show that patients are usually women in their thirties or forties who allege toxic exposure at home or in the workplace, have a high school or college education, and are from middle- to upper-middle-class social groups. Subjects generally are polysymptomatic, with nonspecific complaints. Typical symptoms include fatigue, nausea, headache, malaise, pain, mucosal irritation, disorientation, and dizziness (Black et al. 1990; Terr 1989). Physical and laboratory test abnormalities generally are absent (Simon et al. 1993; Terr 1986). Triggering events identified by patients include toxic fumes at home or in the workplace, exposure to pesticides or insecticides, antibiotic use, exposure to hormones, and psychological stress (Black et al. 1990; Terr 1986, 1989). Clinical ecologists have not reported follow-up data, but Terr (1986) found that all but 2 of 50 patients treated for nearly 2 years by a clinical ecologist remained the same or worse.

Surveys of people whose symptoms have been diagnosed as EI reveal that they develop a deep interest in their illness, join support groups, and read widely about their disorder (Black et al. 1990; Brodsky 1983; Stewart and Raskin 1985). They frequently develop friendships and acquaintances with others who are similarly afflicted. In response to their clinical ecologist's recommendations, they often become less social (mainly to avoid contact with environmental contaminants in social settings), many stop working (at least temporarily) or change occupations, and some relocate to regions they (or their clinical ecologists) believe are less polluted.

Coping with the illness requires a great deal of energy, and Brodsky (1983) observed that patients develop a "lifestyle organized around their illness" (p. 736). Brodsky also observed that they tend to have a history of doctor shopping for evaluation of recurrent physical complaints and often see the same network of clinical ecologists. Many spend significant amounts of time reading about allergies, taking tests for sensitivities, planning diets, and attending to worker's compensation claims.

Psychiatric Disorders

The majority of people who receive a diagnosis of EI exhibit signs or symptoms of a mental disorder (Black et al. 1990, 1993; Brodsky 1983; Fiedler et al. 1992; Pearson et al. 1983; Simon et al. 1990, 1993; Stewart and Raskin 1985; Terr 1986, 1989). Depending on the assessment procedure, the prevalence of mental disorder ranges from 42%–100% (Table 8–1). Mood, anxiety, somatoform, and personality disorders are most frequently identified. In many patients, a history of a mental disorder has preceded the diagnosis of EI by many years (Black et al. 1990; Simon et al. 1993).

One can conclude from the controlled studies that people with a diagnosis of EI exhibit significantly more psychopathology than control subjects. For example, Black and co-workers (1990, 1993) compared 23 patients (of 26 who consented to a diagnostic interview) with a diagnosis of EI with 46 age- and sex-matched control subjects (i.e., 2 control subjects for each case) from the general population; 15 (65%) subjects with a diagnosis of EI met criteria for a mood, anxiety, or somatoform disorder compared with 13 (28%) control subjects, yielding an odds ratio of 4.8 ($P = .003$). Subjects with a diagnosis of EI also had significantly more psychiatric symptoms assessed with the Diagnostic Interview Schedule (Robins et al. 1981) and had a greater number of total lifetime psychiatric diagnoses. The mean number of personality disorders and traits based on DSM-III criteria (Stangl et al. 1985) was also significantly greater among the subjects with a diagnosis of EI. Table 8–2 presents data on the 26 subjects studied by Black and co-workers (1990, 1993).

Researchers have also administered dimensional assessments, such as the Symptom Checklist-90—Revised (Derogatis 1977), the Minnesota Multiphasic Personality Inventory (Graham 1987), and the Illness Behavior Questionnaire (Pilowsky and Spence 1983), which have revealed differences from comparison samples. People with symptoms diagnosed as EI are more likely than control subjects to have mood, anxiety, or other physical or emotional complaints (Black et al. 1990; Simon et al. 1990), to have abnormal elevations on personality profiles (Fiedler et al. 1992), or to affirm dimensions of hypochondriasis (Black et al. 1990; Simon et al. 1990), such as being aware of bodily symptoms, being bothered by many different symptoms, believing that something is seriously wrong with their bodies, and believing that their illness is not being taken seriously by others.

Table 8–1. Review of nine case series of environmentally ill subjects

Investigator	Year published	Location	N	Mean age (year) (range)	% female	% with a diagnosable mental disorder or abnormal psychological test[a]
Brodsky	1983	San Francisco	8	30 to early 50s	88	100
Pearson et al.	1983	Manchester, UK	19	39.1	68	95
Stewart and Raskin	1985	Montreal	18	38	83	100
Terr[b]	1986	San Francisco	50	38.5	78	—
Terr[b]	1989	San Francisco	90	39.5 (20–63)	70	42
Simon et al.	1990	Seattle	13	—	—	92
Black et al.	1990, 1993	Iowa City	26	49.1 (27–78)	88	87[c]
Fiedler et al.	1992	Piscataway, NJ	11	42, men; 43, women (28–57)	73	72
Simon et al.	1993	Seattle	41	46.4	85	75

Note. — = data not presented or absent.
[a]Different methods were used to evaluate subjects but were counted if they yielded a definite diagnosis or significantly abnormal ratings on self-report assessments, such as the Minnesota Multiphasic Personality Inventory (Graham 1987).
[b]Overlapping data sets.
[c]Only 23 of 26 were assessed for symptoms of mental disorders.

Table 8–2. Characteristics of 26 subjects carrying a diagnosis of environmental illness (EI)

Subject no.	Sex	Current age (year)	Age at EI diagnosis (year)	DIS diagnosis	SIDP diagnosis	Clinical[a] diagnosis
1	F	38	38	Social phobia Simple phobia	Histrionic Avoidant Compulsive	—
2	F	75	68	GAD	Paranoid Schizotypal Histrionic Compulsive	Psychoneurosis Neurasthenia
3	F	66	56	None	Schizoid Histrionic Narcissistic Compulsive	—
4	F	52	43	Dysthymia Obsessive-compulsive disorder	Schizotypal Narcissistic	—
5	F	69	47	Somatization	Histrionic Dependent	Panic attacks Possible depression Irritable bowel

					Schizotypal	Somatization
6	F	50	46	None	None	—
7	F	43	38	Not done	Not done	—
8	F	56	51	None	None	—
9	F	34	30	GAD	Histrionic	—
10	M	44	40	None	Avoidant	—
11	F	41	39	Depression Somatization	Compulsive	—
12	F	78	74	Dysthymia Panic disorder Agoraphobia	None	—
13	F	63	59	Panic disorder Agoraphobia	Histrionic Dependent	—
14	F	45	43	None	None	"Hysterical quality"
15	F	41	32	Depression Drug abuse Simple phobia	Dependent	—
16	F	36	34	Not done	Not done	—

(continued)

Table 8–2. Characteristics of 26 subjects carrying a diagnosis of environmental illness *(continued)*

Subject no.	Sex	Current age (year)	Age at EI diagnosis (year)	DIS diagnosis	SIDP diagnosis	Clinical[a] diagnosis
17	F	40	35	Not done	Not done	Obsessive-compulsive disorder
18	F	53	44	Depression Somatization	None	—
19	F	43	35	Depression Simple phobia	Borderline Histrionic Avoidant Passive-aggressive Compulsive	—
20	F	49	43	None	Paranoid Compulsive	—
21	F	45	37	Depression Simple phobia Somatization	Schizotypal Histrionic Narcissistic Dependent Avoidant	—
22	F	39	32	None	Histrionic Dependent Avoidant	—

23	F	54	46	Depression	Histrionic Compulsive	—
24	F	27	25	None	None	Atypical somatoform disorder Conversion disorder
25	M	58	42	Depression	Histrionic	—
26	M	46	43	Panic disorder Agoraphobia GAD Simple phobia	None	Major depression Compulsive personality disorder

Note. EI = environmental illness; DIS = Diagnostic Interview Schedule (Robins et al. 1981); SIDP = Structured Interview for DSM-III Personality Disorders (Stangl et al. 1985); GAD = generalized anxiety disorder. — = charts unavailable.
[a]When medical records were available.

The case of a relatively typical subject with a diagnosis of EI is presented below.

Mrs. J., a 50-year-old homemaker, reported that she had "environmental allergies," a diagnosis made 14 years earlier by a clinical ecologist and later confirmed at a clinic near Chicago specializing in the care of chemically sensitive persons. Mrs. J. believed that her problem with chemicals began 30 years earlier, with the widespread spraying of the pesticide DDT in her rural farming community. She reported a variety of symptoms including weakness, fatigue, poor concentration, and memory impairment, which, she said, worsened when she was exposed to certain foods, perfumes, gasoline fumes, and cooking and other odors. To relieve her symptoms, Mrs. J. had been advised to minimize her contact with the offending chemicals, and, as a result, she seldom left her home, stopped attending church, and rarely went shopping for fear of having a "reaction." She had also given up her work as a schoolteacher and had applied for worker's compensation benefits.

Her clinical ecologist had recommended a special rotation diet and had prescribed alkali salts and calcium carbonate. She was instructed to use sublingual "neutralizing" drops after exposure to exhaust fumes, phenols, formaldehyde, or other offending agents. Because she also had symptoms diagnosed as "yeast disease," she took oral nystatin and received weekly TOE injections (an extract containing three common yeasts and molds) to increase her defenses against *C. albicans*. She turned her bedroom into a "safe" room, which contained only her bed and special air purifiers. When reading newspapers, she wore a charcoal filter mask. More recently, she had discovered that she derived significant relief by holding a pendulum, which she believed, when moving in a clockwise oval, would counterbalance her excessive and abnormal internal magnetic forces.

Before learning of her diagnosis, Mrs. J. was unhappy with her medical care. She told us that she "disliked being thought of as a mental case, a psychological case, or a chronic complainer." She knew something "physical" was wrong. She was relieved when she learned of her chemical sensitivity and pleased at becoming a "co-partner" in her treatment. She became very interested in her condition, read avidly about chemical sensitivity, and joined support groups. Her only dissatisfaction had been with her insurance company, which refused to pay a $15,000 bill for a 1-week stay at an "environmental control unit" in a special hospital near Chicago.

At her interview, Mrs. J. was a neatly dressed and well-groomed woman appearing her age. She reported that her emotional adjustment was excellent and denied significant psychiatric problems. She admitted that she had been psychiatrically hospitalized 20 years earlier for unexplained left arm pain and underwent amobarbital sodium interviews for the apparent conversion disorder. She had been referred to our psychiatrists 3 years earlier to rule out agoraphobia, because she had revealed to a neurologist (who had ruled out multiple sclerosis as a cause of her problems) that her lifestyle was severely constricted. She presented the psychiatrists with a 12-page, typed, single-spaced report on her medical history. The psychiatrists obtained a history of 26 unexplained medical symptoms and 10 organ systems and diagnosed her symptoms as somatization disorder.

Our research evaluation yielded an additional diagnosis of schizotypal personality (this was originally reported in Black 1993).

Our experience and that of others suggest that many, if not most, people with a diagnosis of EI have a history of common psychiatric disorders that cause their high level of symptoms and psychological stress; the symptoms of these disorders partially account for the clinical ecologist's diagnosis of EI. Clinical ecologists would argue that the symptoms directly result from EI, so they must be caused either by mechanisms attributable to EI, such as immune dysfunction or limbic kindling, or by the understandable psychological distress of having to live with a disabling illness. For example, one of our patients had panic disorder, but a clinical ecologist led her to believe that the attacks were reactions to chemical agents.

Physical Disorders

Other people with a diagnosis of EI may have a common physical disorder, such as rheumatoid arthritis, with symptoms (e.g., joint pain, fatigue) that lead the clinical ecologist to diagnose EI (Simon et al. 1993; Terr 1989). In several studies, some people who had symptoms diagnosed as EI had no evidence of physical or psychiatric illness (Black et al. 1990; Simon et al. 1993; Terr 1989). The diagnosis may have been based on minor physical complaints such as chronic nasal congestion. It appears that, almost regardless of the presenting complaint, the clinical ecologist's diagnosis of EI is based on the subject's symptoms and putative history of exposure to environmental contaminants. Because the symptoms of EI are so varied and the historical information used to associate exposure with symptom development so nonspecific, it is relatively easy to attribute almost any physical or psychiatric complaint to EI. People with symptoms diagnosed as EI often come to believe deeply in the diagnosis and are pleased with their clinical ecologist and the treatment offered (Black et al. 1990). The diagnosis may appear sensible to medically unsophisticated people living in a country where media reports of pollution appear almost daily. The clinical ecologist's claims of special expertise in diagnosing and treating patients with EI and its manifestations foster a belief in the illness. The patient's belief in his or her diagnosis is often reinforced by the network of support groups and self-help organizations for patients with EI (Brodsky 1983). Special treatments, avoidance procedures, rotation and other diets, and the self-administration of antigens, all of which require significant cooperation by the patient, further validate the diagnosis for those who see themselves as suffering from this condition.

People with symptoms diagnosed as EI almost uniformly reject psychological explanations for their symptoms (Brodsky 1983; Pearson et al. 1983). They may acknowledge symptoms of anxiety and depression, but they typically attribute them to the neurotoxic effects of chemical exposure. In many cases, the belief in EI appears to have attained the status of an *overvalued idea*, in which a belief is maintained despite evidence to the contrary. People with EI have rejected traditional medicine because physicians were unable to find out "what was wrong" or to provide an explanation that made sense to them; they tend to believe that something is wrong with their body, not their mind. When one of our patients was told at a major university medical center that she had no more allergies than expected, she said that she felt "devastated" by this news (Black et al. 1993). The determination of this woman and others to reject their mainstream physician's judgment shows their considerable investment in EI beliefs.

Personality Profile

Persons who believe they are environmentally sensitive do not appear to have a special personality profile. Most have been influenced at some point by a clinical ecologist (or persons sympathetic to their beliefs) or have learned about the disorder through the media and are highly suggestible. Although exposure to EI theories may be a necessary condition for accepting the diagnosis, it is not sufficient, because most who learn about EI never come to believe that they have it. Other important factors appear to be a history of unexplained symptoms (physical or emotional) and a tendency toward symptom amplification (Simon et al. 1990). A diagnosis of EI is strongly related to overall lifetime histories of psychiatric illness and emotional distress, which vary widely across diagnostic categories. Many, if not most, also meet criteria for a personality disorder, but no specific type predominates (Black et al. 1993). From a standpoint that emphasizes dimensions of personality rather than categories, patients with EI have high levels of neuroticism.

Rosenberg and colleagues (1990) have described the personality style of many EI patients as obsessive/paranoid, that is, people who seek a medical explanation for their physical symptoms and convey their history in a precise, detailed, and fastidious way. They have also identified a histrionic/somatizing type who presents his or her history in a more global, affect-laden, and impressionistic manner. They believe that the difference is important, because the latter type of patient is more willing to explore psychological aspects of the disorder and understands the connection between stress and physical complaints. The former type is more difficult, because such patients demand an explanation that confirms the "reality" of their symptoms.

Some investigators have suggested that persons receiving a diagnosis of EI should be categorized as having a somatoform disorder (Schottenfeld 1987). EI and somatization disorder do in fact have several features in common; both are polysymptomatic, both primarily afflict women, and both involve preoccupation with symptoms. The problem is that most patients with a diagnosis of EI do not meet criteria for somatization disorder, not all are polysymptomatic, and some have an illness onset after age 30 years. Furthermore, the population of persons with EI is heterogeneous. An important subgroup consists of predominantly male industrial workers who have been exposed to potentially toxic chemicals in the workplace (Simon et al. 1990; Sparks et al. 1990).

Many appear to meet criteria for hypochondriasis because they are preoccupied with having an illness whose existence cannot be objectively verified (Black et al. 1990). The illness behavior, however, is largely a result of their clinical ecologist's recommendations reinforcing their belief that they are ill; it is therefore iatrogenic in nature. Other investigators have compared persons with a diagnosis of EI with patients with obsessive-compulsive disorder, because the former appear to have recurrent, anxiety-provoking fears and worries, as well as behaviors (e.g., wearing a mask) that resemble compulsive rituals. Except for a few individuals, the comparison is inappropriate, because the recurrent thoughts associated with EI are generally not intrusive, unwanted, or resisted to any degree. In fact, patients with a diagnosis of EI typically view their beliefs as rational and their behavior as desirable. Thus, whereas most (but not all) people with a diagnosis of EI may have an underlying psychological vulnerability, they do not easily fit a particular psychiatric category.

EVALUATION OF THE PATIENT WITH A DIAGNOSIS OF ENVIRONMENTAL ILLNESS

The relationship among patients, clinical ecologists, and the traditional practitioner can be complicated. Most people who accept a diagnosis of EI continue to receive care from their clinical ecologist (Black et al. 1990). Some patients view their conventional medical practitioners as consultants to their clinical ecologists; others view the clinical ecologist as a consultant to their primary care physician. Some patients may seek conventional medical care once they become disaffected with the clinical ecologist, but they may still adhere to many of the beliefs associated with EI, such as the importance of maintaining a chemical-free environment. Other patients reject the diagnosis of EI or feel that they have been duped by the clinical ecologist. Some patients presenting for care have not consulted a clinical ecologist but have read with interest about EI or have seen presentations in the media. They may believe that they have EI and are seeking confirmation of the diagnosis. Occasionally, a patient may present on the advice of an attorney hoping to file a worker's compensation claim or personal injury lawsuit based on an alleged chemical exposure.

Regardless of how the patient reporting to have EI presents to the mainstream psychiatrist or general physician, the first duty of the physician is to refrain from directly challenging the patient's belief in EI. A premature challenge will undermine the therapeutic relationship. Challenging the patient's belief could also traumatically disrupt the patient's relationship with the clinical ecologist, creating a new psychological stressor that may aggravate the physical symptoms. Patients' beliefs in EI usually are long-standing and firmly held. Even if the beliefs are directly challenged, it is unlikely that the patient will reject them. Physicians do not have to collude with the clinical ecologist and reaffirm the diagnosis of EI, but they do not have to directly challenge it either.

Similar to the procedure used for other patients, physicians begin the comprehensive evaluation of patients with a diagnosis of EI with a thorough history of the illness, followed by a detailed physical examination, and routine laboratory testing (Fiedler et al. 1992; Salvaggio 1991; Simon et al. 1993; Sparks et al. 1994). Because patients report that their symptoms stem from chemical exposures, a detailed occupational and environmental history should be obtained. Consultation with a physician experienced in occupational and environmental medicine should be considered when the history raises the possibility of a bona fide occupational disease or when the patient is one of several similarly afflicted in the same building, neighborhood, or workplace. Industrial hygiene data regarding the patient's exposures may be helpful, and, if exposure occurred in the workplace, relevant material safety data sheets should be obtained from patients or their employers. Many chemicals are well-established causes of symptoms that patients with a diagnosis of EI often describe (e.g., organic solvents causing headache and nausea), although usually not at the low levels of exposure reported by EI patients.

The physician must attempt to exclude medical conditions suggested by the particular patient's symptom profile. The physician should also record detailed information about current and past medical illnesses, previous diagnostic workups and treatments, and the patient's pattern of use of medical care. Obtaining past medical records is useful, particularly when the diagnosis of somatization disorder is suggested by the history.

The evaluation should include routine laboratory tests (e.g., complete blood count, serum electrolytes, serum glucose, urinalysis). Other tests may be appropriate, but their selection will be guided by the patient's reported complaints and symptoms. For example, patients with prominent respiratory tract complaints may need pulmonary function tests to rule out the presence of reactive airway disease. Testing may be useful in some cases to assess exposure to specific chemical substances when a strong correlation is known to exist between exposure and blood or urine levels (e.g., heavy metals). The physician must exercise caution in evaluating the presence of other chemicals that the patient may implicate (e.g., formaldehyde). Because modern laboratory methods allow measurements of parts per billion concentration for many organic solvents and other exogenous chemicals, chemicals found at concentrations that have no clinical relevance may be misinterpreted as evidence of unusual chemical exposure or as an explanation for the symptoms attributed to EI.

If the patient's signs and symptoms appear to be caused by specific allergies, or if the patient indicates that he or she has received a diagnosis of "environmental allergies" or "immune dysregulation," routine skin testing and/or in vitro assays with common allergens can establish the presence or absence of an allergic state, and the humoral and cellular components of the immune system can be evaluated by obtaining an immunoelectrophoresis and subclass quantitation, complement and selected autoantibody assays, and T- and B-cell assays (Salvaggio 1991). These tests provide strong evidence for the normal functioning of the immune system. Currently, no form of immunologic testing has been demonstrated to be diagnostic either of exposure to specific chemicals or of illness caused by exposure in patients with EI. For example, low titers of antibodies to formaldehyde have not been correlated with formaldehyde exposure or with disease attributed to it. Nontraditional tests used by clinical ecologists, such as provocation-neutralization testing, have not been correlated with exposure to chemicals or to disease resulting from specific chemicals (American Academy of Allergy and Immunology 1981; Jewett et al. 1990).

Because psychiatric disorders are so common among people with a diagnosis of EI, psychiatric assessment is essential (Black et al. 1990; Salvaggio 1991; Simon et al. 1993). Patients who reject referral to a psychiatrist must be made aware of the likely benefit from treatment of major mental disorders such as major depression and panic disorder. It may help to point out that the EI can *produce* significant emotional problems (e.g., depression, anxiety, adjustment disorders) requiring careful psychological assessment. Neuropsychological testing, which is dependent on patient cooperation, may occasionally help to rule out other conditions in the differential diagnosis (e.g., dementia in the patient reporting significant problems with concentration and memory). However, neuropsychological testing has not revealed any consistent or diagnostically useful findings in patients with a diagnosis of EI (Simon et al. 1993).

The physical examination and laboratory test results will presumably be normal in most patients and will not confirm the presence of physical illness. Patients can be told the "good news"—that is, that the results were unremarkable and that no other tests are indicated. Physicians can inform patients with a diagnosable psychiatric illness that it is most likely treatable and that the treatment will help to reduce their distressing symptoms. Presenting the existence of a psychiatric condition as a consequence, or a complication, of stress may help the patient to accept recommended psychiatric therapies. This approach avoids directly challenging the patient's illness belief system, yet may facilitate the patient accepting formal psychiatric interventions such as antidepressant medication in the context of a mood disorder.

Patients may request other tests (e.g., neutralization-provocation testing) that they may have read about in EI literature or may seek exotic neuroimaging (e.g., positron-emission tomography) or other tests and procedures that are not indicated. The physician must learn to resist the temptation to comply with these requests unless well-designed and controlled studies demonstrate the clinical utility of such tests in patients alleged to have EI.

Table 8–3 summarizes the evaluation of people with symptoms diagnosed as EI.

TREATMENT RECOMMENDATIONS

Patients whose symptoms have been diagnosed as EI by a clinical ecologist should be reassured, based on the results of the evaluation, that there is no evidence of a verifiable physical disorder, although their symptoms and distress should be acknowledged. These patients will likely have been self-diagnosed, and it is appropriate to discuss the controversial nature of the diagnosis and the lack of data to support its theories and treatment recommendations.

Patients who have developed a strong belief in the diagnosis of EI and who have been or still are under the care of a clinical ecologist can still be helped with their symptoms. Regardless of whether the patient's symptoms are "real," they are still distressing and disabling, despite the absence of observable pathology.

Psychotherapy

Based on a small series of cases, Haller (1993) recommends supportive psychotherapy to help manage the care of patients with EI. Her approach is nonjudgmental and focuses on the goal of enhancing the patient's sense of mastery over workplace or home stressors, including chemical exposures. Control of symptoms does not depend on the patient receiving a specific organic diagnosis or etiology, but on a patient's improved understanding of the role of stress on his or her illness and the acquisition of skills for coping with the impact of EI on daily life. To accomplish these treatment goals, the physician may want to enlist the help of a psychiatrist or other mental health professional who has experience with EI patients.

Environmental Modifications

To reduce stress in the workplace, minor environmental modifications may be helpful, if they are not unreasonable. A person with EI may perceive certain odors (e.g., an exposure to volatile organic compounds) as irritating or noxious. An attempt to reduce and control odors and irritating exposures in the workplace may make sense, even if the current levels of exposure are well below government-mandated

Table 8–3. Medical workup for environmental illness

1. Complete medical and environmental history
   - Focus on exposures at home and in the workplace
2. Thorough physical examination, including neurological examination
3. Mental status examination and formal psychiatric evaluation
4. Routine laboratory studies, which may include
   - Complete blood count, with differential
   - Serum electrolytes
   - Serum glucose
   - Blood urea nitrogen
   - Creatinine
   - Liver function tests
   - Thyroid function tests
   - Urinalysis
   - Electrocardiogram
   - Chest X ray
5. Neuropsychological testing, for patients with cognitive complaints (e.g., memory impairment) or to rule out alternate diagnoses (e.g., dementia)
6. Immunologic tests, for patients reporting immune dysfunction:
   - Skin tests or in vitro assays with common allergens
   - Immunoglobulin levels
   - Complement levels
   - Selected autoantibody assays
   - Simple T- and B-cell assays
7. Other tests will be guided by the patient's complaints (e.g., spirometry for patients whose primary complaints are respiratory, nerve conduction tests for patients with persistent numbness and tingling in the extremities)

or recommended exposure limits. However, complete avoidance of low-level chemical exposure should not be viewed as an option, because this would further contribute to the patient's social and occupational disability; it would probably worsen anxiety or depression and exacerbate the patient's other subjective symptoms (e.g., somatizing). Without minimizing his or her symptoms, the patient should be reassured that this condition is neither progressive nor fatal.

Many patients with EI claim to have an exquisite sense of smell, which enables them to seek out potential environmental dangers, although little evidence supports this claim (Doty et al. 1988). Fear of noxious odors leads many to believe they are being poisoned, although they are not. The immediate solution to allay concern is to remove the odor; however, the long-range goal is to lessen the fear. Patients need to be educated about odors and the fact that smell often has little to do with toxicity. Analogies may be helpful: who, for instance, has not smelled a skunk on a country road half a mile away? Harmless mercaptans with an extremely powerful odor at very low concentrations are responsible for the smell. For this reason, similar compounds are used to give odorless natural gas a smell. The odor itself is nontoxic, but the odorless natural gas is dangerous and potentially lethal.

Avoidance of social and occupational situations for fear of toxic exposure is one of the main sources of disability in patients with EI. Because the recommendation for avoidance can lead to serious and substantial problems (e.g., loss of work and social support), it is important to convince the patient that this recommendation is likely to create more harm than benefit. Rather than being a "friend" to the patient, avoidance behavior should be considered an "enemy" to be conquered.

Behavior Modification Programs

Behavior modification programs that emphasize systematic desensitization may help some patients (Haller 1993; Schottenfeld 1989; Shusterman and Dager 1991). With desensitization, the patient is gradually exposed to odors and fumes found in typical home and work situations. The behavior program should promote an overall increase in physical and social activity as well. It can be patterned after behavior desensitization paradigms used to treat patients with agoraphobia, a condition in which patients learn to avoid specific places and situations for fear of developing a panic attack. In fact, many persons with EI describe "reactions to chemicals" that they experience when exposed to disagreeable odors or fumes that are descriptively similar (or even identical) to panic attacks; the avoidance strongly resembles agoraphobia. Patients may report that they avoid crowded places, such as shopping centers and malls, because of possible chemical exposure from perfumes and deodorants used by other shoppers.

One of our patients described entering a shopping mall and developing a "reaction" characterized by feeling anxious and fearful, heart palpitations, shortness of breath, feelings of dizziness and unsteadiness, and paresthesias. These symptoms generally ceased within minutes of exiting the mall. Her reactions (i.e., panic attacks) were odor triggered; her clinical ecologist encouraged this avoidance behavior (i.e., agoraphobia) because he believed that the panic symptoms were compatible with the diagnosis of EI. In response to the clinical ecologist's recommendations, the patient had learned to avoid places where she might encounter disagreeable odors that she associated with "reactions to chemicals." Thus, the behavior modification approach assumes that an important ingredient to the manifestations of EI is *behavioral conditioning* rather than toxic injury. Patients with this pattern of behavior have been described as "chemophobic" (Terr 1992).

Coexisting Psychiatric Disorders

Treatment of coexisting psychiatric disorders (e.g., major depression, panic disorder) may help to reduce the patient's symptoms of illness and disability (Schottenfeld 1989). Patients whose "reactions" to chemical exposures strongly resemble panic attacks may learn to tolerate exposure to disagreeable odors once the attacks have been pharmacologically blocked. Patients who believe that EI has led to fatigue, lassitude, and dysphoria may find that antidepressant medication relieves these symptoms. On the other hand, patients with somatization disorder can be monitored for the emergence of new symptoms, which can then be placed into context. This will help to reduce unnecessary testing and other medical procedures that may contribute to the patient's ongoing disability. Although many patients with a diagnosis of EI may resist taking "chemicals" to treat their psychiatric disorder, and others will report intolerance to relatively low levels of medication (Schottenfeld 1987), the clinician must be patient, but persistent, in recommending medication when it is deemed appropriate. Treatment should begin at very low doses, because EI patients are very sensitive to changes in their internal milieu. Dosage is gradually increased to a therapeutic range, as tolerated. The rewards of successfully treating depression, anxiety, or other psychiatric disorders are well worth the effort.

Combination of Treatment Measures

Treatment of the patient with EI generally involves a combination of pharmacologic and supportive psychotherapeutic measures (Sparks et al. 1994). In addition to a behavior modification program, individual supportive psychotherapy may be helpful in exploring a patient's feelings of helplessness with his or her "mysterious" illness and feelings of hopelessness about overcoming its symptoms. Supportive psychotherapy can also improve the patient's morale and often low self-esteem. Patients should be encouraged to ventilate their feelings of anger and bewilderment about having developed what they perceive (or have been told) is a chronic disorder and the ongoing "fighting" that they detect among their physicians, some of whom support the diagnosis of EI and some of whom do not. Cognitive restructuring techniques might help patients to reverse some of the maladaptive beliefs that have contributed to their disability (e.g., "If I smell car exhaust, my whole day will be ruined."). Marital and family therapy may be considered for those who have involved their spouse or children in their illness, depending on the amount of dysfunction present and the degree of insight they possess. As with other types of patients with chronic illness behavior, clinicians should assess the extent to which the patient's illness behavior and degree of functional disability is positively reinforced by family members who serve as caretakers. Some patients, for example, may have convinced their close family members that they also have EI. Even when the family members do not believe they have EI, they are often enlisted to participate in unusual dietary regimens or efforts to avoid chemical exposures. Children can be indoctrinated by parents into developing similar illness beliefs.

The following case presentation is of a woman treated in our hospital on a medical-psychiatry unit. The mixed outcome reflects the difficulty in treating patients with EI, particularly those who are fully invested in the diagnosis.

> Ms. E., a 48-year-old single woman, was admitted to the hospital for evaluation of significant weight loss and severe malnutrition. She weighed 80 pounds and had been receiving an elemental diet per nasogastric tube at the referring institution.

On admission, Ms. E. reported a complex medical history. She described having severe "environmental allergy" and "immune dysfunction," which she claimed had been the result of a bout with amebic dysentery 15 years earlier. She had subsequently developed chronic complaints of fatigue, lassitude, dysphoria, and a variety of gastrointestinal problems including flatulence, pain, bloating, and abnormal stools. Because her physical problems failed to diminish, and most physicians told her that her only problem was an "irritable bowel," Ms. E. sought help from nontraditional practitioners including chiropractors, nutritionists, acupuncturists, and, finally, clinical ecologists. Her symptoms were diagnosed as EI, and she was advised to escape the "toxic environment" of her large East Coast city and to begin using rotation diets because several food allergies had been implicated.

She had relocated to Texas and came under the care of a clinical ecologist. Evaluation at a special hospital confirmed the diagnosis of environmental allergies. Because her disorder was believed to be "advanced," she was told to isolate herself by living in a porcelain-lined trailer in a special community. The clinical ecologist also advised her to inject herself with "antigens" before anticipated toxic exposures. Because severe malnutrition had developed, total parenteral nutrition (TPN) was recommended and begun after a central venous catheter was placed.

Ms. E. eventually left Texas and moved in with her parents in a small midwestern community. Although she was a lawyer, her physical complaints had disabled her for many years. She continued to receive TPN, but she developed sepsis twice during the year before hospital admission, probably because of poor catheter care and her insistence on taking several showers a day to wash off spores of *Candida albicans*, which she believed contributed to her poor health.

The patient's life revolved around her illness, and, when living at home, she enlisted her parents' help to cope with her illness. For example, she had her father put aluminum foil on the windows of their home to protect against electromagnetic waves, and she had her mother prepare chard (one of the few foods she could eat) in a special way to reduce its allergenic potential. When her parents failed to comply with her requests, she made them feel guilty by blaming them for her condition.

Ms. E. had an extensive psychiatric history; she first entered psychotherapy 15 years before the hospitalization. She usually sought help from therapists for treatment of depression or problems adjusting to her diagnosis of EI. However, she usually dropped out because she was "environmentally sensitive" to their offices or clothing or because they would not visit her at home and wear special clothing, which she had asked them to do.

The patient presented on admission as a very thin woman with a nasogastric tube in place. She had a low albumin and ferritin and severe anemia with leukopenia. Other laboratory tests were unremarkable. The admitting house officer noted that she was loquacious, circumstantial, and preoccupied with her medical history. She was noted to be intelligent and was more conversant with medical terminology than most patients. She denied having an eating disorder, mood or anxiety symptoms, or psychotic symptoms. She believed that all of her problems stemmed from an "allergy of the stomach" that caused her to be intolerant to foods, which led to considerable gastrointestinal distress and weight loss.

The treatment team had the difficult task of formulating a sensible treatment plan for a patient who was clearly invested in her diagnosis of EI. The main goal was to reverse the patient's continued weight loss, discontinue the elemental feedings that were not medically indicated, and try to improve the patient's social and occupational functioning.

A behavior modification plan was developed to accomplish these goals. The program was explained in detail to her, and she was given a copy of it. The program did not address the controversial nature of EI but focused on her objective behavior. The protocol was specific about what was or was not allowed. For example, she was not allowed to have special mineral water or to select her food; she could only take one shower per day and had to use hospital soap and shampoo. She could wear her own clothing, but could only launder them with hospital detergent. She was not allowed to use the charcoal filter mask that she had been using.

Ms. E. was gradually weaned from her elemental feedings and was required to gradually increase her food intake to meet weight gain targets, similar to what might be expected of a patient with anorexia nervosa. On this plan, she consistently gained weight and was able to tolerate a variety of foods. Failure to comply with the diet resulted in decreased privileges.

During the refeeding period, the patient continued to complain of intermittent abdominal discomfort. She was instructed to call for a physician whenever she experienced problems that she believed were related to her EI. Her physicians could not confirm an allergic response on any occasion.

Ms. E. was told that she must accept the hospital personnel as they were. She could not require them to wash with special soaps or to wear special clothing. During the hospitalization, it became clear that she had no reaction to perfumes, cleaning agents, or foods.

As the patient gained weight, her fatigue lessened and her motivation improved, although she remained mildly anemic. She was allowed to participate in ward activities and voiced an interest in hospital volunteer work. A family therapy session was held, and, with the cooperation of her parents, a recommendation was made that she enter a halfway house where she was urged to continue to participate in a behavior modification program. Because she was no longer believed to be a danger to herself or others, she was discharged at her request.

Although objectively improved, Ms. E. maintained that she was "environmentally sensitive" and said that she would return to her old ways after discharge.

Table 8–4 summarizes treatment recommendations for the management of symptoms in people with a diagnosis of EI.

FUTURE DIRECTIONS

Clinical ecology has emerged as a medical subculture complete with its own practitioners, theories, and treatments. All have developed around the concept of EI, which is rapidly becoming a politically defined illness. Clinical ecologists, and their many patients, have mobilized to seek validation through legislation, administrative fiat, or the courts. The emotion-laden debate is led by persons who genuinely believe that they are chemically sensitive and who have distressing symptoms of EI.

Mainstream physicians are just learning about this medical phenomenon and how best to help reduce disability and distress in people with a diagnosis of EI. Information about clinical ecology and EI is greatly needed. From the standpoint of the medical historian, several questions emerge: How do medical subcultures develop? What leads certain physicians to embrace ideas that put them at odds with their peers? Moreover, what leads a person to accept a controversial diagnosis and the unorthodox treatments that require self-participation? From the standpoint of a mainstream clinician caring for patients with EI, other questions arise: What other illnesses or conditions explain the patient's obvious distress? What is the eventual outcome for persons accepting the diagnosis of EI? How can the physician best help patients to overcome their disabling symptoms? Will psychotropic medication (e.g., serotonin reuptake inhibitors) have any specific effect on the overvalued ideation characteristic of persons with a diagnosis of EI? Finally, how can the physician return the patient to the mainstream medical fold? None of these questions has received serious attention, but researchers have become more attuned to clinical ecology practices. Data are needed to confirm or invalidate the diagnosis of EI and to investigate its relationship to chemical exposure, before medical science becomes irrelevant to social policy decisions relating to EI.

Table 8–4. Recommendations for the management of symptoms in people with a diagnosis of EI

---

1. Do not directly challenge the diagnosis, because it will only backfire.
   - On the other hand, do not reaffirm the diagnosis.
2. Assure the patient that you believe the symptoms are real and not just in the mind.
   - Regardless of etiology, the symptoms are genuine and distressing.
3. Evaluate the patient thoroughly; a careful history and medical evaluation will help rule out other diagnoses that could be responsible for some of the symptoms.
4. Do not ignore the psychiatric evaluation; primary mental disorders are found in the majority of patients with a diagnosis of EI and may partially account for the symptoms reported.
   - Psychiatric treatment (e.g., of depression, panic disorder) could reduce the patient's symptoms.
5. Encourage patients to "fight" the disorder by gradually increasing their exposure to "toxic" agents.
   - This is the only way to reduce the disability that will otherwise ensue.
   - Some patients may need a specific behavior modification program.
   - Cognitive restructuring techniques may help to reverse maladaptive beliefs (e.g., "If I smell car exhaust, my whole day will be ruined").
6. Encourage healthy behavior—the patient has focused exclusively on EI; encourage patients to turn their attention to more important issues (e.g., work, social and family life).
7. The goal of treatment is to give patients a sense of mastery over their symptoms and to enable them to overcome their disability.
8. Family and marital therapy may help those patients with a diagnosis of EI whose marriages or family life have been disrupted.

Note. EI = environmental illness.

SUMMARY

Clinical ecologists have defined a condition that they believe is common and frequently underdiagnosed. Studies show that most people with symptoms diagnosed as EI are middle-aged women with a history of psychological difficulties and who have multiple physical complaints, often occurring in the context of a mood or anxiety disorder. They tend to accept the diagnosis of EI and to become part of a tightly knit group.

When these patients seek care from a mainstream physician, they should receive a thorough evaluation, including a careful history, physical examination, and routine laboratory testing. The physician should refrain from directly challenging the patient's controversial diagnosis. The physician should assist the patient in overcoming the social and occupational disability that may have resulted from the clinical ecologist's treatment recommendations. The physician should also offer long-term supportive care to help improve the patient's morale and low self-esteem.

REFERENCES

Abbey SE, Garfinkle PE: Neurasthenia and chronic fatigue syndrome: the role of culture in making the diagnosis. Am J Psychiatry 148:1638–1646, 1991

American Academy of Allergy and Immunology: Controversial techniques: position statement. J Allergy Clin Immunol 67:333–338, 1981

American Academy of Allergy and Immunology: Clinical ecology: position statement. J Allergy Clin Immunol 78:269–271, 1986

American College of Physicians: Clinical ecology: position statement. Ann Intern Med 111:168–178, 1989

American Medical Association: A report of the Council on Scientific Affairs: clinical ecology. JAMA 268:3465–3467, 1992

Bell IR: Neuropsychiatric and biopsychosocial mechanisms in multiple chemical sensitivity: an olfactory-limbic system model, in Multiple Chemical Sensitivities. Washington, DC, National Academy Press, 1992, pp 89–108

Black DW: Environmental illness and misdiagnosis—a growing problem. Regul Toxicol Pharmacol 18:23–31, 1993

Black DW, Rathe A, Goldstein RB: Environmental illness—a controlled study of 26 subjects with "20th century disease." JAMA 264:3166–3170, 1990

Black DW, Rathe A, Goldstein RB: Measures of distress in 26 "environmentally ill" subjects. Psychosomatics 34:131–138, 1993

Brodsky CM: Allergic to everything: a medical subculture. Psychosomatics 24:731–742, 1983

California Medical Association Scientific Board: Task force on clinical ecology. clinical ecology: a critical appraisal. West J Med 144:239–245, 1986

Crook WG (ed): Chronic Fatigue Syndrome and the Yeast Connection. Jackson, TN, Professional Books, 1992

Cullen MR: The worker with multiple chemical sensitivities: an overview. Occup Med 2:655–667, 1987

Derogatis LR: Symptom Checklist-90-Revised: Administration, Scoring and Procedures Manual. Towson, MD, Clinical Psychometric Research, 1977

Dismukes WE, Wade JS, Lee JY, et al: A randomized, double-blind trial of nystatin therapy for the candidiasis hypersensitivity syndrome. N Engl J Med 323:1717–1723, 1990

Doty R, Deems DA, Frye RE, et al: Olfactory sensitivity, nasal resistance, and autonomic function in patients with multiple chemical sensitivities. Arch Otolaryngol Head Neck Surg 114:1422–1427, 1988

Fiedler N, Maccia C, Kipen H: Evaluation of chemically sensitive patients. J Occup Med 5:529–538, 1992

Gots RE: "Sick-buildings," in Toxic Risks—Science, Regulation, and Perception. Ann Arbor, MI, Lewis Publishers, 1993, pp 187–208

Graham JR (ed): The Minnesota Multiphasic Personality Inventory: A Practical Guide, 2nd Edition. New York, Oxford University Press, 1987

Hall SS: Allergic to the 20th century. Health 7:72–85, 1993

Haller E: Successful management of patients with multiple chemical sensitivities on an inpatient psychiatric unit. J Clin Psychiatry 54:196–199, 1993

Hileman B: Multiple chemical sensitivity. Chemical and Engineering News, July 22, 1991, pp 26–42

Human Ecology Action League: Is EI making you ill? Pamphlet distributed by the Human Ecology Action League, Inc., Chicago, IL

Imboden JB, Canter A, Cluff CE, et al: Brucellosis—psychologic aspects of delayed convalescence. Arch Intern Med 103:406–414, 1959

Jewett DL, Fein G, Greenberg MH: A double-blind study of symptom provocation to determine food sensitivity. N Engl Med 323:429–433, 1990

Levin AS, Byers VS: Environmental illness: a disorder of immune regulation. Occup Med 2:669–681, 1987

Levine SA, Reinhardt JH: Biochemical pathology initiated by free radicals, oxidant chemicals, and therapeutic drugs and the etiology of chemical hypersensitivity disease. Journal of Orthomolecular Psychiatry 12:166–183, 1983

McLellan RK: Biologic interventions in the treatment of patients with multiple chemical sensitivities. Occup Med 2:755–777, 1987

Menzies R, Tamblyn R, Farant JP, et al: The effect of varying levels of outdoor-air supply on the symptoms of sick-building syndrome. N Engl J Med 328:821–827, 1993

Mooser SB: The epidemiology of multiple chemical sensitivities. Occup Med 2:663–668, 1987

Pearson DJ, Rix KJB, Bentley SJ: Food allergy—how much in the mind? clinical and psychiatric study of suspected food hypersensitivity. Lancet 1:1259–1261, 1983

Pilowsky I, Spence ND: Manual for the Illness Behavior Questionnaire, 2nd Edition. Adelaide, Australia, Department of Psychiatry, University of Adelaide, 1983

Randolph TG: Sensitivity to petroleum including the derivatives and antecedents. J Lab Clin Med 40:931–932, 1952

Randolph TG, Moss RW (eds): An Alternative Approach to Allergies. New York, Bantam Books, 1980

Rea WJ, Johnson AR, Ross GH, et al: Considerations for the diagnosis of chemical sensitivity, in Multiple Chemical Sensitivities. Washington, DC, National Academy Press, 1992

Robins LN, Helzer JE, Croughan J, et al: National Institute of Mental Health Diagnostic Interview Schedule: its history, characteristics, and validity. Arch Gen Psychiatry 38:381–389, 1981

Rosenberg SJ, Freedman MR, Schmaling KB, et al: Personality styles of patient asserting environmental illness. J Occup Med 32:678–681, 1990

Rowe AH: Allergic toxemia and migraine due to food allergy. California Western Medicine 33:785–792, 1930

Salvaggio JE: Clinical and immunologic approach to patients with alleged environmental injury. Ann Allergy 66:493–503, 1991

Schluederberg A, Straus SE, Peterson P, et al: Chronic fatigue syndrome research—definition and medical outcome assessment. Ann Intern Med 117:325–331, 1992

Schottenfeld RS: Workers with multiple chemical sensitivities—a psychiatric approach to diagnosis and treatment. Occup Med 2:739–753, 1987

Shusterman DJ, Dager SR: Prevention of psychological disability after occupational respiratory exposures. Occup Med 6:11–27, 1991

Simon GE, Katon WJ, Sparks PJ: Allergic to life: psychological factors in environmental illness. Am J Psychiatry 147:901–906, 1990

Simon GE, Daniell W, Stockbridge H, et al: Immunologic, psychological and neuropsychological factors in multiple chemical sensitivity—a controlled study. Arch Intern Med 118:97–103, 1993

Sparks PJ, Simon GE, Katon WJ, et al: An outbreak of illness among aerospace workers. West J Med 153:28–33, 1990

Sparks PJ, Daniell W, Black DW, et al: Multiple chemical sensitivity syndrome: a clinical perspective. J Occup Med 36:718–737, 1994

Stangl D, Pfohl B, Zimmerman M, et al: Structured Interview for DSM-III Personality Disorders. Arch Gen Psychiatry 42:592–596, 1985

Stewart D, Raskin J: Psychiatric assessment of patients with 20th century disease ("total allergy syndrome"). Can Med Assoc J 133:1001–1006, 1985

Terr AI: Environmental illness: clinical review of 50 cases. Arch Intern Med 146:145–149, 1986

Terr AI: Clinical ecology in the workplace. J Occup Med 31:257–261, 1989

Terr AI: Multiple chemical sensitivity syndrome. Occupational Asthma and Allergies 12:897–908, 1992

Trowbridge JP, Walker M (eds): The Yeast Syndrome. New York, Bantam Books, 1986

Zenz C (ed): Occupational Medicine: Principals and Practical Applications, 2nd Edition. Chicago, IL, Year Book Medical, 1988

Chapter 9

Vulvodynia: Chronic Vulvar Pain Syndromes

Marilynne McKay, M.D.
Julie Farrington, M.D.

Vulvovaginal itching and burning is generally considered to be a relatively commonplace problem, with most women experiencing at least a few episodes at some point in their lives. Infection is the first-line hypothesis for cause, and "cure" is the expected result. Self-medication with over-the-counter preparations is encouraged by television advertising; in many cases, the patient simply calls her doctor's office for a prescription rather than seeking a diagnostic examination. The popular assumption is that vulvovaginal discomfort is a trivial problem that is easy to cure. In most cases this is true, but treatment failures occur for a variety of reasons. Inability to "cure" a genital problem can lead to significant psychological stress, especially when discomfort leads to dyspareunia.

Vulvodynia is a symptom with multiple qualities that make it relevant for a psychiatrist's knowledge base. With influences from cyclic hormonal changes and multiple etiologic factors, some of which (e.g., herpes) are cyclical in and of themselves, vulvodynia can be a complex problem to understand and treat. Medical therapy may also contribute to the patient's symptom pattern, and visible physical findings may be minimal in the doctor's office or laboratory. The ambiguity involved in arriving at a definitive diagnosis (i.e., naming the problem) and effective treatment frustrates both the physician and patient and often leads to a pattern of multiple referrals by physicians and doctor shopping by the patient. The patient begins losing confidence in the medical profession and continues to be plagued with a problem that involves the most personal part of her body, affects sexual intimacy, and carries social stigmata that restrict being able to deal with the symptoms in public or to share concerns and fears with others. To help the patient, the psychiatrist must understand the disorder and the frustrations of both the referring physician and patient. The psychiatrist is also often in the best position to be both an advocate for the patient, by helping coordinate the treatment plan, and the health care profession, by screening for psychiatric problems that may lead to unnecessary medical interventions.

We begin this chapter with a definition of vulvodynia and then list the clinical and social aspects that are important in assessing and treating the patient. There is a paucity of research in this area, but we have cited relevant clinical studies where applicable. We explore psychological factors and their potential role in exacerbating symptoms and/or interfering with treatment. We disavow stereotyping this patient population into having a primary psychiatric diagnosis.

We present differential diagnoses and the topics of itching versus burning symptoms, dysesthesias, interstitial cystitis, urethral syndrome, cutaneous disorders (dermatoses and infections), and dyspareunia. We discuss potential iatrogenic problems before examining patient management options. We conclude this chapter with psychiatric interventions and reviews of the available literature. Specific topics include sexual abuse, chronic pain, substance abuse, somatoform disorders, and the use of psychotropic medication.

DEFINITION AND FEATURES OF VULVODYNIA

Vulvodynia was defined by a task force of the International Society for the Study of Vulvovaginal Disease that was formed in 1981. Young and co-workers (1984) defined vulvodynia as chronic vulvar discomfort, characterized by burning, stinging, irritation, or rawness. In an overview of pruritus vulvae and vulvodynia, McKay (1985) pointed out that the symptom of itching does not seem to alarm patients as much as burning. Itching may be annoying, but scratching pleasurably relieves discomfort, and the patient can usually understand the cause-and-effect relationship between itching and scratching. Vulvodynia, however, is painful, and no consistent method produces relief. The only visible change may be mild erythema, so the patient only knows that she is in pain and "nobody can see anything."

The chronicity of vulvodynia is probably its most important feature. Vulvodynia that has persisted for over 6 months has more in common with chronic pain syndromes than it does with other gynecologic disorders, and the patient's medical evaluation should reflect this observation. Vulvodynia is only a *symptom;* it is not a *disease.* Vulvar burning occurs for a variety of reasons, and recognizable patterns of discomfort respond to different treatment programs (McKay 1988, 1989, 1992).

A COMPLEX AND MULTIFACTORIAL PROBLEM

A thorough evaluation by a knowledgeable examiner is essential for accurate diagnosis of vulvodynia, but the presentation of vulvodynia may be complicated by many factors, including previous therapy. The tendency is to assume that chronic, poorly understood pain in women is psychiatric in nature; this preconception should be rigorously avoided. Many disorders can affect the pelvic floor, and it is very possible that the patient has not consulted an expert "vulvologist." Dermatology, gynecology, urology, neurology, and psychiatry each adds a perspective in understanding the multifactorial nature of chronic vulvar discomfort, and no one specialty seems to have all the answers. In some cases, a nurse practitioner who is experienced in vulvar disease may be a better diagnostician than a highly trained medical specialist. Causes of acute-onset perineal itching or burning include *Candida* infection, irritant and contact dermatitis, urinary tract infection, hemorrhoids, pinworms, and condylomata. Chronic cutaneous symptomatology will be the major focus of this chapter.

There is a notable paucity of scientific research on the topic of vulvodynia, and most publications on this subject are clinical and descriptive, if not anecdotal. The incidence and prevalence of vulvodynia are unknown, for example, and vulvologists are still struggling with definitions of disorders like vulvar vestibulitis, a condition that is routinely treated with surgical excision of the affected area. The relationship of vulvodynia and vaginismus is unknown; it seems likely that pain from the former may be linked to the latter. If there is an organic reason for vaginismus, then psychological counseling may be doomed to failure; however, if vaginismus is caused by an episode of organic pain that has since resolved, then counseling may spare the patient surgery or other treatments even less likely to be effective. Iatrogenic factors are becoming recognized; for instance, the CO_2 laser is not as widely used for nonspecific vulvar pain as it was a few years ago, because experience has shown that it may worsen dyspareunia in certain cases. Basic science research into localized hypersensitivity reactions in skin and mucous membranes is beginning to be applied to vulvodynia, both with regard to nerve endings and inflammatory mediators released by organisms such as *Candida*.

Patients with vulvodynia typically see many physicians. They have usually been given different explanations for their problem, and relief has been temporary at best. Lack of a diagnosis is particularly worrisome; in a series of patients with symptomatic vulvovaginitis, Stewart and colleagues (1990) found much higher stress levels in those patients with undiagnosed symptoms than in those in whom an etiology had been determined. Patients' anxiety increases the longer the problem persists. A spouse or sexual partner may become a focus of resentment or concern. The patient's fears often center around cancer or contagion; patients often seek out multiple specialists and demand "tests" to "find out exactly what I have." Reassurance that infection and cancer have been ruled out can give substantial comfort, but the patient should be advised of the laboratory's limitations. (There are no histologic criteria for vulvar vestibulitis, for example, and a biopsy is relatively useless in this condition.) The patient's fears should be addressed directly, and appropriate testing should be done, but negative results do not mean that the problem is "all in her head." Because there may be few physical signs, many women are told that their problem is primarily psychological, especially when dyspareunia is a major component. P. J. Lynch (1986) and Friedrich (1987) both note that these patients often become resentful, frustrated, and angry, making it difficult for them to find sympathetic care. Simply giving a name to a patient's symptom complex is often a major stress reliever, enabling the patient to relinquish her search for "cure" and concentrate on effective management strategies for her chronic problem. Doctor-patient communication to avoid misunderstanding should be a major therapeutic goal, because vulvodynia is more of a condition than a disease.

PSYCHOLOGICAL ASPECTS OF VULVODYNIA

Twenty-five years ago, much was written on the psychiatric associations of anal and genital symptomatology, but these studies should be evaluated within the context of treatments available at that time. Topical steroids revolutionized the dermatological management of chronic itching (lichen simplex chronicus), and symptoms can now be controlled or even resolved with the use of creams or ointments. In the 1950s, Wittkower and Russell (1953) stated that men with pruritus ani had obsessional personalities, whereas Cormia (1951) thought them depressive; he agreed with Drueck (1945) and Jeffcoate (1949), however, that women with pruritus vulvae were primarily sexually frustrated. Rosenbaum (1945), F. W. Lynch (1952), and Wittkower and Russell (1953) also described hysterical personality characteristics. Reports of personality-linked pruritus declined precipitously after the introduction of topical steroids. Koblenzer (1987), a dermatologist as well as a psychiatrist, adopted the present-day attitude that empathy and reassurance are the most important factors in treating patients of either sex with chronic genital pruritus.

Pain during intercourse focuses attention on the relationship between partners. Sympathy and support are typical when a partner is thought to be experiencing genuine physical discomfort, but when the situation continues for months, frustrations often surface. Because so little is known about perineal pain syndromes, the clinician may diagnose the symptoms as "psychosomatic disease" simply out of ignorance of other diagnostic possibilities. Vulvodynia does not appear to be associated with any one psychiatric diagnosis, so care should be taken in generalizing these patients. Again, these patients have more in common with patients with chronic pain than with patients with "genital disorders." Supportive discussions of stress as a consequence of their disease rather than as a cause are more likely to improve patients' attitudes and outlook. If the disorder appears to have psychiatric comorbidity, then psychiatric consultation may be helpful. In our experience, most patients with vulvodynia are receptive to additional psychological evaluation and even eager to discuss their frustrations and stress.

Caveat: Avoiding "Psychologizing" Symptoms of Vulvodynia

The sexual complications of vulvodynia can be considerable; however, each couple handles dyspareunia differently, and assumptions should not be made. Symptoms vary in severity from patient to patient, as does the ability (or willingness) to tolerate discomfort. Women may be agitated or tearful as they describe frustration with previous physicians or treatments; others seem almost detached. Patients may do their own research, bringing copies of articles and books or bound reports to their consultations. This may be threatening to the health care provider and compromise the therapeutic relationship. Some patients firmly believe that stress worsens the problem; others believe that they could handle stress if only they did not have their chronic pain.

Dodson and Friedrich (1978), P. J. Lynch (1986), and Stewart and associates (1990) have all described the "classic clinical characteristics" of patients with so-called psychosomatic vulvovaginitis (persistent symptoms of long-standing duration, lack of demonstrable pathology, multiple consultations, failure to respond to standard empirical therapies, symptoms out of proportion to objective findings, "allergy" to many common vaginal preparations, reluctance to consider a psychophysiologic cause, and emotional lability). These findings, however, are typical of vulvodynia patients with bona fide physical disorders (McKay 1988), especially those with vulvar vestibulitis, cyclic vulvovaginitis, and dysesthetic vulvodynia or pudendal neuralgia (see "Endogenous Dysesthesias" section below). Interestingly, the same characteristics also describe patients with interstitial cystitis (IC), another poorly understood chronic bladder disorder affecting female patients.

In this chapter, we emphasize the secondary psychiatric *complications* of vulvodynia (such as anxiety and depression) that may amplify the symptomatology or impair the patient's ability to cope with her disease. We do not consider the disorder to be primarily psychogenic or psychiatric in nature.

VULVODYNIA AND THE MEDIA

Although vulvodynia has been defined and studied for over 10 years, it is not a well-known problem. Recently, there has been a flurry of articles in the popular press presenting vulvodynia as a dramatic "disease" that women have heretofore endured in silence. Unfortunately, articles and stories in women's magazines are often biased toward "cure-of-the-month" presentations and anecdotal reports. These articles have done little to increase awareness of the genuine progress that has been made in differential diagnosis and effective treatment of different types of vulvodynia. Patient support groups have been of variable quality: some have touted favorite therapists, whereas others have attempted to provide scientific information. The International Society for the Study of Vulvovaginal Disease (ISSVD, 930 North Meacham Road, Schaumburg, IL 60173-6016) can provide physicians with a list of vulvologists who may be able to assist with referrals of difficult cases.

As a chronic pain syndrome, vulvodynia bears some resemblance to IC as noted earlier. Support groups for IC, however, are much more developed. The Interstitial Cystitis Association (P.O. Box 1553, Madison Square Station, New York, NY 10159) is an outstanding patient support organization that has lobbied Congress and raised money for research. The Interstitial Cystitis Association clearly does not consider this disorder to be psychiatric, although its members are very interested in psychological coping mechanisms for chronic pain. Support groups and the study of vulvodynia are barely beginning to approach the level of awareness and scientific investigation as compared to IC.

ISSUES IN DIFFERENTIAL DIAGNOSIS

Interstitial Cystitis and Urethral Syndrome

IC and urethral syndrome are disorders that also have the potential for being "psychologized." Similar to vulvovaginitis, the complaints are of long-standing duration, there is often lack of demonstrable pathology, the patient has sought multiple consultations, response to treatment has been poor, symptoms seem out of proportion to objective findings, emotional lability may be present, and there may be reluctance to consider a psychophysiologic cause.

Painful micturition is usually a sign of urinary tract infection; local cutaneous inflammation (*Candida,* irritant dermatitis) may also cause stinging with a normal urinary stream. IC is different; it is constant pelvic and bladder pain associated with urinary frequency and mucosal inflammation. There is no precise definition for IC, its etiology and pathogenesis are unknown, and it is considered primarily a diagnosis of exclusion. Urine cultures and cytology studies are negative; cystoscopy may reveal only inflammation of the bladder wall. If no bladder abnormalities are found, the symptoms may be diagnosed as urethral syndrome (Bodner 1988). Irritative voiding symptoms are typical of both IC and urethral syndrome, and Wilkins and others (1989) have proposed that the latter may be an early form of IC.

Two-thirds of IC patients report dyspareunia, with 50% admitting to suicidal ideation. Held and associates (1988) estimated that there are between 20,000 and 90,000 diagnosed IC patients in the United States, 90% of whom are women. Because no uniform criteria exist for diagnosis of the syndrome, it is not unusual for patients to have symptoms undiagnosed for years and to be told that their discomfort is psychological. A small, but significant, percentage of IC patients also have vulvar vestibulitis, raising the possibility of a common neurological pathway.

Itching and Burning

The dermatologist usually has little difficulty distinguishing itchy skin from painful skin; itching is a "hands-on" problem, but burning or pain is a "hands-off" symptom (McKay 1985). When patients rub or scratch, they cause visible changes (excoriation, lichenification, and even ulceration), and the objective signs of pruritus confirm the diagnosis even if the patient denies any skin contact. Itchy mucosal surfaces do not show typical lichenification, and erosions heal quickly, so mild edema or redness may be the only evidence of rubbing. Burning, stinging, or rawness is even more difficult to assess, because patients usually avoid touching the affected skin.

In general, the description of "burning" seems to be applied more often to mucous membrane symptomatology than to that of keratinized epithelium elsewhere on the body. Itching can occur on mucous membranes but seems to be much more common on the conjunctiva, nasal mucosa, or genitalia. Mucosal itching often has a frantic, acute quality, possibly caused by inflammatory mediators. Mucous membranes are treated by different medical specialties (e.g., ophthalmology, otorhinolaryngology, dermatology, allergy, urology, dentistry), so reports of epithelial reactions and disorders may be difficult to compare. *Candida*, for example, is known to be a factor in oral as well as vaginal burning even without typical white mucosal plaques. Witkin (1987) proposed that this may represent a localized mucosal hypersensitivity to *Candida*, an association that may have significance to other mucous membrane symptoms as well. Another cause of mucosal burning is endogenous dysesthesia. Specific nerve roots may affect the entire perineum or localized perineal areas such as the urethra, scrotum, vulva, or anus (or anterior or posterior combinations). Wherever the location, many cutaneous dysesthesias respond well to low-dose tricyclic antidepressants (see "Endogenous Dysesthesias" section below).

Endogenous Dysesthesias

Many terms describe the cutaneous sensation of pain. Neurologists differentiate *neuralgia* (a sharp pain in the distribution of a specific nerve), *dysesthesia* (a disagreeable sensation present with ordinary stimuli), *allodynia* (a sharp pain evoked with light touch), and *causalgia* (a burning pain associated with nerve injury). The neuralgias or dysesthesias (e.g., postherpetic neuralgia) are probably more commonly encountered by nonneurologists. *Dysesthesia* is a useful term for superficial burning related to nerve distribution, because it includes specific neuralgias as well as nonspecific conditions such as reflex sympathetic dystrophy (RSD). The latter is superficial burning pain thought to be related to sympathetic innervation; minor nerve injury sets off hyperesthesia and burning pain that tends to spread beyond the affected dermatome. RSD symptoms are highly variable among individuals and over time, and its pathophysiology is poorly understood, especially as it affects the sacral nerves and pelvic floor.

Innervation of the perineum is primarily sacral in origin, and lateralization of symptoms is not consistent, as midline branches often overlap. At the vagina, the pudendal nerves are the major sensory branches. Further complicating the vulvovaginal neurological examination is the close involvement of internal organs: urethra, bladder, vagina, cervix, and rectum. There are relatively less nerve endings actually inside the vagina, for example, even though patients often complain of "vaginal burning." The vulvar introitus or vestibule is the usual source of this kind of discomfort, and coital stimulation of this area can trigger pain in adjacent areas.

Turner and Marinoff (1991) describe pudendal neuralgia as pain radiating from the vulva to the rest of the perineum, groin, or thighs; cutaneous hyperesthesia in a saddle distribution may extend from the mons pubis to the upper inner thighs and posteriorly across the ischial tuberosities. The diagnosis of pudendal neuralgia comprises a number of symptoms, so it can be difficult to identify a specific syndrome when one patient describes episodic paroxysmal stabbing discomfort, another deep aching, and yet another chronic burning. Sensory loss, as well as hyperacuity, may be another indication that pain is dysesthetic in nature. In some cases, a diagnostic-therapeutic trial of low-dose tricyclic antidepressants is helpful.

Amitriptyline, a tricyclic antidepressant, has proven effective over many years in the management of mucous membrane dysesthesias as well as pudendal and postherpetic neuralgias whether or not depression is present. In a review of the use of antidepressants for pain, France (1987) stated that the recommended dosage is one-half or less than that needed for treatment of depression, and treatment may generally be discontinued when symptoms are controlled. Side effects are common (dry mouth and an initial "tired" feeling), but low doses of 30 to 50 mg at bedtime are usually well tolerated and effective. In older patients, it is best to begin with only 10 mg at bedtime for the first week or two, then increase by 10 mg every week to the dosage required for control of symptoms (50 to 75 mg). Alternative medications with probable equal efficacy and much fewer side effects include nortriptyline, desipramine, trazodone, and clonazepam (a benzodiazepine). Fluoxetine, although well tolerated, has not as yet proven useful for the treatment of neuralgias or dysesthesias. Other neuropharmacologic drugs may also be used; consultation with specialists in neurology or psychiatry (see "Principles of Management" section below) is recommended.

Cutaneous Disorders

Dermatoses

The patient with skin disease at least has a physical change in addition to her symptomatology. She has generally had a more complete workup and is less likely to have been told that her problem is "all in her head." Infections caused by *Candida* or bacteria may be secondary to an underlying dermatitis that has altered the skin's normal barrier function. Table 9–1 summarizes diagnostic considerations described in more detail elsewhere (McKay 1991).

Lichen sclerosus et atrophicus (LS) is probably the most important vulvar dermatosis, not because it is common but because its localization to the vulva may not result in referral to a dermatologist for appropriate diagnosis and therapy. LS is one of three vulvar disorders with "lichen" in the name; the other two, lichen planus and lichen simplex chronicus, usually occur on other areas of the body as well as the vulva. Each disorder is completely different clinically and histologically; a dermatologist can generally recognize each without a biopsy. Unfortunately, gynecologists without the benefit of dermatological training tend to lump "the lichens" into a single group and have traditionally treated them with topical testosterone ointment to "toughen" the skin (a concept with little, if any, scientific basis).

Cutaneous disorders are chronic, and symptoms tend to flare and remit; this may mislead the patient and her physician regarding the efficacy of a particular treatment. Treatment failures may occur for many reasons, including inadequate length of therapy, incorrect potency of medication, incorrect medication, or resistance of the condition to the medication being used. Chronic skin problems should at least be evaluated, if not managed, by a dermatologist, most of whom have at least some experience in genital disease. Dalziel and co-workers (1991) completely changed the concept of LS therapy when they reported the effectiveness of high-potency topical steroids (clobetasol propionate, 0.05%) for this condition, which had previously been almost exclusively treated with topical testosterone. Therapy is maintained on a twice-a-day dosage for the first month or so, then decreased to daily until symptoms are controlled. Maintenance with low-dose steroids is recommended. In prepubertal girls, hydrocortisone cream (1% or 2.5%) is usually sufficient for control of symptoms.

Erosive vulvovaginitis is another complicated problem (see Table 9–1). Patients tend to be treated continually for primary infections, which are actually organisms secondarily invading the eroded mucosal surfaces. Treatment with immunosuppressives such as topical steroids or other agents is often very helpful; workup for systemic disease (i.e., lupus erythematosus) should be considered.

Infections

Candida

Candida is the most important infectious agent to consider in the evaluation of the patient with perineal burning or itching. The organism tends to set up an intense inflammatory reaction in sensitized individuals, and extensive erythema and edema are characteristic. Invasion of dermatitic skin (with a compromised barrier function) is almost a given, and anticandidal therapy should be used liberally. Women, probably because of a vaginal reservoir, seem to be much more likely to develop recurrent candidiasis. Predisposing factors include immunosuppression, systemic antibiotics, and estrogen therapy (oral contraceptives, estrogen replacement).

Cyclic vulvovaginitis may represent the host's immune response to some antigen or cross-reactive substance from the *Candida* organism, because some women remain symptomatic even after vaginal *Candida* has been eliminated by treatment (Ashman and Ott 1989; Witkin 1991). This may be caused by a localized hypersensitivity, with the mucosae

Table 9–1. Cutaneous disorders that may be associated with vulvar symptoms

Vulvar dermatoses	Symptoms	Appearance	Diagnostic test
Irritant dermatitis	Immediate stinging with topical applications; resolves in hours	Diffuse erythema, mild edema	Will not react on intact skin; stop topicals, use bland emollients
Contact dermatitis	48-hour lag between application and itchy rash; lasts 3 weeks	Oozing, weeping, itchy skin; edematous, may blister	Patch testing to ingredient causing allergy; avoid agent in future
Lichen simplex chronicus (LSC)	Intense chronic itching; persists after dermatitis (above)	Thickened skin with scaling and wrinkling	History of scratching; biopsy, KOH for tinea (below)
Lichen sclerosus	May itch or burn; sometimes asymptomatic	White skin, scarring, loss of vulvar folds; progressive without therapy	Biopsy (may occur in childhood)
Lichen planus	Vaginal discharge, soreness	Vulva: purplish papules; vagina and/or mouth: erosions and scarring	Biopsy for histopathology
Psoriasis	May itch or become fissured	Thickened, scaly, fissured skin; lesions on knees, elbows common	History of psoriasis; biopsy, KOH for tinea (below)

	Symptoms	Appearance	Diagnostic test
Seborrheic dermatitis	Mild itching	Intertriginous rash or plaques, no pustules	Appearance; consider KOH for *Candida* or tinea versicolor (below)
Hidradenitis suppurativa	Painful "boils"	Recurrent deep cysts and sinus tracts; scarring and purulent drainage	History; biopsy to rule out cutaneous Crohn's disease
Vulvovaginal erosions	Symptoms	Appearance	Diagnostic test
Aphthosis	Recurrent painful ulcers	"Canker sores," oral/vaginal mucosa	History; culture to rule out herpes
Behçet's syndrome	Recurrent painful ulcers, arthritis, uveitis	Large ulcers, often after trauma	History of systemic involvement; biopsy
Bullous dermatoses	Vulvovaginal erosions and ulcers	Blisters elsewhere on the body	Biopsy for immunofluoresence
Erosive lichen planus	Vaginal discharge, soreness	Vagina and/or mouth: erosions and scarring	Biopsy
Desquamative vaginitis	Vaginal discharge, soreness	Erosions and scarring in vagina, rarely in mouth	Biopsy (may be erosive lichen planus variant)

(continued)

Table 9–1. Cutaneous disorders that may be associated with vulvar symptoms (*continued*)

Infections	Symptoms	Appearance	Diagnostic test
Candida	Itching, burning, swelling; often a secondary infection	Erythema, edema, satellite pustules, ± white vaginal discharge	KOH examination, culture
Herpes simplex	Painful, tiny ulcers; deep "ache"	Single painful papule or grouped blisters	Culture fresh lesion for virus
Herpes zoster	Intense pain, may involve leg	Multiple blisters and erosions	Culture for virus
Streptococcal cellulitis	Persistent soreness and erythema of skin	Erythematous plaque (more common in pediatric patients)	Difficult to culture; prescribe antibiotics
Molluscum contagiosum	Itching or asymptomatic	Umbilicated papules	Biopsy
Staphylococcal furunculosis	Painful pustules	Erythematous pustules and papules at hair follicles; responds to antibiotics	Culture for antibiotic sensitivity; if chronic, consider fungal culture
Tinea	Itching, folliculitis	Rash with scalloped border, may blister or scale	KOH examination
Tinea versicolor	Occasionally itchy	Salmon-colored or pale macules with slight scale	KOH examination

Note. KOH = potassium hydroxide.

exhibiting a persistent allergic reaction that reactivates when only a few *Candida* organisms or antigens are present. Other infectious causes of vaginitis (bacterial vaginosis, *Trichomonas*) have not been associated with chronic burning, although frequent treatment with antibiotics (including oral metronidazole) may precipitate *Candida* superinfection.

Herpes Simplex Virus (HSV)

HSV is a recurrent problem that usually presents with a prodromal ache or itch, followed by the development of painful grouped papules or vesicles that erode, leaving an exposed sore that heals in 7 to 10 days. Some patients have recurrent lesions within a few-centimeters radius, whereas others report that lesions skip locations, even crossing the midline (a pattern similar to oral recurrences). Human immunodeficiency virus (HIV)-positive or immunosuppressed patients may have continuous infections that are resistant to standard therapies. Any persistent cutaneous erosion in these patients should always be cultured for HSV.

Cervical or vaginal lesions may cause symptoms more typical of pudendal neuralgia (episodic discomfort, dysesthesias of the groin or buttock, or sciatica-like pain extending down the back of a thigh). It is very rare for HSV to recur more often than every 3 to 4 weeks; most recurrences are months apart. Pains that are constant, short-lived, or episodic in cycles less than 2 weeks apart are unlikely to be HSV related. For a primary HSV infection, acyclovir is given in a dosage of 200 mg by mouth every 4 hours, five doses daily, for 10 days. Recurrences are treated on the same schedule but for only 5 days. HSV outbreaks can usually be suppressed with 400 mg acyclovir (two tablets) twice daily; some patients do well on 200 mg three times daily.

Herpes Zoster

Herpes zoster (postherpetic neuralgia) is usually diagnosed by the history of a unilateral blistering eruption that often extends to the thigh or leg. Treatment of postzoster neuralgia is the same as that outlined above for pudendal neuralgia, beginning with tricyclic antidepressants. Capsaicin cream, a topical medication that acts on peripheral sensory neurons by depleting substance P, is a relatively new therapeutic agent. Although it has been reported to be effective in postherpetic neuralgia and arthritis elsewhere on the body, drawbacks include the necessity of frequent application and exacerbation of burning discomfort during the first few days of medication use; the latter is a major limitation to its use on mucous membranes at the vaginal introitus.

Streptococcal Cellulitis
Streptococcal cellulitis usually presents as persistent perirectal erythema and irritation, typically over a period of weeks or months (Kokx et al. 1987; Rehder et al. 1988). It is more likely to occur in early childhood and presents with painful defecation and chronic perianal fissures, which may be misdiagnosed as *Candida*. In adults, it is most likely to be seen in immunosuppressed individuals. Long-term antibiotic (erythromycin) therapy may be required.

Human Papillomavirus Infection
Human papillomavirus (HPV; condylomata acuminata) may be symptomatic, especially if extensive lesions make hygiene difficult. Secondary *Candida* infection can complicate the picture, but so-called subclinical HPV is often overdiagnosed as a factor in chronic vulvar burning. The labia minora may become thickened and papillomatous from continuous rubbing and excoriation (lichen simplex chronicus). This condition will gradually resolve as the dermatitis clears. Vestibular papillae are normal in the vulvar vestibule and should not be mistaken for condylomata (Friedrich 1983, 1987, 1988; McKay et al. 1991). Aggressive therapy should be reserved for cervical or vulvar intraepithelial neoplasia, intractable symptoms, or disease recurrence after successful therapy.

Molluscum Contagiosum
Molluscum contagiosum is a disease characterized by flesh-colored umbilicated papules. Tiny lesions may be mistaken for folliculitis, and a grouping may be misdiagnosed as umbilicated vesicles of herpes simplex. Local destruction of lesions (by freezing with liquid nitrogen or by opening lesions with a needle and expressing the contents) is generally effective, but repeated visits may be necessary to treat recurrences.

Staphylococcal Furunculosis
Staphylococcal furunculosis is folliculitis on the mons pubis; pustules at the base of hair follicles are typical of this diagnosis. Pustules not associated with follicles are more likely to be caused by *Candida*; furuncles that do not respond to appropriate antibiotic therapy (dicloxacillin) may be caused by tinea. Topical steroids should be used with caution in the presence of folliculitis, because either bacteria or fungi (and sometimes both) may be present.

IATROGENIC FACTORS

Side Effects of Topical Steroids

The chronic use of potent fluorinated steroids on skin with a high concentration of sebaceous glands (face, vulva) often results in a rebound inflammatory reaction, with erythema and a burning sensation that flares each time the steroid is withdrawn. Because the steroid may have been prescribed for nonspecific symptoms originally, the patient is likely to continue treating the burning and erythema with the agent causing the problem. Tiny pustules are typical of sebaceous hyperactivity and may cause rebound dermatitis that is mistaken for acute candidal infection, and vice versa. High-potency steroids combined with anticandidal drugs may worsen rather than treat the problem. Potent steroids should be reserved for thick and itchy lesions or biopsy-proven vaginal erosive disorders; they should not be used at all on erythematous and/or burning skin.

CO_2 Laser

Removal of the epidermis by CO_2 laser ablation (burning) is a traumatic procedure. Healing by secondary intention is painful in any area, but the genitalia are especially sensitive. Superficial nerve injuries may take months to resolve. In some cases, it seems that vulvar vestibulitis has been initiated by laser therapy. It is not known how this occurs or how it can be avoided; many cases of vestibulitis occur spontaneously, and a few have even been improved with laser therapy, so this does not prove a cause-and-effect relationship. The indications for CO_2 laser are carcinoma in situ (vulvar intraepithelial neoplasia) and extensive condylomata. Treatment of these conditions may warrant the limited risk. Experience has shown that the CO_2 laser is not the treatment of choice for symptomatic vulvar burning.

Alcohol Injections

Gynecologic textbooks have recommended several surgical approaches to the treatment of "intractable pruritus vulvae." Along with vulvectomy or surgical denervation of the vulva (the Mering procedure), one of the best approaches was said to be injecting small aliquots of absolute ethyl alcohol subcutaneously into the entire surface of the vulva. Lichenified skin is relatively resistant to trauma, which might account for the relative success reported, but it should be noted that alcohol injection has never been advocated by dermatologists, who see intractable itching on many areas of the body. Later publications (Clouser and Friedrich 1986; Kaufman et al. 1989) recommended the standard dermatological procedure of injecting intralesional triamcinolone (5 to 10 mg/ml) and, most important, noted that subcutaneous alcohol injection was "of no value" to the patient with vulvar burning. The normal-thickness skin seen in vulvodynia (as opposed to that of lichen simplex chronicus) is far less resistant to trauma; tissue slough is likely, leaving scarring indistinguishable in some cases from atrophic LS.

OVERVIEW OF PRURITUS
VULVAE (ITCHING)

As noted above, chronic genital itching or burning is a perplexing problem for patients and their physicians. With vulvodynia, the search is directed toward possible etiologies and different patterns of pain; pruritus vulvae is an end-stage condition, and the original inciting cause of the itch is unlikely to be found. The key to successful treatment is helping the patient to understand the expectations of therapy: that progress will be slow, and symptom flares do not necessarily mean that the treatment is no longer effective.

Patients often present a long list of medications that have been prescribed by other physicians and complain, "Nothing works." When asked specifically, "Do you mean that the medicine works as long as you use it, or that it doesn't work at all?" the patient often admits that the medication is indeed effective when it is applied but is upset that the symptoms return when it is discontinued. Once the patient understands that therapy must be continued for several weeks, she will be less likely to abandon a potentially effective treatment program when results are not immediately apparent. As dermatologists know well, there are no "miracle cures" or "magic pills" for chronic itching; this may be why patients have been willing to submit to such drastic measures as surgery for conditions that can be successfully treated with time and topical therapy.

Topical steroids are very effective for chronic itching, but the patient should be prescribed only the strength necessary to control symptoms; fluorinated steroids should not be given for normal-thickness skin that is red and burning. Thickened plaques of lichen simplex chronicus may require high-potency steroids, at least initially; betamethasone dipropionate 0.05% or clobetasol propionate 0.05% can be used to treat lichen simplex chronicus for 6 to 8 weeks without complication. On the other hand, much less potent preparations can set off periorificial dermatitis and rebound burning if used on nonlichenified skin (see above section, "Side Effects of Topical Steroids").

In a detailed and well-referenced discussion, Koblenzer (1987) noted that pruritus ani is multifactorial in origin; seborrhea, maceration, hygienic aspects, dietary indiscretions (causing irritating elements in the feces), and secondary infection with bacteria and yeasts all act as potential contributors and exacerbators. A review by Verbov (1984) emphasized the difference between idiopathic and secondary pruritus ani, stating that an underlying cause can be determined in only 30% of women with this disorder. Hanno and Murphy (1987) emphasized that fecal contamination is the most common problem in pruritus ani, mostly acting as an irritant to perineal skin. The influence of psychogenic factors in the etiology of pruritus ani has long been debated. Well-informed professional opinion is currently less likely to consider the symptom of anal itching as a psychiatric symptom, although there is agreement that psychic stresses may be an aggravating or perpetuating factor, as they are in other chronic dermatoses.

The use of tricyclic antidepressants such as nortriptyline or doxepin should be reserved for those cases in which other causes of pruritus ani have been ruled out. Hydroxyzine hydrochloride has been shown to be effective in other pruritic dermatoses and is probably the best first-line systemic medication, especially if the pruritus is thought to be allergy related.

In childhood, genital pruritus is often the result of irritant dermatitis. Young girls may have fecal contamination of the vulva by not wiping front-to-back, may overscrub the genitalia, or may take irritating bubble baths. Pinworms are more common in childhood and typically involve the anus but may also be seen at the vaginal opening. Vaginal or rectal discharge in childhood should be evaluated for evidence of possible sexual abuse (sperm may be identified microscopically), and genital lesions should be examined carefully. LS (see "Cutaneous Disorders" section above) can occur in childhood, and the friable purpuric lesions of this disorder may suggest trauma when they are discovered.

PATTERNS OF VULVODYNIA (BURNING)

Patients who complain of vulvar burning may describe different patterns of discomfort, which, coupled with characteristic physical findings, may give diagnostic clues to the patient's problem (Table 9–2).

INTERMITTENT VULVAR BURNING

Cyclic Vulvovaginitis

This condition is most often seen in women aged 25 to 45 years who produce their own estrogens or who are on estrogen replacement therapy after gynecologic surgery. Patients typically describe recurrent episodes of vulvar burning, often related to a specific time during each menstrual cycle (during ovulation, for example, or just before menses). Dyspareunia is reported as "irritation after intercourse," with inflammation at the introitus. Vaginal discharge is rare, although the introitus is often inflamed; the patient is usually symptom free at other times of the month. Although there does not seem to be a relationship to premenstrual syndrome, physicians and the patient's consort sometimes will assume that cyclic vulvovaginitis is actually a hormonally mediated psychogenic problem. The patient may ascribe postcoital irritation to "allergy," either to condoms or to the partner's semen, but this would be unlikely to occur on an intermittent basis. True allergy to seminal fluid (Matloff 1993) or latex (Task Force 1993) is an immediate (antigen-antibody mediated) reaction; urticaria and itching are typical and occur every time the allergen comes in contact with the sensitized mucosae. In some cases, asthma and even anaphylactic reactions have occurred.

Little is known about the influence of premenopausal hormonal changes on vulvovaginal mucosal symptomatology, but it is likely that several components may be involved. A hyperactive immune response to *Candida* or cross-reactive substances has been postulated as a major factor in this symptom complex. Patients with cyclic vulvovaginitis have almost always had a positive vaginal culture for *Candida* at some point, and they improve temporarily on anticandidal therapy (but usually flare within a month or so after a course of treatment). Sobel (1986) first reported that effective treatment of this group of vulvodynia patients can be based on long-term (4 to 6 months) maintenance therapy with local or systemic anticandidal agents. Either oral fluconazole or an

Table 9–2. Differential diagnosis of vulvodynia

	Symptoms	Physical findings	Therapy
Vulvar dermatoses	See Table 9–1	See Table 9–1	Usually with some form of topical steroid; potency depends on severity of disease.
Cyclic vulvovaginitis	Flare of symptoms with menses; pattern may vary with individual. Dyspareunia: irritation *after* intercourse, often with swelling.	Erythema and edema of mucosae, vaginal discharge rare. History or presence of positive *Candida* cultures. Estrogen: endogenous or replacement.	Long-term, low-dose anticandidals: topical with azoles M-W-F, systemic with fluconazole 1–2 times weekly.
Vulvar vestibulitis	Entry dyspareunia: pain on insertion into vagina; usually posterior, sometimes periurethral as well.	Erythema and tenderness to palpation of ostia of Bartholin's glands at posterior introitus.	Conservative: anticandidals and topical steroids for inflammation, trial of oral hydroxyzine or amitriptyline. Surgery: partial vestibulectomy.
Dysesthetic vulvodynia	Constant unremitting burning, may be improved with lying down. Patients usually postmenopausal. Younger patients often have history of urethral or low back pain.	Minimal; only various degrees of erythema (may be the result of previous therapy).	Low-dose tricyclic antidepressants: amitriptyline, nortriptyline, desipramine; or trazodone, clonazepam. Discontinue with relief of symptoms.

applicator of imidazole or azole vaginal cream may be used, but treatment must continue for several months. This is usually initiated on a twice-daily basis for 2 weeks, then daily for 1 month. After that, one-half applicator of vaginal cream may be used daily for 1 month, decreasing to a half-dose Monday-Wednesday-Friday for another 2 months. Fluconazole, 150 mg orally, seems to be effective as a once- or twice-weekly dosage, is less hepatotoxic than ketoconazole, and does not appear to interact with the antihistamine terfenadine in causing cardiac arrhythmias (see Chapter 2). When *Candida* growth has been suppressed over time, the inflamed mucosa regains its normal barrier function, and medication is no longer required (except prophylactically when the patient must take antibiotics).

CONSTANT VULVAR BURNING

Dysesthetic Vulvodynia

These women are typically postmenopausal and often elderly, and they describe constant vulvar burning in a diffuse pattern, usually over the entire surface of the inner labia minora, sometimes extending onto the labia majora (McKay 1993). The burning is low grade, "always present," and is usually not worsened by touch or wiping. Little can be seen except for a variable erythema, often related to the use of topical medications. Dysesthetic vulvodynia was originally proposed as a diagnosis of exclusion ("essential" vulvodynia) to describe a neurological problem that might relate to damaged sensory nerves or an altered perception of sensation. Patients respond to the same low-dose tricyclic antidepressant regimens used to treat postzoster or pudendal neuralgia (see "Endogenous Dysesthesias" section above).

Urethral or rectal discomfort in addition to vulvar burning may also be part of this symptom complex. These patients are rarely taking estrogen replacements, and, if sexually active, they seldom complain of primary dyspareunia. Tricyclic antidepressant therapy alone (or in conjunction with topical lidocaine 5% ointment) is rarely helpful in vulvodynia patients younger than age 40 years unless they also have symptoms typical of fibromyalgia or urethral syndrome, disorders also reported to respond in some cases to low-dose tricyclic antidepressants (McKay 1993).

Vulvar Vestibulitis

The vestibule is the vulvovaginal area where squamous epithelium changes to mucous membrane. For illustrative purposes, consider the lips and oral cavity; in this model, the labia minora would be equivalent to the lips and the hymenal ring to the gums. Just as the salivary glands lie within the lateral corners of the mouth, the major vestibular glands (Skene's and Bartholin's) as well as the minor glands and the urethra are located in the mucosal vestibule distal to the hymenal ring. For unknown reasons, the vestibular glands may become tender and inflamed. This condition can be acute or chronic, and dyspareunia is the result.

Friedrich (1983, 1987) and Woodruff and Friedrich (1985) were the first to describe what later came to be defined by the International Society for the Study of Vulvovaginal Disease as vulvar vestibulitis (McKay et al. 1991). This is a chronic, persistent clinical syndrome characterized by severe pain on vestibular touch or attempted vaginal entry, tenderness to pressure localized within the vulvar vestibule, and physical findings confined to vestibular erythema of various degrees. Vulvar vestibulitis is a clinical diagnosis; biopsy is rarely of benefit because findings are nonspecific.

Other than vaginismus, pain at or around the vestibular glands is probably the primary cause of entry dyspareunia. In fact, there may well be a continuum between vestibulitis and vaginismus as pain triggers muscle spasms that may recur over months or years. Many investigators have sought an infectious agent in vestibular tissues and glands. Although *Candida* and HPV have been found in a few cases, they have not been present to any significant degree in any study. A definitive histopathological study of vestibular tissue by Pyka and colleagues (1988) revealed only chronic inflammation and local destruction of these glands; damage to nerve endings has also been postulated as a cause of continuing pain.

Episodic entry dyspareunia or vestibulitis seems to have a better prognosis. Remissions occur spontaneously and with conservative therapy. These measures include minimizing local inflammation with regular use of hydrocortisone cream or ointment, avoiding irritating topical medications or high-potency topical steroids, and preventing vaginal yeast infections by using vaginal anticandidal creams or suppositories when taking antibiotics. The idiosyncratic nature of symptom flares makes evaluation of treatment plans difficult; special diets and over-the-counter supplements should be considered experimental. Aggressive destructive therapy such as laser or extensive application of acid solutions for nonspecific findings (e.g., subclinical HPV) may precipitate vulvar vestibulitis in some cases, although this is not predictable. Episodes of entry dyspareunia in the past or worsening of discomfort after local therapy may be indicators of risk.

Vulvar vestibulitis is probably the most important element to evaluate in multifactorial vulvodynia and seems to be the most refractory to treatment (Friedrich 1988). An informal poll of the Committee on Vulvodynia at the 1991 International Society for the Study of Vulvovaginal Disease Congress confirmed that most experts believe that vulvar vestibulitis is probably preventable, although as yet only speculation exists on etiologic or exacerbating factors. If vulvar vestibulitis has persisted for more than 1 or 2 years (i.e., conservative therapy has failed), surgical resection of the affected area may be the only remaining treatment option. Vulvar vestibulectomy consists of removal of a crescent-shaped portion of the affected vestibule, including the adjacent hymenal ring; the vaginal mucosa is undermined and advanced to keratinized skin on the perineum where it is closed primarily. The surgery is low risk with regard to sexual functioning; the anatomic changes do not interfere with clitoral stimulation or orgasm, and, in the sexually mature female, the Bartholin's glands are insignificant in vaginal lubrication in comparison to vaginal secretions. For an excellent overview of vulvar vestibulitis syndrome, including surgical therapy, see Marinoff and Turner (1992).

Patients may be overly optimistic about surgery for vulvodynia, especially if they are impatient for "quick relief." The psychiatrist counseling a patient with vulvodynia and/or dyspareunia should recognize the need for adequate workup and appropriate consultation to confirm the diagnosis. Vulvar vestibulitis is the only condition that responds to surgery; if the patient has not had unremitting entry dyspareunia for 6 to 12 months, the procedure should not be considered. Surgery will not help other patterns of vulvodynia. Treatment of "subclinical" HPV with the CO_2 laser has, in some cases, worsened vulvar vestibulitis. This treatment modality should be used with great caution in patients who already complain of vulvodynia. The success rate of excisional surgery for vulvar vestibulitis is only about 80%–85%, even with experienced surgeons. If the consultant gynecologist is not familiar with the diagnostic nuances of vulvodynia, the success rate is significantly less; in general, the more experienced the surgeon, the better he or she will be able to select patients who are most likely to benefit from vestibulectomy.

When McCormack (1990) reviewed 46 young women with symptoms involving tissues derived from the embryonic urogenital sinus, he found 10 with IC, 25 with focal vulvitis (vulvar vestibulitis), and 11 with both diagnoses, suggesting a possible analogy between certain urethral and vulvovaginal disorders. Cyclic vulvovaginitis and chronic inflammation may be precursors to vulvar vestibulitis in the same way that urethral syndrome may be related to IC. More research remains to be done on both topics.

PRINCIPLES OF MANAGEMENT

Success depends mostly on appropriate diagnosis and therapy, but the relationship between the patient and her physician is a significant factor in her recovery. The clinician's attitude is extremely important in the management of symptoms in patients with vulvodynia. Genital pain is an emotional issue. Although treatment of vulvodynia is successful in most cases, the response is typically slow. Overnight relief is very rare; small increments of improvement occur slowly over time. Regular follow-up appointments to review and emphasize progress encourage both the patient and physician to remain with adequate treatment trials. Between appointments, patients may call physicians with questions about medications, but major therapeutic changes should not be instituted without an office visit. The patient should be discouraged from calling with "emergency" complaints, especially outside of office hours. Symptomatic perineal or genital discomfort does not resolve rapidly, and several weeks or even months of therapy are the rule, not the exception. Episodic flares can be expected and mean very little in the overall course of management. Patients should be warned that these will occur so that they will not panic and interrupt what might otherwise be an effective treatment plan. Flares gradually become less severe, last for a shorter time, and occur less often as the patient recovers. Physicians who calmly explain management strategies for chronic symptomatic problems should be able to develop a pleasant working relationship with these patients who have chronic pain and appreciate genuine caring and concern for their problem.

Indications for Psychiatric Referral

If the patient is refractory to the above principles, a psychiatric referral is warranted. The referral may best be presented as "an augmentation" to treatment; however, some cases may justify making ongoing treatment contingent on psychiatric assessment. The following considerations, combined with clinical judgment, can help in deciding when to make a psychiatric referral. Although the vulvodynia patient population is heterogeneous, the patient presentation is rather uniform. In general, women are eager for improvement, forthcoming and specific with their medical history, and focused on their chief complaint. Patients lacking this typical presentation should raise a flag for psychiatric consultation. Other factors that can help identify the need for consultation are continued demands for specific tests, disbelief in test results, and extensive attempts to make contact outside of appointment times. Patients with additional stressors in their lives (e.g., other medical problems, divorce, loss of a job) are at higher risk for a psychiatric disorder. The degree to which a patient is isolated or lacking a support system will also increase her vulnerability to emotional difficulties. A patient with vulvodynia who has a history of a prior psychiatric disorder is in all likelihood at increased risk for relapse caused by the stress and chronicity of her symptoms. Also, any patient with a suspected personality disorder or even excessive traits, such as histrionic or compulsive individuals, would probably benefit from a psychiatric consultation in establishing a treatment plan to minimize regressive, stress-related behavior and augment positive means of coping with the medical problem.

PSYCHIATRIC ISSUES

General Approach

The typical referred patient with vulvodynia defies a simple categorization, but some general principles can be applied. Based on the multifactorial nature of the problem as well as other factors mentioned later in the chapter (cyclical symptoms, current state of medical knowledge, iatrogenic confounds, societal biases), these patients will probably already have a chronic pain syndrome by the time a psychiatric evaluation is recommended. As with other disorders associated with chronic pain, such as headaches or lower back pain, it is important to address the prior and current treatments, the stress from the symptom(s), and stressors that may be exacerbating the symptoms. At the same time, the patient should be evaluated for complicating comorbid psychiatric disorders. A thorough assessment requires a summary of prior physician contacts, prior treatments, and current treatment plans; verbal contact with the referring physician can also provide a helpful focus before assessing the patient. Once the clinician is satisfied that the patient has received adequate prior medical evaluation and appropriate treatment, the patient's perception of her course of evaluation(s) and treatment(s) can be addressed without discounting her physical symptoms. If the patient believes that the psychiatrist is working in concert with her and the referring physician, the efficiency of treatment is maximized with regard to time course, symptom improvement, and the patient's psychological well-being.

Specific Approaches

A general strategy for the psychiatric evaluation of any patient who believes her primary problem is physical in nature is to look for the possibility of primary and secondary gains. Primary gain may be avoidance of conflict, ranging from absenteeism from a stressful job to decreased sexual activity in an unhappy relationship. Secondary gains may include increased attention, sympathy, and physical rest. It is obvious that establishing rapport and trust is essential in discovering unconscious or repressed conflicts and making appropriate interpretations and interventions. It is also important to inquire about the psychiatric history of both the patient and her family to ascertain the likelihood of increased risk for certain problems.

Sexual Abuse

Historical biases and current societal issues have led to a focus on underlying sexual components for gynecologic symptoms and symptoms involving the lower gastrointestinal tract. Most controlled studies examined populations with chronic pelvic pain and the prevalence of prior sexual abuse (Huber and Roos 1985; Rapkin et al. 1990; Reiter et al. 1991; Walker et al. 1988) as opposed to vulvar pain. Our own preliminary data (M. M., J. F., unpublished, 1994) (with $n = 15$ and $n = 33$) as well as the study by Stewart and colleagues (1990) have not found a higher prevalence of a history of sexual abuse in patients with vulvodynia compared with the general population (Russell 1983). Note, however, that research is limited and potentially confounded by multiple definitions of sexual abuse as well as patients' hesitancy to disclose that part of their history in a screening interview. Prior sexual trauma may be a factor in some patients with vulvodynia; this information is most likely to be elicited in a trusting and supportive setting.

Chronic Pain

Pain is a complex entity in itself, and pain associated with genitalia has added psychological dimensions involving self-image and intimacy. There is a large volume of research on the management of chronic pain syndromes. The Multidimensional Pain Inventory (Kerns et al. 1985) is a psychometric instrument developed to integrate measurements of cognitive, behavioral, and affective dimensions of pain. It provides a helpful categorization of patients into three groups: adaptive copers, interpersonally distressed, and dysfunctional (Walter and Brannon 1991). Patients with vulvodynia are a heterogeneous population whose predominant psychological traits and behaviors could be described using the above categories; the latter two groups are most likely to contain the patients receiving a psychiatric referral. With this conceptual scheme, the therapeutic goal becomes the recategorization of the patient into an "adaptive coper" by defining the areas of distress or dysfunction, exploring alternative behaviors, augmenting coping skills, and managing symptoms. This last aspect of therapy can involve relaxation training, biofeedback, and medication (Portenoy 1993).

Medication

Depending on the clinical presentation of the referred vulvodynia patient, the primary physician may prescribe a low dose of an antidepressant (usually a tricyclic), an anticonvulsant (usually carbamazepine or clonazepam), or hormone-replacement therapy. Patients with dysesthetic vulvodynia are likely to fit into the category of "chronic pain syndrome" and often benefit from tricyclic antidepressants or carbamazepine. Nonsteroidal and narcotic drugs have not been found to be efficacious in treating vulvar pain. If a patient meets diagnostic criteria for a major mood or anxiety disorder, a trial of antidepressant medication at therapeutic levels is warranted. Multiple studies have demonstrated improved pain control with amitriptyline (France 1987) for a variety of disorders including vulvodynia (McKay 1993). Desipramine (Coquoz et al. 1993; Max et al. 1992), nortriptyline (Walker et al. 1991), and moclobemide, a reversible monoamine oxidase inhibitor (not available yet in the United States) (Coquoz et al. 1993), have also been found to augment pain management. To date, the data are mixed on the efficacy of serotonin reuptake inhibitors in pain control (Adly et al. 1992; Coquoz et al. 1993; Diamond and Freitag 1989). Choice of an antidepressant should take into account the patient's sense of pain control and evaluation of any ongoing psychotropic medication, as well as the usual considerations of target symptoms, side-effect profile, concurrent medical conditions, drug interactions, pregnancy and menopausal status, and birth control. Response and compliance are enhanced by including the patient and referring physician in treatment planning.

Substance Abuse, Somatoform Disorders

Substance abuse may develop in response to the chronicity of pain or stress. It is underdiagnosed in women (Brady et al. 1993; Cyr and Moulton 1993) because the majority of past research has defined male patterns of abuse. Somatoform disorders can be missed when a patient is referred from a specialist focusing on one medical problem. The psychiatrist should obtain a complete medical history and further screen for somatoform disorders as clinically indicated. Our clinical impression is that somatization disorder is not strongly associated with the vulvodynia syndrome.

SUMMARY

The psychiatrist who has an interest in working with vulvodynia patients can also gain insight by appreciating the physician-patient dynamic in relation to the different medical specialists who may refer these patients. Consultation services may need to be modified according to the expectations the patient has developed as a result of interaction with her physician(s). Some medical specialties have more appeal to certain personality types than others, and a few general comments may be useful in this context. Gynecologists and urologists are surgically oriented. Patient problems are approached in a direct fashion, and most are considered "curable." In fact, most gynecologic problems are treated by surgical procedures of some type (cancer, infertility), antibiotics or antifungals, and adjustment or replacement of hormones. The gynecologist can frequently "take the problem away" for the patient, and this is part of this specialty's appeal to those who choose it.

Patients with complex, painful problems are unusual and may be perceived as fascinating or annoying, depending on the patient's ability to form a relationship with the physician. Almost every gynecologist has a handful of patients with recalcitrant vulvovaginal symptoms; it is unfortunate that there are not enough of these patients for most physicians to see patterns to their complaints, and these patients do not respond to exactly the same management plans.

Patients may feel extreme loyalty to a gynecologist who has been there for them through pregnancies and emergencies; they may persistently follow their doctor's directions even when they do not seem to be particularly sensible to the outside observer. At the other end of the spectrum, healthy patients who have seen the gynecologist only for yearly Papanicolaou smears may have little loyalty to one over another. They will change treatment plans in midstream, often based on advice from a friend or a women's magazine. They want quick results and cures and will seek a physician who claims to be able to provide them. A patient who has performed her own literature search and has many questions may intimidate the physician to the point that she is perceived as having "unreasonable" demands. An assertive patient may be referred to a psychiatrist more readily than the passive, compliant patient who does not "cause trouble," even though it may be the latter patient who is clinically depressed and more in need of consultation.

The dermatologist or neurologist is more comfortable dealing with chronic, symptomatic discomfort. Dermatologists especially are accustomed to prolonged treatment trials, flares and remissions of disease (especially stress exacerbated), and, most important, the psychological effects of altered body image. Relatively few skin diseases are curable, and dermatology patients are frequently anxious, upset, frightened, angry, or otherwise difficult to manage. Dermatologists recognize that accurate assessment of the patient's personality traits is essential to their ability to treat skin problems successfully; the patient must cooperate in managing chronic and nonemergent disease. When a patient has both skin and psychiatric disorders, the dermatologist may or may not recognize personality disorders that will prevent the patient from following a treatment plan successfully. Like neurological problems, many skin diseases are multifactorial, and these specialists are trained to approach problems methodically and rationally, believing more in objective than subjective evidence. The nonsurgeon's gratification, then, depends less on "curing" the patient than on the correct identification of the problem and the establishment of an effective treatment plan. If the patient is unwilling or unable to cooperate with the physician in a rational plan, the psychiatrist's consultation may be sought.

The psychiatrist can become a valued colleague to any specialist treating vulvodynia patients. The problem is complex; the relative newness of the disorder makes it fertile territory for systematic clinical research. Significant clinical experience has shown vulvodynia patients to be diagnostically challenging but responsive to informed and methodical medical management. In our clinical experience, psychiatric interventions are likewise usually received positively, and "resistant" patients present no greater obstacles than any psychiatric population. Successful treatment of a patient with chronic pain is an extremely rewarding experience; there is much to be gained by working in an area in which so much can be learned.

AREAS OF FUTURE RESEARCH

More studies ascertaining the prevalence of comorbid psychiatric disorders need to be undertaken. The results would direct further research regarding the efficacy of various psychiatric interventions and the determination of the choice of intervention. Specifically, questions are 1) Is outcome, in terms of response to treatment and efficiency of treatment (number of physicians, cost, time course) improved by psychiatric intervention? and 2) What type of interventions (medication, individual therapy, group therapy) are effective? The high prevalence and chronicity of vulvodynia, coupled with its multiple emotional factors, make it a fruitful area of psychiatric research.

REFERENCES

Adly C, Straumanis J, Chesson A: Fluoxetine prophylaxis of migraine. Headache 32:101–104, 1992

Ashman RB, Ott AK: Autoimmunity as a factor in recurrent vaginal candidosis and the minor vestibular gland syndrome. J Reprod Med 34:264–266, 1989

Bodner DR: The urethral syndrome. Urol Clin North Am 15:699–704, 1988

Brady KT, Grice DE, Dustan L, et al: Gender differences in substance use disorders. Am J Psychiatry 150:1707–1711, 1993

Clouser JK, Friedrich EG Jr: A new technique for alcohol injection in the vulva. J Reprod Med 31:971–972, 1986

Coquoz D, Porchet HC, Dayer P: Central analgesic effects of desipramine, fluoxamine, and moclobemide after single oral dosing: a study in healthy volunteers. Clin Pharmacol Ther 54:339–344, 1993

Cormia FE: Basic concepts in the production and management of the psychosomatic dermatoses. Br J Dermatol 63:83–92, 1951

Cyr MG, Moulton AW: The physician's role in prevention, detection, and treatment of alcohol abuse in women. Psychiatric Annals 23:454–462, 1993

Dalziel KL, Millard R, Wojnarowska F: The treatment of vulval lichen sclerosus with a very potent topical steroid (clobetasol propionate 0.05%) cream. Br J Dermatol 124:461–464, 1991

Diamond S, Freitag FG: The use of fluoxetine in the treatment of headache (letter). Clin J Pain 5:200–201, 1989

Dodson MG, Friedrich EG Jr: Psychosomatic vulvovaginitis. Obstet Gynecol 51 (suppl 1): 23S–25S, 1978

Drueck CJ: Pruritus vulvae and repressed sexual urge. Neurologic Cutaneous Reviews 49:306–308, 1945

France RD: The future for antidepressants: treatment of pain. Psychopathology 20 (suppl 1):99–113, 1987

Friedrich EG Jr: The vulvar vestibule. J Reprod Med 28:773–777, 1983

Friedrich EG Jr: Vulvar vestibulitis syndrome. J Reprod Med 32:110–114, 1987

Friedrich EG Jr: Therapeutic studies on vulvar vestibulitis. J Reprod Med 33:514–518, 1988

Hanno R, Murphy P: Pruritus ani: classification and management. Dermatol Clin 5:811–816, 1987

Held P, Hanno PM, Wein AJ, et al: A study of women with painful bladder syndrome, NIH workshop on interstitial cystitis, 1987. J Urol 140:203–206, 1988

Huber J, Roos C: Effects of spouse abuse and/or sexual abuse in the development and maintenance of chronic pain in women, in Advances in Pain Research and Therapy, Vol 9. Edited by Fields HL. New York, Raven, 1985, pp 889–895

Jeffcoate TNA: Pruritus vulvae. BMJ 2:1196–1200, 1949

Kaufman RH, Friedrich EG Jr, Gardner HL: Non neoplastic epithelial disorders of the vulvar skin and mucosa, in Benign Diseases of the Vulva and Vagina, 3rd Edition. Chicago, IL, Year Book Medical, 1989, p 319

Kerns RD, Turk DC, Rudy TE: The West Haven-Yale Multidimensional Pain Inventory. Pain 23:345–356, 1985

Koblenzer CS: Pruritus ani, in Psychocutaneous Disease. Orlando, FL, Grune & Stratton, 1987, pp 220–226

Kokx NP, Comstock JA, Facklam RR: Streptococcal perianal disease in children. Pediatrics 30:659–663, 1987

Lynch FW: Pruritus vulvae as seen in dermatologic practice. JAMA 150:14–18, 1952

Lynch PJ: Vulvodynia: a syndrome of unexplained vulvar pain, psychologic disability and sexual dysfunction. J Reprod Med 31:773–779, 1986

Marinoff SC, Turner MLC: Vulvar vestibulitis syndrome. Dermatol Clin 10:435–444, 1992

Matloff SM: Local intravaginal desensitization to seminal fluid. J Allergy Clin Immunol 91:1230–1231, 1993

Max MB, Lynch SA, Muir J, et al: Effects of desipramine, amitriptyline, and fluoxetine on pain in diabetic neuropathy. N Engl J Med 326:1250–1256, 1992

McCormack WM: Two urogenital sinus syndromes: interstitial cystitis and focal vulvitis. J Reprod Med 35:873–876, 1990

McKay M: Vulvodynia versus pruritus vulvae. Clin Obstet Gynecol 28:123–133, 1985

McKay M: Subsets of vulvodynia. J Reprod Med 33:695–698, 1988

McKay M: Vulvodynia: a multifactorial problem. Arch Dermatol 125:256–262, 1989

McKay M: Vulvar dermatoses. Clin Obstet Gynecol 34:614–629, 1991

McKay M: Vulvodynia: diagnostic patterns. Dermatol Clin 10:423–433, 1992

McKay M: Dysesthetic ("essential") vulvodynia: successful treatment with amitriptyline. J Reprod Med 38:9–13, 1993

McKay M, Frankman O, Horowitz BJ, et al: Vulvar vestibulitis and vestibular papillomatosis: report of the ISSVD committee on vulvodynia. J Reprod Med 36:413–415, 1991

Portenoy RK: Chronic pain management, in Psychiatric Care of the Medical Patient. Edited by Stoudemire A, Fogel BS. New York, Oxford University Press, 1993, pp 341–363

Pyka RE, Wilkinson EJ, Friedrich EG Jr, et al: The histopathology of vulvar vestibulitis syndrome. Int J Gynecol Pathol 7:249–257, 1988

Rapkin AJ, Kames LD, Drake LL, et al: History of physical and sexual abuse in women with chronic pain. Obstet Gynecol 76:92–96, 1990

Rehder PA, Eliezer ET, Lane AT: Perianal cellulitis: cutaneous group A streptococcal disease. Arch Dermatol 124:702–704, 1988

Reiter RC, Shakerin LR, Gambone JC, et al: Correlation between sexual abuse and somatization in women with somatic and nonsomatic chronic pelvic pain. Am J Obstet Gynecol 165:104–109, 1991

Rosenbaum M: Psychosomatic factors in pruritus. Psychosom Med 7:52–57, 1945

Russell DEH: The incidence and prevalence of intrafamilial and extrafamilial sexual abuse of female children. Child Abuse Negl 7:133–146, 1983

Sobel J: Recurrent vulvovaginal candidiasis: a prospective study of the efficacy of maintenance ketoconazole therapy. N Engl J Med 315:1455–1458, 1986

Stewart DE, Whelan CI, Fong IW, et al: Psychosocial aspects of chronic, clinically unconfirmed vulvovaginitis. Obstet Gynecol 76:852–856, 1990

Task Force on Allergic Reactions to Latex: Committee report. J Allergy Clin Immunol 92:16–18, 1993

Turner ML, Marinoff SC: Pudendal neuralgia. Am J Obstet Gynecol 165:1233–1236, 1991

Verbov J: Pruritus ani and its management: a study and reappraisal. Clin Exp Dermatol 9:46–52, 1984

Walker EW, Katon W, Harrop-Griffiths J, et al: Relationship of chronic pelvic pain to psychiatric diagnoses and childhood sexual abuse. Am J Psychiatry 145:75–80, 1988

Walker EW, Roy-Byrne PP, Katon WJ, et al: An open trial of nortriptyline in women with chronic pelvic pain. Int J Psychiatry Med 21:245–252, 1991

Walter L, Brannon L: A cluster analysis of the multidimensional pain inventory. Headache 31:476–479, 1991

Wilkins EGL, Payne SR, Pead PJ, et al: Interstitial cystitis and the urethral syndrome: a possible answer. Br J Urol 64:39–44, 1989

Witkin SS: Immunology of recurrent vaginitis. Am J Reprod Immunol 15:34–37, 1987

Witkin SS: A controlled trial of nystatin for the candidiasis hypersensitivity syndrome (letter). N Engl J Med 324:1593, 1991

Wittkower E, Russell B: Emotional Factors in Skin Disease. London, Cassell, 1953, pp 74–83

Woodruff D, Friedrich EG Jr: The vestibule. Clin Obstet Gynecol 28:134–141, 1985

Young AW, Azoury RS, McKay M, et al: Burning vulva syndrome: report of the ISSVD Task Force. J Reprod Med 29:457, 1984

Chapter 10

Psychiatric Aspects of Bone Marrow Transplantation

Lynna M. Lesko, M.D., Ph.D.

Mythological, ancient, and recent history is replete with accounts of transplantation. Ancient mythology speaks of the *chimera* (a term still used today), consisting of a serpent's tail and lion's head, in addition to tales of two-headed dogs. Probably one of the earliest clinical examples of transplantation is the medieval tale of Saints Damien and Cosmos. This mythical surgical feat entailed grafting a leg from an Ethiopian Moor to a Roman soldier. As we know today, this miraculous operation far surpassed immunological problems quite unresolvable until current transplant medicine. In the past 20 years, major advances have occurred in the area of solid organ transplantation (i.e., kidney, heart, lung, and pancreas). Bone marrow transplantation (BMT) has followed in the last 15 years and is rapidly changing from a controversial research procedure with high morbidity and mortality to a widely used modality offering potential and realistic cure. This dramatic change is a consequence of more advanced techniques in tissue typing, better understanding of the immune system (particularly the introduction of antithymocyte globulin) and the biological response

The author acknowledges and greatly appreciates the Leukemia Society of America for their continued grant support throughout her early career (Fellow's, Special Fellow's, Scholar's Grants and the 1989 Stohlman Scholars Award). The author also wishes to thank Linda Maxwell, Melody Owens, and Lauren Mundy, who provided excellent skills and personal dedication in the preparation of this chapter.

415

modifiers (such as the colony-stimulating factors), and better support-ive care (central line catheter placement, newer antibiotics, and more aggressive and intensive peritransplant care) (Santos 1983; Sullivan et al. 1989).

BMT has become an important innovative treatment of hemato-logical malignancies, solid tumors, immunodeficiency diseases, and metabolic disorders. It has evolved over the last decade from a contro-versial research procedure to a standard therapeutic modality that pro-longs remission in some patients and cures others (Lenfant and Quesenberry 1993). Historically, the BMT procedure is divided into several stages, each of which has accompanying emotional problems. In providing psychological care for transplant recipients, donors, and families, caregivers must be familiar with the psychological stages of the procedure, such as issues involving body image and rebirth, and the patient's mechanisms of coping with the extreme stress. BMT's complex medications, high-dose chemotherapy, total-body irradiation (TBI), germ-free environment, graft-versus-host disease (GvHD), Broviac or Hickman line catheterization, and total parenteral nutrition (TPN) can precipitate significant psychological sequelae, with immedi-ate and long-term consequences. In response to their illness, transplant patients may also develop anxiety, depression, agitation, noncompli-ance, and suicidal ideation.

In this chapter, I provide information about 1) the biology, epide-miology, history, and economics of BMT; 2) informed consent issues; 3) psychological and social assessment of patients and families before BMT; 4) the psychological and pharmacological care of patients during BMT; 5) special issues concerning donation of marrow, donor registries, family issues, children as patients, and prevention of staff burnout; and 6) the psychosocial adjustment and quality of life of BMT patients as they convalesce and reenter normal daily routines. I also present recent research that investigates the role of psychosocial factors in predicting post-BMT outcome.

TRANSPLANT BIOLOGY

Biological Setting

BMT emerged in the early 1980s as a treatment of choice for severe aplastic anemia, severe combined immunodeficiency disease, some congenital hematological disorders such as Fanconi's anemia and Wiskott-Aldrich syndrome, and radiation accidents. Over the past 10 years, it has been used with increasing and encouraging success for acute leukemia and is now being used for patients with chronic leukemia, paroxysmal nocturnal hemoglobinuria, lymphomas, solid tumors sensitive to radiation (breast, testicular cancer, neuroblastoma), and genetic disorders of bone marrow such as thalassemia, Hurler's syndrome, and sickle cell anemia (O'Reilly 1983; Parr et al. 1991; Santos 1990). It is unfortunate that the advances made with such innovative therapy have been tempered by complications of toxicity of cytoreductive preparatory regimens, acute and chronic GvHD, and unavailability of immunocompetent marrow donors (Parr et al. 1991).

The marrow transplantation procedure comprises several stages, each of which makes psychological demands on the patient; these are described in the next section, "Stages of BMT." First, the patient's immunologically deficient or malignant bone marrow or solid tumor is destroyed by high-dose chemotherapy (cyclophosphamide, etoposide [VP-16], methotrexate, and other agents), alone or in combination with TBI. This marrow is then replaced by an infusion of marrow from an immunologically compatible donor (a *syngeneic transplant* from a monozygotic twin; an *allogeneic transplant* or *allograft* from a parent, sibling, or unrelated [registry] donor) or by the patient's own marrow (an *autologous transplant* or *autograft*). In the latter case, the patient's marrow is harvested before chemoradiation and then "purged" or chemotherapeutically cleansed of malignant cells by additional chemotherapeutic agents, if necessary. The allogeneic procedure requires extensive medical evaluation with human lymphocyte antigen (HLA)-histocompatibility and mixed lymphocyte culture (MLC) testing.

The HLA loci are located on chromosome 6 and include several classes of antigens (HLA-A, HLA-B, HLA-C, HLA-D, HLA-DR, HLA-DP, and HLA-DQ). HLA-A, B, C, D, and DR are most commonly used today to detect histocompatibility. Incompatibility of these loci may cause GvHD, an acute or chronic condition in which immunologically active new marrow rejects its recipient. Most individuals are only guaranteed a 25% chance of HLA histocompatibility with each sibling. The percentage of finding an unrelated donor through the marrow registers is discussed later in this chapter in the section "Donor Registries." Both allogeneic and autologous transplants necessitate 2 to 3 months of hospitalization in a reverse-isolation room or laminar–air flow (sterile) unit.

Complications may arise from immediate and delayed effects including infection, GvHD (allogeneic transplant), infertility, endocrine and gonadal dysfunction, cataracts, growth and maturation problems, cognitive (central nervous system [CNS]) dysfunction, interstitial pneumonia, pulmonary fibrosis, and relapse.

Despite an approximate 50% morbidity rate (subsequent BMT-related sequelae) with the allogeneic BMT procedure, 2- to 10-year long-term survival and even cure have been reported to be 50%–75%. These survival rates depend on the age of the patient, type of disease, extent of disease (first year, subsequent remissions), acute and chronic complications, relapse, and type of transplant (allogeneic versus autologous). In contrast, standard or conventional chemotherapy results in 5-year disease-free survival in about 20%–30% of adults with acute leukemia who usually relapse within 12 to 24 months (Appelbaum 1988; O'Reilly 1983; Santos 1990).

Allogeneic marrow transplantation is the only currently available effective therapy for chronic myelogenous leukemia and severe aplastic anemia. Patients on hydroxyurea or other standard treatment for chronic myelogenous leukemia develop fatal blast crisis within 1 to 3 years of diagnosis, whereas BMT provides a 50%–60% possibility of cure (Goldman et al. 1986; Santos 1990; Thomas et al. 1986). The mortality in severe cases of aplastic anemia treated with conventional therapy is over 95%; most patients will die within 12 months. Allogeneic BMT has resulted in 1- to 6-year survival rates of 50%–60% in aplastic anemia patients, with complete hematological restoration (O'Reilly 1983). Both allogeneic and autologous transplantation are the treatments of choice for patients with lymphoma that has disseminated (stage IV) or that recurs often with use of aggressive conventional chemotherapy. Again, in patients who undergo a transplant earlier in the course of their illness or while in remission, survival rates at 3 years increase to 45% from 18% (the rate of survival in patients transplanted during relapse) (Appelbaum 1988).

A newer alternative technique of autologous BMT has renewed clinicians' enthusiasm, particularly for those patients with hematological malignancies who have no donors and for those with solid tumors. Autoharvest of bone marrow, peripheral blood, and stem cells; purging; and subsequent reinfusion could offer a cure and provide an opportunity to administer higher doses of chemotherapy and radiation. Autologous BMT for testicular cancer actually requires a double bone marrow transplant (two autologous transplants separated by 1 to 2 months of convalescence); this procedure is done at most transplant centers that perform transplants for testicular tumors. Advantages of autologous BMT include not having to rely on a very small, unrelated donor pool, which may produce GvHD, and a usually shorter hospital stay. Disadvantages include inadequate purging techniques to free the host marrow of malignant cells and the possibility (although circumstantial in humans) that GvHD itself has a direct antitumor effect (Burnett 1988). Autologous BMT is now being used for patients with poor-prognosis Hodgkin's disease, non-Hodgkin's lymphomas, acute leukemia (those with no related or unrelated match), late-stage neuroblastoma (in children), breast cancer, and testicular cancer. Within the last few years, protocols have begun for small-cell lung cancer, chronic leukemia, myeloma, and malignant brain tumors. Readers are directed to an excellent review article by Cheson and colleagues (1989) for extensive information on autologous BMT.

The possibility of using very high and toxic dosages of radiation and chemotherapy to eradicate malignant disease with marrow rescue is no longer an experimental or research dream. Today, clinicians who perform transplants have new goals and concerns for 1) developing newer purging techniques for autologous harvests; 2) eliminating GvHD with the use of prophylactic regimens (steroids, cyclosporine, antithymocyte globulin) and T-cell-depleted marrows (using lectins or monoclonal antibodies); 3) reducing hospital stay by using various colony-stimulating factors to enhance early proliferation of patients' white blood cell (WBC) counts before discharge; 4) mediating viral infections via prophylaxis; and 5) improving the margin of safety of BMT in the geriatric population.

A guide is urgently needed for the referring physician, patient, and family 1) to determine whether to use autologous or allogeneic transplantation in patients with various hematologic disorders (thalassemia, sickle cell anemia, aplastic anemia, acute and chronic leukemia, multiple myeloma, lymphomas), solid tumors (testicular, lung, breast neuroblastoma), immunodeficiency disorders, and metabolic disorders (lipid storage diseases); and 2) to report 2- to 5-year survival rates and ranges for age and stages of illness. This critical guide does not exist, probably because the field changes so rapidly, week by week, with advancing technology, and such guides are out-of-date before they are printed. One example is the rising age cutoff for transplants in older patients. Determining which patients are appropriate for BMT is so dependent on age, stage of illness, expertise of the center performing the transplant, and protocol offered that guides are virtually impossible. The best approach is for the patient and family to gather information from federal organizations such as the National Cancer Institute; from others such as the American Cancer Society, Leukemia Society of America, and Cancer Care; and from several transplantation centers. Family physicians can also use the same resources as well as information from their local medical societies.

The International Bone Marrow Transplant Registry (IBMTR) conducted a survey during 1985 to 1987 to determine the number of allogeneic BMT centers and their activity (Bortin and Rimm 1989). Data reported by 258 transplant centers in 41 countries revealed that 10,887 patients received a BMT during 1985 to 1987 (73% for leukemia, 11% for other malignancies, 9% for aplastic anemia, 3% for severe combined immunodeficiency disease [SCID], 2% for thalassemia, and 2% for metabolic, genetic, or other disease); more than 50% had transplants in only 37 centers. Of the total, 46% were performed in North America and 42% in western Europe. In 1978, 199 transplants were performed, and, in 1987, the number increased to 3,964; thus, in 1995, the projected number of transplants is at least 7,600. Not included in these impressive figures is the burgeoning field of autologous BMT, particularly for breast and testicular cancers. Currently, more than 12,000 individuals in the United States are potential candidates for allogeneic BMT, and 40,000 to 50,000 individuals are potential candidates for autologous BMT (Vaughn et al. 1986). With the advances made in increasing the National Bone Marrow Registry (NBMR) donor pool, improved methods of autologous BMT, colony-stimulating factor use leading to decreased hospital stay, and partial and full insurance coverage (particularly for breast cancer in late 1990), many more individuals may opt for this chance for cure.

Cost

The current average cost of BMT per patient is between $130,000 and $200,000 (Durbin 1988; Leukemia Society of America, personal communication, January 1992). In the early 1970s, the National Institutes of Health (NIH) usually assumed all patient care costs. In addition, by 1986, allogeneic BMT was covered by Medicaid in 45 states. Autologous BMT financing has been slow to follow, with Medicaid approval only in 1989. Third-party payer reimbursement is now mandatory and universal. Considering the likely future complexity of rising costs for

BMT hospitalization, the potential of more candidates, and the resistance by insurance companies for BMT payment, a financial struggle could result in the near future.

Donor Registries

At least 60% of individuals opting for BMT will not have a suitably matched sibling donor, necessitating advanced methodology for autologous BMT or investigation of possible HLA-matched BMT by unrelated donors. Since the first unrelated donor marrow transplant in 1979, approximately 110 unrelated donor transplants have been performed as of April 1989 (National Marrow Donor Program, personal communication, June 1989). By February 1990, 300 unrelated donor transplants were performed, and the National Marrow Donor Program (NMDP) had a pool of 87,037 volunteers. The NMDP is a federally funded organization that began in 1987; it involves 50 donor centers and more than 20 transplant centers. According to their statistics, the chances of finding an unrelated match range from 1 in 1,000 to 1 in 1,000,000. Odds increase when donors are within the patient's ethnic group; finding a match for a Caucasian with another Caucasian is, on average, approximately 1 in 20,000. Matching for histocompatibility, when possible, requires 2 to 6 months. It is still premature to present the number of successful matches found, successfully completed unrelated transplants, and survival rates of these individuals (Bealty et al. 1989; McCullough et al. 1989).

STAGES OF BONE MARROW TRANSPLANTATION

The BMT procedure encompasses several stages of medical treatment, each with its own psychological effects (Brown and Kelly 1976; Futterman et al. 1989; Haberman 1988; Lesko 1989a). Figure 10–1 shows the medical stages of BMT, and I describe the corresponding psychological states throughout various sections of this chapter.

The decision to undergo the transplantation procedure is often made in a place many miles from the transplantation center, in an atmosphere of chronic illness and, at times, organ failure. Patients may have experienced months of feeling ill and may have endured radiation, chemotherapy, medications, and transfusions to prolong survival. During this time, fears of death and uncertainty, coupled with the hope of possible cure, pervade. Because of these urgent medical complications affecting the physical status of the patient (remission, relapse) and the availability of a bed, the decision to have a transplant often must be made quickly.

In contrast to leukemia or lymphoma patients, patients with severe aplastic anemia often develop symptoms suddenly and are unacquainted with chronic illness and hospitalization. Regardless of whether the onset of cancer is rapid, the decision of patients and families to accept the recommendation for transplant is always accompa-

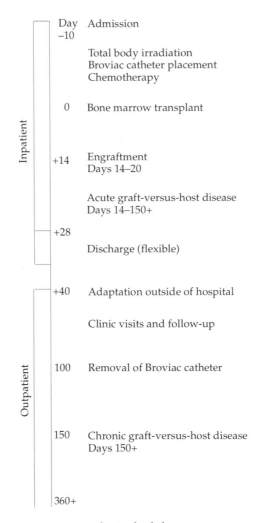

Figure 10–1. Bone marrow transplant schedule.

nied by the stresses associated with the batteries of physical tests, tissue typing of family members, or application to a donor registry to determine whether the transplantation is feasible. If potential donors are found within the nuclear family, rivalry may ensue. The compatible donor may be vulnerable to pressure from within the family to donate, once and even twice, and must cope with personal and family guilt if they refuse the procedure or if the transplant is unsuccessful. Occasionally, when a family member is not a histocompatible donor, a sense of family guilt or shame may develop. Another psychologically difficult step is the decision to find an unrelated donor through a registry. Some families spend tremendous amounts of energy in this search, particularly in organizing tissue typing drives in their communities and places of worship. For individuals whose ethnic background is not common among the donors to the NMDP, families organize drives in communities where their ancestors had lived or in distant racial and ethnic communities. This emotional energy in searching often tempers the family's sense of helplessness; however, issues of how far and how long to search arise. When an unrelated donor is found, blinding euphoria can mask future concerns of actual hospitalization, hidden costs, disruption in family schedules, and the possibility of graft rejection and the need for another donor search. Some transplant centers discourage, and even prohibit, patients from contacting the unrelated donor for a second harvest and subsequent donation. Most believe that it may be too stressful or painful to know that the first transplant was unsuccessful, and the donor may worry that the second transplant may also be unsuccessful.

Psychological and Psychosocial Assessment Concerns

Oncologists and mental health care professionals have become increasingly concerned with the identification of psychiatric, psychological, or social factors that might promote patient compliance or that may affect the family's adjustment during BMT hospitalization. To date, few studies have evaluated patients and families before BMT. However, long-standing guidelines from the psychiatric consultation literature as well as literature and research on solid organ transplants (lung, heart, liver, kidney) strongly suggest that all pretransplant patients undergo evaluations for history of psychiatric illness, such as psychosis, delirium, or depression; mental retardation; alcohol or recreational substance abuse; history of poor compliance with medical care; impulsivity; and poor coping skills, especially during long hospitalizations or separations from families. This evaluation may allow staff to develop patient-specific programs for compliance after the transplantation.

The BMT literature takes another stance regarding preevaluation. Most, if not all, patients are accepted for BMT irrespective of any psychological and social obstacles. Patients are usually declined a transplant only if their medical state is rapidly declining or if they lack a donor. However, preevaluation of patients and families provides valuable information for staff to institute programs for each patient and to be prepared for any psychological distress during the long BMT hospitalization. Research is needed to determine whether psychological intervention improves patient and family compliance with BMT and whether that translates to improved health outcome. BMT staff usually request that family members visit daily, which often imposes a demanding schedule of support. Consequently, family members should also be questioned about past psychiatric illness, coping strategies, drug abuse, social supports, financial situation, and their availability to visit the patient so that the staff have realistic expectations. Any ethnic or religious concerns that may complicate medical care should also be evaluated.

Futterman and colleagues (1989) and Futterman and Wellisch (1990) proposed a three-level schema of psychosocial adjustment to BMT based on the characteristics of the patient, the family, and life experiences. They retrospectively evaluated psychiatric history, quality of social and family support, coping history (particularly to medical issues), quality of affect, present and past mental status, and how patients reacted to anticipatory phenomena. They concluded that level I patients needed the fewest psychiatric consultation interventions (approximately 60 to 120 minutes per week); these interventions included relaxation training, short-term crisis management, and general support. Level II patients needed to be seen two to three times per week and required much more support from staff and family. Patient interventions included cognitive-behavior therapy to improve coping strategies and to reframe negative experiences, often along with the adjunctive administration of anxiolytics. Level III patients required intensive psychiatric follow-up. Level III patient issues tended to involve impulsivity, regression, and mood disturbances. Interventions consisted of educational and psychological support with no dynamic or interpretative materials. Staff were usually overwhelmed and needed support in caring for this group. The investigators believe that this coding system can reliably identify patients who need care before transplantation. It is unclear whether these investigators provided such care free of charge because patients were on a research protocol or whether patients were charged by time or type of intervention schedule. Most BMT units provide psychosocial interventions that 1) may be covered by a research grant, 2) could be entirely free, or 3) are most likely billed by social work, nursing, or psychiatric services. The reader is directed to Futterman's work for a more complete description of the interventions they used, which is beyond the scope of this chapter.

Psychiatric consultation data during 12 months on an 11-bed autologous BMT unit at Memorial Sloan-Kettering Cancer Center revealed that, of 23 patients who eventually received a psychiatric consultation (46% of patients who received an autologous BMT for that year), only 1 had been seen before the transplant (Die-Trill and Lesko 1990). Of the 23 patients receiving psychiatric consults, 56% had a previous psychiatric diagnosis, but only 9% reported a history of alcohol or drug abuse. One cannot conclude on this basis that the other 22 patients should have been evaluated before BMT, but it would be interesting to determine whether their psychiatric problems (39% adjustment disorder, 12% major mental disorders) could have been detected before BMT. On this particular unit, not every patient or family was evaluated because of the lack of a consultant solely dedicated to autologous BMT and the large numbers of patients admitted monthly. A social worker preliminarily evaluated all patients. However, actual psychiatric evaluation (e.g., for medication, psychiatric diagnosis, stress reduction, coping issues, pain) occurred only when recommended by the autologous BMT oncologist.

The question of whether all patients should be evaluated before hospitalization remains unanswered. A brief session with a nurse, clinician, or social worker is the norm in many centers; preevaluation is quite a luxury in most institutions. Often, psychosocial support staff are funded by their own departments and patient reimbursement. In an ideal world, all BMT units would have a separate psychosocial team available to patients, staff, and families, but, currently, resources to support such staff are not readily available from BMT programs.

To date, the only other research that has examined the psychological distress of patients and parents of children during admission for BMT (i.e., within the first 48 hours of hospitalization) is that reported by Lesko and associates (Dermatis and Lesko 1990, 1991; Lesko et al.

1989). Adult patients (n = 39) and parents of pediatric patients (n = 61) were assessed on admission using the Brief Symptom Inventory (Derogatis and Spencer 1982) to measure various domains of psychological distress. (This inventory measures distress and is not a diagnostic tool such as DSM-IV [American Psychiatric Association 1994]; it has been used in nonpsychiatric control populations to develop normative controls.) Mothers (n = 46) and fathers (n = 15) of pediatric patients were one standard deviation above the mean level of psychological distress compared with a nonpatient reference group (P < .01). Seventy-two percent of mothers and 60% of fathers exhibited clinically significant levels of anxiety (similar to levels of anxiety in patients presenting at an outpatient clinic), and 70% of the mothers demonstrated clinically significant levels of depressive distress. Sixty percent of mothers and 47% of fathers exhibited significant psychological distress of a generalized nature. In general, mothers were more distressed than fathers (P < .05) during the initial 48 hours of admission. The level of parents' distress was unrelated to characteristics of their childs' disease or treatment milieu (reverse isolation versus laminar air flow) or to the parents' recall of BMT informed consent information.

Certain coping strategies and better communication between physicians and parents were related to decreased psychological distress. The investigators believe that at least 50% of parents would benefit from psychosocial interventions during the initial periadmission phase of BMT when informed consent is a major issue.

Dermatis and Lesko (1991) studied the psychological distress in adult patients during the first 48 hours of BMT hospitalization. Mean distress scores for men and women were again one standard deviation above the mean for a nonpatient reference group (P < .01). (In general, men were more distressed than women, compared with control subjects.) Married patients exhibited lower global psychological distress (P < .01). It is interesting that distress was not related to coping style or perceived quality of communication between patient and doctor.

Informed Consent

Informed consent has been described as a continual process of mutual decision making between the patient and the physician (Ford 1990; Lasagna 1983; Lesko and Hawkins 1983; Lesko et al. 1989). Informed consent should represent the voluntary nature of consent (i.e., freedom to withdraw and the research nature of the treatment) and comprehension of the information in the consent document. Physicians treating adult patients thought that the information provided in most consent forms was overly technical and excessive, although most patients did not agree. Penman and co-workers (1984) reported a similar pattern of divergent perceptions regarding information presented in the consent document among physicians and their patients consenting to investigational chemotherapy.

Several recommendations might improve the referral and general informed consent process for BMT. First, the referring oncologist, a key professional in the patient's care, should be familiar with several BMT institutions and their protocols. The oncologist should encourage families to evaluate several transplant centers to select the best one for the patient (each transplant center has its own protocol and patient requirements). An example of a determining factor would be the requirement that both families and patients stay geographically close to the center for 6 to 9 months. Second, patients and families should be required to visit the transplant center, including the BMT unit, to meet the staff before making a decision. Patients should have a psychological evaluation in addition to their medical evaluation to determine their ability to comply with the rigors of the hospitalization and convalescent period. Third, the patient and family should meet a former BMT patient and family. Data have suggested that such patient-to-patient meetings will not "dissuade" a patient from undergoing BMT and will actually improve the quality of a potential candidate's decision (Chauvenet and Smith 1988; Patenaude et al. 1986a, 1986b).

Finally, it is suggested that oncologists can facilitate the informed consent process by

- Offering support and reassurance to patients regarding their right to make their own decision, without assuming that patients think autonomous decision making is sanctioned by their physicians
- Training oncology staff to anticipate and respond to questions from patients and concerned members and friends of their families regarding the medical treatment
- Providing opportunities for patients to discuss the treatment with other patients who have consented to treatment as well as with health-care professionals
- Evaluating a patient's readiness to assimilate information (particularly treatment-related risks and side effects) by eliciting discussion during the BMT consultation and including, if necessary, a review of

the material in a subsequent consultation with the patient
- Ascertaining how the patient regards the consent form and determining its use as a tool for reinforcing information on an individual basis.

All of these suggestions are global in nature and must be tailor-made for a particular center's patient population by the available staff.

Ethical and Legal Issues

Organ transplantation always involves many complex moral, ethical, and legal issues. BMT is being presented as a treatment option to patients at much earlier stages of their disease, especially when individuals must weigh long-term potential cure and high morbidity against current quality of life and less aggressive treatment. It has therefore become more important to evaluate attendant moral and ethical issues earlier in the course of an illness. The ethical issues associated with BMT are not new; they involve previous questions, such as

- How are quality of life and extension of life defined, particularly "do not resuscitate" decisions?
- How do certain BMT centers select candidates, based on protocol requirements (age, stage of diseases, type of disease)?
- How are donors selected, and what are donors' rights (particularly unrelated donors, minor donors, newborn umbilical cord donations, and the procreation of new potential infant donors within a family)?
- How are scarce resources allocated (blood products, intensive medical and nursing care, investigational chemotherapeutic agents), based on the global welfare of individuals and society?
- How are aggressive and experimental research protocols instituted?
- Is the patient competent?
- How are decision makers selected?

Many of these ethical issues have been historically reviewed in connection with kidney dialysis, kidney transplant patients, and, most recently, with other solid organ recipients.

Determining how therapeutic and/or experimental an innovative treatment is poses many questions. Currently, many physicians disagree on the experimental versus routine or conventional quality of transplantation. The dilemma of providing therapeutic, but innovative and experimental, care halted cardiac transplantation in the early 1970s and questioned the removal of cytotoxic T cells during BMT in the late 1980s.

Legal issues in BMT are fortunately few, unlike in other transplant settings. These cases may result from issues surrounding transplanting a "liquid regenerative organ" (i.e., marrow) versus a "solid non-regenerative organ" (i.e., heart, lung, pancreas, liver, kidney). Holder (1990) reviewed legal issues that may arise in the BMT process. Malpractice actions could arise as a result of inappropriate medical care by the health-care professional or donated marrow that was inappropriately matched or screened for cytomegalovirus (CMV), hepatitis, syphilis, or acquired immunodeficiency syndrome (AIDS). Today, these situations are limited, because screening is standardized. However, at our institution, we have had potential histocompatible family donors with histories of drug abuse, human immunodeficiency virus (HIV), and hepatitis. In these cases, the most conservative and medically appropriate choice is to seek another family member or unrelated donor registry match. Again, total disclosure is mandatory when donating marrow through the National Registry.

The sale of bone marrow is mentioned in the National Organ Transplant Act (PL 98-507, 1984) because, although regenerative, marrow is one of the organs that cannot be bought or sold. Fines mandate $50,000 and/or incarceration for 5 years.

Marrow donation, although considered a minor, possibly 1-day, hospital surgical procedure with minimal risk of anesthesia, has potential legal ramifications. Donation by minors (even children as young as 6 months) is commonplace. Institutions usually see no need to ask for court permission in donations from minors; the parent usually grants permission. A minor unwilling to donate would not currently be compelled to do so. In a celebrated case in Chicago (New York Times, July 1990; Curran 1991), the father of a 12-year-old boy with leukemia went through the court system to request testing of his son's twin half-brothers. Their biological mother, estranged from her common-law husband, refused HLA testing for their leukemic son. The court system upheld her wishes. In donations through the National Marrow Registry, the court usually has upheld the wishes of a potential donor. In another case, a terminally ill man from Iowa (*Head v. Colloton*) tried to sue the director of a National Marrow Registry to release the name of a woman who was a potential donor but who had subsequently declined to donate her marrow. The Iowa Supreme Court upheld that releasing her name was an invasion of her privacy. No doubt the future will bring many more legal issues concerning procurement of bone marrow, especially that from infant donors, the elderly at risk of medical complications, and the uncharted territory of unrelated marrow donation. These ethical and legal questions challenge whether informed, voluntary consent is truly informed and truly voluntary. For a more in-depth review of ethical issues in allocation of marrow, reimbursement by insurance companies, and cost-effective analysis of the procedure (which are all beyond the scope of this chapter), the reader is directed to articles by Langedoen (1993), Kelahan (1993), and Welch (1993), respectively.

Very few patients and families decline a BMT procedure, either before or after their exhaustive evaluation and screening period. Virtually no data or articles are available on why patients decline further treatment. It can only be surmised that financial issues, distance from home, lack of family support, insurance coverage, and extensive medical problems are contributing factors.

Hospitalization

As mentioned earlier in this chapter, the transplant process can be divided into several physical stages (Figure 10–1), each accompanied by a particular emotional tone (Brown and Kelly 1976; Lesko 1989a); it has been suggested that many of these stages overlap (Haberman 1988). The actual admission, hospitalization, and preparation for the transplant require more tests; patients experience feelings of anxiety and hope. Patients enter the sterile or reverse-isolation room immediately to avoid infection. They then undergo a 10-day pretransplant conditioning regimen consisting of high-dose immunosuppressive drugs and hyperfractionated TBI (given for several days in multiple sessions per day at levels lethal to bone marrow: 1,200 to 1,400 rads; autologous procedures entail a shorter preconditioning regimen and may not involve TBI). The oncologic rationale for the preconditioning therapy is that it provides space in the marrow cavity for new marrow, allows destruction of remaining tumor cells, and impairs the host immune system to allow engraftment of new donor marrow (Holmes 1990). Chemotherapy drugs used are cyclophosphamide, busulfan, carmustine, etoposide, cytarabine hydrochloride, used alone or in combination, to achieve total bone marrow ablation. (The reader is referred to Massie and Lesko [1989] for the psychotoxocity of these drugs.) A Broviac or Hickman catheter is placed using local anesthesia. This is a central venous line that allows the drawing of blood samples and administration of blood products, medications, antibiotics, and TPN without frequent punctures of the patient's skin. During this time, patients have mixed feelings of anxiety and hope and episodes of nausea, vomiting, and fatigue, secondary to the irradiation and chemotherapy.

For many leukemia patients, this preparation or cytoreductive regimen is familiar; it is similar in some respects to their induction chemotherapy. For the aplastic or chronic leukemia patient with newly diagnosed symptoms, this environment and toxic drug regimen are new, and the side effects are more intolerable. The patient's blood counts begin to fall as a result of the cytoreductive procedure. This is "the point of no return," because, unlike kidney transplantation, there is no dialysis to fall back on. However, it is similar to a cardiac transplant in that graft rejection heralds a possible "second try."

The transplant is brief and anticlimactic compared with the lengthy pretransplant treatment and the convalescent period. It is usually uncomplicated and is paradoxically undramatic for patients, involving only an infusion of concentrated bone marrow. The donor, however, undergoes general anesthesia to harvest his or her marrow by multiple aspirations of both iliac crests, similar to a bone marrow biopsy. Usually the donor is admitted to the hospital the night before and leaves the day after the procedure. Donors can return to a normal routine within a few days, experiencing only minor hip soreness and discomfort. Many centers are now harvesting marrow in a day-hospital setting.

In the immediate convalescent period, the BMT recipient is concerned about marrow engraftment, transplant rejection, continuation of immunosuppressive drugs, the risk of infection, high fever, mucositis, problems and side effects consequent to prolonged exposure to multiple antibiotics, nausea, anorexia, relief of pain, and the possibility of GvHD (Holmes 1990). This latter "turning of the transplant" against the recipient is poorly understood and causes great distress to the recipient, the donor, and staff when it occurs. Fortunately, researchers are virtually eliminating patients' risk of developing GvHD by employing newer techniques of T-cell-depleted grafts.

The requisite in-hospital convalescent period for both allogeneic and autologous BMT is usually 1 to 2 months, during which the patient must undergo weeks of hyperalimentation and antibiotic administration. Pain, isolation, restricted activities, and very regimented or structured care can routinely lead to regressive behavior, anxiety over very minor events, mild depression, noncompliance, excessive demands on staff, and sleep disturbances (Ford 1990). The unpredictability of the BMT course appears to be the major psychological stressor for high levels of anxiety and psychological distress. Noncompliance, even in the best patient, is the norm, particularly with mouth care and mouth hygiene, eating, and medications for gut sterilization. Often staff must provide behavioral interventions and creative/flexible solutions to deal with these non–life threatening, but nevertheless frustrating, issues. It is a trying time for the patient as well as for the families, who are usually asked to visit daily to provide important emotional support. Family disruption may be quite obvious at this time, when the stresses of the seemingly endless procedure do not relent.

Preparation for discharge begins 1 to 2 months after the transplant, when the marrow is functioning adequately (WBC count > 1,000) and the likelihood of infection is low. Patients have renewed hope of resuming their lives where they left off and a heightened interest in the world outside the hospital. When patients are physically stable, they may begin physical therapy, which may include a favorite hobby, riding a stationary bicycle, or "working on their computer from home." Patenaude (1990) describes patients using binoculars or telescopes to bring the outside environment into their rooms. However, as they begin to learn the self-care procedures that will be necessary at home (Broviac or Hickman catheter care and medication regimens), the excitement over the anticipated discharge is mixed with fears of leaving the security of the isolation room and transplant unit. At this time, patients commonly have difficulty with appetite, particularly as they are being weaned from hyperalimentation. This transition period can also be complicated by side effects secondary to GvHD.

The number of days a patient is hospitalized for BMT varies greatly, depending on the type of transplant (allogeneic-unrelated donor, allogeneic-related donor, or autologous). Patients may expect to stay 3 to 4 months, 2 months, or less than 1 month in the respective transplant situations. Longer, more medically arduous hospitalizations are associated with a clinical impression of increased rates of depression, particularly in adult patients.

Posthospitalization

Adaptation and convalescence outside the hospital are protracted and can last almost 6 months. Transplantation does not guarantee total restoration of previous health status; thus, the transplant patient requires considerable support from staff throughout the discharge and convalescence period. Weekly visits to the transplant clinic occur for at least the first 2 to 4 months. Over time, patients turn their concerns from "living as a patient" to "living as a survivor." They have profound fatigue and may show signs of difficulty or actual inability to "reenter" normal activities related to home and work space. Currently, several investigators are beginning to study the potential comparison of these symptoms with a more classic posttraumatic stress disorder in adults and children (K. Smith, personal communication, June 1992; M. Steuber, personal communication, February 1992). Young mothers who have undergone BMT may especially need help in managing their small, active children. Rehabilitation is as much a psychological process as a physiological process; the two must proceed simultaneously. Children, as compared with adults, resume normal life more rapidly. This phase is discussed in the following section.

IMMEDIATE SIDE EFFECTS AND COMPLICATIONS OF THE BONE MARROW TRANSPLANTATION PROCEDURE

BMT demands a high level of commitment and extraordinary cooperation from patients. It is clear from our clinical experience that having adequate information about illness and treatment reduces stress and improves most patients' ability to cope (Lesko et al. 1989). It is therefore important for the mental health provider to give an accurate explanation of the disease, a careful description of the BMT treatment and its desired effect, and adequate information about side effects that must be tolerated to obtain the treatment's benefits.

Immediate toxic complications of the cytoreductive regimen of chemotherapy and radiation include mucositis, bleeding, infection, nausea, and vomiting. Stomatitis, esophagitis, and gastroenteritis result in oropharyngeal ulcers, severe pain, decreased food intake, and the need for continuous intravenous narcotic drips. Most, if not all, medications must be given parenterally. Intramuscular and rectal administration are contraindicated because the patients' platelet counts are dangerously low (11,000–20,000) as a result of the chemotherapy and radiation treatments. Again, sublingual administration is not usually attempted because of the patients' severe stomatitis and mouth ulcers and difficult mouth hygiene. Bacterial, viral, and fungal infections are common during the hospitalization and require multiple intravenous medications that can secondarily cause anorexia and diminished hearing. Other toxicities of the cytoreductive conditioning regimen include cyclophosphamide-induced cardiomyopathy, hemorrhagic cystitis and veno-occlusive disease (an inflammation and fibrosis resulting in obliteration of the small hepatic venules), hepatomegaly, weight gain, abdominal pain, and elevated liver function tests in approximately 22% of BMT patients (N. Kernan, S. Gulathi, L. M. Lesko, personal communication, April 1991).

General systemic transient side effects of BMT are nausea and vomiting during the few weeks before the BMT infusion, usually as a result of the cytoreductive regimen, and pain secondary to stomatitis during the 2 weeks post-BMT infusion. This period is also marked by fatigue, malaise from high fevers, and anorexia from pain, stomatitis, and antibiotics. Nausea and vomiting are controlled by a potent combination of prochlorperazine, hydroxyzine, lorazepam, and metoclopramide or ondansetron. Pain is routinely assessed by nurses and patients with visual analogue scales and managed by narcotics administered by intravenous push, drip, or a patient-controlled analgesia (PCA) program. Traditionally, PCA programs are usually administered by a pain, neurology, or anesthesia service, not typically by a psychiatrist. The latter form of administration allows better pain management and avoids the anxiety experienced by patients who must ask and then wait for pain relief (thus increasing the need for more drug). It is common for many BMT settings to use PCA even in children and adolescents. Chapman and Hill (1990) have written an elegant article on the physical and psychological issues of PCA in the transplant setting. This means of narcotic administration has been used extensively with children; it does not pose an increased risk for psychological narcotic dependence, it provides patient control over pain, and it eliminates "tense negotiations" between staff and patients.

Chemotherapy

The acute toxic side effects of high-dose chemotherapy for BMT usually involve transient fatigue, nausea and vomiting, hair loss, stomatitis, hemorrhagic cystitis from cyclophosphamide, and complete bone marrow suppression that renders the patient immunologically incompetent. Cardiomyopathy may develop within days of starting the cytoreductive regimen (cyclophosphamide), which is monitored by a drop in voltage on the electrocardiogram (ECG). High-dose steroids are used as immunosuppressive agents and antiemetics. Acute and chronic administration may produce cushingoid symptoms, weight gain, insomnia, elevated glucose, muscle atrophy, fatigue, and a wide variety of psychiatric symptoms such as emotional lability, depression, and psychosis. Late effects of chemotherapeutic agents, particularly in high doses (in conjunction with pre-BMT chemotherapy), include cardiomyopathy, infertility, and risk of secondary malignancies.

TBI

Patients may receive immunologically and hematologically lethal doses of TBI, in the range of 800 to 1,300 rads (usually divided into 12 hyperfractionated treatments over 3 to 4 days). Toxic acute complications can include stomatitis, radiation burns, nausea, and vomiting. Late effects involve possible thyroid dysfunction, cataracts, pulmonary fibrosis, sterility, and premature menopause in women, as well as growth and maturation complications in very young children. I discuss the sexual and endocrine issues in detail in the section below, "Donor, Family, and Staff Concerns." The effects of this irradiation on the CNS may lead to transient or delayed neuropsychological sequelae. Transient impairment of intellectual function may include sedation, somnolence, and difficulty concentrating. This impairment is thought to be caused by increased intracranial pressure secondary to radiation-induced changes in the blood-brain barrier.

The long-term neuropsychological effects of exposure to cranial irradiation in combination with chemotherapy have been studied by Meadows and associates (1981), Rowland and colleagues (1984), and others. These investigators found that children who receive cranial irradiation and intrathecal methotrexate as part of their CNS prophylaxis for leukemia developed mild learning and intellectual disabilities.

An "early-delayed encephalopathy" may begin 1 to 4 months after radiation treatment but has been reported earlier and later. Symptoms consist of lethargy, headache, nausea, and vomiting. In children who receive whole brain radiotherapy (RT) prophylactically for leukemia, the picture is usually one of generalized somnolence and headache. Patients who receive more focal RT to the brain can present with symptoms of focal neurological disease suggestive of tumor recurrence. The cause of early-delayed radiation encephalopathy is unknown but may be related to radiation-induced edema or demyelination. Improvement in symptoms usually occurs spontaneously in 1 to 6 weeks. Steroids may help treat symptoms and can be used as prophylaxis before RT.

A "late-delayed encephalopathy" (usually severe and permanent) may develop 6 months to 3 years (average 12 months) after radiation therapy. This syndrome is usually seen only in patients who receive large doses of CNS radiation. It is characterized by symptoms that suggest a focal neurological lesion (e.g., necrosis), accompanied by personality change and headache. Patients may complain of cognitive problems involving concentration, attention, and memory. Seizures can also complicate the picture. Differential diagnosis includes recurrent tumor, infarct, or abscess. Computed tomography (CT) scan of the brain usually reveals a hypodense lesion in the white matter. Brain biopsy shows necrosis. Steroids can help symptomatically, but surgical resection of the necrotic mass is often necessary.

Little research has been published concerning long-term cognitive deficits secondary to BMT TBI. Ringden and others (1988) reported little neuropsychological impairment in 31 children 1 to 6 years post-BMT. However, children who received a transplant at an earlier age appeared to have more deficits. Andrykowski and co-workers (1990) reported that 30 adult BMT recipients, with a mean of 4 years post-BMT, demonstrated increased cognitive dysfunction, independent of concurrent psychological or affective illness, with increased TBI dose. The investigators used the Confusion Scale of the Profile of Mood States (McNair et al. 1971) and the Alertness Behavior Scale of the Sickness Impact Profile (Bergner et al. 1976), measures not usually employed in more rigorous neuropsychological studies. Rebeta and colleagues (1990) compared adult patients undergoing conventional chemotherapy for acute leukemia with those who had an additional bone marrow transplant. Results from this study indicate that there is little cognitive decline with the additional radiation of BMT in adult survivors compared with acute leukemia patients with or without their original CNS radiation. The paucity of research on the long-term neuropsychiatric sequelae of BMT now mandates extensive study.

Broviac or Hickman Catheterization and TPN

Dudrick and colleagues introduced TPN in 1969, and it is currently used routinely in all BMT patients in the transplant setting. The continuous intravenous infusion of a hypertonic solution of protein hydrolysates, glucose, vitamins, minerals, and lipids requires an indwelling catheter placed in the large vessels and right atrium. The catheters are also used as a route of administration for blood products, immunosuppressive drugs, and other medication. Patients may be maintained indefinitely on TPN, but it is generally discontinued 2 weeks before discharge. However, the catheters may stay in place after transplantation to maintain a venous access for amphotericin or platelets.

Hickman or Broviac line catheterization can occasionally cause anxiety, depression, fear, and negative body image. On the positive side, however, this special type of venous access decreases anxiety related to the multiple painful venipunctures that would otherwise be necessary. TPN-related adjustment problems of transplant are minor and consist of four major areas: 1) the temporary loss of the basic function of eating and controlling nutrition; 2) the psychological dependence on the line itself for food and fluids; 3) dependence on nurses for TPN care, resulting in separation anxiety on discharge; and 4) the high level of technical care for maintenance of the catheter for home use. Patients are often expected to have adequate caloric intake before being weaned from TPN, which, in itself, suppresses appetite. Struggles usually develop between patient and staff over actual oral intake and weaning of TPN. As patients begin oral feedings, learned food aversions developed before chemotherapy resurface. Bernstein (1989) and Lesko (1989b) have written on learned food aversions and cancer-related anorexia, respectively. While the patient is hospitalized and on TPN because of stomatitis and side effects of chemotherapy and radiation, most medications can be given parenterally. Sublingual use of psychotropics is useless in such patients who have little tolerance for medication instructions; aversions to food, tastes, and smells; and severe stomatitis.

GvHD

Engraftment of donor bone marrow in the patient is a sign of partial success, but, paradoxically, it sometimes brings the life-threatening problem of acute or chronic GvHD, which results when the engrafted competent cells recognize the host antigens and react immunologically against them. Because recipients are immunologically suppressed, they are incapable of rejecting the engrafted cells. Such a "turning of the transplanted organ against the recipient" is unique to BMT. Approximately 50% of recipients develop mild to moderate GvHD; it is fatal in 15%–50% of patients (N. Kernan, S. Gulathi, L. M. Lesko, personal communication, March 1990). GvHD has the clinical manifestations of an acute immune disease: enteritis, serositis, malar erythema, skin eruptions, polymyositis, and elevated liver enzymes. Chronic GvHD may develop after 150 days, with chronic skin pigmentation, dysphagia, dry mucous membranes, obstructive liver dysfunction, malabsorption, an insidious deterioration in cell-mediated and humoral immunity, and debilitating contractures. It occurs in 17%–22% of long-term survivors and may be secondary to the development of a nonspecific subgroup of suppressor T cells (Parr et al. 1991). Both the acute and chronic forms add to the uncertainty of chronic illness, physical deformity, long-term medication, and altered lifestyle. Today, progress is being made in preventing GvHD by better selection of donors and purging marrow with monoclonal antibodies and/or lectins to remove cytotoxic T cells thought to initiate such reactions. Other research approaches have been to use thalidomide or ricin conjugation monoclonal antibodies once GvHD has developed.

PSYCHOLOGICAL COMPLICATIONS

BMT is used in patients who usually already have a severe, chronic, or life-threatening disease. Usual coping mechanisms and psychological techniques (conscious and unconscious) to master stresses, such as regression, repression, displacement, and rationalization, are also means by which the individual copes with the transplant environment. Very central to successful adaptation (not necessarily good physical prognosis) is the ability of patients to delegate temporarily much of their control and authority to others and the capacity to establish a close, trusting relationship with the staff (Viederman 1974).

Anxiety, Delirium, and Depression

During the pretransplant period, most patients are anxious about their hospitalization and its outcome. Anxiety is the major psychological syndrome during the BMT hospitalization and is usually precipitated by new procedures, an inadequate base of knowledge about a procedure, or preexisting anxiety over diagnostic procedures. Anticipatory anxiety can develop similarly to anticipatory nausea and vomiting (i.e., nausea and vomiting that is "conditioned" and develops before receiving the next dose of chemotherapy). Patient knowledge, anxiolytics, and behavioral techniques are appropriate interventions. Anxiety and sleep disturbances are treated with short-acting anxiolytics such as lorazepam or alprazolam in a similar fashion to other cancer settings. Pretransplant, these are usually taken as oral medications, with no modification in regular dosages used in a healthy, non–medically ill group of patients (Massie and Lesko 1989).

Delirium is rare during pre-BMT evaluations or post-BMT, unlike patients undergoing solid organ (lung, liver) transplantations (Surman 1989). Delirium may be precipitated by narcotic medications for pain relief or may indicate an electrolyte imbalance, sepsis, viral encephalitis, or multiorgan dysfunction. Isolation in a protected or germ-free environment never precipitates delirium.

During convalescence, anxiety and depression are by far the most common psychiatric sequelae of the transplantation procedure and the associated stresses of frequent outpatient visits; prophylactic medication for GvHD and infections; repeated blood tests and bone marrow biopsies; fatigue; decreased stamina; and concerns about relapse, disability, integration of home responsibilities, and job status. Many patients become disillusioned as they attempt to make the necessary philosophical transition from living "one day at a time" to anticipating the future. Adapting to the immediate stresses of relapse by "not looking beyond tomorrow" and aiming at short-term goals can result in depression and difficulties in dealing with longer-term goals after discharge. Clinicians should meet noncompliance with an attempt to understand the patients' motivations, to respect their wishes for control, and to avoid power struggles. Although studies are needed to assess the adjustment of these patients, it is encouraging to note that patients in our BMT unit have exhibited little noncompliance. This contrasts with reports from other transplant settings for solid organ transplants.

Antidepressants

The use of antidepressants in the BMT setting is quite controversial. No studies have examined their efficacy and side-effect profile. From clinical experience, any of the older- and newer-generation antidepressants would be useful in treating depression in the transplant setting. However, most BMT oncologists are vehemently concerned about the possibility of bone marrow suppression secondary to any medication. Other psychotropic drugs are often an equal target, along with antibiotics and cimetidine, because of concern about immune suppression. Consequently, current clinical practice mandates the prohibition of any antidepressant, except, possibly, stimulants such as methylphenidate, during the BMT hospitalization period. No clinical reports or clinical trials have explored the immunosuppressive capacity of any antidepressant or stimulant in this setting. I have treated one allogeneic-transplant hospitalized patient for severe depression between his first rejection and second transplant. However, the patient had virtually no marrow, and medical staff were thus unconcerned about the potential for marrow suppression. On the other hand, antidepressants can be given with a margin of safety during the convalescence period (3 to 6 months postdischarge) without fear of bone marrow suppression. Selection of a particular antidepressant or stimulant, its schedule, and dosing should follow good clinical practice, similar to that in patients with advanced medical illness or cancer (Massie and Lesko 1989). Further research is clearly needed to study their side-effect profile during BMT hospitalization itself.

Over the last few years, systematic data have been collected from consultation to the autologous BMT service at Memorial Sloan-Kettering Cancer Center (DieTrill and Lesko 1990; Levenson and Lesko 1989). Psychiatric consultations were requested for 50%–80% of patients, depending on the integration of routine psychiatric services. Initially, 79% of patients (19 of 24) were followed for a 6-month period. Five patients were evaluated for prominent psychiatric symptoms of anxiety or depression secondary to poorly controlled pain; 7 had symptoms diagnosed as adjustment disorders, of which 5 occurred in a setting of prolonged hospital stay; 5 had preexisting psychiatric diagnoses; and 2 developed delirium secondary to narcotic pain medications. Levenson and Lesko (1989) concluded that patients at risk for psychiatric and social evaluation

- Had a history of substance abuse
- Required maintenance of psychotropics during autologous BMT hospitalization
- Had a history of an anxiety disorder or severe depression early in autologous BMT
- Were noted in preevaluation to have a rigid coping style given the medical and psychological demands of autologous BMT
- Had poor family support
- Were adolescents

Clinical Issues

Several clinical issues emerged with staff and patients. First, adolescent control struggles developed in a setting of enforced dependence, and compliance with regimented treatments and emotional reactions decreased among young house and nursing staff caring for such adolescents. Second, pain and analgesia-induced psychiatric symptoms were usually missed by the consultee. Those who received both chemotherapy and radiation experienced more severe pain. Patient's altered mental status responded to lowering doses of opiates (using ones with shorter half-lives) and to the use of a neuroleptic agent (intravenous haloperidol is the most commonly used agent). Third, management of depression became challenging as a result of the consultant's inability to use pharmacotherapy because of its potential to interfere with engraftment of infused marrow. Depression was more common in patients with prolonged stay and medical complications. Ongoing family support tended to prevent severe demoralization during a lengthy stay.

As the autologous BMT service grew, the psychiatric liaison became more integrated into weekly rounds and day-to-day care, and 51% of patients were seen for initial consultation (25 of 49). Of these patients, 44% had no psychiatric diagnosis made at initial consultation, 39% had adjustment disorders, and the rest had major psychiatric syndromes. Interestingly, 9% of patients and 22% of family reported a history of psychiatric illness or alcohol abuse. The number of psychiatrist visits ranged from 1 to 16 (mean 5) during a 6- to 12-week hospitalization. The frequency of interventions varied: 13% received one type of intervention, 35% received two, 26% received three, and 13% received four interventions. These interventions included individual counseling, family counseling, administration of benzodiazepines, behavioral interventions, sleeping medication, no psychiatric intervention, referral to other medical services, pain control, and patient education.

Psychological Themes and Conflicts

Investigators have noted rebirth, changed body image, and psychological integration and/or rejection of the new organ as psychological themes expressed by transplant patients. Such themes are quite common in the transplantation of all solid organs. Fantasies that one may take on physical or psychological characteristics of the donor are less common after receiving a bone marrow transplant. However, a typical fantasy or wish was illustrated by a young male recipient on our BMT unit who hoped he would acquire some of his donor brother's athletic skills and good looks with the transplanted marrow. His mother added, on the transplantation day, that she hoped her recipient son would acquire the donor son's even-tempered personality. One obvious and striking difference between BMT and other transplants such as kidney is that the organ being transplanted is fluid and thus becomes integrated into the body; solid organs do not. This must have implications for patients' psychological adaptation to BMT and helps to explain why BMT patients have few of the difficulties in "integrating or assimilating" the organ as described in studies of kidney recipients.

Psychological conflicts regarding sexual identity, noted in cases of kidney transplantation from a donor of the opposite sex, have not been seen with BMT. BMT patients have expressed feelings of being reborn, of having a "new lease on life," or "of having a second chance" and newly developed phobias concerning germs. Readers are referred to Lesko and Hawkins (1983) for clinical examples of such themes and to Futterman and Wellisch (1990) who have written a comprehensive manuscript on their clinical experiences concerning psychodynamic themes during BMT. They include patient regression, spouse/partner dynamics, and donor/recipient relationships.

Psychiatric Illness

Any BMT patient with a history of psychiatric illness is at risk of having a recurrence of that illness during the course of transplantation (preevaluation to long-term convalescence). Presence of a major psychiatric disorder, such as schizophrenia, bipolar disorder, suicidal ideation, or psychotic depression, are mandatory indications for a psychiatric consultation before admission for transplantation. Severely disturbed patients may not be able to comply with the rigors of the transplantation procedure. However, the psychological abnormality must be severe, and it is very rare for a patient to be denied transplantation on this basis. We have found that even very disturbed patients can be maintained through the procedure with adequate psychiatric consultation, although input must be extensive in some cases. The use of psychopharmacological agents is often critical to management in this situation.

Other patients with certain personalities, methods of coping, or character disorders adapt very poorly to transplantation. Common problems include excessive dependence, regressed behavior, excessive demands, manipulation of staff and family, and hostility toward staff. Management of these issues is discussed in the following section.

PROTECTED AND GERM-FREE ENVIRONMENTS

Optimal care for patients with some types of BMT requires germ-free environments. Currently, reverse isolation (requiring staff and visitors to use cap, mask, gown, and gloves) is used more often than sterile laminar–air flow rooms. Although therapeutically useful to decrease the risk of infection and bone marrow suppression, laminar–air flow environments require prolonged physical isolation of the patient from staff and family.

Much of the research on the psychological consequences of isolation has been done in pediatric populations, and opinions differ concerning the effects of isolation on the pediatric patient. Although patients may, at times, exhibit symptoms of regression as well as affective, sensory, and behavioral changes, many researchers believe that these symptoms tend to be transient and that isolation environments do not fundamentally interfere with normal development (Kellerman et al. 1980). Others, however, have found that children in isolation exhibit a high level of anxiety, depression, and behavioral problems (Powezak et al. 1978).

Most research on psychological aspects of adaptation of adults to protected environments was initiated with the expectation that severe psychological disturbances might result from prolonged isolation, a natural extension from earlier work on sensory deprivation and intensive care unit (ICU) psychosis. Indeed, depression, anxiety, irregular sleep, regression, withdrawal from one's surroundings, and occasional disorientation have been noted in adults in isolation (Kellerman et al. 1977). However, researchers found that, although most patients were anxious and apprehensive before entering isolation, all adapted well despite the serious nature of their illnesses, their unusual environments, and their very different personalities. Cognitive and perceptual disturbances such as those described in sensory deprivation experiments were not found, nor was it necessary in any of these studies to remove a patient from the germ-free environment for psychological reasons. Only the severity of the patients' physical debilitation or the presence of a delirium, rather than isolation itself, had a profound influence on their psychological equilibrium. The loss of opportunities to touch and have physical contact was also a consideration in patients' adjustment.

Holland and co-investigators (1977) carried out the first major systematic study of cancer patients treated in isolation. Using a nurses' rating scale of patients' daily behavior, psychological state, and mood, they studied 50 leukemic patients undergoing chemotherapy in germ-free laminar–air flow rooms. They found that patients adapted well to their protected environment and, ironically, complained of overstimulation, along with the lack of physical touching. Patients can withstand the emotional stress of germ-free isolation; their behavioral changes are related to the severity of their illness rather than to the isolation itself (Gordon 1975; Holland et al. 1977; Lesko 1989c; Lesko et al. 1984).

Environmental manipulations to prevent disorientation and reduce anxiety are suggested from the ICU literature and adult and child isolation literature. Access to windows, natural light, clocks, and calendars; wearing street clothes; and personal belongings (stereo, hobbies, posters, paintings) from home are believed to be very helpful. A stable daily schedule and maintenance of the usual day and night cycle are recommended. Mobility should be encouraged; thus, equipment limiting movement should be minimized. The use of monitoring equipment should clearly be indicated, and it should be kept outside the patient's room. Exposure to other patients' distress should be eliminated; therefore, private rooms are suggested. Monotonous noises such as paging systems and air conditioning units should be minimized, and stimulus variety should be provided by patient-operated televisions and radios. Regression is discouraged by the patients' participation in their own care. Liberal visiting privileges for family and friends of the patient will help to maintain the necessary object ties and contacts with the outside world.

In summary, many clinicians and researchers have speculated about the psychological problems created by germ-free environments. In the past, they hypothesized that responses to this therapy would be similar, if not identical, to behavior associated with sensory deprivation, social isolation, and parent-child separation paradigms. This has not been borne out. When it occurs, psychopathological behavior is usually a consequence of the underlying physical illness rather than an effect of the environment. Few patients require neuroleptics, and it is very rarely mandatory to discontinue isolation therapy for psychological reasons. Most researchers agree that a protected environment gives most patients a positive feeling of being attentively cared for, and, in some, it promotes feelings of becoming a privileged, "special" patient during the hospitalization. The belief that isolation environments are adversely psychologically stressful may be more a reflection of the medical staff's projected reaction to this environment than of any real consequences of the treatment to the patient. Extensive guidelines that are beyond the scope of this chapter (Lesko 1989c; Lesko et al. 1984) offer ways to minimize any adverse sequelae for both patients and caregivers.

DONOR, FAMILY, AND STAFF CONCERNS

Donation

Unlike donors of solid organs, the donor of bone marrow provides a body product that is easily regenerated within a few weeks. Donor selection is made purely on histocompatibility and not on donor self-selection or the "family subsystem" of donor selection governed by family dynamics. In the case of BMT, once the genetically potential donors have been tissue-typed, the power of the family system to influence the medical selection process diminishes greatly.

Too often the "healthy" BMT donor receives little psychological attention. This is unfortunate because donor relatives do sometimes experience problems in connection with their donation. Left unaddressed, these problems may provide the seed for future psychological morbidity or may lead to difficulties in interpersonal relationships between the donor, patient, and other family members. The psychiatrist needs to prepare bone marrow donors for donation by helping them understand the regenerative nature of the marrow and that the loss of such an organ will not have psychological consequences. Other issues that the psychiatrist needs to keep in mind when working with donors are their psychological stability, their degree of ambivalence, possible family pressure for donation, motivation for the donation (ostracized family members who are often "black sheep" try to redeem themselves by giving a lifesaving organ) (Abram 1978), and personality structure (for hospital management of the donor). In summary, the liaison psychiatrist may be asked to assist the team in screening and selecting the appropriate donor, to prepare the donor for harvest, and to attend to the donor's concerns, feelings, and fantasies after the transplantation. Unlike some other organ donations, donation takes on a more serious note because there is no fallback such as being kept alive on a dialysis machine.

Donors are hospitalized for less than 2 days. Harvesting, which is performed under general anesthesia, is completed within 2 hours, and discharge follows 24 hours later. In some institutions, donor harvest is performed in a surgical day-hospital within a 6- to 12-hour period. Unlike other organ donors, these donors do not become depressed, mourn the loss of a body part, or usually resent those who suggested participation.

However, the long-term psychiatric or psychosocial repercussions of donating bone marrow have received very little attention in the clinical or research literature. In one of the few research studies on BMT-related donors, Wolcott and colleagues (1986a) reported from a mail questionnaire on the psychological consequences of donation to BMT patients who survived their transplant. These 18 BMT donors demonstrated some psychological sequelae as a result of their donation. Of the 12 donor-recipient matched pairs, the current quality of donor-recipient relationship was correlated with the recipient's health status and a few psychological variables. This study and clinical experience demonstrate that the psychological outcome of the donation and the donor's few medical complications help to determine the physical and psychosocial resiliency of the donor post-BMT.

To date, virtually no psychological data about the unrelated donor have been collected. Anonymous donation, which is standard procedure after a match is found, can certainly alleviate some of the face-to-face personal issues between donors and recipients. However, one could imagine the feelings of importance and moral pride from being able to contribute a unique and scarce resource. Of course, donors may question: "Will my marrow succeed in helping this person?" "Will I in some way be responsible for the GvHD or death if it is not successful?" "What will the donation do to me physically?" "Will I be able to function and get back to work?" And, most important, "Will I be asked to donate again?" It is unknown whether unrelated donors should be approached for second donations if the bone marrow did not engraft in their matched recipient. Unfortunately, at many centers, it is unresolved who is responsible for covering which medical expenses and whether to provide any psychosocial support for donors after their donation. Total anonymous donations through a registry program should alleviate some of these issues. This area of psychological evaluation, follow-up, and research in unrelated donors will no doubt expand in the next few years.

Family

Transplantation can be very difficult for the rest of the family as well as for the patient and donor. The repeated disappointment, uncertainty about the future, and stress of chronic chemotherapy are shared by parents, spouses, siblings, and children. Anxiety increases because BMT itself is still somewhat innovative and because morbidity and mortality can be very high. When the patient is a child, families must make difficult, critical decisions about BMT as a cohesive, smoothly running family unit. Each family brings to the transplantation its own marital conflicts, financial problems, school problems, and psychological concerns. Some research suggests that even the most untroubled families experience the pressures of chronic illness, the transplant procedure, and dislocation from home and friends (Patenaude et al. 1986a). Families often must travel hundreds of miles to a specialized unit, set up a new home away from home, and periodically take children out of school. Even if the transplant center is in the same city, families may feel dislocated because they are encouraged, if not expected, to participate actively in caring for the patient, which often requires all-day trips to the unit. Family adjustment during the BMT experience depends on their previous experience with medical illness; dislocations from home, family, and friends; preexisting family and economical problems; religious or ethnic background; and educational background. It is often thought that the "ideal family" (e.g., educated, well informed, and middle class) adjusts well. However, the ideal family with no problems and no need for psychological support does not truly exist.

On many transplant services, a psychiatrist or social worker and a nurse meet weekly with the patients' families. Meetings are often held away from the BMT unit to provide family members with a safe environment in which to air concerns and a geographical gap from the patient. These professionals can assist families with 1) an introduction to the BMT unit (its personnel, procedures, medical terminology, staff expectations), 2) airing concerns about donor selection, 3) rearranging their lifestyles (e.g., managing dislocation from home and friends and relocation to the transplant center), 4) managing preexisting marital or family problems, 5) coping with the strain of having the wage earner or the mother figure incapacitated, 6) developing an identity with the medical team to promote better communication, and 7) learning how to best help and motivate the patient during the hospitalization. Dealing with signs of graft rejection, a transition into a terminal phase of illness, or preparation for discharge are also discussed (Patenaude et al. 1986a). Our transplant team and others have recognized that a patient's positive response to hospitalization and treatment can be jeopardized if the patient returns to an unstable marital or family situation.

A BMT family support group satisfies various needs that are often not addressed in individual supportive psychotherapy. Patenaude and associates (1986a) summarize these needs as 1) providing a common geographical area and time for family members to meet and share their unique experience; 2) creating a safe place to share feelings, decrease a sense of isolation, and normalize their family BMT experience; and 3) reducing a sense of helplessness by becoming empowered with medical knowledge and new coping skills.

Staff and Liaison Issues

It is surprising that many BMT centers do not routinely offer psychosocial services. Rappaport (1988) reported that, based on the response to a brief questionnaire mailed to 57 BMT programs, 29% of the 52 respondents had no regular psychosocial services for patients or staff. Seventy-one percent had "some regular consultation-liaison psychiatric contact," with services provided by psychiatrists (8%); nonphysicians, such as psychologists, social workers, and nurses (78%); or a team of psychiatric and nonpsychiatric consultants (14%). Seventy-five percent of these BMT centers that had some type of psychosocial component did not use a psychiatrist for any regular service such as individual consults or staff support. Psychiatric liaison to a bone marrow transplant unit is ideal and, when in place, works well (Fawzy et al. 1977; Patenaude and Rappeport 1984; Rappaport 1988; Wellisch et al. 1978). Models vary from pure psychiatric consultation to a pure liaison model solely working with staff. At Memorial Sloan-Kettering Cancer Center, we have a five-member psychosocial team composed of the unit-based nurse clinician trained in psychosocial aspects of patient care, a psychiatrist (L.M.L.), a psychiatric psychooncology fellow, a psychiatric nurse clinician, and a social worker. This team meets weekly with the BMT nurses to discuss psychosocial care plans; a member of the Memorial Sloan-Kettering Cancer Center ethics committee or a neuropsychologist may attend when particular patients are discussed. The psychiatric nurse leads a weekly support group for the nurses and provides nurse-to-nurse psychiatric consultation for patients and families. These consultations are referred to the psychiatrist and/or fellow for further psychiatric evaluations if necessary. These formal consultations usually entail discussions of medical and legal issues, patients with previous psychiatric diagnosis or with current psychiatric syndromes requiring medication, noncompliance, ethical or "do not resuscitate" issues, and routine pre-BMT consultation for patients at risk for psychosocial problems. The social worker routinely provides day-to-day general support of the patient and family. The BMT unit–based nurse clinician, as coordinator of this team, initiates when and how each team member becomes involved in patient care and also coordinates the weekly psychosocial rounds. Weekly psychosocial care plans are logged in a notebook and then followed or changed. The team, not the BMT attending, initiates any psychosocial or psychiatric intervention, a highly unusual consultation-liaison model.

The mental health professional may help members of the transplant team cope with the psychologically stressful tasks they must perform. Because BMT teams must work closely with patients and families, an unusual sense of intimacy develops. This intimacy may lead the staff to 1) become overly protective and possessive of their patients (especially when the patients are transferred back to the referring physician), 2) take on too many parental responsibilities in caring for their patients, 3) become angry when a transplant patient does not return to a productive life, 4) feel guilty and disappointed when a patient dies despite their efforts, and 5) develop hostility toward patients who withdraw from posttransplant care even when the quality of care available to them is adequate. Staff meetings should review stressful and nonconstructive emotional reactions as part of patient care rounds.

Regular staff meetings with a team psychiatrist or psychologist usually focus on ethical aspects of decisions, management of the patient's psychological symptoms, and communication with patients and families. The consultant may interpret a patient's anger and maladaptive behavior for the staff. When conflicts arise among the members of the staff, the psychiatrist must balance the roles of participant, consultant, and arbitrator. A consultant skilled in group therapy may be asked to help resolve unusual team conflicts. Using psychotherapeutic skills requires precise judgment and balance by the BMT mental health professional. The psychiatrist must recognize signs of major psychological distress in a team member to make early referral to another psychiatrist for consultation.

Bloom (1981) summarized the function of the liaison mental health professional as "witness, bystander, and translator of emotional events" and "catalyst in promoting the best and most adaptive ways of interpersonal functioning." One liaison professional on a pediatric bone marrow unit views her role as a "lightening rod" (Patenaude et al. 1979). The presence of a psychologically minded team member legitimizes certain topics that would otherwise be discussed less often or not at all. The role of a mental health professional (psychiatrist, psychologist, social worker, or psychiatric nurse clinician) should ideally include

- Assisting the team in predicting the psychological implications and effects of the organ transplant on the donor, family, and recipient.
- Determining patients' coping styles, predicting their emotional response, and thus preventing the development of complicated and severe emotional disturbances.
- Supporting patients and families throughout the preparation, transplant, and convalescent period.
- Helping the team in the psychological management of patients' symptoms during treatment.
- Providing psychotherapy and medication (by psychiatrist) when serious disturbances develop.

Programs have been developed for nurses on BMT units to prevent "burnout" (Sarantos 1988) and stress related to the closing of a unit (Zevon et al. 1990). These have involved "psych" rounds, hospital workshops, in-service educational programs on the BMT floor, weekly support meetings, staff support ("buddy") systems between new and experienced staff nurses, informal and personal conversations with peers, and formal consultations with mental health providers regarding specific patient care issues. One model, similar to the Memorial Sloan-Kettering Cancer Center model, is described below.

The Fred Hutchinson Marrow Transplant Center developed a comprehensive psychosocial program for their nurses (Sarantos 1988). It is unique in that it is staff directed and cost-effective and provides crisis and prevention services. Previous experience with a psychiatric nurse clinician consulting on their unit had led to the development of a unique staff-directed psychosocial committee and staff program coordinator. This coordinator acted as a resource to mobilize psychiatric consultation; directed behavioral or social interventions; provided day-to-day support to patients and families; and taught fellow nurses communication skills training, clinical problem solving, stress management, and therapeutic massage. In addition, a therapist was hired, oriented by this nurse coordinator to provide individual counseling to nurses experiencing crisis at work or in their personal lives.

Smaller BMT units may have other effective models. However, when developing consultation and liaison services to a BMT unit, the practitioner should follow appropriate clinical practices that apply to any oncology unit. For example, being flexible and available, avoiding use of psychiatric jargon, visiting staff and patients daily but briefly, attending essential BMT medical conferences, and providing services that the staff can easily implement.

LATE PHYSICAL SEQUELAE OF BONE MARROW TRANSPLANTATION

Convalescence often requires 6 to 12 months (Nims 1991). Weekly, or occasionally twice-weekly, visits to the BMT clinic are mandatory for the first 3 months after discharge. During these "maintenance" visits, blood counts, engraftment, and infection are monitored. Bearman and colleagues (1988) developed a regimen-related toxicity (RRT) scale (stage I to IV) to predict actual survival. Retrospective examination of 195 BMT patients revealed that all patients developed at least grade I toxicity in at least one organ. RRT was more common in relapse versus remission, allogeneic- versus autologous-transplant patients, and those receiving > 1,500 versus 1,200 cGy of TBI. They concluded that those patients who developed grade II to IV toxicity during post-BMT were unlikely to survive beyond 100 days.

Many late sequelae may occur months and years after discharge, including infection, delayed reconstitution of the immune system, chronic GvHD, cataracts, cardiomyopathy from anthracycline and radiation, pulmonary interstitial pneumonitis relapse, rare second malignancies occurring 10 to 15 years post-BMT, particularly lymphoma (Witherspoon et al. 1989), infertility, sexual dysfunction, and growth/maturation failure in children. Pot-Mees (1989) found nonsignificant cognitive decline in young patients secondary to BMT. However, the BMT children demonstrated a lower intelligence quotient (IQ) in general, compared with healthy children or a comparison group of cardiac surgery patients; effects of behavioral, affective disturbances, and absence from school could not be ascertained.

Despite these numerous potential late sequelae, patients are reported to have good performance status. Lesko and co-workers (1992) reported 94% of their cohort of BMT survivors (5 years after BMT) had Karnofsky ratings of 90 or above. In another study, 93% of BMT patients could perform normal activities without any or minor physical problems and reported Karnofsky score > 80% 4 years after transplantation (Wingard et al. 1991a). Only 25% of another cohort of BMT survivors 3.5 years after transplantation (n = 25) reported ongoing medical problems (Wolcott et al. 1986b); however, the impact of these medical problems (colds, pneumonia, infections) was not connected to actual physical performance.

Unlike the other areas of transplantation psychiatry, BMT research has concentrated mainly on psychological adjustment posttransplant, rather than pretransplant evaluation or comorbidity issues in selecting "good-risk" transplant candidates. Several survivor studies are noteworthy (Andrykowski et al. 1989a, 1989b; Baker et al. 1991; Hengeveld et al. 1988; Jenkins et al. 1991; Lesko et al. 1992; Syrjala et al. 1988; Wingard et al. 1991a, 1991b; Wolcott et al. 1986b). In general, most research studies of BMT survivors 1) share common methodological strategies and findings, 2) are retrospective and cross-sectional, 3) evaluate adult survivors (ages 19 to 50 years) 1 to 4 years after BMT, and 4) combine cancer and noncancer diagnoses (e.g., aplastic anemia and metabolic disorders) and combine allogeneic- and autologous-transplant procedures. Information is gathered by mail survey or an interview format. The latter format usually combines an interview with commonly used psychometrically sound psychosocial inventories. However, research in this area is still somewhat unsophisticated in that only one source of information is used (often a mail survey) rather than two or three sources or numerous methods (interview, video, questionnaires) gathered at several points in time. None of these methods tests any intervention; they provide basic prevalence information on quality-of-life issues. The only studies that have compared a population of BMT survivors with other transplant survivors and conventionally treated cancer patients are by Andrykowski and colleagues (1990), Altmaier and others (1991), and Lesko and associates (1992).

Results from these studies reveal that patients who have successfully survived their transplant biologically are doing extremely well in their physical performance and psychological well-being. However, most of these patients were at least 1 to 2 years post-BMT; this disregards the issue of crucial adjustment during the first 12 months after discharge. In general, these survivors were from "traditional" populations in which men worked and women were homemakers. Poorer psychological adjustment was found in areas where one was concentrating on their reentry issues (i.e., men at work and women at home with their nuclear or extended families). Infertility and psychosexual rehabilitation appeared to be the most problematic reentry and survivor issues. Such resilient BMT survivors understand the importance of visiting and sharing their recovery with patients currently undergoing this procedure.

Psychosexual Adjustment

To date, little has been written about the ovarian and testicular function of patients undergoing autologous BMT. For now, we must extrapolate crucial information on endocrine and gonadal function, fertility and pregnancy, and psychosexual function from the few allogeneic-transplant studies. Again, we must exert caution in extrapolating these data to all autologous patients, particularly those patients who have undergone treatment for testicular cancer.

Chemotherapeutic agents, singly or in combination, have a profound impact on male and female gonadal function. For men, several agents produce a dose-related depletion of germinal epithelium lining, resulting in decreased testicular volume, oligospermia, azoospermia, and possible infertility. Low sperm count and elevated follicle-stimulating hormone (FSH) levels are physiological indicators of such germinal aplasia. Testosterone levels remain within normal range (Sherins and Mulvihill 1989). Additional chemotherapy during allogeneic or autologous BMT severely complicates gonadal recovery, as does retroperitoneal lymph node dissection. Chemotherapeutic agents are not known to directly affect the sexual response cycle (desire, arousal, ejaculation/orgasm) of men.

Ovarian failure has been documented in women receiving single-agent and combination chemotherapy. Alkylating agents appear to be the most notorious cause of ovarian failure, particularly in the older patient. Such failure is evident by dysfunction of ova and follicles, ovarian fibrosis, low estradiol levels, and elevated serum FSH and luteinizing hormone (LH) levels, resulting in amenorrhea and menopausal symptoms of estrogen deficiency (e.g., hot flashes, vaginal dryness, vaginitis, dyspareunia, irritability, decreased libido, vaginal epithelium atrophy, and endometrial hypoplasia). The cumulative dose of the chemotherapeutic agent and the age of the patient influence the frequency and duration of amenorrheic symptomatology. It appears that older women are less able to tolerate larger cumulative drug doses before amenorrhea develops and have a greater likelihood of permanent dysfunction when treatment is stopped. As in men, combination chemotherapy can cause gonadal dysfunction in women. Unlike gonadal dysfunction in men, ovarian failure and subsequent low estradiol levels can directly and indirectly affect the sexual response cycle in women. The estrogen deficiency symptoms of decreased libido, vaginal atrophy, decreased vaginal secretions, and dyspareunia can all deleteriously affect desire, arousal, and orgasm. Unlike the research on the gonadal toxicity of chemotherapeutic agents, information is known about the adverse effects of RT (Sherins and Mulvihill 1989).

The testes are very radiosensitive; damage (both to germinal epithelium and Leydig cells) and recovery appear to be dose dependent. Temporary azoospermia develops after 150 to 2,000 cGy, and men who receive 2,000 to 3,000 cGy require at least 3 years to recover. Permanent sterility results at 6,000 cGy. Unfortunately, adolescents and young men receiving higher doses of radiation to the testes as prophylaxis for gonadal relapse of acute lymphoblastic leukemia have demonstrated germinal aplasia as well as Leydig cell dysfunction, resulting in testosterone deficiencies. RT may also cause erectile and ejaculatory difficulties, thereby affecting the male sexual response cycle.

For women, gonadal dysfunction and infertility after RT are dose related, but they are also age dependent (unlike in men). Loescher and co-workers (1989) found permanent infertility occurred in 60% of women aged 15 to 40 and in 100% over age 40, after 25 to 500 cGy.

Particularly in lymphoma therapy, the ovary may be shielded from radiation by oophorectomy (surgically placing the ovaries midline behind the uterus). This procedure appears to lower the risk of ovarian failure to 50% of women receiving pelvic radiation (Loescher et al. 1989). Radiation may also alter vasocongestive mechanisms of female genital arousal, decrease vaginal lubrication during the excitement phase, and cause dyspareunia as a result of vaginal stenosis, atrophy, and fibrosis and vaginitis. Thus, radiation may adversely affect all phases of the female sexual cycle.

An extensive follow-up of patients by Sanders and colleagues (1987, 1988) reveals the following: first, after receiving a high-dose alkylating agent such as cyclophosphamide alone for BMT, most prepubertal children develop normally through puberty and have normal gonadotropin levels (LH and FSH). Of course, those children with symptoms diagnosed as aplastic anemia received no gonadal toxic treatments before BMT. Second, the majority of prepubertal children with acute leukemia who received cyclophosphamide and TBI as a preconditioning regimen had delayed puberty and abnormal gonadotropin levels. However, a few girls did achieve menarche, which suggests that radiation to the ovary of the prepubertal girl may not result in permanent damage. Testosterone or estrogen/progesterone supplementation may be necessary. Third, the majority of adults who received a cyclophosphamide-only regimen regained normal gonadal function. Approximately 50% of women had return of their menstrual cycles 6 to 18 months post-BMT; however, recovery was transient for some (2 to 6 years), with development of menopausal symptoms, low estradiol levels, and elevated gonadotropin levels. All men had normal testosterone levels post-BMT and a majority (88%) had normal LH levels (FSH was elevated in 76% of patients). Most regained normal gonadotropin levels. Limited data were available on semen analysis. Sixty-seven percent of patients appeared to have detectable sperm counts. Fourth, primary gonadal dysfunction appears to occur in all patients who are postpubertal at transplant after a combination of cyclophosphamide and TBI. All of these patients had leukemia and received prior cytoreductive therapy. Women had primary ovarian failure, amenorrhea, and elevated gonadotropin levels. Recovery of ovarian function occurred in less than 10% of women 3 to 7 years after transplantation; all were age 26 years and younger at BMT. Menopausal symptomatology (i.e., amenorrhea, vaginitis, decreased vaginal lubrication, osteoporosis, vasomotor instability, and dysphoria) was evident in at least 75% of women who were older than age 26 years at BMT. Hormonal replacement in women appeared to be efficacious in relieving menopausal symptoms.

Sanders and co-investigators (1987) estimated a 35% probability of developing ovarian failure at 7 years for women who received cyclophosphamide alone and 100% at 1 year for those who received cyclophosphamide and TBI. Women receiving cyclophosphamide only had a 92% probability of ovarian recovery at 7 years, and those receiving cyclophosphamide and TBI had a 24% probability of recovery. They concluded that both greater patient age and TBI were significantly correlated with a greater probability of ovarian failure.

Given the complex etiology and manifestations of sexual and reproductive problems, a multidisciplinary approach is often necessary. Interventions include hormone-replacement therapy, sperm banking, and pharmacologic and surgical means of protecting fertility during treatment. Hormone replacement may be effective in several instances when patients are undergoing BMT. For example, some adolescent or prepubertal boys receiving radiation may need testosterone replacement to promote the development of secondary sexual characteristics, and all women who have undergone premature menopause after BMT need hormone replacement. Low-dose estrogen and progesterone combinations and topical estrogen ameliorate most of the menopausal symptomatology. Nonhormonal drug therapies (e.g., clonidine) may help to relieve menopausal symptoms in women who refuse initial estrogen replacement. (Dosing regimens for hormonal replacement are beyond the scope of this chapter.) Patients and families are strongly encouraged to seek out an endocrinologist who primarily treats oncological patients and who has a special interest in the long-term sequelae of cancer treatment.

It has been suggested that hormone replacement during chemotherapy may suppress germ-cell proliferation, thereby preventing antineoplastic therapy–associated gonadal toxicity. Gonadal protection during chemotherapy has included administering testosterone in men, oral contraceptives in women, and gonadotropin-releasing hormone (GnRH) analogues in both sexes. Unfortunately, results from preliminary studies have not proved efficacious.

An appropriate and relatively effective method of protecting fertility in men undergoing BMT is sperm banking. Unfortunately, semen from pretreated cancer patients and treated patients about to undergo BMT may reveal low sperm count and poor or inadequate sperm mobility. Approximately one-half of the men with testicular cancer or lymphoma have abnormal sperm specimens that prevent sperm banking before any cancer treatment. However, cryobanking should be encouraged for all men, even if sperm counts are low. Multiple ejaculate samples can increase the total number of viable sperm for storage. Few data are available on how many BMT patients choose sperm banking. Mumma and colleagues (1992) noted in a small study of male BMT patients that, of the four (36%) who were offered the option of sperm banking, three chose to do so.

In summary, this procedure involves sensitive encouragement by BMT staff for patients to bank sperm, a receptive patient who has undergone little or relatively nontoxic cancer treatment, the availability of a local sperm banking facility because most BMT units do not provide this service on site, and enough time for travel (in some cases, many miles) and banking. The last two factors are critical and often unavailable. Many insurance companies do not reimburse the costs associated with this procedure, and financial constraints may present a barrier for some men who want to take advantage of this technique.

An experimental option available to women before BMT is in vitro fertilization. Several fertility centers have developed highly innovative programs in which women ending chemotherapy for their cancers are stimulated with hormonal therapy to collect ovum for fertilization and then storage. Possible use of these fertilized ovum after transplantation is a new and highly ethically and emotionally charged area of patient concern, particularly for the potential father of a child when the woman has unsuccessfully proceeded through the transplantation procedure and died.

There have been a few reports of pregnancies and deliveries of healthy children in women with severe aplastic anemia treated with allogeneic BMT (Card et al. 1980; Deeg et al. 1983; Hinterberger-Fischer et al. 1991; Jacobs and Dubovsky 1989; Sanders et al. 1987, 1988). Even though healthy infants were delivered 15 to 24+ months post-transplantation, success must be tempered by the fact that these female patients, unlike other patients undergoing BMT, had no preconditioning chemotherapy regimens, received only high-dose cyclophosphamide as a preparatory regimen for their BMT (i.e., no TBI), and, in general, most were young at time of transplant; all of these conditions led to probably less gonadal dysfunction. I do not know of any reports of failed pregnancies and deliveries, but it would be interesting to determine what percentage are normal.

A thorough review of the literature reveals a relative absence of empirical studies examining the impact of BMT on psychosexual functioning. (See Ostroff and Lesko [1991] for a comprehensive chapter on psychosexual function in BMT patients.) These authors delineate the specific sexual disorders possible after transplantation and suggest phase-appropriate clinical and pharmacological interventions aimed at improving sexual functioning.

Further clarification of the incidence, nature, and risk factors associated with sexual dysfunction among BMT patients is needed to develop and refine prevention and rehabilitation efforts geared toward maintenance of sexual health among cancer survivors treated with BMT. For instance, Mumma and colleagues (1992) compared the psychosexual functioning of acute leukemia survivors treated with either conventional chemotherapy alone or conventional chemotherapy followed by allogeneic BMT. They found no significant differences in sexual desire, satisfaction, and body image between these two subgroups of long-term leukemia survivors. They concluded that leukemia survivors treated with BMT experienced no greater psychosexual sequelae than their conventional treatment counterparts who noted significant decline in sexual satisfaction. This research protocol was also conducted with chronic leukemia patients treated with either conventional chemotherapy alone or followed by allogeneic BMT, and the results were similar, in that BMT patients fared no worse in terms of their sexual health. Compared with physically healthy control subjects, women survivors generally reported decreased sexual frequency and satisfaction, whereas both men and women survivors reported poorer body image. Longer time since completing cancer treatment predicted more frequent sexual activity in women but poorer body image for both men and women. Those survivors who reported decreased sexual frequency, decreased satisfaction, and poorer body image reported greater psychological distress and decreased energy. Results indicate that psychosexual sequelae in survivors of leukemia occur frequently and warrant intensive investigation, particularly to address the need for intervention in those most distressed.

Wingard and associates (1991b) also retrospectively studied sexual satisfaction in BMT survivors. One hundred thirty-five adults were surveyed 6 to 149 months posttransplantation for sexual satisfaction. Sixty-five percent revealed a moderate level of sexual satisfaction. Factors associated with greater satisfaction included younger age at transplantation, a satisfying relationship with a partner, satisfaction with body image/appearance, noncancer versus cancer diagnosis, and general overall life satisfaction. Several gender-specific gonadal psychological issues arise from these studies (Mumma et al. 1992; Ostroff et al. 1991; Wingard et al. 1991b). Ninety percent of women had reported irregular or aberrant menses in the study by Mumma and others (1992), which also noted poor endocrine follow-up. As mentioned before, these women reported decreased sexual drive and satisfaction and had poor body image that did not improve with time. In another study of 57% of women receiving estrogen-replacement therapy, only 40% had regular menses (Wingard et al. 1991b). Another study suggests implications for psychosocial follow-up, citing that 50% of women were prematurely menopausal secondary to cancer treatment and were on estrogen-replacement therapy (but had not undergone BMT) met criteria for a sexual disorder, despite high levels of marital satisfaction (Ostroff et al. 1991). Future studies are needed to randomize women to several doses of estrogen replacement to evaluate the psychological interplay between sexual dysfunction and infertility.

Men, irrespective of sperm banking and normal testosterone levels, may be vulnerable to sexually related issues. Implications could be generalized to male BMT survivors from a provocative study by Lesko and co-workers (L. M. Lesko, D. Cella, S. Tross, et al., unpublished data, 1994) of 126 men who had undergone curative treatment of Hodgkin's disease, acute leukemia, BMT, and testicular cancer. Subjects were classified as low risk or high risk for subsequent infertility. *Low* risk included benign testicular biopsy or acute leukemia, and *high* risk included Hodgkin's disease, testicular cancer, or BMT. Patients were also classified by marital status. A multivariate analysis of variance examined the effect of infertility risk, marital status, and the infertility risk plus marital status interaction. Body image was significantly more disturbed in the married group ($P < .05$), and there was a significant group and marital status effect ($P < .05$) on body image and sexual satisfaction. Specifically, within the high-risk infertility group, the married men showed more impairment than the unmarried counterparts. Within the low-risk infertility group, the unmarried subgroup showed more impairment than the married subgroup. No effects were observed for sexual dysfunction or sense of masculinity. Within the married times high-risk subgroup, pretreatment sperm banking failed to protect individuals from impairment. The results suggest that, among cancer survivors at high risk for infertility, being married may have a disruptive rather than an enhancing effect on body image and sexual satisfaction, in contrast to the positive effects of being married that are usually observed among physically healthy individuals. Clinically, one could generally surmise that the young male BMT survivor who is married or has a close relationship may be confronted with more stress than his unattached counterpart. He more readily needs to face these issues when discharged because he is returning to a family and spouse and may feel more pressure to return to an active psychological and sexual relationship. In the study by Wingard and associates (1991b), 24% ($n = 43$) of men had some difficulty with erection and ejaculation that was significantly associated with decreased sexual satisfaction, despite all men having normal testosterone levels.

Clinically, in summary, BMT patients who report fewer psychosexual issues after convalescence are usually those who are younger, have a nonmalignant disease, had no pre-BMT sexual problems, currently have a satisfying sexual relationship with a significant other, report no body image concerns, and are generally satisfied with their lives.

CONCLUSION

Future areas of psychological research in the area of BMT survivorship should include the careful assessment of long-term effects of BMT treatment (chemotherapy and radiation) on intellectual and sexual development; the longitudinal study of immediate and delayed impact of BMT on psychological adaptation of patients; and the development and testing of materials to enhance information to reduce distress and facilitate re-entry. Multicentered collaborative research, now in its infancy for BMT, will be mandatory to collect enough data for meaningful information. The future of such psychiatric research lies in collaboration with multiple centers and researchers. Comparison of BMT patients' adjustment with other transplant patients (liver, cardiac, renal) has not provided important data. Careful comparisons are needed between treatment options and adjustment to such treatment options for patients (e.g., patients with chronic myelogenic leukemia who choose conventional chemotherapy versus those who choose BMT). The next decade promises to be quite exciting.

REFERENCES

Abram HS: Renal transplantation, in Massachusetts General Hospital Handbook of General Hospital Psychiatry. Edited by Hackett TP, Cassem NH. St Louis, MO, CV Mosby, 1978, pp 365–379

Altmaier EM, Gingrich RD, Fyfe MA: Two year adjustment of bone marrow transplant survivors. Bone Marrow Transplant 7:311–316, 1991

American Psychiatric Association: Diagnostic and Statistical Manual of Mental Disorders, 4th Edition. Washington, DC, American Psychiatric Association, 1994

Andrykowski MA, Henslee PJ, Farall MG: Physical and psychological functioning of adult survivors of allogeneic bone marrow transplantation. Bone Marrow Transplant 4:65–71, 1989a

Andrykowski MA, Henslee-Downey J, Barnett RL: Longitudinal assessment of psychological functioning of adult survivors of allogeneic bone marrow transplantation. Bone Marrow Transplant 4:505–509, 1989b

Andrykowski MA, Altmaier EM, Barnett RL, et al: Quality of life in adult survivors of allogeneic bone marrow transplantation: correlates and comparison with matched renal transplant recipients. Transplantation 50:399–406, 1990

Anonymous: Cancer economics. Cancer Lett Suppl July 1990, pp 1–2

Appelbaum FR: Marrow transplantation for hematologic malignancies: a brief review of current status and future prospects. Semin Hematol 25 (suppl 3):16–22, 1988

Baker F, Cubow B, Wingard JR: Role retention and quality of life of bone marrow transplant survivors. Soc Sci Med 32:697–704, 1991

Bealty PG, Hansen JA, Anasetti C, et al: Marrow transplantation from unrelated HLA-matched volunteer donors. Transplant Proc 21:2993–2941, 1989

Bearman SI, Appelbaum FR, Buckner CD, et al: Regimen-related toxicity in patients undergoing bone marrow transplantation. J Clin Oncol 6:1562–1568, 1988

Bergner M, Bobbilt RA, Pollard WE: Sickness Impact Profile: validation of a health status measure. Med Care 14:57–61, 1976

Bernstein I: Learned food aversions as a factor in the nutritional management of cancer patients. Nutrition 5:116–118, 1989

Bloom V: Functions of liaison psychiatrist in a kidney center: personal reflections. Dialysis and Transplantation 10:51–55, 1981

Bortin MM, Rimm AA: Increasing utilization of bone marrow transplantation. Transplantation 48:453–458, 1989

Brown HN, Kelly MJ: Stages of bone marrow transplantation: a psychiatric perspective. Psychosom Med 38:439–446, 1976

Burnett AK: Autologous bone marrow transplantation in acute leukemia. Leuk Res 12:531–536, 1988

Card RT, Holmes IH, Sugarman RG, et al: Successful pregnancy after high dose chemotherapy and marrow transplantation for treatment of aplastic anemia. Exp Hematol 8:57–60, 1980

Chapman CR, Hill HF: Patient-controlled analgesia in a bone marrow transplant setting, in Advances in Pain Research and Therapy, Vol 16. Edited by Foley KM. New York, Raven, 1990, pp 231–247

Chauvenet AR, Smith NM: Referral of pediatric oncology patients for marrow transplantation and the process of informed consent. Med Pediatr Oncol 16:40–44, 1988

Cheson BD, Lacerna L, Leyland-Jones B, et al: Autologous bone marrow transplantation. Ann Intern Med 110:51–65, 1989

Curran WF: Bone marrow transplantation among half-siblings. N Engl J Med 324:1818–1819, 1991

Deeg HJ, Kennedy MS, Sanders JE, et al: Successful pregnancy after marrow transplantation for severe aplastic anemia and immunosuppression with cyclosporine. JAMA 250:647, 1983

Dermatis H, Lesko LM: Psychological distress in parents consenting to child's bone marrow transplantation. Bone Marrow Transplant 6:411–417, 1990

Dermatis H, Lesko LM: Psychosocial correlates of physician-patient communication at time of informed consent for bone marrow transplantation. Cancer Invest 9:621–628, 1991

Derogatis LP, Spencer MS: The Brief Symptom Inventory (BSI): Administration, Scoring, and Procedures Manual. Baltimore, MD, Clinical Psychometric Research, 1982

Die-Trill M, Lesko LM: Psychiatric consultation in cancer patients undergoing autologous bone marrow transplantation (abstract). Presented at the Academy of Psychosomatic Medicine meeting, 1990

Durbin M: Bone marrow transplantation: economic, ethical, and social issues. Pediatrics 82:774–783, 1988

Fawzy FI, Wellisch D, Yager J: Psychiatric liaison to bone marrow transplant project, in The Family in Mourning: A Guide for Health Professionals. Edited by Hollingsworth CE, Pasnau RC. New York, Grune & Stratton, 1977, pp 181–189

Ford RE: Psychosocial and ethical issues in bone marrow transplantation, in Bone Marrow Transplantation: A Nursing Perspective. Edited by Kasprisin CA, Snyder EL. Arlington, VA, American Association of Blood Banks, 1990, pp 129–151

Futterman AD, Wellisch DK: Psychodynamic themes of bone marrow transplantation. Hematol Oncol Clin North Am 4:699–709, 1990

Futterman AD, Bond G, Wellisch DK: The psychosocial levels system: identifying patients at risk for emotional complications during bone marrow transplantation (abstract). Psychosom Med 51:265, 1989

Goldman JM, Apperley JF, Jones L, et al: Bone marrow transplantation for patients with chronic myeloid leukemia. N Engl J Med 314:202–208, 1986

Gordon AM: Psychological adaptation to isolation therapy in acute leukemia. Psychosomatics 26:132–139, 1975

Haberman MR: Psychosocial aspects of bone marrow transplantation. Semin Oncol Nurs 4:55–59, 1988

Head v Colloton (1983)

Hengeveld MD, Houtman RB, Zwaan FE: Psychological aspects of bone marrow transplantation: a retrospective study of 17 long-term survivors. Bone Marrow Transplant 3:69–75, 1988

Hinterberger-Fischer M, Kier P, Kalhs P, et al: Fertility, pregnancies and offspring complications after bone marrow transplantation. Bone Marrow Transplant 7:5–9, 1991

Holder AR: Legal issues in bone marrow transplantation. Yale J Biol Med 63:521–525, 1990

Holland J, Plumb M, Yates J, et al: Psychological response of patients with acute leukemia to germ free environments. Cancer 40:871–879, 1977

Holmes W: Preparing the patient for bone marrow transplantation: nursing care issues. Yale J Biol Med 63:487–494, 1990

Jacobs P, Dubovsky DW: Bone marrow transplantation followed by normal pregnancy. Am J Hematol 11:209–212, 1989

Jenkins PL, Livingston A, Whittaker JA: A retrospective study of psychosocial morbidity in bone marrow transplant recipients. Psychosomatics 32:65–71, 1991

Kelahan AM: View from a third party insurance representative (letter). Leukemia 7:110, 1993

Kellerman J, Rigler D, Sigel SE: The psychological effects of isolation in protected environments. Am J Psychiatry 134:563–565, 1977

Kellerman J, Siegel SE, Rigler D: Special treatment modalities: laminar airflow rooms, in Psychological Aspects of Childhood Cancer. Edited by Kellerman J. Springfield, IL, CC Thomas, 1980, pp 128–154

Langedoen K: Ethical issues in the allocation and reimbursement of bone marrow transplantation. Leukemia 7:1117–1121, 1993

Lasagna L: The professional-patient dialogue. Hastings Cent Rep 13:9–11, 1983

Lenfant C, Quesenberry PJ: The status of bone marrow transplantation for hematologic diseases: LSA symposium. Leukemia 7:1074–1129, 1993

Lesko LM: Bone marrow transplantation, in Handbook of Psychooncology: The Psychological Care of the Patient With Cancer. Edited by Holland JC, Rowland JR. New York, Oxford University Press, 1989a, pp 163–173

Lesko LM: Anorexia, in Handbook of Psychooncology: The Psychological Care of the Patient With Cancer. Edited by Holland JC, Rowland JR. New York, Oxford University Press, 1989b, pp 434–443

Lesko LM: Protected environments, in Handbook of Psychooncology: The Psychological Care of the Patient With Cancer. Edited by Holland JC, Rowland JR. New York, Oxford University Press, 1989c, pp 174–179

Lesko LM, Hawkins DR: Psychological aspects of transplantation medicine, in New Psychiatric Syndromes: DSM-III and Beyond. Edited by Akhtar S. New York, Jason Aronson, 1983, pp 265–309

Lesko LM, Kern J, Hawkins DR: Psychological aspects of patients in germ-free isolation: a review of child, adult and patient management literature. Med Pediatr Oncol 12:43–49, 1984

Lesko LM, Dermatis H, Penman D, et al: Patients', parents', and oncologists' perceptions of informed consent for bone marrow transplantation. Med Pediatr Oncol 17:181–187, 1989

Lesko LM, Ostroff JS, Mumma GH, et al: Long term psychological adjustment of acute leukemia survivors: impact of bone marrow transplantation vs. conventional chemotherapy. Psychosom Med 54:30–47, 1992

Levenson J, Lesko LM: The role of the consultation-liaison psychiatrist on an autologous bone marrow transplantation service (abstract). Presented at the Academy of Psychosomatic Medicine meeting, 1989

Loescher LL, Welch-McCaffrey D, Leigh SA, et al: Surviving adult cancers, part I: physiologic effects. Ann Intern Med 111:411–432, 1989

Massie MJ, Lesko LM: Psychopharmacological management, in Handbook of Psychooncology: The Psychological Care of the Patient With Cancer. Edited by Holland JC, Rowland JR. New York, Oxford Press, 1989, pp 470–491

McCullough J, Hansen J, Perkins H, et al: The national marrow donor program: how it works, accomplishments to date. Oncology 3:63–74, 1989

McNair DM, Lorr M, Droppleman LF: EdITS Manual for the Profile of Mood States. San Diego, CA, Educational and Industrial Testing Service, 1971

Meadows A, Massan DJ, Gordon J, et al: Declines in IQ scores and cognitive dysfunctions in children with acute myelocytic leukemia treated with cranial radiation. Lancet 2:1015–1018, 1981

Mumma GH, Mashberg D, Lesko LM: Long term psychosexual adjustment of acute leukemia survivors: impact of marrow transplantation vs. conventional chemotherapy. Gen Hosp Psychiatry 14:43–55, 1992

National Organ Transplant Act, PL 98-507 (1984)

Nims JW: Survivorship and rehabilitation, in Bone Marrow Transplantation: Principles, Practice and Nursing Insights. Edited by Whedon MB. Boston, MA, Jones & Bartlett, 1991, pp 334–345

O'Reilly RJ: Allogeneic bone marrow transplantation: current status and future directions. Journal of the American Society of Hematology 62:941–964, 1983

Ostroff JS, Lesko LM: Psychosexual adjustment and fertility issues, in Bone Marrow Transplantation: Principles, Practices and Nursing Insights. Edited by Whedon MB. Boston, MA, Jones & Bartlett, 1991, pp 312–333

Ostroff J, Stern V, Dukoff R, et al: The psychosexual adjustment of prematurely menopausal cancer survivors treated with hormone replacement therapy (abstract). Presented at the American Psychosomatic Society meeting, 1991

Parr MD, Messino MJ, Mcintyre W: Allogeneic bone marrow transplantation: procedures and complications. Am J Hosp Pharm 48:127–137, 1991

Patenaude AF: Psychological impact of bone marrow transplantation: current perspectives. Yale J Biol Med 3:515–519, 1990

Patenaude AF, Rappeport JM: Collaboration between hematologists and mental health professionals on a bone marrow transplant team. Journal of Psychosocial Oncology 2:81–92, 1984

Patenaude AF, Syzmansi L, Rappaport J: Psychological costs of bone marrow transplantation in children. Am J Orthopsychiatry 49:409–422, 1979

Patenaude AF, Levinger L, Baker K: Group meetings for parents and spouses of bone marrow transplant patients. Soc Work Health Care 12:51–65, 1986a

Patenaude AF, Rappeport JM, Smith BR: The physicians' influence on informed consent for bone marrow transplantation. Theor Med 7:165–179, 1986b

Penman D, Holland J, Bahna G, et al: Informed consent for investigational chemotherapy: patients' and physicians' perceptions. J Clin Oncol 2:849–855, 1984

Pot-Mees CC (ed): The Psychosocial Effects of Bone Marrow Transplantation in Children. Delft, Eburon Publishers, 1989

Powezak M, Groff JR, Schyung J: Emotional reactions of children to isolation in a cancer hospital. J Pediatr 92:834–837, 1978

Rappaport BS: Evolution of consultation liaison services in bone marrow transplantation. Gen Hosp Psychiatry 10:346–351, 1988

Rebeta J, Ostroff J, Zazula T, et al: The effect of methotrexate upon neuropsychological functioning in acute leukemia patients (abstract). Presented at the First Consultation Liaison Psychiatry Research Forum, New York. American Psychiatric Association, May 1990

Ringden K, Bolme P, Persson A, et al: Psychomotor skills in children after bone marrow transplantation (letter). Bone Marrow Transplant 3 (suppl 1):292, 1988

Rowland J, Olidwell O, Sibley R, et al: Effects of different forms of central nervous system prophylaxis on neuropsychological function in childhood leukemia. J Clin Oncol 2:1327–1335, 1984

Sanders JE, Buckner CD, Amos D, et al: Ovarian and testicular function following marrow transplantation. Paper presented at the International Conference on Reproduction and Human Cancer, National Cancer Institute, Bethesda, MD, May 1987

Sanders JE, Buckner CD, Amos D, et al: Ovarian function following bone marrow transplantation for aplastic anemia or leukemia. J Clin Oncol 6:813–818, 1988

Santos GW: History of bone marrow transplantation. Baillieres Clin Haematol 12:611–639, 1983

Santos GW: Bone marrow transplantation in hematologic malignancies: current status. Cancer 5:786–791, 1990

Sarantos S: Innovations in psychosocial staff support: a model program for the marrow transplant nurse. Semin Oncol Nurs 4:69–73, 1988

Sherins RJ, Mulvihill JJ: Gonadal dysfunction, in Cancer, Principles and Practice of Oncology. Edited by Devita VT, Helman S, Rosenberg SA. Philadelphia, PA, JB Lippincott, 1989, pp 2170–2181

Sullivan KM, Witherspoon RP, Storb R, et al: Long-term results of allogeneic bone marrow transplantation. Transplant Proc 21:2926–2928, 1989

Surman OS: Psychiatric aspects of organ transplantation. Am J Psychiatry 146:972–982, 1989

Syrjala KL, Chapko MK, Cummings C, et al: Physical and psychological functioning in the first year after bone marrow transplantation: a prospective study (abstract). Presented at the Society of Behavioral Medicine Scientific Sessions, 1988

Thomas ED, Clift RA, Fefer A, et al: Marrow transplantation for the treatment of chronic myelogenic leukemia. Ann Intern Med 104:155–163, 1986

Vaughn WP, Purtillo RB, Butler CD, et al: Ethical and financial issues in autologous marrow transplantation: a symposium sponsored by the University of Nebraska Medical Center. Ann Intern Med 105:134–135, 1986

Viederman M: Adaptive and maladaptive regression in hemodialysis. Psychiatry 37:68–77, 1974

Welch HG: Marrow transplantation, cost effectiveness analysis and setting units. Leukemia 7:1108–1111, 1993

Wellisch DK, Fawzy F, Yager J: Life in venus' flytrap: psychiatric liaison to patients undergoing bone marrow transplantation, in Contemporary Models in Liaison Psychiatry. Edited by Faguet RA, Fawzy FI, Wellisch DK, et al. California, SP Medical & Scientific Books, 1978, pp 39–51

Wingard JR, Curbow B, Baker F, et al: Health, functional status and employment of adult survivors of bone marrow transplantation. Ann Intern Med 114:113–118, 1991a

Wingard JR, Curbow B, Baker F, et al: Sexual satisfaction in bone marrow transplant (BMT) survivors (abstract). Proceedings of the American Society of Clinical Oncology 10:322, 1991b

Witherspoon RP, Fisher LD, Schoch G, et al: Secondary cancers after bone marrow transplantation for leukemia or aplastic anemia. N Engl J Med 321:784–789, 1989

Wolcott DL, Wellisch DK, Fawzy FI, et al: Psychological adjustment of adult bone marrow transplant donors whose recipients survived. Transplantation 41:484–488, 1986a

Wolcott DL, Wellisch DK, Fawzy FI, et al: Adaptation of adult bone marrow transplant recipient long term survivors. Transplantation 41:478–483, 1986b

Zevon MA, Donnelly JP, Starkey EA: Stress and coping relationships in the medical environment: a natural experiment. Journal of Psychosocial Oncology 8:65–77, 1990

Index

*Page numbers printed in **boldface** refer to tables or figures.*

Absorption of drugs, 1–9, **4**
  in cardiac disease, 26
  characteristics of site for, 2
  factors influencing, 1–2, **4**
  first-pass effect and, 2
  in gastrointestinal disease, 2, **6**, 21–22
  lag time for, 2, **4**
  rate of, 2–3, **4**
  related to route of administration, 2–3, 22
  in renal disease, 49
Acebutolol, **186**
Acetylation, 15
α_1-Acid glycoprotein (AAGP) binding of drugs, 10–12, **11**
Acquired immunodeficiency syndrome (AIDS), 257. *See also* Human immunodeficiency virus infection
  "AIDS belt" of Africa, 261
  AIDS dementia complex, 268–277
  AIDS Education Project, 258
  Centers for Disease Control case definition of, 259
  chemical, 347. *See also* Environmental illness
  early history of, 259–260
  incidence of, 257
  search for causative agent in, 260–261
Acrivastine, 103
Activated partial thromboplastin time (APPT), 40
Acyclovir
  for chronic fatigue syndrome, 239, **242**

neuropsychiatric side effects of, 304
Adjustment disorders, associated with HIV infection, 267, **270**
Age effects
  on prognosis after head injury, 319
  on psychopharmacokinetics, 1
Agitation
  felbamate-induced, 118
  risperidone-induced, 114
Agranulocytosis, drug-induced, 117
  carbamazepine, 120–121
  clozapine, 106–107, 168
  felbamate, 117
Akathisia, selective serotonin reuptake inhibitor–induced, 91, 92
Alanine aminotransferase (ALT), tacrine effects on, 134–136
Albumin binding of drugs, 10–12, **11**
Alcohol injections, vulvar, 397–398
Allergies
  chronic fatigue syndrome and, 233
  environmental illness and, 347, 350, 352, 368
Allodynia, 389
Alprazolam
  for bone marrow transplant recipient, 439
  formulations of, **8**
  half-life of, **19**, 284
  interaction with fluoxetine, **87**
  interaction with nefazodone, 97
  metabolism of, **9**
    by cytochrome P_{450}-3A4, 36, 85

Alprazolam *(continued)*
  onset of action of, 3
  use in liver disease, 42
  use in renal disease, **54–55**
Alzheimer's disease
  tacrine for, 133–136
  zolpidem for insomnia in, 133
Amantadine
  for head-injured patient, 329,
    330, 335
  for Parkinson's disease, **155,** 156,
    162
Amenorrhea, after bone marrow
    transplantation, 454,
    458–459
Amiflamine, **82**
Amikacin (Amikin), 304
p-Aminosalicylate, **186**
Aminosalicylic acid, **186**
Amitriptyline
  for fibromyalgia, **246–248**
  formulations of, **8**
  for head-injured patient, **331**
  interaction with fluvoxamine, **87**
  interaction with valproate,
    105–106
  metabolism of, 45, **85**
    by cytochrome P_{450}-2D6,
      36, **82**
  for mucous membrane
    dysesthesias, 389–390
  side effects of, 390
  use in liver disease, 45
  use in renal disease, **64–65**
  for vulvodynia, 408
Amoxapine
  formulations of, **8**
  use in renal disease, **54–55**
Amphetamines, protein binding of,
    10
Amphotericin B, 304
Angiotensin-converting enzyme
    (ACE) inhibitors, interaction
    with lithium, 113

Anorexia
  after bone marrow
    transplantation, 434
  venlafaxine-induced, 93
Antacids, drug interactions with, 21
Antiarrhythmics
  metabolism by cytochrome
    P_{450}-2D6, **83**
  use after myocardial infarction,
    97–98
Antibiotics
  for bone marrow transplant
    recipient, 431
  environmental illness and, 351
  interactions with valproate, 130
Antibodies
  anticardiolipin, **198,** 204–205
  antineuronal, **198,** 203–206
  antinuclear, 184, **187,** 188, 193,
    195, **197**
  antiphospholipid, 204–206
  antiribosomal P protein, **198,**
    203–206
  to HIV, 263
  in systemic lupus
    erythematosus, 184, **187,**
    188, 195, **197, 198,**
    202–206
Anticholinergic drugs
  effect on drug absorption, 2
  for Parkinson's disease, **155,** 156,
    161
  psychotoxicity of, 161
Anticonvulsants. *See* Antiepileptic
    drugs
Antidepressants. *See also* specific
    drugs
  for bone marrow transplant
    recipient, 439–440
  for chronic fatigue syndrome, 241
  for fibromyalgia, 241, **246–248**
  formulations of, **8**
  for head-injured patient,
    331–333, 335–337

for HIV-infected persons,
280–282
metabolism of, **9,** 14
for mucous membrane
dysesthesias, 389–390
for persons with environmental
illness, 372
for pruritus ani, 399
use in gastrointestinal disease,
23–24
use in renal disease, 53, **54–55,** 66
use in systemic lupus
erythematosus, 207, 208
for vulvodynia, 408–409
Antidepressants, tricyclic (TCAs),
79. *See also* specific drugs
for children, 100–101, **102**
dialyzability of, 53
drug interactions with
carbamazepine, 45, 124, 339
cholestyramine, 105
felbamate, 118
sertraline, **89**
valproate, 105–106, 339
for head-injured patient, **331,**
335–336
high-fiber diet and, 105
for HIV-infected persons,
281–282
metabolism of, 44–45
by cytochrome P$_{450}$-2D6, **82**
parenteral, 281
pharmacology in medical
patients, 97–101
protein binding of, 10
rectal administration of, 104–105
side effects of, 281
cardiac effects, 97–101
sudden death in children,
100–101, **102**
use in cardiac disease, 30–31,
97–99
use in gastrointestinal disease,
23–24

use in liver disease, 39, 41,
44–45
use in renal disease, 53, **62–65,** 66
Antiepileptic drugs, 116–130. *See
also* specific drugs
carbamazepine, 120–125
felbamate, 116–119
gabapentin, 119–120
for head-injured patient, **333,**
337–339
for HIV-related mania, 283
valproate, 125–130
for vulvodynia, 408
withdrawal from, 119
Antihypertensive agents, **82**
Antinuclear antibodies (ANA)
conditions associated with, **197**
screening for, 193
in systemic lupus
erythematosus, 184, **187,**
188, 195, **197**
Antiparkinsonian drugs, 153–156,
154–155
differential psychotoxicity of,
161–162
"drug holidays" from, 163
psychosis induced by, 151,
156–176
differential diagnosis of,
156–158
epidemiology of, 158
phenomenology of, 158–160
treatment of, 162–176
Antipsychotics. *See* Neuroleptics
Antithymocyte globulin, 415
Anxiety
associated with HIV infection,
267–268, **269–270**
in bone marrow transplant
recipient, 431–432, 439–440
environmental illness and, 356,
358–361
gabapentin-induced, 120
postconcussional, 315

Anxiety *(continued)*
　related to protected isolation
　　environment, 443
　risperidone-induced, 114
　in systemic lupus
　　erythematosus, 192, 207
Anxiolytics
　for bone marrow transplant
　　recipient, 424, 438–439
　formulations of, **8**
　for HIV-infected persons, 284
　use in gastrointestinal disease, 22
　use in liver disease, 42–43
　use in renal disease, 52–53,
　　54–59
Aphthosis, vulvar, **392**
Aplastic anemia, bone marrow
　transplantation for, 415–460
Arrhythmias
　clozapine-induced tachycardia,
　　107
　desipramine-related, in children,
　　100–101
　sotalol for, 104
　terfenadine-induced, 102–103
Arthralgias, in chronic fatigue
　syndrome, 221
Ascites, 35
Aspirin, interaction with valproate,
　130
Astemizole
　interaction with nefazodone, 97
　metabolism of, **85**
Ataxia
　gabapentin-induced, 120
　zolpidem-induced, 133
Atenolol, **186**
　interaction with fluvoxamine, **87**
　interaction with sertraline, **89**
Atovaquone, 303
Attention
　HIV-associated deficits in, 269
　postconcussional deficits in, 315
　testing for, 324, **326**

tacrine-induced improvements
　in, 134–135
Attention-deficit hyperactivity
　disorder (ADHD), head injury
　and, 319, 322
Azithromycin, 304
AZT. *See* Zidovudine

Bactrim. *See* Trimethoprim/
　sulfamethoxazole
Barbiturates
　protein binding of, 10
　use in renal disease, **54–55**
Behavior modification, for
　environmental illness, 371–372
Behçet's syndrome, **392**
Bender Gestalt test, 199
Benzodiazepines. *See also* specific
　drugs
　absorption of, 3
　achieving steady state of, 17
　active metabolites of, 18, **19,** 52
　formulations of, **8**
　half-lives of, 18, **19,** 284
　for head-injured patient, **334,** 339
　for HIV-infected persons, 284
　intramuscular, 3
　measuring serum concentrations
　　of, 52
　metabolism of, **9,** 14–15
　protein binding of, 10, 42
　use in cardiac disease, 27
　use in gastrointestinal disease, 22
　use in liver disease, 42–43
　use in renal disease, 52, **54–59**
Benztropine, use in liver disease, 44
Betapace. *See* Sotalol
Biaxin. *See* Clarithromycin
Bilirubin, 40
Bioavailability of drugs, **5,** 9, 39
　in liver disease, 32–33, 39
Bipolar disorder
　carbamazepine for, 120
　valproate for, 125

Bleeding tendencies
  fluoxetine-induced, 90
  valproate-induced, 126–127
β-Blockers
  for head-injured patient, **334**
  lupus induced by, **186**
  metabolized by cytochrome
    P$_{450}$-2D6, **82**
Body temperature alterations, in
  chronic fatigue syndrome, 221
Bone marrow transplantation
  (BMT), 415–460
  allogeneic, 417–418
    for aplastic anemia, 418
    for chronic myelogenous
      leukemia, 418
    human lymphocyte antigen
      histocompatibility
      testing for, 417
  autologous, 417–419
  biological setting for, 416–420
  centers performing, 420
  convalescent period after,
    431–432, 451
  cost of, 420–421
  data on incidence of, 420
  donors for, 417, 445–447
    anonymous, 446–447
    children as, 429, 430
    guilt felt by, 423
    harvesting marrow from, 431,
      446
    long-term psychological
      effects in, 446
    psychological preparation of,
      445
    registries of, 421
    search for, 423
    selection of, 445
  ethical and legal issues related
    to, 428–430
  family concerns about, 424–426,
    447–448
  future research related to, 460

  goals of, 419
  guide for decision making about,
    419–420
  history of, 416–417
  hospitalization for, 417,
    430–432
    protected and germ-free
      environments, 417,
      443–445
  indications for, 416–417
  informed consent for, 426–428
  Karnofksy score after, 452
  pain management after, 434
  patient refusal of, 430
  patient selection for, 419
  posthospitalization support
    after, 432–433
  procedure for, 417, 431
  psychiatric liaison services for
    staff on unit for, 448–451
  psychological and psychosocial
    assessment for, 423–426
  psychological complications of,
    438–443
    antidepressants for, 439–440
    anxiety, delirium, and
      depression, 438–439
    clinical issues related to, 441
    psychiatric illness, 442–443
    psychological themes and
      conflicts, 441–442
    risk factors for, 440
  psychosexual adjustment after,
    453–460
    chemotherapy-induced
      gonadal dysfunction,
      453–455
    hormone-replacement
      therapy, 456
    pregnancy, 457
    problems in men, 459–460
    radiotherapy-induced
      gonadal dysfunction,
      454–456

Bone marrow transplantation
(BMT) *(continued)*
psychosexual adjustment after
sperm banking, 456–457
studies of, 457–459
in vitro fertilization, 457
routes of medication
administration after, 433,
437
side effects and complications of,
418, 431, 433–438
chemotherapy-related,
434–435
general systemic transient
side effects, 434
graft-versus-host disease,
416–419, 431–432,
437–438
immediate toxic
complications, 433–434
late physical sequelae, 451–453
related to Broviac or Hickman
catheterization and total
parenteral nutrition,
436–437
total-body irradiation–related,
435–436, 454
stages of, 416, 421–423, **422,**
430–432
survival after, 418, 419, 451–452
regimen-related toxicity scale
for prediction of,
451
syngeneic, 417
third-party reimbursement for,
420
Brain imaging
in AIDS dementia complex,
276
for head-injured patient,
311–313, **321,** 325–328
in systemic lupus
erythematosus, **198,**
199–202

Brain injury. *See* Head injury
Brain tumors, bone marrow
transplantation for, 419
Breast cancer, bone marrow
transplantation for, 417, 419
Brief Psychiatric Rating Scale
(BPRS), 159, 166–167
Bromocriptine, for Parkinson's
disease, 153, **154**
Bromperidol, use in renal disease,
58–59
Brotizolam, use in renal disease,
54–55
Broviac catheter–related problems,
436–437
Brucellosis, chronic, 217, 348. *See
also* Chronic fatigue syndrome
Bufarolol, **82**
Bullous dermatoses, vulvar, **392**
Bupropion
for chronic fatigue syndrome,
241, **244**
formulations of, **8**
for head-injured patient, **333,** 337
for HIV-infected persons, 282
use in cardiac disease, 30–31
use in renal disease, **54–55**
Burns, effect on albumin binding of
drugs, 10
Buspirone
formulations of, **8**
for head-injured patient, **334,**
339–340
for HIV-infected persons, 282, 284
metabolism of, **9**
use in liver disease, 43
use in renal disease, 53, **58–59**
Busulfan, before bone marrow
transplantation, 430
Butterfly rash, 183, 184

Calcium channel blockers
for AIDS dementia complex,
275–276

interaction with imipramine, 105
interaction with lithium, 112–113
L-Canavanine, **186**
Cancer patients
    bone marrow transplantation
        for, 415–460
    dextroamphetamine for, 113
Candidiasis
    chronic, 217. *See also* Chronic
        fatigue syndrome
    sensitivity to, 347–348, 351, 354.
        See also Environmental
        illness
    vulvar, 391, **394,** 395
        treatment of, 400, 402
    vulvodynia and, 383–384, 400
Capastat. *See* Capreomycin
Capreomycin, 304
Captopril, **186**
Carbamazepine, 79, 120–125
    for bipolar disorder, 120
    drug interactions with, 123–124
        felbamate, 117–118
        fluoxetine, **87**
        fluvoxamine, **87**
        paroxetine, **88**
        selective serotonin reuptake
            inhibitors, 336, 339
        tricyclic antidepressants, 45,
            124, 339
        valproate, 48–49, 117, 127,
            129–130
    environmental effects on
        stability of, 125
    formulations of, **8,** 25
    generic preparations of, 124
    for head-injured patient, **333,**
        338–339
    for HIV-related mania, 283
    metabolism of, **9**
    overdose of, 122–123
    in pregnancy, 123
    rectal administration of, 104–105
    for refractory depression, 120

reintroduction after
        discontinuation of, 124
    side effects of, 120–122, 338
        lupus, 122, **186**
    switching between preparations
        of, 124–125
    therapeutic index for, 124
    use in gastrointestinal disease, 25
    use in liver disease, 33, 47–48
    for vulvodynia, 408
    withdrawal from, 119
Carbon dioxide laser therapy,
        vulvar, 397
Cardiac Arrhythmia Suppression
    Trials (CASTs), 97–99
Cardiac catheterization, 99
Cardiac disease, 26–32
    guidelines for drug dosing in,
        28–30
    pharmacokinetic effects of, 26–28
        absorption, 26
        distribution, 26–27
        excretion, 27–28
        metabolism, 27
    use of antidepressants in, 30–31
        selective serotonin reuptake
            inhibitors, 92–93
        tricyclics, 97–99
        venlafaxine, 95
    use of antipsychotics in, 31
    use of lithium in, 31–32, 112
Cardiac effects
    of cyclophosphamide, 434
    of imipramine, 96
    of intravenous haloperidol,
        103–104
    of nefazodone, 96
    of selective serotonin reuptake
        inhibitors, 80, 92–93
    of stimulants, 113–114
    of terfenadine, 86
    of tricyclic antidepressants,
        97–101
        for chest pain, 99–100

Cardiac effects *(continued)*
  of tricyclic antidepressants
    sudden death in children,
      100–101
  of venlafaxine, 95
Carmustine, before bone marrow
    transplantation, 430
Cataracts, in bone marrow
    transplant recipient, 435, 451
Catatonia, in systemic lupus
    erythematosus, 193
Causalgia, 389
CD3 cells, 260
CD4 cells, 259–262
CD8 cells, 260
Celiac disease, 2, 10
Center for Epidemiologic
    Studies—Depression Scale
    (CES-D), 278
Cerebral blood flow (CBF)
  in congestive heart failure, 29
  in systemic lupus
    erythematosus, 201–202
Cerebrospinal fluid (CSF) analysis,
    in AIDS dementia complex, 276
"Chemical sensitivity" syndromes,
    347–378. *See also*
    Environmental illness
Chemotherapy
  before bone marrow
    transplantation, 417, 430,
    434–435
  gonadal dysfunction due to,
    453–455
Chest pain, imipramine for, 99–100
Children
  as bone marrow donors, 429, 430
  tricyclic antidepressants for
    guidelines for monitoring
      cardiac toxicity, **102**
    sudden death and, 100–101
Chimera, 415
Chloral hydrate, use in renal
    disease, **58–59**

Chlordiazepoxide
  achieving steady state of, 17
  clearance of, 17
  formulations of, **8**
  half-life of, 17, **19**
  metabolism of, **9**
  metabolites of, 18
  use in liver disease, 42
  use in renal disease, **56–57**
  volume of distribution of, 13, 17
Chlorpromazine
  formulations of, **8**
  for HIV-infected persons, 285
  lupus induced by, 184
  protein binding of, 12
  use in gastrointestinal disease, 23
  use in liver disease, 43–44
  use in renal disease, **62–63**
Chlorprothixene, **8**
Chlorthalidone, **186**
Cholestyramine, interaction with
    tricyclic antidepressants, 105
Chronic fatigue syndrome (CFS),
    215–250
  case definitions of, 216, 221,
    222–226
  conceptual models for, 216,
    218–219
  conflicting data about, 216
  diagnosis of, 235–239
    approach to patient, 235–237
    patient evaluation, 238
    viral serologies, 238–239,
      240
  differentiation from
    environmental illness,
    349–350
  as disorder of immune
    regulation, **218**, 232–233
    cellular immunity, 233
    humoral immunity, 232–233
  epidemiology of, 223–229
    community studies, 223,
      227–228

primary care studies, 228–229,
230
tertiary care studies, 229, **231**
history of, 216–221, **220**
as infectious disease, 216, **218,**
230–232
medical and psychiatric
disorders associated with,
230–231
as muscle disorder, **218,** 234
persons providing treatment for,
216
as psychiatric disorder, **219,** 235
relationship to fibromyalgia, 234,
236
signs and symptoms of, 221,
227–228
as sleep disorder, **218,** 233–234
terminology for, 217, 221
treatment of, 239–241
cognitive-behavior strategies,
241, **244,** 249, **249**
general approach, 239
lessons from fibromyalgia
literature, 241, **246–248**
pharmacological strategies,
239–241, **242–245**
Chronic obstructive pulmonary
disease (COPD), use of
zolpidem in, 132
Cimetidine
cytochrome P_{450} inhibition by,
37, **85,** 86
drug interactions with, 21
carbamazepine, 123
clozapine, 108
paroxetine, **88**
terfenadine, 103
venlafaxine, 95
Ciprofloxacin (Cipro)
interaction with terfenadine, 103
neuropsychiatric side effects of,
304
Cirrhosis. *See* Liver disease

Clarithromycin
interaction with carbamazepine,
123
neuropsychiatric side effects of,
305
Clearance of drugs, **5,** 15–16
calculation of, 15
in cardiac disease, 27–28
disease effects on, **7,** 18
factors influencing, 15
hepatic, 39, 41–42
relationship to maintenance
dose, 15–16
renal, 41–42
steady state and, 17
systemic, 41
Clinical ecology, 347–378. *See also*
Environmental illness
Clinical Global Impression Severity
(CGIS), 167
Clinical interview, after head injury,
321, 322–323
Clofazimine, 305
Clomipramine
for fibromyalgia, **247**
formulations of, **8**
metabolism of, **82**
Clonazepam
drug interactions with, 89–90
fluoxetine, 37, **88**
half-life of, **19**
for HIV-infected persons, 284
metabolism of, **9,** 89
for mucous membrane
dysesthesias, 390
use in liver disease, 90
use in renal disease, **56–57**
for vulvodynia, 408
Clonidine
for chest pain, 99–100
for clozapine-induced
hypersalivation, 164–165
Clorazepate
active metabolite of, 3, 15

Clorazepate *(continued)*
    formulations of, **8**
    half-life of, **19**
    metabolism of, **9**
    onset of action of, 3
    use in gastrointestinal disease, 22
    use in liver disease, 42
    use in renal disease, **56–57**
Closed head injury. *See* Head injury
Clozapine, 79, 106–109
    for atypical parkinsonism, 168–169
    drug interactions with, 108
        cimetidine, 108
        fluoxetine, **88,** 108
        phenytoin, 108
    for elderly patients, 108, 168
    mechanism of action of, 164
    for Parkinson's disease, 106
        motoric effects, 167–168
        for psychosis, 165–169, **166**
    pharmacology of, 164–165
    for schizophrenia, 165
    side effects of, 106–109, 168
        agranulocytosis, 106–107, 168
        neuroleptic malignant
            syndrome, 108–109
        seizures, 107
    for tardive dyskinesia and
        dystonia, 109
Codeine, **83**
Cognitive effects
    of bone marrow transplantation,
        435–436, 451–452
    of head injury, 314
        neuropsychological
            assessment for, 323–325
        testing for, 324, **326**
    of HIV infection, 268–277
    of posttraumatic stress disorder,
        317–318
    of rheumatoid arthritis, 192, 193
    of systemic lupus
        erythematosus, 188,
        191–194

Cognitive-behavior therapy (CBT)
    for bone marrow transplant
        recipient, 424
    for chronic fatigue syndrome,
        241, **244,** 249, **249**
Compensation neurosis, 315
Computed tomography (CT)
    after head injury, 313, **321,**
        325–328
    in AIDS dementia complex, 276
    in systemic lupus
        erythematosus, **198,** 199
Concentration deficits
    due to total-body irradiation, 435
    in HIV infection, 269
    postconcussional, 315
Condylomata acuminata, 396
Confusion
    in chronic fatigue syndrome, 221
    clozapine-induced, 164
    in Parkinson's disease, 157
Congestive heart failure (CHF),
        26–32
    cerebral blood flow in, 29
    drug absorption in, 26
    drug distribution in, 26–27
    drug excretion in, 27–28
    drug metabolism in, 27
    guidelines for drug dosing in,
        28–30
    use of antidepressants in, 30
    use of antipsychotics in, 31
    use of lithium in, 31–32
Constipation, nefazodone-induced,
        96
Contrecoup injury, 311
Contusions, brain, 310–312
Coping skills, of bone marrow
        transplant candidate, 423–424
Coronary angiography, 99
Corticosteroids
    for bone marrow transplant
        recipient, 434–436
    psychiatric effects of, 208

for systemic lupus
erythematosus, 189, 194,
207
for vulvar itching, 398–399
lichen simplex chronicus, 384
rebound inflammatory
reaction, 397
Counseling, before and after HIV
testing, 265–266
Creatinine clearance, 51–52
lithium effects on, 110
Crohn's disease
effect on protein binding of
drugs, 10
use of chlorpromazine in, 23
Cryoprecipitate, 127
Cyclophosphamide
before bone marrow
transplantation, 417, 430, 434
gonadal dysfunction due to, 455
Cycloserine, 305
Cyclosporine
interaction with fluoxetine, **88**
interaction with midazolam, 37
metabolism by cytochrome
P$_{450}$-3A4, 85
Cyclothymia, valproate for, 125
Cystitis
hemorrhagic, 434
interstitial, 386, 387–388
Cytarabine hydrochloride, before
bone marrow transplantation,
430
Cytochrome P$_{450}$ (CyP$_{450}$), 14,
36–37, **38,** 80–86
CyP$_{450}$-3A4, 36–37, 85–86
drugs metabolized by, 85, **85**
inhibition of, **85,** 86
CyP$_{450}$-2D6, 36–37, 81
drugs metabolized by,
82–83
selective serotonin reuptake
inhibitor inhibition of,
36–37, 83–85, **84**

disease effects on drug
metabolism by, 40
isoenzymes of, 36–37, 80
levels in liver biopsies, 40
subfamilies of, 36–37, 80
Cytomegalovirus (CMV), chronic
fatigue syndrome and,
231–232
Cytovene. *See* Ganciclovir

Dapsone, 303
DATATOP study, 156
ddC. *See* Zalcitabine
ddI. *See* Didanosine
Dealkylation, 14
Deamination, 14
Debrisoquin, **82**
Delirium
after head injury, 314
associated with HIV infection,
269, 285–286
in bone marrow transplant
recipient, 423, 439
induced by lithium and
diltiazem, 112–113
induced by tricyclic
antidepressants, 281
Delusions, in Parkinson's disease,
160
Dementia
after head injury, 314
AIDS dementia complex,
268–277. *See also* Human
immunodeficiency virus
infection
tacrine for, 133–136
valproate for, 125
Demoxepam, **19**
Depression
after traumatic brain injury,
309–310, 315
associated with HIV infection,
267–268, **269–270,**
277–278

Depression (continued)
  in bone marrow transplant
    recipient, 423, 431,
    438–441
  chronic fatigue and, 235
  DSM-IV criteria for major
    depressive episode vs.
    mood disorder due to
    general medical condition,
    309–310, **311**
  poststroke, 113
  related to protected isolation
    environment, 443
  in systemic lupus
    erythematosus, 188, 192,
    207–208
  treatment of. See also
    Antidepressants
  carbamazepine, 120
  methylphenidate, 113
  selective serotonin reuptake
    inhibitors, 80
Desalkylflurazepam, **19**
N-Desalkyl-2-oxoquazepam, **19**
Desipramine
  drug interactions with
    fluoxetine, **87**, 89
    fluvoxamine, **87**, 89
    propafenone, 106
    selective serotonin reuptake
      inhibitors, 85
  electrocardiographic effects of,
    100–101
  formulations of, **8**
  for head-injured patient, **331**, 336
  for HIV-infected persons, 281,
    282
  metabolism of, 45
    by cytochrome P450-2D6, 36, **82**
  for mucous membrane
    dysesthesias, 390
  sudden death in children and,
    100–101
  use in renal disease, **64–65**

for vulvodynia, 408
Desmethylchlordiazepoxide, 18, **19**
N-Desmethyldiazepam, 3, 15, 18, **19**
Desmethylsertraline, 36
O-Desmethyl-venlafaxine, 93
Desmopressin (DDAVP), 127
Desmoxazepam, 18
Desulfuration, 14
Dextroamphetamine
  for cancer patients, 113
  for head-injured patients, **330,**
    335
  for HIV-infected persons,
    282–283
Dextromethorphan
  for AIDS dementia complex,
    275
  metabolism by cytochrome
    P450-2D6, **83**
Dextropropoxyphene, **83**
DHPG. See Ganciclovir
Diabetes mellitus, effect on drug
    absorption, 2
Diagnostic Interview Schedule
    (DIS), 223, 356, **358–361**
Dialysis, 51
Dialyzable leukocyte extract, 239,
    245
Diazepam
  achieving steady state of, 17
  clearance of, 17
  distribution of, 12–13
  formulations of, **8**
  half-life of, **19**
  interaction with fluoxetine, **87**
  metabolism of, **9**
  onset of action of, 3
  use in liver disease, 33, 42
  use in renal disease, **56–57**
  volume of distribution of, 13, 17
Didanosine (ddI), 303
Diet
  environmental illness and, 352,
    354

tricyclic antidepressants and
fiber in, 105
Diffuse axonal injury, 310–311,
313–314
Diflucan. *See* Fluconazole
Digit Span test, **326**
Diltiazem
interaction with carbamazepine,
123
interaction with imipramine,
105
interaction with lithium, 112–113
Disinhibition, after head injury, 312,
314
Distribution of drug, **5,** 9–14
in cardiac disease, 26–27
diseases affecting, **6–7**
factors influencing, 9–10
protein binding and, 10–12, **11**
two-compartment model and, 13
volume of, **5,** 12–14
Disulfiram, interaction with
terfenadine, 103
Divalproex sodium, **8**
Dizziness
drug-induced
clozapine, 107
felbamate, 118
gabapentin, 120
nefazodone, 96
venlafaxine, 93
postconcussional, 315
"Do not resuscitate" orders, 428
Dopamine, tacrine effects on, 136
Dopamine agonists
for head-injured patient, 329,
330, 335
for Parkinson's disease, 153, **154,**
162
psychotoxicity of, 162
Dopamine antagonists, for
head-injured patient, 329,
330–331
Dothiepin, for fibromyalgia, **247**

Doxepin
formulations of, **8**
for HIV-infected persons, 281
metabolism of, 45
for pruritus ani, 399
rectal administration of, 104–105
use in cardiac disease, 30
use in renal disease, **64–65**
Dronabinol, 305
Droperidol, **8**
Drowsiness
clozapine-induced, 107
zolpidem-induced, 133
"Drug holidays," from
antiparkinsonian drugs, 163
Drug interactions
with antacids, 21
with carbamazepine, 123–124, 339
with clonazepam, 89–90
with clozapine, 108
with fluoxetine, **87–88**
with fluvoxamine, **87**
kinetics and, 20
with lithium, 112–113
with nefazodone, 97
with paroxetine, **88**
with propafenone, 106
related to cytochrome P_{450}
subfamilies, 37
with selective serotonin reuptake
inhibitors, 86, **87–89,** 336
with sertraline, **89**
with terfenadine, 102–103
with valproate, 127–130, 339
with venlafaxine, 95
Dry mouth
nefazodone-induced, 96
tricyclic antidepressant–induced,
281
venlafaxine-induced, 93
DSM-IV
criteria for major depressive
episode vs. mood disorder
due to general medical
condition, 309–310, **311**

DSM-IV *(continued)*
    criteria for personality change
        due to general medical
        condition, 310, **312**
    diagnoses associated with
        traumatic brain injury, **309,**
        309–310
    research criteria for
        postconcussional
        syndrome, **316**
Dysesthesias, endogenous, 389–390
Dyskinesia, selective serotonin
    reuptake inhibitor–induced, 91
Dyspareunia
    due to vulvodynia, 385
    entry, 403–404
    in interstitial cystitis, 385
    postcoital, 400
Dystonia, selective serotonin
    reuptake inhibitor–induced, 91

Ecchymoses, fluoxetine-induced, 90
Ecologic illness, 347. *See also*
    Environmental illness
Elderly persons
    clozapine for, 108, 168
    gabapentin for, 119
    prevalence of Parkinson's
        disease in, 158
    risperidone for, 115–116
    systemic lupus erythematosus
        in, 188–189
    tacrine for Alzheimer's disease
        in, 133–136
    zolpidem for, 131–133
Electrocardiography (ECG)
    desipramine effects on, in
        children, 100–101
    imipramine effects on, 96
    intravenous haloperidol effects
        on, 103–104
    lithium effects on, 112
    nefazodone effects on, 96
    risperidone effects on, 115

terfenadine effects on, 86, 103
    venlafaxine effects on, 95
Electroconvulsive therapy (ECT)
    for HIV-infected persons, 283
    for Parkinson's disease, 170–172
    use in systemic lupus
        erythematosus, 208
Electroencephalography (EEG)
    in Lennox-Gastaut syndrome,
        116
    in systemic lupus
        erythematosus, 196–199,
        198
Elimination of drugs, 9, 14–18
    in cardiac disease, 28–29
    clearance, **5,** 15–16
    half-life, **5, 16,** 16–18
    phase I reactions, **9,** 14–15, 36
    phase II reactions, **9,** 15, 36
Enalapril, interaction with lithium,
    113
Encainide
    metabolism by cytochrome
        P$_{450}$-2D6, **83**
    use after myocardial infarction,
        98
Encephalitis
    benign myalgic, 217, **220.** *See also*
        Chronic fatigue syndrome
    subacute, 268
Encephalopathy
    HIV, 268
    related to total-body irradiation,
        435–436
        early-delayed, 435–436
        late-delayed, 436
Enterovirus, chronic fatigue
    syndrome and, 232
Environmental illness (EI), 347–378
    clinical description of persons
        with, 355–366
        personality profile, **358–361,**
            364–366
        physical disorders, 363–364

psychiatric disorders,
356–363, **357–361**
clinical ecologist and, 348–349
definition of, 351
diagnosis of, 351–352
differential diagnosis of,
349–350
evaluation of patient with
diagnosis of, 366–369, **370**
future directions in, 376–377
history of, 348
lack of acceptance by
mainstream medical
community, 349
prevalence of, 348
putative causes of, 351
support groups for people with,
351, 355
terminology for, 347–348
theories of, 352–353
bipolarity phenomenon, 353
spreading phenomenon, 353
switch phenomenon, 353
total body load concept, 353
treatment of, 369–376
behavior modification,
371–372
case example of difficulty of,
373–376
by clinical ecologists, 353–354
for coexisting psychiatric
disorders, 372–373
combination treatment
measures, 373
environmental modifications,
370–371
psychotherapy, 369–370
recommendations for, **377**
Environmental sensitivity, 217. *See
also* Chronic fatigue syndrome
Enzyme-limited drugs, 32–33, 39
Enzyme-linked immunosorbent
assay (ELISA), for HIV
infection, 264

Eosinophilia, clozapine-induced,
108
Epidemiologic Catchment Area
(ECA) study, 223, 227, 266
Epidemiology
of chronic fatigue syndrome,
223–229
of HIV infection, 258–259
of Parkinson's disease, 158
Epoetin alfa, 305
Epstein-Barr virus (EBV) infection,
chronic, 217, 230–232, 238–239,
240. *See also* Chronic fatigue
syndrome
Erythromycin
inhibition of cytochrome
P$_{450}$-3A4 by, **85**, 86
interaction with carbamazepine,
123
interaction with terfenadine, 86,
103
interaction with valproate, 130
Esophageal motility testing, 99
Esophagitis, in bone marrow
transplant recipient, 433
Essential fatty acids, for chronic
fatigue syndrome, 239, **242**
Estazolam
formulations of, **8**
half-life of, **19**
metabolism of, **9**
Estrogen deficiency
after bone marrow
transplantation, 453–454
symptoms of, 453–454
Estrogen replacement therapy
after bone marrow
transplantation, 456
for vulvodynia, 408
Ethambutol, 305
Ethanol, zero-order kinetics and,
19–20
Ethchlorvynol, use in renal disease,
58–59

Ethical issues, related to bone
marrow transplantation,
428–430
Ethosuximide, **186**
Etoposide, before bone marrow
transplantation, 417, 430
Executive function deficits after
head injury, 312
testing for, **326–327**
Extrapyramidal side effects
clozapine for, 109
in HIV-infected persons, 283–285
risperidone and, 115–116
selective serotonin reuptake
inhibitor-induced, 91–92

Fanconi's anemia, 417
Fansidar. *See* Sulfadoxine/
pyrimethamine
Fatigue, 215
after bone marrow
transplantation, 434
chemotherapy-induced, 431
chronic, 215–250. *See also*
Chronic fatigue syndrome
epidemiology of, 223
gabapentin-induced, 120
postconcussional, 315
psychiatric comorbidity with,
215
Febricula, 217. *See also* Chronic
fatigue syndrome
Felbamate, 116–119
dosage of, 117
drug interactions with, 117–118
antidepressants, 118
carbamazepine, 117–118
valproate, 118
efficacy for seizures, 117
indications for, 116
mechanism of action of, 116
side effects of, 117–118
Fever, in chronic fatigue syndrome,
221

Fibromyalgia, 217, 234, **236**. *See also*
Chronic fatigue syndrome
treatment of, 241, **246–248**
First-order kinetics, 18–19
First-pass effect, 2
Flecainide
metabolism by cytochrome
P_{450}-2D6, **83**
use after myocardial infarction,
98
Flow-limited drugs, 32–33, 39
Fluconazole, 86
neuropsychiatric side effects of,
304
for vulvar candidiasis, 400, 402
Fluoxetine
achieving steady state of, 17
cytochrome P_{450} inhibition by,
36, 46, **84**, 84–85
drug interactions with, **87–88**
carbamazepine, 123–124
clonazepam, 37
clozapine, 108
desipramine, 85
terfenadine, 86
warfarin, 90
formulations of, **8**, 23
half-life of, 17, 336
for head-injured patient, **332**, 336
for HIV-infected persons,
280–281
side effects of
akathisia, 92
bradycardia, 80
hematologic effects, 90–91
use in gastrointestinal disease, 23
use in liver disease, 45–46, 92
use in renal disease, **54–55**, 66, 92
use in systemic lupus
erythematosus, 208
Fluphenazine
formulations of, **8**
for head-injured patient, **330**
for HIV-related mania, 283

metabolism by cytochrome
P$_{450}$-2D6, **82**
Flurazepam
formulations of, **8**
half-life of, **19**
metabolism of, **9**
use in liver disease, 42
use in renal disease, **56–57**
Fluvoxamine
drug interactions with, **87**
imipramine, 86, 89
warfarin, 90
use in liver disease, 92
Follicle-stimulating hormone (FSH),
in bone marrow transplant
recipients, 453, 455
Formaldehyde "off-gassing," 350,
353
Foscarnet (Foscavir), 304
Frontal lobe syndromes, 312, 314
Fungizone IV. *See* Amphotericin B

Gabapentin, 119–120
advantage of, 119
for elderly patients, 119
side effects of, 120
use in liver disease, 119
use in renal disease, 119
Galactorrhea, risperidone-induced,
114
Galveston Orientation and Amnesia
Test (GOAT), **320, 321,** 322, **326**
Ganciclovir, 304
Gastrointestinal disease, 21–26
effect on drug absorption, 2, 3, **6,**
21–22
gastroenteritis in bone marrow
transplant recipients, 433
use of antidepressants in, 23–24
use of antipsychotics in, 22–23
use of anxiolytics in, 22
use of carbamazepine in, 25
use of lithium in, 24–25
use of valproate in, 25–26

Gastrointestinal effects
of nefazodone, 96
of zolpidem, 131
Gay Men's Health Crisis, 288
Gender effects
on prevalence of fatigue, 223, 228
on prevalence of HIV infection,
258–259
on psychopharmacokinetics, 1
Genetics, psychopharmacokinetics
and, 1
Germ-free hospital environment,
417, 443–445
Glasgow Coma Score (GCS), **320,**
322, **326**
Glucuronidation, 14
in liver disease, 37–39
in renal disease, 52
Glutethimide, use in renal disease,
58–59
Gold salts, **186**
Graft-versus-host disease (GvHD),
416–419, 431–432, 437–438
chronic, 438, 451
clinical features of, 438
prevalence after bone marrow
transplantation, 437, 438
prevention of, 438
Griseofulvin, **186**
Group therapy, for HIV-infected
persons, 287–288
Growth disorders, in bone marrow
transplant recipients, 435,
451
Guanoxan, **82**
Gynecomastia,
risperidone-induced, 114

Halazepam
formulations of, **8**
half-life of, **19**
metabolism of, **9**
use in liver disease, 42
Half-life, **5, 16,** 16–18

Half-life *(continued)*
  apparent volume of distribution
    and, 17, 34
  of benzodiazepines, 18, **19,** 284
  calculation of, 17
  disease effects on, 18
  of metabolites, 18, **19**
Hallucinations
  in Parkinson's disease, 159–160
  zolpidem-induced, 133
Haloperidol
  first-pass metabolism of, 2
  formulations of, **8**
  for head-injured patient, 329, **330**
  for HIV-infected persons, 283,
    285–286
  interaction with fluoxetine, **87**
  intravenous, 103–104, 286
  torsades de pointes induced by,
    103–104, 286
  use in liver disease, 44
  use in renal disease, 53, **60–61**
Hamilton Anxiety Scale, 268
Hamilton Rating Scale for
    Depression (Ham-D), 113, 268,
    278, 323, **327**
Head injury, 307–340
  brain imaging after, 311–313,
    321, 325–328
  classification of severity of,
    308–309
  clinical interview and
    neuropsychiatric mental
    status examination after,
    321, 322–323
  deaths due to, 307
  depression after, 309–310, **311**
  DSM-IV diagnoses associated
    with, **309,** 309–310
  history taking for patient with,
    319–322, **320–321**
  peritraumatic history, 319–322
  pretraumatic or premorbid
    history, 319

incidence of, 307
mild, 307–340
neuropsychiatric assessment of
    patient with, 318, **320–321**
neuropsychological testing of
    patient with, 323–325,
    326–327
  clinically driven testing,
    323–324
  forensically driven testing,
    324
  test domains, 324–325
pathophysiology of, 310–314
  clinical significance of, 314
  contusions and lacerations,
    310–312
  diffuse axonal injury, 310–311,
    313–314
  indirect damage, 312–313
  shear damage, 312–313
personality change after, 310,
    312, **312**
postconcussional disorder after,
    314–317, **316**
posttraumatic stress disorder
    after, 317–318
prognosis for, 319, 321–322
psychotropic medications for
    persons with, 328–340,
    330–334
  antidepressants, 335–337
  antiepileptic drugs, 337–339
  benzodiazepines, 339
  buspirone, 339–340
  dopamine agonists, 329, 335
  dopamine antagonists, 329
  lithium, 337
  psychostimulants, 335
types of, 308
Headache
  in chronic fatigue syndrome, 221
  felbamate-induced, 117
  postconcussional, 315
  risperidone-induced, 114

Hematologic disorders, bone
marrow transplantation for,
415–460
Hematologic effects
of carbamazepine, 120–121
of fluoxetine, 90–91
of valproate, 125–127
of zidovudine, 283
Hematomas, brain, 310–311
Hemodialysis, 51
Hemoglobinuria, paroxysmal
nocturnal, 417
Hemophilia, HIV infection and, 260
Hepatic blood flow (HBF), 32–33
in congestive heart failure, 28
diseases affecting, 33
Hepatic metabolism of drugs, 2, 9,
9, 14–15
in cardiac disease, 27
in liver disease, 36–40
Herpesviruses
chronic fatigue syndrome and,
231–232
vulvar herpes simplex virus
(HSV), **394**, 395
vulvar herpes zoster, **394**, 395
Hexobarbital, use in renal disease,
54–55
Hickman catheter–related
problems, 436–437
Hidradenitis suppurativa, vulvar,
392
HIV. *See* Human immunodeficiency
virus (HIV) infection
Hivid. *See* Zalcitabine
Hodgkin's disease, bone marrow
transplantation for, 419
Homosexuality, HIV infection and,
258–260
Homovanillic acid (HVA), tacrine
effects on, 136
Hormone-replacement therapy,
after bone marrow
transplantation, 456

Human Ecology Action League
(HEAL), 351
Human herpes virus 6, chronic
fatigue syndrome and,
231–232
Human immunodeficiency virus
type 1 (HIV-1), 261
type 2 (HIV-2), 261
Human immunodeficiency virus
(HIV) infection, 257–290
AIDS dementia complex,
268–277
brain imaging in, 276
cerebrospinal fluid analysis
in, 276
clinical features of, 269–270
diagnosis of, **271–274**, 276
neuropsychological testing
for, 276–277
pathogenesis of, 274–276
prevalence and incidence of,
270, 274
staging of, 270, **275**
terminology for, 268–269
treatment of, 286
assessing immunologic status in,
260
Centers for Disease Control
classification system for,
259, 260
depression and, 267–268,
269–270, 277–278
diagnostic criteria for central
nervous system disorders
in, **271–274**
incidence of, 257
among injecting drug users,
258–260, **267**, 269–270, 289
manic syndromes and, 279–280
maternal-to-infant transmission
of, 262
mechanisms of infection and
virology in, 261–262
outcome of, 262

Human immunodeficiency virus
(HIV) infection *(continued)*
prevalence of psychiatric
morbidity in, 266–268,
269–270
psychopharmacologic and
somatic therapies for,
280–286
antidepressants, 280–282
antimanic drugs, 283–284
anxiolytics, 284
delirium, 285–286
dementia, 286
electroconvulsive therapy, 283
neuroleptics, 284–285
neuropsychiatric side effects
of drugs, 303–305
stimulants, 282–283
psychotherapy for, 286–288
role of psychiatrist in
management of, 257–258
search for causative agent in,
260–261
among severely mentally ill
patients, 288
shifting demographics of,
258–259
suicidality and, 268, 279, 287
testing for, 262–265
antibody responses, 263
counseling before and after,
265–266
distress related to, 264–265
enzyme-linked
immunosorbent assay,
264
tuberculosis and, 289–290
screening for, 290
Human lymphocyte antigen (HLA)
histocompatibility testing, 417
Human papillomavirus (HPV)
infection, 396
Human T-lymphotropic virus
(HTLV), 260–261

Hurler's syndrome, bone marrow
transplantation for, 417
Hydralazine, 27, **186**
lupus induced by, 184
Hydrazine, **186**
Hydrolysis, 15
Hydroxychloroquine, 208
3-Hydroxydiazepam, **19**
N-1-Hydroxyethylflurazepam, **19**
5-Hydroxyindoleacetic acid
(5-HIAA), tacrine effects on, 136
1-Hydroxymethylmidazolam, **19**
9-Hydroxy-risperidone, 114
Hydroxyzine, 434
Hyperammonemia,
valproate-induced, 128
Hyperamylasemia,
valproate-induced, 128
Hyperbilirubinemia, 34
Hypercalcemia, lithium-induced,
111–112
Hypercholesterolemia,
carbamazepine-induced, 121
Hyperlipidemia,
carbamazepine-induced, 121
Hyperparathyroidism,
lithium-induced, 111–112
Hyperprolactinemia,
risperidone-induced, 114
Hypersalivation,
clozapine-induced, 164
Hypertension
clozapine-induced, 107
venlafaxine-induced, 94
Hypochondriasis, 356, 365
Hypoglycemia, 217. *See also*
Chronic fatigue syndrome
Hyponatremia
carbamazepine-induced, 122
risperidone-induced, 114
Hypothyroidism
carbamazepine and, 122
effect on albumin binding of
drugs, 10

ICU psychosis, 443
Illness Behavior Questionnaire, 356
Imipramine
    cardiac effects of, 96
    for chest pain in patients with
        normal coronary
        angiograms, 99–100
    drug interactions with
        diltiazem, 105
        fluoxetine, **87,** 89
        fluvoxamine, 86, **87,** 89
        labetalol, 105
        verapamil, 105
    formulations of, **8**
    metabolism of, 45, **85**
        by cytochrome P_{450}-2D6, 36, **82**
    use in cardiac disease, 30
    use in renal disease, 53, **64–65**
    volume of distribution of, 13
Immune system
    bone marrow transplantation for
        dysfunction of, 415–460
    chronic fatigue syndrome and,
        218, 232–233
    environmental illness and, 347,
        352–353, 368
    in HIV infection, 257–290
Immunoglobulin G (IgG), chronic
    fatigue syndrome and,
    232–233, 239, **243**
Immunosuppressive agents
    before bone marrow
        transplantation, 417, 430,
        434–435
    for systemic lupus
        erythematosus, 189,
        207–208
Immunotherapy, for environmental
    illness, 354
Impulse control problems
    after head injury, 314
    assessing bone marrow
        transplant candidate for,
        423–424

In vitro fertilization, before bone
    marrow transplantation,
    456–457
Informed consent, for bone marrow
    transplantation, 426–428
Insomnia. *See also* Sleep
    disturbances
    felbamate-induced, 117
    risperidone-induced, 114
    venlafaxine-induced, 93
    zolpidem for, 132–133
Interferon-α, for chronic fatigue
    syndrome, 241, **245**
Interferon alfa-2a, 305
International Bone Marrow
    Transplant Registry (IBMTR),
    420
International Society for the Study
    of Vulvovaginal Disease, 386,
    403
Interstitial cystitis, 386, 387–388
Interstitial Cystitis Association, 387
Interstitial pneumonitis
    in bone marrow transplant
        recipient, 451
    carbamazepine-induced, 122
Intracranial pressure elevation, due
    to total-body irradiation, 435
Irritability, postconcussional, 315
Isoniazid, **186**
    interaction with valproate, 130
    neuropsychiatric side effects of,
        305
Isoquinazepan, **186**
Itching, vulvar, 381–382, 388,
    398–399. *See also* Vulvodynia
Itraconazole
    cytochrome P_{450} inhibition by, **85**
    neuropsychiatric side effects of,
        304

Kaposi's sarcoma, 259
Karnofksy score, after bone marrow
    transplantation, 452

Ketoconazole
    cytochrome P$_{450}$-3A4 inhibition
        by, 36–37, **85,** 86
    for environmental illness, 354
    interaction with terfenadine, 86
    neuropsychiatric side effects of,
        304
Kindling, 352

Labetalol, interaction with
        imipramine, 105
Laboratory tests
    for AIDS dementia complex, 276
    for environmental illness, 352,
        367, **370**
    liver function tests, 40
    to measure drug blood
        concentration, 12, 18
    for systemic lupus
        erythematosus, 195,
        197–198
Lacerations, brain, 310–311
Laminar-air flow rooms, 417,
        443–445
Lamprene. *See* Clofazimine
Language testing, after head injury,
        324, **326**
LE cell test, 195
Legal issues
    neuropsychological testing of
        brain-injured patient, 323,
        324
    related to bone marrow
        transplantation, 428–430
Legionnaire's disease, 350
Lennox-Gastaut syndrome, 116
Lentiviruses, 261
Lethargy, in HIV infection, 270
Leukemia, bone marrow
        transplantation for, 415–460
Leukopenia, use of carbamazepine
        in, 121
Levodopa, for head-injured patient,
        329

Levodopa/carbidopa, **154**
    for Parkinson's disease, 152–153,
        161–162
    psychotoxicity of, 161–162
    visual hallucinosis induced by,
        151
Lewy bodies disease, 168
Lichen planus, **392, 393**
Lichen sclerosus et atrophicus, 390,
        392, 399
Lichen simplex chronicus, 384, **392,**
        398–399
Lidocaine
    metabolism by cytochrome
        P$_{450}$-3A4, 85
    use in cardiac disease patients, 26
Lightheadedness,
        nefazodone-induced, 96
Linear kinetics, 18–19
Lipid solubility of drugs, 12–14
Lipid storage diseases, bone
        marrow transplantation for, 419
Lisinopril, interaction with lithium,
        113
Lithium, 79, 110–113
    cardiac effects of, 31
    distribution of, 13
    drug interactions with, 112–113
        valproate, 127–128
    excretion of, 36
    formulations of, **8, 24**
    for head-injured patient, **333,**
        337, 337
    for HIV-infected persons, 282,
        283
    lupus induced by, **186**
    parathyroid function and,
        111–112
    renal failure and, 110–111
    side effects of, 283
    use in cardiac disease, 27, 31–32,
        112
    use in gastrointestinal disease,
        24–25

use in liver disease, 33, 46–47
use in renal disease, **60–61,**
       66–67, 111
volume of distribution of, 13
Liver disease, 32–49
   ascites and, 35
   hyperbilirubinemia and, 34
   pharmacokinetic effects of, **7,**
          32–35
      bioavailability, 32–33, 39
      drug metabolism, 36–40, **38**
      flow-limited and
             enzyme-limited drugs,
             32–33, 39
      hepatic blood flow and, 32–33
      hepatic clearance, 39
      preservation of
             glucuronidation
             reaction, 37–39
      protein binding of drugs, 10,
             34–35
      systemic availability, 39–40
   recommendation for drug
          dosing in, 40–42
   renal disease and, 41–42
   use of antidepressants in, 44–46
      fluoxetine, 45–46, 92
      sertraline, 46
      trazodone, 45
      tricyclics, 39, 41, 44–45
      venlafaxine, 94
   use of antipsychotics in, 43–44
   use of anxiolytics in, 42–43
   use of carbamazepine in, 47–48
   use of felbamate in, 49
   use of gabapentin in, 119
   use of lithium in, 46–47
   use of valproate in, 48–49, 126,
          128
   use of zolpidem in, 131
Liver extract-folic acid-
       cyanocobalamin (LEFAC), for
       chronic fatigue syndrome, 239,
       242

Liver function tests, 40
Loratadine, 103
Lorazepam
   achieving steady state of, 17
   for bone marrow transplant
          recipient, 439
   clearance of, 17
   formulations of, **8**
   half-life of, 17, **19,** 284
   for head-injured patient, **334,** 339
   for HIV-infected persons, 284,
          286
   interaction with fluvoxamine, **87**
   interaction with valproate, 127,
          129
   intramuscular, 3
   metabolism of, **9,** 14–15, 52
   for nausea and vomiting, 434
   onset of action of, 3
   use in cardiac disease, 27
   use in liver disease, 39, 42
   use in renal disease, **56–57**
   volume of distribution of, 13, 17
Loss of consciousness (LOC), **320**
   diffuse axonal injury indicated
          by, 313
   severity of brain injury based on,
          308–309
Loxapine, **8**
Lumbar puncture, in systemic
       lupus erythematosus, 196, **198**
Lung cancer, bone marrow
       transplantation for, 419
Lupus, discoid, 184, 187
Lupus, drug-induced, 184
   clinical features of, 184, **187**
   differentiating from systemic
          lupus erythematosus, 184
   drugs associated with, **186**
      carbamazepine, 122
      chlorpromazine, 184
      hydralazine, 184
      procainamide, 184
      valproate, 129

Lupus, drug-induced *(continued)*
    laboratory features of, 184, **187**
    treatment of, 184
Lupus anticoagulant (LA), 204
Luteinizing hormone (LH), in bone
    marrow transplant recipients,
    454, 455
Lymphadenopathy, in chronic
    fatigue syndrome, 221
Lymphomas, bone marrow
    transplantation for, 415–460

Magnesium, for chronic fatigue
    syndrome, 241, **243**
Magnetic resonance imaging (MRI)
    after head injury, 313, **321,**
    325–328
    in AIDS dementia complex, 276
    in systemic lupus
        erythematosus, **198,**
        199–201
Malaise, in chronic fatigue
    syndrome, 221
Malnutrition, effect on albumin
    binding of drugs, 10
Mania, HIV-related, 279–280
MAOIs. *See* Monoamine oxidase
    inhibitors
Maprotiline
    for fibromyalgia, **247**
    formulations of, **8**
    for HIV-infected persons, 282
    use in renal disease, **54–55**
Marinol. *See* Dronabinol
Melena, fluoxetine-induced, 90
Memory deficits
    in chronic fatigue syndrome,
        221
    in HIV infection, 269
    postconcussional, 312, 315
        testing for, 324–325, **326**
    among Vietnam veterans with
        posttraumatic stress
        disorder, 317–318

Menopause
    dysesthetic vulvodynia after,
        402
    premature, due to total-body
        irradiation, 435
Mental retardation
    assessing bone marrow
        transplant candidate for,
        423
    valproate for persons with, 125
Mental status examination, after
    head injury, **321,** 322–323
Mental Status Examination in
    Neurology, **326**
Mephenytoin, **186**
Meprobamate, use in renal disease,
    60–61
Mepron. *See* Atovaquone
Mering procedure, 397
Mesoridazine, **8**
Methadone, interaction with
    rifampin, 290
Methamphetamine, **83**
Methaqualone, use in renal disease,
    60–61
Methimazole, **186**
Methotrexate, 417, 435
Methoxyphenamine, **82**
N-Methyl-D-aspartate (NMDA)
    receptors, role in AIDS
    dementia complex, 275
Methylation, 15
Methyldopa, **186**
Methylphenidate
    for bone marrow transplant
        recipient, 440
    formulations of, **8**
    for head-injured patients, **330,**
        335
    for HIV-infected persons,
        282–283
    for poststroke depression, 113
Methylthiouracil, **186**
Methysergide, **186**

Metoclopramide, 2, 434
Metoprolol, **186**
    interaction with fluoxetine, **88**
    metabolism of, **82**
Michaelis-Menten kinetics, 19–20
β_2-Microglobulin
    in AIDS dementia complex, 276
    in renal disorders, 51
Midazolam
    formulations of, **8**
    half-life of, **19**
    interaction with cyclosporine, 37
    intramuscular, 3
    metabolism of, **9**
        by cytochrome P_{450}-3A4, 36, 85
    use in liver disease, 43
    use in renal disease, **58–59**
    volume of distribution of, 13
Mini-Mental State Exam (MMSE), 134, 277
    for head-injured patient, 322, **326**
Minnesota Multiphasic Personality Inventory (MMPI), 323, **327,** 356
Moclobemide, for vulvodynia, 408
Molindone
    formulations of, **8**
    for head-injured patient, **331**
    for HIV-infected persons, 285
Molluscum contagiosum, **394,** 396
Monoamine oxidase inhibitors (MAOIs), 79
    for head-injured patient, **332,** 335–337
    for HIV-infected persons, 282
    metabolized by cytochrome P_{450}-2D6, **82**
    use in gastrointestinal disease, 23
    use in renal disease, **62–63**
Mood disorders. *See also* Bipolar disorder; Depression; Mania
    after head injury, 309–310, **311,** 314, 315

associated with HIV infection, 267–268
    due to general medical condition, 309–310, **311**
    environmental illness and, 356, **358–361,** 372
    gabapentin-induced, 120
    in systemic lupus erythematosus, 188, 191, 192
Mood stabilizers. *See also* specific drugs
    for head-injured persons, 337–339
    use in gastrointestinal disease, 24–26
    use in liver disease, 46–49
Moricizine, 98
Motor deficits, in HIV infection, 269
Mucositis, 433
Multidimensional Pain Inventory, 408
Multiple chemical sensitivity, 347–349, 351. *See also* Environmental illness
Multiple myeloma, bone marrow transplantation for, 419
Myalgias, chronic fatigue syndrome and, 234
Myambutol. *See* Ethambutol
Myelopathy, associated with HIV infection, **272–273**
Myocardial infarction
    drug protein binding and, 10, 27
    use of antiarrhythmics after, 97–98

Naproxen, for fibromyalgia, **247**
National Bone Marrow Registry (NBMR), 420
National Marrow Donor Program (NMDP), 421
National Organ Transplant Act (PL 98-507), 429

Nausea and vomiting
 in bone marrow transplant
  recipient, 431, 433–435
 drug-induced
  felbamate, 117
  nefazodone, 96
  venlafaxine, 93, 281
  zolpidem, 131
 medications for, 434
Nefazodone, 79, 95–97
 cytochrome P_{450}-3A4 inhibition
  by, **85,** 86
 cytochrome P_{450}-mediated
  biotransformation of, 36
 drug interactions with, 97
 mechanism of action of, 95
 pharmacology in medical
  patients, 97
 side effects of, 95–97
Nephrotic syndrome, 10, 50
Nervous exhaustion, 217. *See also*
 Chronic fatigue syndrome
Nervousness
 felbamate-induced, 118
 venlafaxine-induced, 93
Neural tube defects, 123
 antenatal diagnosis of, 123
 carbamazepine exposure and,
  123
Neuralgia, 389
 postherpetic, 395
 pudendal, 389–390
Neurasthenia, 217, 348. *See also*
 Chronic fatigue syndrome
Neurobehavioral Rating Scale
 (NBRS), **321,** 322, **327**
Neuroblastoma, bone marrow
 transplantation for, 417, 419
Neuroleptic malignant syndrome
 (NMS)
 clozapine-induced, 108–109
 neuroleptic treatment after, 109
Neuroleptics. *See also* specific drugs
 formulations of, **8**

for head-injured patient, 329,
 330–331
for HIV-infected persons,
 284–285
 for mania, 283–284
interaction with valproate,
 127–128
metabolism of, **9,** 14
 by cytochrome P_{450}-2D6, **82–83**
parenteral, 22–23
for psychosis in Parkinson's
 disease, 163–164
use after neuroleptic malignant
 syndrome, 109
use in cardiac disease, 31
use in gastrointestinal disease,
 22–23
use in liver disease, 43–44
use in renal disease, 53
use in systemic lupus
 erythematosus, 207, 208
Neurological examination, in HIV
 infection, 276
Neuropsychological testing
 in AIDS dementia complex,
  276–277
 of bone marrow transplant
  recipients, 436
 of head-injured patients,
  323–325, **326–327**
 in systemic lupus
  erythematosus, 194, **198,**
  199
Neurotransmitters
 clozapine effects on, 164–165
 tacrine effects on, 136
Neutropenia,
 carbamazepine-induced, 121
New York's Gay Men's Health
 Crisis, 288
Nicotine, protein binding of, 10
Nifedipine, 85
Nimodipine, for AIDS dementia
 complex, 275

Nitrazepam
  metabolism of, 90
  use in liver disease, 42
  use in renal disease, **58–59**
Nitrofurantoin, **186**
Nizoral. *See* Ketoconazole
Noncompliance, of bone marrow
  transplant recipient, 423,
  431–432, 439
Nonlinear kinetics, 19–20
Norfluoxetine. *See also* Fluoxetine
  cytochrome P$_{450}$ inhibition by,
    36, 84, **84**
  half-life of, 17, 85
Nortriptyline
  drug interactions with
    carbamazepine, 124
    fluoxetine, **87**
    quinidine, 37
    valproate, 106
  formulations of, **8,** 23
  for head-injured patient, **331,** 336
  for HIV-infected persons, 281,
    282
  metabolism of, 45
    by cytochrome P$_{450}$-2D6, 36,
      37, **82**
  for mucous membrane
    dysesthesias, 390
  for pruritus ani, 399
  use in cardiac disease, 30
  use in renal disease, **64–65,** 66
  volume of distribution of, 13
  for vulvodynia, 408
Nystatin, for candidiasis, 354, 362

Occupational medicine, 367
Olivopontocerebellar atrophy, 169
Ondansetron, for psychosis in
  Parkinson's disease, 169
Opioids
  after bone marrow
    transplantation, 433–434,
    441

interaction with carbamazepine,
  124
Oral contraceptives, **186**
  interaction with carbamazepine,
    124
Orbitofrontal lobe syndromes, 312,
  314
Organ transplantation, 415. *See also*
  Bone marrow transplantation
Organic Aggression Scale (OAS),
  321, 322, **327**
Organic mental syndromes,
  associated with HIV infection,
  267, **269–270**
Oropharyngeal ulcers, 433
Orthostatic hypotension
  drug-induced
    clozapine, 107
    imipramine, 96
    nefazodone, 96
    risperidone, 116
  in head-injured patient, 329
Ovarian failure,
  chemotherapy-induced,
  453–455
Oxazepam
  formulations of, **8**
  half-life of, **19,** 284
  for head-injured patient, **334,** 339
  metabolism of, **9,** 14–15, 52
  use in cardiac disease, 27
  use in liver disease, 33, 39, 42
  use in renal disease, **58–59**
  volume of distribution of, 13
2-Oxoquazepam, **19**
Oxprenolol, **186**
Oxyphenisatin, **186**

Paced Auditory Serial Addition
  Test, **326**
Pain
  chronic, 408
  management after bone marrow
    transplantation, 434

Pain *(continued)*
  vulvodynia, 381–411
Pancreatitis
  clozapine-induced, 107
  effect on albumin binding of
      drugs, 10
  effect on drug absorption, 2
  valproate-induced, 128
Panic disorder, valproate for, 125
Parathyroid hormone (PTH), in
    patient on lithium, 111–112
Parkinsonism
  atypical, clozapine for,
      168–169
  compared with Parkinson's
      disease, 152
  selective serotonin reuptake
      inhibitor–induced, 91
Parkinson's disease (PD)
  age at onset of, 158
  compared with parkinsonism,
      152
  exacerbated by selective
      serotonin reuptake
      inhibitors, 91
  pathophysiology of, 152
  treatment of, 152–156,
      154–155
    amantadine, 156
    anticholinergics, 156
    clozapine, 106, 164–169
    dilemma in, 151
    dopamine agonists, 153
    electroconvulsive therapy,
        170–172
    levodopa, 152–153
    selegiline, 153, 156
Parkinson's disease–associated
    psychosis, 156–176
  differential diagnosis of,
      156–158
  differential psychotoxicity of
      antiparkinsonian drugs,
      161–162

epidemiology of, 158
phenomenology of, 158–160
  delusions, 160
  hallucinations, 159–160
  sleep disturbances, 160
risk factors for, 158
treatment of, 162–176
  adjustment of
      antiparkinsonian drugs,
      162–163
  approach to, 172–175, **173**
  case reports of, 175–176, **177**
  clozapine, 164–169, **166**
  electroconvulsive therapy,
      170–172
  hospitalization, 174–175
  ondansetron, 169
  risperidone, 169
  typical neuroleptics, 163–164
Paroxetine
  cytochrome P_{450} inhibition by,
      36, 46, 84, **84,** 280
  drug interactions with, **88**
    valproate, 130
    warfarin, 91
  formulations of, **8**
  half-life of, 17
  for head-injured patient, **333,**
      336
  for HIV-infected persons, 280
  use in cardiac disease, 31
  use in gastrointestinal disease, 23
  use in liver disease, 92
Patient-controlled analgesia (PCA),
    434
Pemoline
  formulations of, **8**
  for head-injured patients, 335
  for HIV-infected persons, 282
Penicillamine, **186**
Penicillin, **186**
Pentamidine (Pentam), 303
Pentobarbital, use in renal disease,
    54–55

Pergolide, for Parkinson's disease, 153, **154**
Perhexiline, **83**
Perineal pain, 385, 389–390
Peritoneal dialysis, 51
Perphenazine
  formulations of, **8**
  interaction with fluoxetine, 87
  metabolism by cytochrome
    P₄₅₀-2D6, 36, **82**
Personality changes
  after brain injury, 310, 312, **312,**
    314
  due to general medical
    condition, 310, **312**
Personality disorders
  associated with HIV infection,
    269–270
  chronic fatigue and, 235
  environmental illness and, 356,
    358–361, 364–366
Petechiae, fluoxetine-induced, 90
Pharmacokinetics. *See*
  Psychopharmacokinetics
Pharyngitis, in chronic fatigue
  syndrome, 221
Phase I reactions, **9,** 14–15, 36
Phase II reactions, **9,** 15, 36
Phenelzine
  for head-injured patient, **332**
  use in renal disease, **62–63**
Phenformin, **83**
Phenobarbital
  interaction with paroxetine, 88
  use in renal disease, **54–55**
Phenothiazines
  protein binding of, 10
  use in renal disease, 53, **62–63**
Phenylbutazone, **186**
Phenylethylacetylurea, **186**
Phenytoin
  interaction with clozapine, 108
  interaction with fluoxetine, **88**
  interaction with paroxetine, **88**

lupus induced by, **186**
protein binding of, 10
withdrawal from, 119
zero-order kinetics and, 19–20
Physician-patient relationship,
  chronic fatigue syndrome and,
  215, 239
Pimozide
  formulations of, **8**
  interaction with fluoxetine, **88**
  use in cardiac disease, 31
Pinworms, 399
Platelet abnormalities
  carbamazepine-induced, 121
  fluoxetine-induced, 90
  valproate-induced, 126–127
Pneumonia
  effect on albumin binding of
    drugs, 10
  Pneumocystis carinii, 259
    neuropsychiatric effects of
      drugs used for, 303
Polyserositis, clozapine-induced,
  108
Positron-emission tomography
  (PET)
  in AIDS dementia complex, 276
  in systemic lupus
    erythematosus, 194, 202
Postconcussional disorder, 307–308,
  314–317, **316.** *See also* Head
  injury
  duration of, 316–317
  symptoms of, 315–317
  terminology for, 315
Posttraumatic stress disorder
  (PTSD)
  after head injury, 317–318
  zolpidem for, 131
Practolol, **186**
Prazepam
  active metabolite of, 3, 15
  formulations of, **8**
  half-life of, **19**

Prazepam (continued)
   metabolism of, **9**
   onset of action of, 3
   use in liver disease, 42
   use in renal disease, **58–59**
Pregnancy
   after bone marrow
      transplantation, 457
   carbamazepine in, 123
   effect of zidovudine on
      maternal-to-infant HIV
      transmission in, 262
   systemic lupus erythematosus
      and, 206
Priapism, clozapine-induced, 107
Primidone, **186**
Procainamide, lupus induced by, 184
Prochlorperazine
   formulations of, **8**
   for nausea and vomiting, 434
Procrit. See Epoetin alfa
Profile of Mood States, 436
Prokine. See Sargramostim
Propafenone
   drug interactions with, 106
   metabolism of, **82**
Propantheline, 2
Propranolol
   for akathisia, 92
   for head-injured patient, **334**
   interaction with fluvoxamine, **87**
   metabolism of, **82**
   use in HIV-infected persons, 284
   volume of distribution of, 13
Propylthiouracil, **186**
Protein binding of drugs, 9–12
   in cardiac disease, 29
   dialyzability and, 51
   diseases affecting, 10–12, **11**
   effect on laboratory
      measurement of
      therapeutic range, 12
   in liver disease, 10, 34–35
   myocardial infarction and, 27

in renal disease, 10, 50
Prothrombin time (PT), 40
Protriptyline
   formulations of, **8**
   for HIV-infected persons, 281
   metabolism of, 45
   use in renal disease, **64–65**
Pruritus ani, 385, 399
Pruritus vulvae, 385, 398–399. See
   also Vulvodynia
Psoriasis, vulvar, **392**
Psychopharmacokinetics, 1–67,
   4–5
   absorption, 1–9, **4**
   bioavailability, **5,** 9
   clearance, **5,** 15–16
   disease effects on, **6–7,** 20–67
      cardiac disease, 26–32
      gastrointestinal disease,
         21–26
      liver disease, 32–49
      renal disease, 41–42, 49–67
   distribution, **5,** 9–14
   drug metabolites, 3, **9,** 15, 18
   elimination, 9, **9,** 14–18
   factors influencing, 1
   half-life, **5, 16,** 16–18, **19**
   lipid solubility, 12–14
   pharmacokinetic models, 18–20
      first-order kinetics, 18–19
      zero-order kinetics, 19–20
   protein binding, 9–12, **11**
   steady state, **5**
   volume of distribution, **5,** 12–14
Psychosis
   assessing bone marrow
      transplant candidate for,
      423
   drug-induced
      buspirone, 284
      corticosteroids, 208
      gabapentin, 120
   in HIV-infected persons, 284–285
   ICU, 443

in Parkinson's disease, 151–176. *See also* Parkinson's disease–associated psychosis
in systemic lupus erythematosus, 191, 192, 207, 208
Psychostimulants. *See* Stimulants
Psychotherapy
for chronic fatigue syndrome, 241, **244,** 249, **249**
for environmental illness, 369–370, 373
for HIV-infected persons, 286–288
for systemic lupus erythematosus, 206
Psychotropic drugs
dosage of
calculating loading dose, 14
in cardiac disease, 28–30
kinetics affecting increases in, 20
in liver disease, 40–42
related to route of administration, 2
in renal disease, 51–52
formulations of, **8**
for HIV-infected persons, 280–286
intramuscular, 3
measuring blood concentration of, 12, 18
metabolized by cytochrome P_{450}-2D6, **82–83**
onset of action of, 3
parenteral, 3, **8,** 22–23
for patients with mild traumatic brain injury, 328–340, **330–334**
PTSD. *See* Posttraumatic stress disorder
Pudendal neuralgia, 389–390

Pulmonary fibrosis, due to total-body irradiation, 435
Pyrazinamide, 305

Quazepam
formulations of, **8**
half-life of, **19**
metabolism of, **9**
Quinidine
cytochrome P_{450} inhibition by, 36, 37
interaction with nortriptyline, 37
interaction with venlafaxine, 95
lupus induced by, **186**
metabolism by cytochrome P_{450}-3A4, 85
use after myocardial infarction, 98
Quinine, interaction with carbamazepine, 123

Racial effects, on psychopharmacokinetics, 1
Radiation accidents, 417
Ranitidine, 21
Recombinant granulocyte colony-stimulating factor (rG-CSF), 107
Reflex sympathetic dystrophy (RSD), 389
Renal blood flow (RBF), 50–51
in congestive heart failure, 27–28
Renal disease
lithium and, 110–111
liver disease and, 41–42
pharmacokinetic effects of, **7,** 49–52, **54–65**
absorption, 49
dialysis, 51
fluid shifts and protein binding, 10, 50
recommendations for drug dosing in, 51–52

Renal disease (continued)
    use of antidepressants in, 53,
        54–55, 66
        fluoxetine, 66, 92
        nortriptyline, 66
        tricyclics, 53, 62–65, 66
        venlafaxine, 94–95
    use of anxiolytics in, 52–53
    use of gabapentin in, 119
    use of lithium in, 60–61, 66–67,
        111
    use of zolpidem in, 131
Reserpine, 186
Respiratory effects, of zolpidem,
    131–132
Retrovir. See Zidovudine
Retroviruses, 261–262
Rheumatoid arthritis
    cognitive impairment in, 192, 193
    effect on protein binding of
        drugs, 10
    environmental illness and, 363
Rifampin (Rifadin, Rimactane)
    interaction with methadone, 290
    neuropsychiatric side effects of,
        305
Risperidone, 79, 114–116
    active metabolite of, 114
    for elderly patients, 115–116
    formulations of, 8
    half-life of, 114
    for head-injured patient, 329, 331
    for HIV-infected persons, 284,
        285
    mechanism of action of, 114
    metabolism by cytochrome
        P450-2D6, 115
    for psychosis in Parkinson's
        disease, 169
    for schizophrenia, 114
    side effects of, 114–116
Roferon-A. See Interferon alfa-2a

San Francisco Shanti Project, 288

Sargramostim, 305
Scale for the Assessment of Positive
    Symptoms (SAPS), 159
Schizoaffective disorder, associated
    with HIV infection, 269
Schizophrenia
    associated with HIV infection,
        267, 269–270
    clozapine for, 165
    risperidone for, 114–116
Seborrheic dermatitis, vulvar, 392
Secobarbital, use in renal disease,
    54–55
Sedation
    due to total-body irradiation, 435
    risperidone-induced, 114
    venlafaxine-induced, 93
Seizures
    clozapine-induced, 107
    felbamate for, 116–117
    gabapentin for, 119
    in systemic lupus
        erythematosus, 191, 196,
        207
    venlafaxine-induced, 95
Selective Reminding Test, 318
Selective serotonin reuptake
    inhibitors (SSRIs), 80–93. See
    also specific drugs
    achieving steady state of, 17
    dopamine inhibition by, 91
    drug interactions with, 86,
        87–89, 336
        carbamazepine, 336
        clozapine, 108
        desipramine, 85
        felbamate, 118
        trazodone, 83
        warfarin, 90
    half-lives of, 17
    for head-injured patient,
        332–333, 335–336
    for HIV-infected persons,
        280–282

inhibition of cytochrome
P$_{450}$-3A4 by, **85,** 86
inhibition of cytochrome
P$_{450}$-2D6 by, 36–37, 46,
83–85, **84**
metabolism of, **9**
pharmacology in medical
patients, 80–93
side effects of, 80, 336
cardiac effects, 80, 92–93
extrapyramidal symptoms,
91–92
hematologic effects, 90–91
surgery in patients on, 91
use in cardiac disease, 30–31,
92–93
use in gastrointestinal disease, 23
use in liver disease, 92
use in renal disease, 92
Selegiline
mechanism of action of, 153
neuroprotective effect of, 153
for Parkinson's disease, 153, **154,**
156, 162
Seromycin. *See* Cycloserine
Serotonin (5-HT)
nefazodone effects on, 95
tacrine effects on, 136
Sertraline
cytochrome P$_{450}$ inhibition by,
36, 46, **84,** 84–85
drug interactions with, **89**
desipramine, 85
felbamate, 118
warfarin, 90–91
formulations of, **8**
half-life of, 17
for head-injured patient, **332,**
336
for HIV-infected persons, 280
metabolism of, **85**
use in gastrointestinal disease, 23
use in liver disease, 46
Serum creatinine, 51–52

Serum glutamic-oxaloacetic
transaminase (SGOT), 40
Serum glutamic-pyruvic
transaminase (SGPT), 40
Severe combined
immunodeficiency disease,
416, 420
Sexual abuse
vaginal or rectal discharge due
to, 399
vulvodynia and, 407–408
Sexual dysfunction
after bone marrow
transplantation, 453–460
chemotherapy-induced,
453–455
radiotherapy-induced, 454–456
treatment of, 456–457
dyspareunia, 385
hypoactive sexual desire
disorder in HIV-infected
women, 268
nefazodone-induced, 96
selective serotonin reuptake
inhibitor–induced, 336
venlafaxine-induced, 93–94
Short bowel syndrome, 2
Sialorrhea, clozapine-induced, 107
Sick-building syndrome, 349–350
Sickle cell anemia, bone marrow
transplantation for, 417, 419
Sickness Impact Profile, 436
Sinemet. *See* Levodopa/carbidopa
Single photon-emission computed
tomography (SPECT)
after head injury, **321,** 327–328
in AIDS dementia complex, 276
in systemic lupus
erythematosus, **198,**
201–202
Skin biopsy, in systemic lupus
erythematosus, 195
Skin disorders
carbamazepine-induced, 122

Skin disorders *(continued)*
  discoid lupus, 184, 187
  drug-induced lupus, 184,
    186–187
  systemic lupus erythematosus,
    183–209
  vulvar, 390–396, **392–394**
Sleep disturbances. *See also*
  Insomnia
  in bone marrow transplant
    recipient, 432, 439
  in chronic fatigue syndrome,
    218, 221, 233–234
  in Parkinson's disease, 160
  related to protected isolation
    environment, 443
  in systemic lupus
    erythematosus, 192
Sodium nitroprusside, 27
Somatization disorder
  chronic fatigue and, 235
  environmental illness and, 356,
    358–360, 372
  vulvodynia and, 409
Somnolence
  due to total-body irradiation, 435
  gabapentin-induced, 120
  nefazodone-induced, 96
Sotalol, torsades de pointes induced
  by, 104
Sperm banking, before bone
  marrow transplantation,
    456–457
Sporanox. *See* Itraconazole
SSRIs. *See* Selective serotonin
  reuptake inhibitors
Staphylococcal furunculosis, **394,**
  396
Steady state, **5**
  relation to half-life, 17–18
Sterility, due to total-body
  irradiation, 435
Stimulants, 79, 113–114
  cardiac effects of, 113–114

formulations of, **8**
for head-injured patient, **330,**
  335
for HIV-infected persons,
  282–283
Stomach resection, 2
Stomatitis, in bone marrow
  transplant recipient, 433–435
Streptococcal cellulitis, **394,** 396
Streptomycin, **186**
Stress, effect on protein binding of
  drugs, 10
Structured Clinical Interview for
  DSM-III-R (SCID), 323, **327**
Structured Interview for DSM-III
  Personality Disorders, **358–361**
Substance use disorders
  assessing bone marrow
    transplant candidate for,
    423
  associated with HIV infection,
    258–260, **267,** 269–270,
    289
  vulvodynia and, 409
Suicidality, associated with HIV
  infection, 268, 279, 287
Sulfadoxine/pyrimethamine, 303
Sulfonamides, **186**
Support groups
  for environmental illness, 351,
    355
  for families of bone marrow
    transplant recipients, 448
  for interstitial cystitis, 387
  for systemic lupus
    erythematosus, 206
  for vulvodynia, 386
Surgery
  drug-induced bleeding
    tendencies and
    selective serotonin reuptake
    inhibitors, 91
  valproate, 126–127
  effect on drug absorption, 22

effect on protein binding of
drugs, 10
Sweating, venlafaxine-induced, 93
Symptom Checklist-90—Revised,
356
Syndrome of inappropriate
secretion of antidiuretic
hormone, risperidone-induced,
114
Systemic lupus erythematosus
(SLE), 183–209
autoantibodies in, 184, **187,** 188,
195, **197**
search for specific antibodies
in neuropsychiatric
lupus, **198,** 202–206
causes of death in, 189
clinical course of, 189
clinical features of, 183–184, **185,**
187, 187, **190, 196**
cognitive impairment in, 188,
191–194
diagnosis of, 188–189
brain imaging, **198,** 199–202
computed tomography, 199
magnetic resonance
imaging, 199–201
positron-emission
tomography, 194, 202
single photon-emission
computed
tomography, 201–202
electroencephalogram,
196–199, **198**
issues and problems in,
194–195
lumbar puncture, 196, **198**
neuropsychological testing,
194, **198,** 199
serology and chemistry tests,
195, **197–198**
skin biopsy, 195
differential diagnosis of,
184–187, **186,** 193

discoid lupus, 184, 187
drug-induced lupus, 184,
186–187
in elderly persons, 188–189
epidemiology of, 184
immune abnormalities in, **187**
neuropsychiatric symptoms and
psychopathology in, 188,
191–192, **192**
prevalence of, 184
prognosis for, 189
psychiatric presentations of,
192–193
psychiatrist's role in, 191
support groups for patients
with, 206
treatment of, 189, 206–209, **207**
drug therapy for
neuropsychiatric
syndromes, 206–208
guidelines for, 208–209
psychiatric effects of
medications used for, 208

T lymphocytes, in HIV infection,
259, 260
Tachycardia, clozapine-induced, 107
Tacrine, 79, 133–136
alanine aminotransferase
elevation due to, 134–136
effects on neurotransmitters, 136
efficacy studies of, 134
guidelines for termination of, 135
improvement in attention vs.
memory due to, 134–135
indications for, 133–134
patient selection for, 136
predicting responsiveness to, 135
side effects of, 134–136
Tardive dyskinesia
clozapine for, 109
risperidone for, 115
Tardive dystonia, clozapine for, 109
Tartrazine, **186**

Tegretol. *See* Carbamazepine
Temazepam
    formulations of, **8**
    half-life of, **19**
    for head-injured patient, **334,** 339
    metabolism of, **9,** 15, 52
    use in cardiac disease, 27
    use in liver disease, 39, 42
Temporal lobe syndromes, 312, 314
Terfenadine, 102–103
    drug interactions with, 102–103
        cytochrome P$_{450}$-3A4
            inhibitors, 86
        nefazodone, 97
    metabolism by cytochrome
        P$_{450}$-3A4, 85
    overdose of, 103
Terfenadine carboxylate, 102–103
Testicular cancer, bone marrow
    transplantation for, 417–419
Testosterone, in bone marrow
    transplant recipients, 453, 455
Tetracycline, **186**
Thalassemia, bone marrow
    transplantation for, 417, 419,
    420
Theophylline, interaction with
    fluvoxamine, **87**
Therapeutic range, 12
Thiopental, use in renal disease,
    54–55
Thioridazine
    cytochrome P$_{450}$-2D6 inhibition
        by, 84
    formulations of, **8**
    metabolism by cytochrome
        P$_{450}$-2D6, 36, **83**
    use in cardiac disease, 31
Thiothixene, **8**
Thrombocytopenia
    carbamazepine-induced, 121
    valproate-induced, 126
Thyroid dysfunction, due to
    total-body irradiation, 435

Thyroid-stimulating hormone
    (TSH), in patient on lithium, 111
Timolol, **82**
Tinea infections, vulvar, **394**
Tolazamide, **186**
Tolbutamide, interaction with
    paroxetine, **88**
Torsades de pointes, 86, 101–104
    astemizole-induced, 103
    intravenous
        haloperidol–induced,
        103–104, 286
    sotalol-induced, 104
    terfenadine-related, 102–103
Total parenteral nutrition (TPN)
    for bone marrow transplant
        recipient, 416, 431
    complications related to,
        436–437
Total-body irradiation (TBI)
    before bone marrow
        transplantation, 416, 430,
        435–436
    gonadal dysfunction due to,
        454–456
    long-term neuropsychological
        effects of, 435–436
    toxic acute complications of, 435
Trail Making test, **326**
Tranylcypromine, for head-injured
    patient, **332**
Trauma
    effect on albumin binding of
        drugs, 10
    head injury, 307–340
Trazodone
    formulations of, **8**
    for head-injured patient, **333,** 337
    for HIV-infected persons, 282
    interaction with selective
        serotonin reuptake
        inhibitors, 83
    for mucous membrane
        dysesthesias, 390

use in cardiac disease, 30–31
use in liver disease, 45
Tremor. *See also* Parkinsonism
gabapentin-induced, 120
in HIV infection, 269
Triazolam
formulations of, **8**
half-life of, **19**
interaction with nefazodone, 97
metabolism of, **9**
by cytochrome P_{450}-3A4,
36, 85
use in liver disease, 42–43
use in renal disease, **58–59**
Tricyclic antidepressants (TCAs).
See Antidepressants, tricyclic
Trifluoperazine, **8**
Trifluperidol, **82**
Triiodothyronine (T_3), for
HIV-infected persons, 282
Trimethadione, **186**
Trimethoprim/sulfamethoxazole,
303
Trimipramine, **8**
Tuberculosis, HIV infection and,
289–290
Tumors
bone marrow transplantation
for, 415–460
effect on albumin binding of
drugs, 10
Twentieth century disease, 347. *See
also* Environmental illness
Two-compartment model, 13

Uremia. *See* Renal disease
Urethral syndrome, 387–388
Urinary retention, tricyclic
antidepressant–induced, 281

Valproate, 79, 125–130
benefits of, 129
drug interactions with,
127–130

carbamazepine, 48–49, 117,
127, 129–130
clozapine, 108
felbamate, 118
fluoxetine, **88**
lorazepam, 127, 129
paroxetine, **88**
tricyclic antidepressants,
105–106, 339
effects on coagulation, 126–127
formulations of, **8, 25**
for head-injured patient, **333,**
338–339
for HIV-related mania, 283
indications for, 125
metabolism of, **9**
protein binding of, 10–12
rapid loading of, 129
side effects of, 125–126, 128–129,
338
use in gastrointestinal disease,
25–26
use in liver disease, 48–49, 126,
128
use in systemic lupus
erythematosus, 208
volume of distribution of, 13
withdrawal from, 119
Vasodilators, 27
Venlafaxine, 79, 93–95
active metabolite of, 93
dosage of, 93
dosing schedule for, 94
drug interactions with, 95
formulations of, **8**
half-life of, 93–95
for head-injured persons, 337
for HIV-infected persons, 281
metabolism by cytochrome
P_{450}-2D6, 95
protein binding of, 10, 93
side effects of, 93–94, 281
use in cardiac disease, 95
use in liver disease, 94

Venlafaxine (continued)
  use in renal disease, 94–95
Verapamil
  interaction with carbamazepine,
    123
  interaction with imipramine,
    105
Videx. See Didanosine
Vietnam veterans, cognitive
  impairment in, 317–318
Vinblastine, 83
Viral infections
  chronic fatigue syndrome and,
    230–232
  vulvar, 394, 395–396
Visual blurring,
  nefazodone-induced, 96
Visual hallucinosis,
  antiparkinsonian
  drug–induced, 151, 159–160
Vitamin supplementation, for
  environmental illness, 354
Volume of distribution, 5, 12–14
  disease effects on, 18
  half-life and, 17, 34
von Willebrand's factor, valproate
  effects on, 127
VP-16. See Etoposide
Vulvodynia, 381–411
  areas of future research on, 411
  chronicity of, 382–383
  clinical features of, 382–383
  complexity of, 383–384
  definition of, 382
  differential diagnosis of,
    387–396, 401
  cutaneous disorders, 390–396,
    392–394
  candidiasis, 391, 395
  dermatoses, 390–391
  herpes simplex virus, 395
  herpes zoster, 395
  human papillomavirus
    infection, 396

  molluscum contagiosum,
    396
  staphylococcal
    furunculosis, 396
  streptococcal cellulitis, 396
  endogenous dysesthesias,
    389–390, 402
  interstitial cystitis and urethral
    syndrome, 387–388
  itching and burning, 388
  iatrogenic factors in, 397–398
  alcohol injections, 397–398
  CO_2 laser, 397
  side effects of topical steroids,
    397
  itching in, 381–382, 388, 398–399
  management of, 405–406, 409–411
  by dermatologist, 410
  by gynecologist, 409–410
  psychiatric referral, 405–406, 411
  surgical therapy, 404
  media attention to, 386–387
  patterns of, 400, 401
  cyclic vulvovaginitis, 400–402
  dysesthetic vulvodynia,
    389–390, 402
  vulvar vestibulitis, 403–405
  psychiatric issues related to,
    406–409
  approach to patient, 406–407
  chronic pain, 408
  medication, 408–409
  primary and secondary gains,
    407
  sexual abuse, 407–408
  somatoform disorders, 409
  substance abuse, 409
  psychological aspects of, 384–386
  relationship with vaginismus,
    383

Warfarin
  interaction with carbamazepine,
    124

interaction with selective
  serotonin reuptake
  inhibitors, **87–89,** 90–91
Weakness
  in chronic fatigue syndrome, 221
  nefazodone-induced, 96
Wechsler Adult Intelligence
  Scale—Revised (WAIS-R), 199,
  318, **326**
Wechsler Memory Scale, 318
Weight change
  felbamate-induced, 117
  risperidone-induced, 114
Wisconsin Card Sorting Test, **326**
Wiskott-Aldrich syndrome, 417
"Worried well," 258, 287

Yeast disease, 348, 362

Zalcitabine, 303
Zero-order kinetics, 19–20

Zidovudine
  effect on maternal-to-infant HIV
    transmission, 262
  neuropsychiatric side effects of,
    303
  to reduce progression of
    AIDS-dementia complex,
    286
Zithromax. *See* Azithromycin
Zolpidem, 79, 131–133
  dosage of, 131
  for elderly persons, 131–133
  half-life of, 131
  metabolism of, 131
  respiratory effects of, 131–132
  side effects of, 131–133
  use in liver disease, 131
  use in renal disease, 131
Zovirax. *See* Acyclovir

Cumulative Index for Volumes 1–3

Page numbers printed in **boldface** *refer to tables or figures.*

Abandonment, II:562
Abbreviated Boston Naming Test, **II:420**
Abbreviated Hooper Visual Organization Test, **II:420**
Abbreviated Token Test, **II:420**
Abortion, II:237, II:308
Abscess, epidural, II:339, II:370
Absorption of drugs, III:1–9, **III:4**
  in cardiac disease, III:26
  characteristics of site for, III:2
  factors influencing, III:1–2, **III:4**
  first-pass effect and, III:2
  in gastrointestinal disease, III:2, **III:6,** III:21–22
  lag time for, III:2, **III:4**
  rate of, III:2–3, **III:4**
  related to route of administration, III:2–3, III:22
  in renal disease, III:49
Acebutolol, **III:186**
Acetaminophen, for low-back pain, **II:356,** II:366
Acetazolamide
  administered during SPECT scanning, II:149–150
  effect on cerebral blood flow, II:149
Acetylation, III:15
Acetylcholine
  estrogen effects on, II:239
  in Huntington's disease, II:473
  in Parkinson's disease, II:450
Achondroplastic dwarfism, II:180

α_1-Acid glycoprotein (AAGP)
  binding of drugs, III:10–12, **III:11**
Acne, I:297–298
Acoustic neuroma, I:414–415, II:175
Acquired immunodeficiency syndrome (AIDS), II:309, III:257. *See also* Human immunodeficiency virus infection
  "AIDS belt" of Africa, III:261
  AIDS dementia complex, I:245–246, I:248, I:254–256, III:268–277
  AIDS Education Project, III:258
  AIDS-related complex, II:53
  Centers for Disease Control case definition of, III:259
  chemical AIDS, III:347. *See also* Environmental illness
  early history of, III:259–260
  impact on medical decision making, II:538
  incidence of, III:257
  search for causative agent in, III:260–261
Acrivastine, III:103
Activated partial thromboplastin time (APPT), III:40
Acupuncture, II:49
  cigarette smoking and, I:576
Acyclovir
  for chronic fatigue syndrome, III:239, **III:242**

Acyclovir *(continued)*
    neuropsychiatric side effects of,
        III:304
Adenoma sebaceum, II:175
Adenosine, for supraventricular
        tachycardia, II:205
Adenosine diphosphate, II:216
Adjustment disorders
    associated with HIV infection,
        III:267, **III:270**
    in Huntington's disease patients,
        II:498
    postpartum blues, II:250–252
    secondary to medical illness, II:20
Adoption studies, II:185
Adrenal medullary implants, for
        Parkinson's disease, II:464
Adrenochrome, II:215
Adrenocorticotropic hormone
        (ACTH), for multiple sclerosis,
        II:416, II:436
Adrenoleukodystrophy, II:177
    genetic testing for, II:177
        genetic linkage analysis,
            II:177
        measuring very long chain
            fatty acids, II:177
    phenotypes of, II:177, II:179
Adrenomyeloneuropathy, II:177,
        II:179
Advance medical treatment
        directives, II:537–559
    durable power of attorney for
        health care, II:553–556
    ethical issues related to,
        II:557–559, **II:558**
    legal principles relevant to,
        II:538–541
    competency, II:539–540
    doctrine of consent, II:539
    incompetency, II:540–541
    refusal of consent, II:539
    living will declarations,
        II:552–553

Patient Self-Determination Act,
        II:548–552
    right-to-die cases, II:542–548
Affective disorder, I:514
Age effects
    on prognosis after head injury,
        III:319
    on psychopharmacokinetics, III:1
Age progression and regression,
        under hypnosis, II:42
Agitation, I:379–380
    in critical care setting, II:113
    felbamate-induced, III:118
    parenteral neuroleptics for, II:113
        combined with
            benzodiazepines,
            II:123–125
    postoperative, II:403–404
    preceding ventricular
        arrhythmias, II:217
    risperidone-induced, III:114
Agnosia, in Alzheimer's disease,
        II:173
β-Agonists, for stress-related vagal
        response, II:205
Agranulocytosis, drug-induced,
        III:117
    carbamazepine, III:120–121
    clozapine, III:106–107, III:168
    felbamate, III:117
Akathisia
    buspirone-induced, II:83
    depot neuroleptic–induced, II:120
    fluoxetine-induced, II:74
    intramuscular
        haloperidol–induced, II:118
    selective serotonin reuptake
        inhibitor–induced, III:91,
        III:92
Akinesia, in Parkinson's disease,
        II:448, II:451
Akinetic mutism, I:371
Alanine aminotransferase (ALT),
        III:40

sertraline effects on, II:75
tacrine effects on, II:97,
    III:134–136
Albumin binding of drugs,
    III:10–12, **III:11**
Alcohol injections, vulvar,
    III:397–398
Alcohol use
    cigarette smoking and, I:545
    EEG detection of, I:171
    frontal lobe dysfunction and,
        I:366–367
    among organ transplant
        recipients, I:318–321
    psoriasis and, I:292
Alcohol withdrawal
    bupropion-induced seizures
        during, II:79
    buspirone for symptoms of,
        II:81
Alcoholism
    bupropion use in, II:79–80
    cerebral blood flow studies in,
        II:158–159
    genetics of, II:185
    Huntington's disease and, **II:476,**
        II:479–480
Alcoholism Prognosis Scale,
    I:319–321
Alfentanil, II:394
"Algogens," II:371, **II:373**
Alkaline phosphatase, sertraline
    effects on, II:75
Allergies
    chronic fatigue syndrome and,
        III:233
    environmental illness and,
        III:347, III:350, III:352,
        III:368
Allodynia, III:389
Alopecia, I:296–297, I:299
Alprazolam, I:625
    for bone marrow transplant
        recipient, III:439

buspirone for symptoms of
    withdrawal from, II:80
    formulations of, **III:8**
    half-life of, **III:19**, III:284
    interaction with fluoxetine,
        III:87
    interaction with nefazodone,
        III:97
    metabolism of, **III:9**
        by cytochrome P_{450}-3A4,
            III:36, III:85
    onset of action of, III:3
    for patient with low-back pain,
        II:367
    for premenstrual syndrome,
        II:263
    use in liver disease, III:42
    use in renal disease, **III:54–55**
Altered mental status, I:169–171
Alzheimer's disease, **II:493**
    age at onset of, II:173
    definition of, II:173
    extrapyramidal symptoms of,
        II:448, II:449
    frontal lobe dysfunction and,
        I:351–352
    genetic testing for, II:167,
        II:173–174
        genetic linkage analysis, II:174
        mutations, II:174
    inheritance of, II:173
    neuropathology of, II:173
    olfactory acuity in, I:363
    selegiline for, I:372, II:98
    SPECT evaluation of, II:152–153
        physostigmine activation
            studies, II:153
    tacrine for, II:69, II:94–97,
        III:133–136
    zolpidem for insomnia in, III:133
Amantadine
    for head-injured patient, III:329,
        III:330, III:335
    for Huntington's disease, II:498

Amantadine *(continued)*
    for "nerve fiber fatigue" of
        multiple sclerosis, II:437
    for Parkinson's disease,
        II:454–455, **III:155**, III:156,
        III:162
Amenorrhea, II:265, II:268
    after bone marrow
        transplantation, III:454,
        III:458–459
American Fertility Society (AFS),
    II:309–310
American Society of Clinical
    Hypnosis, II:61
Amiflamine, **III:82**
Amikacin (Amikin), III:304
gamma-Aminobutyric acid (GABA)
    estrogen effects on, II:239
    in Huntington's disease, II:473
p-Aminosalicylate, **III:186**
Aminosalicylic acid, **III:186**
Amitriptyline, I:403
    for fibromyalgia, **III:246–248**
    formulations of, **III:8**
    for head-injured patient, **III:331**
    for Huntington's disease, II:497
    interaction with fluvoxamine,
        III:87
    interaction with valproate,
        III:105–106
    for low-back pain patients, **II:359**
    metabolism of, III:45, **III:85**
        by cytochrome P_{450}-2D6,
            III:36, **III:82**
    for mucous membrane
        dysesthesias, III:389–390
    parenteral, **II:115**, II:125–129
        dosage of, II:128
    side effects of, III:390
    use in liver disease, III:45
    use in renal disease, **III:64–65**
    for vulvodynia, III:408
Amnesia. *See* Memory deficits
Amniocentesis, II:101

Amoxapine
    formulations of, **III:8**
    use in renal disease, **III:54–55**
Amphetamine, I:477, **II:493**
    iodine-123-labeled, II:146–148,
        II:147
    for Parkinson's disease patients,
        II:460
    protein binding of, III:10
Amphotericin B, III:304
Amyloid gene, II:174
Anafranil. *See* Clomipramine
Analgesia, II:46
    hypnotic, II:42, II:46–47, II:49–50
    interview about use of,
        II:343–345
    for low-back pain, **II:356–359**
        acute, II:339
    patient-controlled, III:434
Androgens, II:238–239
    added to estrogen replacement
        therapy, II:275
    conversion to estrogens in brain,
        II:239
    elevated β-endorphins and,
        II:267
    for endometriosis, II:308
    functions of, II:238–239
    libido and, II:239
        in postmenopausal women,
            II:275, II:276
    in polycystic ovarian disease,
        II:265–268
Anesthesia, II:389–404
    awareness during, II:397–399
        causes of, II:397
        complete paralysis with,
            II:398–399
        definition of, II:397
        drugs associated with,
            II:397–398
        posttraumatic stress disorder
            related to, II:398

prevalence of, II:398
psychiatric treatment for
    patients experiencing,
    II:398
total spinal anesthesia and,
    II:398–399
cardiopulmonary monitoring
    during, II:390
drug interactions with,
    II:399–402, **II:401**
cyclic and atypical
    antidepressants,
    II:400–401
lithium, II:402
monoamine oxidase
    inhibitors, I:61, I:109,
    II:399–400
neuropsychiatric effects, II:403
electroconvulsive therapy and,
    I:99–135
historical overview of, II:389–390
hypnosis for, II:42
malpractice claims related to use
    for electroconvulsive
    therapy, II:576–578
neuropsychiatric effects of,
    II:402–403
for outpatient surgery, II:395–397
postoperative agitation and
    delirium, II:403–404
postoperative anxiety, II:392
preanesthetic anxiety, II:390–392
    factors affecting, II:391
    needle and intravenous
        catheter phobia,
        II:390–391
    prevalence of, II:390
    related to general versus
        regional anesthesia,
        II:391
    temporal component of,
        II:391–392
    types of fears, II:390–391
    in women versus men, II:391

prevalence of use of, II:389
purposes of, II:389–390
treatment of anxiety related to,
    II:392–395
audiovisual aids, II:392–393
induction room, II:395
medications, II:393–394
preanesthetic interview,
    II:394–395
wakefulness and, II:397
Anger
associated with cardiac arrest,
    II:220
of medically ill patients, II:16
preceding ventricular
    arrhythmias, II:217
related to infertility, II:310
Angina pectoris, II:70, II:199, II:201
electroconvulsive therapy and,
    I:128–129
during sexual activity, II:229
tacrine use in, II:97
Angiotensin-converting enzyme, in
    Huntington's disease, II:473
Angiotensin-converting enzyme
    inhibitors, interaction with
    lithium, III:113
"Animal magnetism," II:40
Anorexia
after bone marrow
    transplantation, III:434
venlafaxine-induced, III:93
Anorgasmia, fluoxetine-induced,
    II:74
Anosognosia, II:418
Antacids, drug interactions with,
    III:21
Anthropological studies of sudden
    death, II:227–229
Antiarrhythmics
metabolism by cytochrome
    P450-2D6, **III:83**
use after myocardial infarction,
    III:97–98

Antibiotics
    for bone marrow transplant
        recipient, III:431
    environmental illness and, III:351
    interactions with valproate,
        III:130
Antibodies
    anticardiolipin, **III:198,**
        III:204–205
    antineuronal, **III:198,** III:203–206
    antinuclear, III:184, **III:187,**
        III:188, III:193, III:195,
        III:197
    antiphospholipid, III:204–206
    antiribosomal P protein, **III:198,**
        III:203–206
    to HIV, III:263
    in systemic lupus
        erythematosus, III:184,
        III:187, III:188, III:195,
        III:197, III:198, III:202–206
Antibody-capture enzyme
    immunoassay test, I:269–270
Anticholinergic agents, I:444
    drug interactions with, **II:401**
    effect on drug absorption, III:2
    for Parkinson's disease,
        II:454–455, II:462, **III:155,**
        III:156, III:161
    for premedication, II:396
    psychotoxicity of, III:161
    use in Huntington's disease,
        II:493, II:498
Anticipatory excitement, preceding
    ventricular arrhythmias, II:217
Anticoagulant malingering,
    I:231–232
Anticonvulsants. *See* Antiepileptic
    drugs
Antidepressants, II:46. *See also*
    specific drugs
    for bone marrow transplant
        recipient, III:439–440
    buspirone, II:81

for chronic fatigue syndrome,
    III:241
for cigarette cessation treatment,
    I:570–572
for depressed multiple sclerosis
    patients, II:434
for fibromyalgia, III:241,
    III:246–248
formulations of, **III:8**
for head-injured patient,
    III:331–333, III:335–337
for HIV-infected persons,
    III:280–282
for Huntington's disease, **II:496,**
    II:497
interaction with anesthetics,
    II:400–401, **II:401**
metabolism of, **III:9,** III:14
for migraine headache, I:402–403
for mucous membrane
    dysesthesias, III:389–390
for persons with environmental
    illness, III:372
for persons with mental
    retardation, I:522–523
pregnancy and, I:624
for premenstrual syndrome,
    II:264
for pruritus ani, III:399
second-generation, II:69–80
    bupropion, II:77–80
    fluoxetine, II:69–74
    paroxetine, II:76
    selective serotonin reuptake
        inhibitors, II:76–77
    sertraline, II:74–75
side effects of, I:300–302
use in gastrointestinal disease,
    III:23–24
use in renal disease, III:53,
    III:54–55, III:66
use in systemic lupus
    erythematosus, III:207,
    III:208

for vulvodynia, III:408–409
for woman undergoing
        infertility treatment, II:324
Antidepressants, tricyclic (TCAs),
        I:30–38, III:79. *See also* specific
        drugs
analgesic properties of, I:466
for anxiety disorders in
        Parkinson's disease
        patients, II:460
for children, I:464–467,
        III:100–101, **III:102**
for chronic low-back pain, **II:359,**
        II:366, II:378
contraindications to, I:468
for depression, I:335
dialyzability of, III:53
drug interactions with
    carbamazepine, III:45, III:124,
            III:339
    cholestyramine, III:105
    enflurane, II:400–401, **II:401**
    felbamate, III:118
    fluoxetine, II:71
    sertraline, II:75, **III:89**
    valproate, III:105–106, III:339
electroconvulsive therapy and,
        I:111–112
for head-injured patient, **III:331,**
        III:335–336
high-fiber diet and, III:105
for HIV-infected persons, I:255,
        III:281–282
mechanism of action of, II:126
metabolism of, III:44–45
    by cytochrome P_{450}-2D6, **III:82**
methylphenidate as adjunct to,
        II:129
parenteral, II:125–129, III:281
    advantages of, II:125
    dosage of, II:128
    effect on downregulation of
            β-adrenergic receptors,
            II:125, II:126
effect on pharmacological
        action, II:125–126
guidelines for administration
        of, **II:115**
indications for, II:125
preparations of, II:128
recommendations for use of,
        II:127–128
side effects of, II:127
pharmacology in medical
        patients, III:97–101
pregnancy and, I:625
protein binding of, III:10
rectal administration of,
        III:104–105
side effects of, I:30, I:38, I:255,
        I:467–469, III:281
    cardiac effects, III:97–101
    seizures, II:78, II:79
    sudden death in children,
            III:100–101, **III:102**
    syndrome of inappropriate
            antidiuretic hormone
            secretion, II:74
use in cardiac disease, II:214,
        III:30–31, III:97–99
use in gastrointestinal disease,
        III:23–24
use in liver disease, III:39, III:41,
        III:44–45
use in renal disease, III:53,
        III:62–65, III:66
withdrawal from, I:470
Antiepileptic drugs, I:71–81, II:69,
        II:493, III:116–130. *See also*
        specific drugs
breast-feeding and, II:101
carbamazepine, III:120–125
effect on folate metabolism, II:100
felbamate, III:116–119
fluoxetine interaction with, II:73
gabapentin, III:119–120
for head-injured patient, **III:333,**
        III:337–339

Antiepileptic drugs *(continued)*
  for HIV-related mania, III:283
  for persons with mental
    retardation, I:524
  prophylactic, for patient taking
    bupropion, II:79
  teratogenicity of, II:98–101
  use during breast-feeding,
    II:101
  use in pregnancy, II:98–101
  valproate, III:125–130
  for vulvodynia, III:408
  withdrawal from, III:119
Antihypertensive agents, **III:82**
Antinuclear antibodies (ANA)
  conditions associated with,
    III:197
  screening for, III:193
  in systemic lupus
    erythematosus, III:184,
    III:187, III:188, III:195,
    III:197
Antiparkinsonian drugs,
    III:153–156, **III:154–155**
  differential psychotoxicity of,
    III:161–162
  "drug holidays" from, III:163
  psychosis induced by, III:151,
    III:156–176
    differential diagnosis of,
      III:156–158
    epidemiology of, III:158
    phenomenology of, III:158–160
    treatment of, III:162–176
Antipsychotics. *See* Neuroleptics
Antithymocyte globulin, III:415
Anxiety
  associated with HIV infection,
    III:267–268, **III:269–270**
  in bone marrow transplant
    recipient, III:431–432,
    III:439–440
  in children and adolescents, I:461
  chronic low-back pain and, II:367

environmental illness and,
    III:356, **III:358–361**
  gabapentin-induced, III:120
  generalized anxiety disorder in
    women, II:237
  in Huntington's disease, II:476
  hypnosis for, II:43
  organ transplant recipients,
    I:324–325, I:327
  in Parkinson's disease, II:459,
    II:460
  in persons with mental
    retardation, I:515–516
  postconcussional, III:315
  postoperative, II:392
  postpartum depression and, II:254
  preanesthetic, II:390–392
  pregnancy and, I:616–617,
    I:624–626
  related to protected isolation
    environment, III:443
  risperidone-induced, III:114
  in systemic lupus
    erythematosus, III:192,
    III:207
  treatment of, I:336–337
Anxiolytics
  benzodiazepines, II:84–90
  for bone marrow transplant
    recipient, III:424,
    III:438–439
  buspirone, I:52, II:80–84
  formulations of, **III:8**
  for HIV-infected persons, III:284
  for postoperative anxiety, II:392
  preanesthetic, II:391, II:393–394
  for premenstrual syndrome,
    II:263–264
  use in gastrointestinal disease,
    III:22
  use in liver disease, III:42–43
  use in renal disease, III:52–53,
    III:54–59

Aortic aneurysm, I:107–108,
  I:131
Apathy, in Huntington's disease,
  II:478–479
Aphasia
  in Alzheimer's disease, II:173
  competency determination for
    patient with, II:529–533
Aphthosis, vulvar, **III:392**
Aplastic anemia, bone marrow
  transplantation for, III:415–460
Apoplexy, II:199
Apraxia, in Alzheimer's disease,
  II:173
Arachnoiditis, II:370
Arm levitation, II:43–44
Arrhythmias. *See also* Sudden
  cardiac death
  atrial, II:205–207
    placebo effect on, II:206–207
    role of fatigue and sleep
      deprivation in, II:206
    stress-related, II:200, II:201,
      II:205–206
    triggers for, II:205, II:206
  bupropion effect on, II:78
  clozapine-induced tachycardia,
    III:107
  desipramine-related, in children,
    III:100–101
  effect of reassurance on, II:225
  fluoxetine and, II:70
  induced by diving, II:212
  mesoridazine-induced, II:118
  role of catecholamines in,
    II:215–216
  sexual activity and, II:229–230
  sotalol for, III:104
  terfenadine-induced, III:102–103
  ventricular, II:213–230
    evoked reflex activity and,
      II:213
    learned voluntary control of,
      II:225

provoked during
  psychological stress
  testing, II:218–220, **II:219**
during sexual activity,
  II:229–230
stress-related, II:214–218
sympathetic withdrawal and,
  II:224–227
circadian variation,
  arrhythmias, and
  death, II:225–227
effects of sleep and
  meditation,
  II:224–225, **II:226**
Artane. *See* Trihexyphenidyl
Arthralgias, in chronic fatigue
  syndrome, III:221
Artificial insemination with donor
  sperm (AID), II:309–310
  donor's anonymity for, II:312,
    II:318
  motivations for, II:311
  number of babies born by, II:309
  psychiatric evaluation before,
    II:321, II:322
  religious prohibitions against,
    II:311
  selection and screening of
    donors for, II:309–310
  for single women, II:312–313
Ascites, III:35
"Ash leaf patches," II:175
Aspartate aminotransferase (AST),
  III:40
  sertraline effects on, II:75
Aspirin
  interaction with valproate, I:79,
    III:130
  for low-back pain, **II:357**
Assertion training, II:361
Astemizole
  interaction with nefazodone,
    III:97
  metabolism of, **III:85**

Asthma, hypnotic desensitization
    for, II:53–54
Astrocytoma, II:579
Asystole, II:211, II:212, II:216
Ataxia
    cerebellar, **II:493**
    drug-induced
        flurazepam, II:87
        gabapentin, III:120
        quazepam, II:87
        triazolam, II:89
        zolpidem, III:133
Atenolol, **III:186**
    interaction with fluvoxamine,
        III:87
    interaction with sertraline, II:75,
        III:89
    to prevent ventricular fibrillation
        after myocardial
        infarction, II:216
Ativan. *See* Lorazepam
Atovaquone, III:303
Atrial fibrillation
    fluoxetine and, II:70
    stress-related, II:205–206
    triggers for, II:206
Atrial flutter
    fluoxetine and, II:70
    stress-related, II:205–206
Atrial premature beats,
    stress-related, II:205
Atrioventricular block
    fluoxetine and, II:70
    transient stress-related, II:204
Atropine, II:205
Attention
    HIV-associated deficits in, III:269
    postconcussional deficits in,
        III:315
    testing for, III:324, **III:326**
    tacrine-induced improvements
        in, III:134–135
Attention-deficit hyperactivity
    disorder (ADHD), I:352, II:185

head injury and, I:365–366,
    III:319, III:322
    treatment of, I:373–374, I:475–476
Audiovisual aids, to relieve
    preanesthetic anxiety,
    II:392–393
Auditory As, **II:420**
Auditory Trials A, **II:420**
Autism
    buspirone for, I:52
    due to fragile X syndrome,
        II:175–176
    genetics of, II:185
Autoerythrocyte sensitization,
    I:230–231
Autonomy
    beneficence and, II:587–588
    effect of manifest and latent
        content on, II:591–599
    refusal of treatment and,
        II:599–600
    respect for, II:587
    truth telling and, II:590–591
Azathioprine, II:417
Azithromycin, III:304
Azoospermia, II:306, II:309
AZT. *See* Zidovudine

Babinski reflex, II:346
Baclofen
    for Huntington's disease, II:495
    for muscle spasm, II:371
Bactrim. *See* Trimethoprim/
    sulfamethoxazole
Barbiturates
    drug interactions with, **II:401**
        paroxetine, II:76
    electroconvulsive therapy and,
        I:118–121
    electroencephalographic
        detection of, I:171
    overdose of, II:121
    protein binding of, III:10
    use in renal disease, **III:54–55**

Basal body temperature (BBT)
chart, **II:305,** II:305–306
Basal ganglia
infarction of, **II:493**
tumor of, **II:493**
Battery, II:562
case study of claim of,
II:569–570, II:572
defenses to charge of, II:562
definition of, II:562
restraint of patient as, II:562,
II:569–570, II:572
"Battle fatigue," II:41
Beck Depression Inventory (BDI),
II:376
for multiple sclerosis patients,
II:431, II:433, II:435
for Parkinson's disease patients,
II:458
Behavior
of children and adolescents,
I:492–493
frontal lobe dysfunction and,
I:355–357, I:375–376
of persons with mental
retardation, I:513–514
Behavior modification
for environmental illness,
III:371–372
for smoking cessation, I:572–577
Behçet's syndrome, **III:392**
Belief systems, I:493–494, I:602
Bender-Gestalt Visual Motor
Retention Test, II:218, III:199
Beneficence, II:587–588, II:598–599
autonomy and, II:587–588
paternalism and, II:588
Benzamide, labeled with iodine-123
(IBZM), II:158, II:159
Benzodiazepine receptor
antagonist, II:69, II:90. *See also*
Flumazenil
Benzodiazepine receptors, in
Huntington's disease, II:473

Benzodiazepine withdrawal
bupropion-induced seizures
during, II:79
buspirone for symptoms of, II:80
flumazenil-induced, II:92, II:93
triazolam-induced, II:89
Benzodiazepines. *See also* specific
drugs
absorption of, III:3
achieving steady state of, III:17
active metabolites of, II:122,
III:18, **III:19,** III:52
for anxiety in Parkinson's
disease, II:460
buspirone compared with, II:80
for children and adolescents,
I:461–464
clinical effects of, II:120–121
drug interactions with
barbiturates, **II:401**
paroxetine, II:76
sertraline, II:75
electroconvulsive therapy and,
I:121
electroencephalography and,
I:171–172
flumazenil for overdose of,
II:91–93
formulations of, **III:8**
half-lives of, II:121–122, III:18,
III:19, III:284
for head-injured patient, I:370,
III:334, III:339
for HIV-infected persons, III:284
for Huntington's disease, **II:496**
hypnotics, II:84–90
estazolam, II:85–86
quazepam, II:86–88
selection for medically ill
patients, II:89–90
triazolam, II:88–89
measuring serum concentrations
of, II:121–122, III:52
metabolism of, **III:9,** III:14–15

Benzodiazepines *(continued)*
    for muscle spasm, II:371–372
    parenteral, II:120–123
        absorption of, II:121–122
        blood levels of, II:121
        combined with neuroleptics,
            II:123–125
        distribution of, II:121–122
        elimination half-life of,
            II:121–122
        guidelines for administration
            of, **II:114–115**
        intramuscular, II:123, III:3
        intravenous, II:123
        metabolism of, II:122–123
        use in elderly patients and
            children, II:125
        use in respiratory disease,
            II:124
    for persons with mental
        retardation, I:525
    for postanesthesia emergence
        reactions, II:403
    for preanesthetic anxiety, II:391,
        II:393
    pregnancy and, I:625
    for premenstrual syndrome,
        II:263, II:264
    protein binding of, III:10, III:42
    side effects of, I:370, I:463–464
        delirium, I:169–170
    therapeutic index for, II:121
    use in cardiac disease, III:27
    use in elderly patients, II:122
    use in gastrointestinal disease,
        III:22
    use in liver disease, II:122,
        III:42–43
    use in renal disease, III:52,
        III:54–59
Benztropine
    for Parkinson's disease, II:455
    use in liver disease, III:44
"Best interest" standard, II:543

Betapace. *See* Sotalol
Biaxin. *See* Clarithromycin
Bilirubin, III:40
Bioavailability of drugs, **III:5,** III:9,
    III:39
    in liver disease, III:32–33, III:39
Biofeedback, for low-back pain,
    II:360
Biogenic amine hypothesis of
    depression, II:240
Biomechanical assessment, II:347
Biopsychosocial model, II:332–335,
    II:333, II:336
Bipolar disorder
    carbamazepine for, III:120
    duty to treat patient with,
        II:603–604
    endometriosis and, II:269
    genetic linkage studies of,
        II:187–188
    in Huntington's disease, **II:476,**
        II:477–478
    mental retardation and, I:514
    in multiple sclerosis, II:435–436
        clinical reports of, **II:430–433**
        drug-related, II:436
        prevalence of, II:435
        treatment of, II:436
    phenotypes of, II:179, II:180
    pregnancy and, I:616, I:620–623
    valproate for, III:125
Birth control pills. *See* Oral
    contraceptives
Bleeding tendencies
    fluoxetine-induced, II:73,
        III:90
    valproate-induced, III:126–127
Blockade therapy, I:571–572
α-Blockers, for chronic pain, II:371
β-Blockers
    for head-injured patient, I:372,
        III:334
    for long Q-T syndrome, II:214
    lupus induced by, **III:186**

metabolized by cytochrome
P$_{450}$-2D6, **III:82**
for migraine headache, I:402,
I:405
for persons with mental
retardation, I:525–526
to prevent stress-related
ventricular arrhythmias,
II:215–216
for supraventricular tachycardia,
II:205
timing for administration of,
II:227
Blood pressure. *See also*
Hypertension
morning surge in, II:227
during sexual activity, II:229
stress-related elevation of, II:202
Blues, postpartum ("maternity
blues," "baby blues"),
II:250–252. *See also* Postpartum
depressions
Body temperature. *See also* Fever
alterations in chronic fatigue
syndrome, III:221
basal body temperature chart,
II:305, II:305–306
Bone marrow transplantation
(BMT), III:415–460
allogeneic, III:417–418
for aplastic anemia, III:418
for chronic myelogenous
leukemia, III:418
human lymphocyte antigen
histocompatibility
testing for, III:417
autologous, III:417–419
biological setting for, III:416–420
centers performing, III:420
convalescent period after,
III:431–432, III:451
cost of, III:420–421
data on incidence of, III:420
donors for, III:417, III:445–447

anonymous, III:446–447
children as, III:429, III:430
guilt felt by, III:423
harvesting marrow from,
III:431, III:446
long-term psychological
effects in, III:446
psychological preparation of,
III:445
registries of, III:421
search for, III:423
selection of, III:445
ethical and legal issues related
to, III:428–430
family concerns about,
III:424–426, III:447–448
future research related to, III:460
goals of, III:419
guide for decision making about,
III:419–420
history of, III:416–417
hospitalization for, III:417,
III:430–432
protected and germ-free
environments, III:417,
III:443–445
indications for, III:416–417
informed consent for, III:426–428
Karnofksy score after, III:452
pain management after, III:434
patient refusal of, III:430
patient selection for, III:419
posthospitalization support
after, III:432–433
procedure for, III:417, III:431
psychiatric liaison services for
staff on unit for, III:448–451
psychological and psychosocial
assessment for, III:423–426
psychological complications of,
III:438–443
antidepressants for, III:439–440
anxiety, delirium, and
depression, III:438–439

Bone marrow transplantation
  (BMT) *(continued)*
  psychological complications of
    clinical issues related to, III:441
    psychiatric illness, III:442–443
    psychological themes and
      conflicts, III:441–442
    risk factors for, III:440
  psychosexual adjustment after,
    III:453–460
    chemotherapy-induced
      gonadal dysfunction,
      III:453–455
    hormone-replacement
      therapy, III:456
    pregnancy, III:457
    problems in men, III:459–460
    radiotherapy-induced
      gonadal dysfunction,
      III:454–456
    sperm banking, III:456–457
    studies of, III:457–459
    in vitro fertilization, III:457
  routes of medication
    administration after,
    III:433, III:437
  side effects and complications of,
    III:418, III:431, III:433–438
    chemotherapy-related,
      III:434–435
    general systemic transient
      side effects, III:434
    graft-versus-host disease,
      III:416–419, III:431–432,
      III:437–438
    immediate toxic
      complications,
      III:433–434
    late physical sequelae,
      III:451–453
    related to Broviac or Hickman
      catheterization and total
      parenteral nutrition,
      III:436–437
    total-body irradiation–related,
      III:435–436, III:454
  stages of, III:416, III:421–423,
    III:422, III:430–432
  survival after, III:418, III:419,
    III:451–452
    regimen-related toxicity scale
      for prediction of, III:451
  syngeneic, III:417
  third-party reimbursement for,
    III:420
Bone scanning, spinal, II:347
Bradycardia
  fluoxetine-induced, II:70
  sertraline-induced, II:75
  stress-related, II:204–205
Bradykinesia
  in Huntington's disease, II:475,
    II:486, II:487
  in Parkinson's disease, II:448
Brain, estrogen and progesterone
  receptors in, II:238
Brain electrical activity mapping
  (BEAM), I:21–22, I:180,
  II:492
Brain imaging, I:3–24
  in AIDS dementia complex,
    III:276
  for head-injured patient,
    III:311–313, **III:321,**
    III:325–328
  in HIV infection, I:253–254
  interpretation of, I:14–15
  in systemic lupus
    erythematosus, **III:198,**
    III:199–202
Brain implants, for Parkinson's
  disease, II:463–464
Brain injury. *See* Head injury
Brain tumors, II:579
  bone marrow transplantation
    for, III:419
  electroconvulsive therapy and,
    I:104–105

Breast cancer
  bone marrow transplantation
      for, III:417, III:419
  estrogen replacement therapy
      and, II:274
  oral contraceptives and, II:245
Breast-feeding, I:626–627
  antiepileptic drug use during,
      II:101
  oral contraceptive use during,
      II:244
  postpartum blues and, II:251
  psychotropic drug use during,
      II:249, II:254
Bretylium, for long Q-T syndrome,
      II:214
Brief Psychiatric Rating Scale
      (BPRS), II:81, III:159, III:166–167
Brief psychodynamically informed
      therapy, II:3–33
  central principles in, II:9, **II:10,**
      II:33
  cost efficiency of, II:8
  decreased use of medical
      services related to, II:8
  done "by design" rather than
      "by default," II:9
  effectiveness of, II:7–8, II:33
  focus of, II:12
  for medically ill patients, II:14–33
      attention to narcissistic injury,
          II:16
      clinical issues, II:14–17
      effectiveness, II:17–18
      focus on denial, II:16
      short-term dynamic therapy
          of stress response
          syndromes, II:27–33
      time-limited dynamic
          psychotherapy, II:18–27
      what it means to be ill, II:16
  most patients receiving, II:7–8
  number and duration of sessions
      for, II:10–11

  patient selection for, II:12–14,
      II:13
      exclusion criteria, **II:13,** II:14
  for psychiatric reactions to
      illness or trauma, II:14–15
  psychodynamic
      improvement-attendance
      relationship, **II:7,** II:7–8
  social and economic factors
      favoring, II:9
  training in, II:9
  variety of techniques for, II:6
  viewpoint for, II:3–6
Briquet's syndrome, II:266
Bromocriptine, I:443
  effect on occurrence of hot
      flushes, II:271
  for ovulation induction, II:307
  for Parkinson's disease,
      II:453–454, II:462, III:153,
      III:154
  for polycystic ovarian disease,
      II:266, II:268
Bromperidol, use in renal disease,
      III:58–59
Bronchodilators, II:54
Bronchospasm, hypnosis for,
      II:53–54
Brotizolam, use in renal disease,
      III:54–55
Broviac catheter–related problems,
      III:436–437
Brucellosis, chronic, III:217, III:348.
      See also Chronic fatigue
      syndrome
Bufarolol, **III:82**
Bullous dermatoses, vulvar, **III:392**
Bupropion, II:77–80
  cardiovascular effects of,
      II:77–78, III:30–31
      compared with imipramine,
          II:78
      in hypertensive patients, II:78
      safety, II:78

Bupropion *(continued)*
  for chronic fatigue syndrome,
    III:241, **III:244**
  contraindicated for psychotic
    patients, II:77
  drug interactions with
    anesthetics, II:400
    enflurane, **II:401**
    fluoxetine, II:72
  formulations of, **III:8**
  half-life of, II:77
  for head-injured patient, **III:333,**
    III:337
  for HIV-infected persons, III:282
  for Parkinson's disease patients,
    II:460
  seizures due to, II:69, II:78–80
    in alcoholic patients, II:79–80
    anticonvulsant prophylaxis
      for, II:79
    dosage and, II:79
    prevalence of, II:78–79
    risk factors for, II:79
  side effects of, I:47–50
  use in cardiac disease, III:30–31
  use in renal disease, **III:54–55**
Burns, effect on albumin binding of
  drugs, III:10
Buserelin, for premenstrual
  syndrome, II:264
Buspirone (BuSpar), I:50–53, I:571,
  II:69, II:80–84
  cognitive effects of, II:82–83
  compared with benzodiazepines,
    II:80
  effect on sleep, II:82
  emerging indications for,
    II:80–81
    aggression and anxiety
      reduction in mental
      retardation and organic
      mental disorders, II:81
    alcohol withdrawal, II:81
    antidepressant, II:81

  benzodiazepine withdrawal,
    II:80
  obsessive-compulsive
    disorder, II:81
  schizophrenia, II:81
  smoking cessation, II:80–81
extrapyramidal effects of,
  II:83–84
formulations of, **III:8**
for head-injured patient, **III:334,**
  III:339–340
for HIV-infected persons, III:282,
  III:284
metabolism of, **III:9**
neuroendocrine effects of, II:83
pharmacokinetics of, II:84
for premenstrual syndrome,
  II:263
respiratory effects of, II:82
use in liver disease, III:43
use in medically ill patients,
  II:82–84
use in renal disease, III:53,
  III:58–59
variation in steady state blood
  levels of, II:84
Buspirone-prolactin test, II:83
Busulfan, before bone marrow
  transplantation, III:430
"But for" rule, II:566
Butterfly rash, III:183, III:184
Butyrophenones, for Huntington's
  disease, II:494–495

Café-au-lait spots, II:175
Caffeine
  effect on cerebral blood flow,
    II:148
  premenstrual syndrome and,
    II:262
Calcium, II:275
Calcium channel antagonist
  receptors, in Huntington's
  disease, II:473

Calcium channel blockers
  for AIDS dementia complex,
    III:275–276
  interaction with imipramine,
    III:105
  interaction with lithium,
    III:112–113
California Verbal Learning Test,
  II:420
L-Canavanine, **III:186**
Cancer
  associated with estrogens, II:245
  bone marrow transplantation
    for, III:415–460
  dextroamphetamine use in,
    III:113
  hypnosis to mitigate side effects
    of chemotherapy for,
    II:55–56
  hypnotic analgesia for pain of,
    II:49
  use of visualization in, II:55–56
Candidate genes, II:187
Candidiasis
  chronic, III:217. *See also* Chronic
    fatigue syndrome
  sensitivity to, III:347–348, III:351,
    III:354. *See also*
    Environmental illness
  vulvar, III:391, **III:394**, III:395
    treatment of, III:400, III:402
    vulvodynia and, III:383–384,
    III:400
Capastat. *See* Capreomycin
Capreomycin, III:304
Captopril, **III:186**
Carbamazepine, **II:493,** III:79,
  III:120–125
  for bipolar disorder, III:120
  dosage, I:75–76
  drug interactions with,
    III:123–124
    felbamate, III:117–118
    fluoxetine, II:72, **III:87**

    fluvoxamine, **III:87**
    oral contraceptives, II:99
    paroxetine, **III:88**
    selective serotonin reuptake
      inhibitors, III:336, III:339
    tricyclic antidepressants,
      III:45, III:124, III:339
    valproate, III:48–49, III:117,
      III:127, III:129–130
  environmental effects on
    stability of, III:125
  formulations of, **III:8**, III:25
  generic preparations of, III:124
  for head-injured patient, I:372,
    III:333, III:338–339
  for HIV-related mania, III:283
  metabolism of, **III:9**
  for multiple sclerosis patients,
    II:436
  overdose of, III:122–123
  for persons with mental
    retardation, I:524
  in pregnancy, III:123
    neural tube defects related to,
      II:99, II:100
  prophylactic, for patient taking
    bupropion, II:79
  rectal administration of,
    III:104–105
  for refractory depression, III:120
  reintroduction after
    discontinuation of, III:124
  side effects of, I:71–76,
    III:120–122, III:338
    lupus, III:122, **III:186**
  switching between preparations
    of, III:124–125
  for symptoms of benzodiazepine
    withdrawal, II:80
  therapeutic index for, III:124
  use in gastrointestinal disease,
    III:25
  use in liver disease, III:33,
    III:47–48

Carbamazepine *(continued)*
    for vulvodynia, III:408
    withdrawal from, III:119
Carbohydrates, premenstrual
    craving for, II:262
Carbon dioxide laser therapy,
    vulvar, III:397
Cardiac Arrhythmia Suppression
    Trials (CASTs), III:97–99
Cardiac catheterization, III:99
Cardiac disease, III:26–32. *See also*
    Arrhythmias; Sudden cardiac
    death
    arrhythmias provoked during
        psychological stress
        testing in patients with,
        II:218–220, **II:219**
    clinical cardiac syndromes, II:201
    guidelines for drug dosing in,
        III:28–30
    methylphenidate use in, II:129
    pharmacokinetic effects of,
        III:26–28
        absorption, III:26
        distribution, III:26–27
        excretion, III:27–28
        metabolism, III:27
    use of antidepressants in,
        III:30–31
        fluoxetine, II:70
        selective serotonin reuptake
            inhibitors, III:92–93
        tricyclics, III:97–99
        venlafaxine, III:95
    use of antipsychotics in, III:31
    use of lithium in, III:31–32, III:112
Cardiac effects
    of anesthesia, I:122
    of bupropion, I:48–49
    of carbamazepine, I:73–79
    of cyclophosphamide, III:434
    of electroconvulsive therapy,
        I:100–102, I:106–107,
        I:128–133

    of imipramine, III:96
    of intravenous haloperidol,
        III:103–104
    of Lyme disease, I:271
    of nefazodone, III:96
    of selective serotonin reuptake
        inhibitors, III:80, III:92–93
    of stimulants, III:113–114
    of terfenadine, III:86
    of tricyclic antidepressants,
        I:35–36, III:97–101
        for chest pain, III:99–100
        sudden death in children,
            III:100–101
    of venlafaxine, III:95
Cardiac innervation, II:212–213
Cardiomyopathy, catecholamine,
    II:215
Cardiovascular responses to stress,
    II:202–207, **II:203**
    type I response, II:202, II:204
    type II response, II:204–207
        adrenergic, II:205–207
        vagal, II:204–205
    type III response, II:207
Carmustine, before bone marrow
    transplantation, III:430
Cataracts, in bone marrow
    transplant recipient, III:435,
    III:451
Catatonia, I:434–435
    in systemic lupus
        erythematosus, III:193
Catecholamines
    effect of increased levels on
        pregnancy outcome, II:246
    estrogen effects on, II:239
    morning surge in, II:227
    in polycystic ovarian disease,
        II:266, II:267
    role in arrhythmias, II:215–216
Cauda equina syndrome, II:339
Causalgia, III:389
Causation, II:566

in cases of missed diagnosis,
II:579–580
in fact (direct), II:566
"but for" rule and, II:566
legal (proximate), II:566
CD3 cells, III:260
CD4 cells, II:411, III:259–262
CD8 cells, II:411, III:260
Celiac disease, III:2, III:10
Center for Epidemiologic
Studies—Depression Scale
(CES-D), II:241, II:253, II:381,
III:278
Central nervous system diseases,
I:243–277
Cerebral blood flow (CBF), I:14–16
acetazolamide effects on, II:149
age effects on, II:148
in alcoholism and substance
abuse, II:158–159
in Alzheimer's disease,
II:152–153
caffeine effects on, II:148
in CNS lupus, II:154
in congestive heart failure, III:29
in dementia, II:152–153
in depression, II:157–158
effect of mental activity on,
II:149
in epilepsy, II:156
in HIV infection, II:155
psychotropic drug effects on,
II:148
in schizophrenia, I:14, II:149,
II:158
SPECT imaging of, II:141–160.
See also Single
photon-emission
computed tomography
in stroke, II:151
in systemic lupus
erythematosus, III:201–202
in women versus men, II:148–149
Cerebral palsy, I:352

Cerebrospinal fluid (CSF) analysis,
I:263–265, I:268–271
in AIDS dementia complex,
III:276
to diagnose multiple sclerosis,
II:414, **II:414**
Cerebrovascular problems and
electroconvulsive therapy,
I:102–103, I:105–106, I:127
Charcot-Marie-Tooth disease, II:180
Cheese reaction, II:400
"Chemical sensitivity" syndromes,
III:347–378. *See also*
Environmental illness
Chemotherapy
before bone marrow
transplantation, III:417,
III:430, III:434–435
gonadal dysfunction due to,
III:453–455
Chest pain, imipramine for,
III:99–100
Children
as bone marrow donors, III:429,
III:430
conceived through technology,
II:311–312, II:317
developmental stages in,
I:491–492
with disabilities, I:606
eczema in, I:292–293
effect of mother's postpartum
depression on, II:247
family therapy for, I:483–503
in female-headed families,
II:313
headaches in, I:420–421
hemophilia in, I:199–200
of homosexual women, II:313
hypnotic analgesia for, II:49
hypnotizability of, II:43
legal issues related to, I:458–459
medical disorder characteristics
of, I:490

Children *(continued)*
  parenteral benzodiazepine use
    in, II:125
  psychotropic drugs for, I:456–478
  sickle cell disease in, I:204–206
  social relationships of, I:487
  stress-related ventricular
    arrhythmias in, II:214
  tricyclic antidepressants for,
    I:464–467
    guidelines for monitoring
      cardiac toxicity, **III:102**
    sudden death and, III:100–101
Chimera, III:415
Chloral hydrate, use in renal
  disease, **III:58–59**
Chlordiazepoxide
  achieving steady state of, III:17
  clearance of, III:17
  formulations of, **III:8**
  half-life of, III:17, **III:19**
  intramuscular, II:121
  metabolism of, II:122, **III:9**
  metabolites of, III:18
  use in liver disease, III:42
  use in renal disease, **III:56–57**
  volume of distribution of, III:13,
    III:17
Chlorothiazide, fluoxetine
  interaction with, II:72
Chlorpromazine, I:518–519
  formulations of, **III:8**
  for HIV-infected persons,
    III:285
  intramuscular, **II:114,** II:118
  lupus induced by, III:184
  protein binding of, III:12
  use in gastrointestinal disease,
    III:23
  use in liver disease, III:43–44
  use in renal disease, **III:62–63**
Chlorprothixene, **III:8**
  intramuscular, **II:114**
Chlorthalidone, **III:186**

Cholecystokinin, in Huntington's
  disease, II:473
Cholestyramine, interaction with
  tricyclic antidepressants,
    III:105
Choline magnesium trisalicylate,
  for low-back pain, **II:357**
Chorea
  differential diagnosis of,
    II:492–494, **II:493**
  drugs for suppression of, II:495
  in Huntington's disease,
    II:474–475, II:486
  senile, **II:493**
  Sydenham's, **II:493**
Chorea-acanthocytosis, **II:493**
Chromatographic methods of drug
  testing, I:151–152, I:154
Chromosomes
  abnormalities of, II:179–180
  long *(q)* and short *(p)* arms of,
    II:170
Chronic fatigue syndrome (CFS),
    III:215–250
  case definitions of, III:216,
    III:221, **III:222–226**
  conceptual models for, III:216,
    III:218–219
  conflicting data about, III:216
  diagnosis of, III:235–239
    approach to patient,
      III:235–237
    patient evaluation, III:238
    viral serologies, III:238–239,
      III:240
  differentiation from
    environmental illness,
      III:349–350
  as disorder of immune
    regulation, **III:218,**
      III:232–233
    cellular immunity, III:233
    humoral immunity, III:232–233
  epidemiology of, III:223–229

community studies, III:223,
III:227–228
primary care studies,
III:228–229, **III:230**
tertiary care studies, III:229,
III:231
history of, III:216–221, **III:220**
as infectious disease, III:216,
III:218, III:230–232
laboratory tests for, I:274–275
medical and psychiatric
disorders associated with,
III:230–231
as muscle disorder, **III:218,**
III:234
persons providing treatment for,
III:216
as psychiatric disorder,
I:275 276, **III:219,**
III:235
relationship to fibromyalgia,
III:234, **III:236**
signs and symptoms of, III:221,
III:227–228
as sleep disorder, **III:218,**
III:233–234
symptoms of, I:272–274
terminology for, III:217, III:221
treatment of, I:276, III:239–241
cognitive-behavior strategies,
III:241, **III:244,** III:249,
III:249
general approach, III:239
lessons from fibromyalgia
literature, III:241,
III:246–248
pharmacological strategies,
III:239–241, **III:242–245**
Chronic obstructive pulmonary
disease (COPD)
buspirone use in, II:82
estazolam use in, II:86
evaluating patients for carbon
dioxide retention, II:89–90

quazepam use in, II:88
tacrine use in, II:97
triazolam use in, II:89
zolpidem use in, III:132
Cigarette smoking. *See also* Nicotine
cessation of, II:80–81
epidemiology of, I:542–543
headaches and, I:416
psychiatric disorders and,
I:543–545, I:579–582
treatment of, I:556–582
approach to, I:578–583
nonpharmacologic, I:572–578
pharmacologic, I:556–572
Cimetidine
cytochrome P_{450} inhibition by,
III:37, **III:85,** III:86
drug interactions with, III:21
carbamazepine, III:123
clozapine, III:108
fluoxetine, II:72
paroxetine, **III:88**
sertraline, II:75
terfenadine, III:103
venlafaxine, III:95
Ciprofloxacin (Cipro)
interaction with terfenadine,
III:103
neuropsychiatric side effects of,
III:304
Circadian variations, arrhythmias
and, II:225–227
Circulation, II:199
Cirrhosis, I:45–46, I:51. *See also*
Liver disease
accumulation of active
metabolites of midazolam
in, II:122
benzodiazepine use in, II:122–123
fluoxetine metabolism in
patients with, II:71
Clarithromycin
interaction with carbamazepine,
III:123

Clarithromycin *(continued)*
  neuropsychiatric side effects of,
    III:305
Clearance of drugs, **III:5,** III:15–16
  calculation of, III:15
  in cardiac disease, III:27–28
  disease effects on, **III:7,** III:18
  factors influencing, III:15
  hepatic, III:39, III:41–42
  relationship to maintenance
    dose, III:15–16
  renal, I:460, III:41–42
  steady state and, III:17
  systemic, III:41
Climacteric, II:269
Clinical ecology, III:347–378. *See also*
  Environmental illness
Clinical Global Impression Severity
  (CGIS), III:167
Clinical interview, after head injury,
  III:321, III:322–323
Clofazimine, III:305
Clomiphene citrate (Clomid)
  adverse psychiatric effects of,
    II:307, II:324
  mechanism of action of, II:307
  multiple pregnancies due to,
    II:307
  for ovulation induction, II:307
  for polycystic ovarian disease,
    II:268
Clomipramine
  for fibromyalgia, **III:247**
  formulations of, **III:8**
  for Huntington's disease, II:497
  intravenous, **II:115,** II:125–129
    dosage of, II:128
    effect on sleep, II:126–127
    side effects of, II:127
    tolerance to oral therapy after,
      II:127
  metabolism of, **III:82**
  for postpartum depression,
    II:254

for premenstrual syndrome,
    II:264
Clonazepam, I:80–81
  drug interactions with, III:89–90
    fluoxetine, III:37, **III:88**
  half-life of, **III:19**
  for HIV-infected persons,
    III:284
  for Huntington's disease, II:495,
    II:497
  metabolism of, **III:9,** III:89
  for mucous membrane
    dysesthesias, III:390
  for patient with low-back pain,
    II:367
  pregnancy and, I:625–626
  use in liver disease, III:90
  use in renal disease, **III:56–57**
  for vulvodynia, III:408
Clonidine, I:526, I:569–570, I:579
  for chest pain, III:99–100
  for clozapine-induced
    hypersalivation, III:164–165
  labeled with iodine-123, II:159
  for opiate detoxification, II:365
  for preanesthetic anxiety, II:394
Clorazepate
  active metabolite of, III:3, III:15
  formulations of, **III:8**
  half-life of, **III:19**
  metabolism of, **III:9**
  onset of action of, III:3
  use in gastrointestinal disease,
    III:22
  use in liver disease, III:42
  use in renal disease, **III:56–57**
Closed head injury. *See* Head injury
Clozapine, I:53–56, III:79, III:106–109
  for atypical parkinsonism,
    III:168–169
  drug interactions with, III:108
    cimetidine, III:108
    fluoxetine, **III:88,** III:108
    phenytoin, III:108

for elderly patients, III:108,
    III:168
for Huntington's disease,
    II:497
mechanism of action of,
    III:164
for Parkinson's disease,
    II:456–457, III:106
    motoric effects, III:167–168
for psychosis, III:165–169,
    III:166
pharmacology of, III:164–165
for schizophrenia, III:165
side effects of, III:106–109, III:168
    agranulocytosis, III:106–107,
        III:168
    neuroleptic malignant
        syndrome, III:108–109
    seizures, III:107
for tardive dyskinesia and
    dystonia, III:109
Cluster headaches, I:409–410
Cocaine dependence, II:159
Codeine, **III:83**
    for low-back pain, **II:357**
Cogentin. *See* Benztropine
Cognex Access Program, II:94
Cognitive assessment
    computed tomography for, I:5
    frontal lobe dysfunction and,
        I:355–362
    for organ transplant recipients,
        I:313–316
    types of tests for, I:359–360
Cognitive effects
    of Alzheimer's disease
        selegiline for, II:98
        tacrine for, II:95
    of bone marrow transplantation,
        III:435–436, III:451–452
    of buspirone, II:82–83
    of estazolam, II:86
    of flurazepam, II:86
    of head injury, III:314

neuropsychological assessment
    for, III:323–325
    testing for, III:324, **III:326**
    of HIV infection, III:268–277
    of Huntington's disease,
        II:480–481
    of multiple sclerosis, II:417–419
        therapy and management of,
            II:419–421
    of Parkinson's disease, II:450,
        II:460–464
    of posttraumatic stress disorder,
        III:317–318
    premenstrual, II:259–260
    of rheumatoid arthritis, III:192,
        III:193
    of systemic lupus
        erythematosus, III:188,
        III:191–194
    of triazepam, II:86
    of triazolam, II:88
Cognitive rehabilitation, II:420–421
Cognitive retraining, I:374–375
Cognitive-behavior therapy (CBT)
    for bone marrow transplant
        recipient, III:424
    for chronic fatigue syndrome,
        III:241, **III:244,** III:249,
        III:249
    for depressed multiple sclerosis
        patients, II:434
    for patients with low-back pain,
        II:354, II:369
Commission for the Control of
    Huntington Disease and Its
    Consequences, II:503
Communication skills
    of anesthesiologists, II:394
    for competency determinations,
        II:524
    of interdisciplinary team
        members, II:601
    training for low-back pain
        patients, II:361

Compensation neurosis, II:377–378,
    III:315
Competency determinations,
    II:515–533
  for aphasic patient, II:529–533
  assessment for, II:521–533
  behavioral observations for,
    II:533
  change from notion of
    competence to capacity,
    II:518, II:540
    implications for competency
    assessment, II:518–519
  communication skills required
    for, II:524
  competency to consent to
    treatment, II:525–533,
    II:539–540
    assessment procedures,
    II:527–528, **II:528**
    case study, II:529–533
    necessary functional abilities,
    II:526–527, **II:527**
  domains of, II:521–522, **II:522**
  historical views of
    "incompetency," II:516–517
  for involuntary commitment,
    II:519–521
  as legal construct, II:516
  misconceptions about, II:515–516
  obstacles to, II:522–525
    clinician's lack of familiarity
      with patient, II:524
    generic types of disagreement,
    II:523–524
    lack of absolute criteria,
    II:522–523
    patients' neurological
      impairments, II:525
  for patient executing advance
    care directive, II:551–552
  recent legislation affecting,
    II:516–521
  subjectivity of, II:533

Computed tomography (CT)
  after head injury, III:313, **III:321,**
    III:325–328
  in AIDS dementia complex,
    III:276
  applications of, I:5–9
  brain electrical activity mapping
    and, I:22
  compared with SPECT, II:141
  in dementia, II:152
  to evaluate headache, I:394–395
  to evaluate stroke, II:151
  in Huntington's disease,
    II:490–491
  indications for, I:7
  interpretation of, I:5–6
  magnetic resonance imaging
    and, I:8, I:10–12
  mechanism of, I:5
  of spine, II:347
  in systemic lupus
    erythematosus, II:154,
    III:198, III:199
Computer techniques
  dipole localization method,
    I:181–182
  evoked potentials, I:177–180
  topographic EEG mapping,
    I:173–177
Concentration deficits
  due to total-body irradiation,
    III:435
  in HIV infection, III:269
  postconcussional, III:315
Conduct disorder, in Huntington's
    disease, II:476, **II:476,** II:477
Condylomata acuminata, III:396
Confidentiality, of genetic testing,
    II:190
Confusion
  in chronic fatigue syndrome,
    III:221
  clozapine-induced, III:164
  in Parkinson's disease, III:157

Congenital anomalies
    antiepileptic drugs and neural
        tube defects, II:99–101
    associated with oral
        contraceptive use in
        pregnancy, II:245
Congestive heart failure (CHF),
    I:129–130, II:70, III:26–32. *See
    also* Cardiac disease
    cerebral blood flow in, III:29
    drug absorption in, III:26
    drug distribution in, III:26–27
    drug excretion in, III:27–28
    drug metabolism in, III:27
    guidelines for drug dosing in,
        III:28–30
    use of antidepressants in, III:30
    use of antipsychotics in, III:31
    use of bupropion in, II:78
    use of lithium in, III:31–32
Consent to treatment. *See also*
    Informed consent
    battery and, II:562
    competency for, II:539–540. *See
        also* Competency
        determinations
    assessment of, II:525–533
    implied, II:562
    incompetency and, II:516–517,
        II:540–541
    informing patients of rights
        regarding, II:549
    legal doctrine of consent, II:539
    "rule of consent," II:539
    "rule of informed consent,"
        II:539
    refusal of, II:539. *See also* Refusal
        of treatment
Constipation, nefazodone-induced,
    III:96
Consultation-liaison psychiatry,
    II:237
Contraception. *See also* Oral
    contraceptives

during postpartum psychosis,
    II:256
Contrecoup injury, III:311
Controlled Oral Word Association
    Test, **II:420**
Contusions, brain, III:310–312
Conversion disorder, I:611, II:377
    hypnosis for assessment of,
        II:44–45, II:57–58
Coordination and frontal lobe
    dysfunction, I:364
Coping
    assessing for bone marrow
        transplant candidate,
        III:423–424
    effect of medical illness on, II:39
Coping Health Inventory for
    Parents, I:493
Copolymer I, for multiple sclerosis,
    II:417
Coronary angiography, III:99
Coronary artery bypass grafting,
    II:393, II:394, II:595
Coronary artery disease, II:222
    arrhythmias provoked during
        psychological stress
        testing in patient with,
        II:218–220, **II:219**
    silent ischemia due to mental
        stress in patient with, II:220
Correlativity thesis, II:586
Corticosteroids
    affective side effects of, II:416,
        II:436
    for bone marrow transplant
        recipient, III:434–436
    for multiple sclerosis, II:416,
        II:417
    psychiatric side effects of, II:242,
        III:208
    for systemic lupus
        erythematosus, III:189,
        III:194, III:207
    for vulvar itching, III:398–399

Corticosteroids *(continued)*
for vulvar itching
lichen simplex chronicus,
III:384
rebound inflammatory
reaction, III:397
Cortisol, II:240
buspirone effects on secretion of,
II:83
Cotinine assays, I:561
Counseling, before and after HIV
testing, III:265–266
Countertransference, II:5, II:39
with Huntington's disease
patients, II:500–501
in time-limited dynamic
psychotherapy, II:19
Cranial neuralgia, I:419
Creatinine clearance, II:71, III:51–52
lithium effects on, III:110
Creutzfeldt-Jakob disease, I:173,
II:157, **II:493**
Crohn's disease
effect on protein binding of
drugs, III:10
use of chlorpromazine in, III:23
Cryoprecipitate, III:127
CT. *See* Computed tomography
Culture
death and, II:227
menarche and, II:241–242
postpartum depression and,
II:248
Curare, II:390, II:397
Cyclophosphamide
before bone marrow
transplantation, III:417,
III:430, III:434
gonadal dysfunction due to,
III:455
for multiple sclerosis, II:417
Cycloserine, III:305
Cyclosporine, I:329–332
interaction with fluoxetine, **III:88**

interaction with midazolam,
III:37
for multiple sclerosis, II:417
Cyclothymia, valproate for, III:125
Cylert, I:373–374
Cysteamine, for Huntington's
disease, II:495
Cystitis
hemorrhagic, III:434
interstitial, III:386, III:387–388
Cytarabine hydrochloride, before
bone marrow transplantation,
III:430
Cytochrome P450 (CyP450), III:14,
III:36–37, **III:38,** III:80–86
buspirone and, II:84
CyP450-3A4, III:36–37, III:85–86
drugs metabolized by, III:85,
III:85
inhibition of, **III:85,** III:86
CyP450-2D6, III:36–37, III:81
drugs metabolized by,
III:82–83
selective serotonin reuptake
inhibitor inhibition of,
III:36–37, III:83–85, **III:84**
disease effects on drug
metabolism by, III:40
fluoxetine and, II:71
isoenzymes of, III:36–37, III:80
levels in liver biopsies, III:40
sertraline and, II:75
subfamilies of, III:36–37, III:80
Cytomegalovirus (CMV), II:154–155
chronic fatigue syndrome and,
III:231–232
Cytovene. *See* Ganciclovir

Daily Rating Form, II:259, II:261,
II:293–300
Damages, II:566–567
Danazol, II:308
"Dangerousness," II:521
Dantrolene, I:443–444

Dapsone, III:303
Darier's disease, I:299–300
DATATOP study, III:156
Day treatment programs, for
    Huntington's disease patients,
    II:502
ddC. *See* Zalcitabine
ddI. *See* Didanosine
De Motu Cordis, II:199
Deafferentation pain, I:419
Dealkylation, III:14
Deamination, III:14
Death
    psychophysiological, II:227
    related to bereavement,
        II:222–223
    self-willed, II:227
    sudden cardiac, II:199–231. *See
        also* Sudden cardiac death
    by suggestion, II:227
    voodoo, II:211–212, II:227
Debrisoquin, **III:82**
Dehydroepiandrosterone sulfate
    (DHAS), II:266
Delirium
    after head injury, III:314
    associated with HIV infection,
        III:269, III:285–286
    in bone marrow transplant
        recipient, III:423, III:439
    in children and adolescents, I:473
    in critical care settings, II:113,
        II:116
    electroencephalography and, I:169
    haloperidol for, I:332–333
    induced by lithium and
        diltiazem, III:112–113
    induced by tricyclic
        antidepressants, III:281
    in organ transplant recipients,
        I:325, I:327
    postoperative, II:403–404
Delusions
    in Parkinson's disease, III:160

postpartum, II:255
Dementia. *See also* Cognitive effects
    after head injury, III:314
    AIDS dementia complex,
        II:155–156, III:268–277. *See
        also* Human
        immunodeficiency virus
        infection
    Alzheimer's. *See* Alzheimer's
        disease
    "apathetic," II:479
    electroencephalography and,
        I:172–173
    in Huntington's disease, II:475,
        II:476, II:480–481
    impact on medical decision
        making, II:537–538
    multi-infarct, I:172–173, II:153
    in multiple sclerosis, II:418
    in Parkinson's disease, II:460–464
    SPECT evaluation of, II:152–153
        activation procedures during,
            II:149–150
        AIDS dementia complex,
            II:155, II:156
    subcortical, I:246–247, II:418,
        II:475, II:481
    tacrine for, III:133–136
    valproate for, III:125
Demoxepam, **III:19**
Demyelination, II:411–412
Denial
    in medically ill patients, II:16
        adaptive and maladaptive
            effects of, II:30
    as phase of stress response
        syndromes, II:28–30, **II:29**
Dentate nucleus lesion, **II:493**
Deontology, II:586
Depo-Provera. *See*
    Medroxyprogesterone
Deprenyl. *See* Selegiline
Depression
    after myocardial infarction, II:223

Depression *(continued)*
  before and after puberty, II:241
  after traumatic brain injury,
      III:309–310, III:315
  associated with HIV infection,
      III:267–268, **III:269–270,**
      III:277–278
  biogenic amine hypothesis of,
      II:240
  in bone marrow transplant
      recipient, III:423, III:431,
      III:438–441
  cerebral blood flow studies in,
      II:157–158
  chronic fatigue and, III:235
  cigarette smoking and, I:543–545
  disability and, I:604–605
  DSM-IV criteria for major
      depressive episode vs.
      mood disorder due to
      general medical condition,
      III:309–310, **III:311**
  early-onset, II:241
  fibromyalgia and, II:374
  Huntington's disease and, II:172,
      II:476, II:476–478
  low-back pain and, II:341, II:366,
      II:378–379, II:381–382
  "masked," II:378
  in medically ill patients, II:16–17
  mental retardation and, I:513
  migraine headaches and,
      I:404–405
  in multiple sclerosis, II:423,
      II:428–435, **II:430–433**
      biological explanation for,
          II:428–429
      clinical reports of, **II:430–433**
      prevalence of, II:428
      problems with studies of,
          II:434–435
      severity of, II:428
      suicide and, II:428
      treatment for, II:434
  in organ transplant recipients,
      I:324, I:326–327
  in Parkinson's disease, II:457–460
  pathophysiology of, II:240
  poststroke, I:368, III:113
  preceding ventricular
      arrhythmias, II:217
  in pregnancy, I:623–624
  reactive, II:423
  related to protected isolation
      environment, III:443
  SPECT evaluation of, in elderly
      patients, II:157
  sudden cardiac death and,
      II:222
  in systemic lupus
      erythematosus, III:188,
      III:192, III:207–208
  treatment of, I:58, I:334–336. *See
      also* Antidepressants
    carbamazepine, III:120
    electroconvulsive therapy in
        medical patients,
        II:575–578
    intravenous clomipramine,
        II:125–127
    methylphenidate, II:129–130,
        III:113
    selective serotonin reuptake
        inhibitors, III:80
  in women, II:237
    oral contraceptive–related,
        II:238, II:242–245
    postpartum, II:238, II:246–257.
        See also Postpartum
        depressions
    during pregnancy, II:254
    premenstrual syndrome and,
        II:260
    related to menopause,
        II:272–274
    undergoing infertility
        treatment, II:324–325
Dermatitis, I:292–298

Dermatologic conditions. *See* Skin disorders
Desalkylflurazepam, II:87, **III:19**
N-Desalkyl-2-oxoquazepam, **III:19**
Desensitization
   hypnotic, for asthma, II:53–54
   for phobias, II:56
   systematic, II:391
Desipramine, I:30, II:125
   for depressed multiple sclerosis patients, II:434
   drug interactions with
      fluoxetine, **III:87,** III:89
      fluvoxamine, **III:87,** III:89
      propafenone, III:106
      selective serotonin reuptake inhibitors, III:85
   electrocardiographic effects of, III:100–101
   formulations of, **III:8**
   for head-injured patient, **III:331,** III:336
   for HIV-infected persons, III:281, III:282
   for Huntington's disease, II:497
   inhibition of norepinephrine uptake by, II:126
   metabolism of, III:45
      by cytochrome P$_{450}$-2D6, III:36, **III:82**
   for mucous membrane dysesthesias, III:390
   sudden death in children and, III:100–101
   use in renal disease, **III:64–65**
   for vulvodynia, III:408
Desmethylchlordiazepoxide, III:18, **III:19**
Desmethylclomipramine, II:127
Desmethyldiazepam, II:122, III:3, III:15, III:18, **III:19**
Desmethylimipramine. *See* Desipramine
Desmethylsertraline, III:36

O-Desmethyl-venlafaxine, III:93
Desmopressin (DDAVP), III:127
Desmoxazepam, III:18
Desulfuration, III:14
Desyrel. *See* Trazodone
Deterrent therapy, I:572
Developmental stages of children, I:491–492
Dextroamphetamine (Dexedrine), I:373
   for cancer patients, III:113
   for head-injured patients, **III:330,** III:335
   for HIV-infected persons, III:282–283
   use in Huntington's disease, II:497–498
Dextromethorphan
   for AIDS dementia complex, III:275
   for Huntington's disease, II:495
   metabolism by cytochrome P$_{450}$-2D6, **III:83**
Dextropropoxyphene, **III:83**
DHPG. *See* Ganciclovir
Diabetes mellitus
   drug absorption in, III:2
   fluoxetine use in, II:73
   Huntington's disease and, II:490
   lithium use in, I:41
   time-limited dynamic psychotherapy for patient with, II:20–33
Diagnostic Interview Schedule (DIS), III:223, III:356, **III:358–361**
Diagnostic Net, II:332–334, **II:333, II:336,** II:339
Dialysis, III:51
Dialyzable leukocyte extract, III:239, **III:245**
Diamox. *See* Acetazolamide
Diazepam, I:462
   achieving steady state of, III:17

Diazepam (continued)
    active metabolite of, II:122
    clearance of, III:17
    distribution of, III:12–13
    formulations of, **III:8**
    half-life of, II:122, **III:19**
        in elderly patients, II:122
    interaction with fluoxetine, II:72,
        III:87
    metabolism of, II:122, **III:9**
    onset of action of, III:3
    parenteral, **II:114–115**, II:116,
        II:122, II:123
        intramuscular, II:123
        intravenous, II:123
        use in respiratory disease,
            II:124
    for patient with low-back pain,
        II:367
    pharmacokinetics of, II:122
    for postanesthesia emergence
        reactions, II:403
    for preanesthetic anxiety,
        II:393–394
    respiratory effects of, II:82
    use in liver disease, III:33, III:42
    use in renal disease, **III:56–57**
    volume of distribution of, III:13,
        III:17
Diazepam binding inhibitor (DBI),
    II:473
Didanosine (ddI), III:303
Diet
    environmental illness and,
        III:352, III:354
    for patient on selegiline, II:98
    for patient on tacrine, II:97
    for premenstrual syndrome,
        II:262
    tricyclic antidepressants and
        fiber in, III:105
Diethylstilbestrol (DES), II:270
Diffuse axonal injury, III:310–311,
    III:313–314

Diflucan. See Fluconazole
Diflunisal, for low-back pain,
    II:357
Digit Span test, **III:326**
Digoxin
    interaction with fluoxetine, II:72
    interaction with paroxetine, II:76
    interaction with sertraline, II:75
    for supraventricular tachycardia,
        II:205
Diisopropylphenol, I:121–123
Diltiazem
    interaction with carbamazepine,
        III:123
    interaction with imipramine,
        III:105
    interaction with lithium,
        III:112–113
Dipole localization method,
    I:181–182
Disability
    in children, I:606
    documentation of, I:608–611,
        I:619
    psychological adjustment to,
        I:603–607
    psychological tests for, I:607–608
    work and, I:598–603, I:609–611
Disinhibition, after head injury,
    III:312, III:314
Disk herniation, II:339, II:340, II:346,
    II:370, II:374
Diskitis, II:339, II:370
Dissociation, under hypnosis, II:40,
    II:42
Distribution of drug, **III:5**, III:9–14
    in cardiac disease, III:26–27
    diseases affecting, **III:6–7**
    factors influencing, III:9–10
    protein binding and, III:10–12,
        III:11
    two-compartment model and,
        III:13
    volume of, **III:5**, III:12–14

Disulfiram, interaction with
  terfenadine, III:103
Diuretics, for premenstrual
  syndrome, II:263
Divalproex sodium, **III:8**
Dive reflex, II:212
Dizziness
  drug-induced
    clozapine, III:107
    felbamate, III:118
    gabapentin, III:120
    nefazodone, III:96
    venlafaxine, III:93
  postconcussional, III:315
"Dodo bird verdict," II:8
"Do-not-resuscitate" orders, II:546,
  III:428
Dopamine
  dopaminergic function,
    I:370–372, I:439, I:441
  electroconvulsive therapy and,
    I:445
  in Huntington's disease, II:473
  oxidative metabolism of, II:453
  in Parkinson's disease, II:450
  in polycystic ovarian disease,
    II:266–268
  tacrine effects on, III:136
Dopamine agonists, I:441
  for head-injured patient, III:329,
    III:330, III:335
  for Parkinson's disease,
    II:453–454, III:153, **III:154,**
    III:162
  psychotoxicity of, III:162
Dopamine antagonists
  for head-injured patient, III:329,
    III:330–331
  for Huntington's disease,
    II:494–495
Doral. *See* Quazepam
Dorsal horn "pain neurons," II:371
Dothiepin, for fibromyalgia, **III:247**
Down syndrome, II:179

Doxepin, I:304
  formulations of, **III:8**
  for HIV-infected persons, III:281
  for low-back pain patients, **II:359**
  metabolism of, III:45
  for pruritus ani, III:399
  rectal administration of,
    III:104–105
  use in cardiac disease, III:30
  use in renal disease, **III:64–65**
Dronabinol, III:305
Droperidol, **II:114,** II:117, **III:8**
Droperidol-fentanyl, agitation due
  to, II:402
Drowsiness
  clozapine-induced, III:107
  zolpidem-induced, III:133
Drug Enforcement Agency (DEA),
  II:364
"Drug holidays," from
  antiparkinsonian drugs, III:163
Drug interactions, I:435–436
  with anesthetics, II:399–402,
    II:401
    cyclic and atypical
      antidepressants,
      II:400–401
    lithium, II:402
    monoamine oxidase
      inhibitors, II:399–400
  with antacids, III:21
  with buspirone, I:51–52
  with carbamazepine, I:33–34,
    I:75, III:123–124, III:339
  with clonazepam, I:81, III:89–90
  with clozapine, III:108
  with fluoxetine, I:45–46, II:71–73,
    III:87–88
  with fluvoxamine, **III:87**
  with histamine blockers, I:38
  kinetics and, III:20
  with lithium, I:42–44, III:112–113
  with monoamine oxidase
    inhibitors, I:68–70

Drug interactions *(continued)*
  with nefazodone, III:97
  with nicotine, I:552–553
  with over-the-counter drugs,
    I:68–70
  with paroxetine, II:76, **III:88**
  with propafenone, III:106
  with quazepam, II:87
  related to cytochrome P$_{450}$
    subfamilies, III:37
  with selective serotonin reuptake
    inhibitors, III:86, **III:87–89,**
    III:336
  with selegiline, II:98
  with sertraline, II:75, **III:89**
  with tacrine, II:96–97
  with terfenadine, III:102–103
  with tricyclic antidepressants,
    I:38
  with valproate, I:78–79,
    III:127–130, III:339
  with venlafaxine, III:95
Drug testing
  cost and accuracy of, I:156
  informed consent for, I:147
  interpreting results of,
    I:158–159
  NIDA certification for, I:157
  procedure for, I:146–147,
    I:150–156
  sample management for,
    I:148–156
Dry mouth
  nefazodone-induced, III:96
  tricyclic antidepressant–induced,
    III:281
  venlafaxine-induced, III:93
DSM-III-R, II:435
  classification of pain in, II:379
  late luteal phase dysphoric
    disorder in, II:257, II:258
  postpartum blues in, II:250–251

  postpartum psychosis in, II:255
DSM-IV, II:380
  criteria for major depressive
    episode vs. mood disorder
    due to general medical
    condition, III:309–310,
    III:311
  criteria for personality change
    due to general medical
    condition, III:310, **III:312**
  diagnoses associated with
    traumatic brain injury,
    III:309, III:309–310
  research criteria for
    postconcussional
    syndrome, **III:316**
Durable power of attorney for
    health care, II:537, II:553–556.
    See also Advance medical
    treatment directives
  application of, II:554–555
  background for development of,
    II:553–554
  compared to living wills,
    II:555–556
  language required for, II:555
  legal recognition of, II:554
  patient's decision controls and,
    II:556
Duty of reasonable care, II:565
Duty to treat, II:602–604
Dynorphin, in Huntington's
    disease, II:473
Dysarthria, in Huntington's
    disease, II:475, II:487
Dysesthesias, endogenous,
    III:389–390
Dyskinesia
  fluoxetine-induced, II:74
  intravenous lithium–induced,
    II:132
  selective serotonin reuptake
    inhibitor–induced, III:91
Dyspareunia, II:269, II:303

due to vulvodynia, III:385
entry, III:403–404
in interstitial cystitis, III:385
postcoital, III:400
Dysphagia, II:487
Dysphasia, II:475
Dysthymia, **II:476,** II:476–478
Dystonia
buspirone-induced, II:83
in Huntington's disease, II:486,
II:487
parenteral haloperidol–induced,
II:117
selective serotonin reuptake
inhibitor–induced, III:91

Eating disorders, II:237
Ecchymoses, fluoxetine-induced,
II:73, III:90
Ecologic illness, III:347. *See also*
Environmental illness
ECT. *See* Electroconvulsive therapy
Eczema
in children, I:292–293
hypnosis for, II:52
Edema, triazolam-induced, II:89
Education and training
in brief psychotherapy, II:9
for families of medically ill
children, I:497–500
in hypnosis, II:61
in time-limited dynamic
psychotherapy, II:19
work ethic and, I:602
Egg donation, II:310, II:312
psychological issues in donors,
II:318–319
Egoism, II:586
Ejaculation
difficulties in multiple sclerosis,
II:437
premature, II:303
retrograde, II:306
Eldepryl. *See* Selegiline

Elderly persons
benzodiazepines for, II:122
parenteral, II:125
clozapine for, III:108, III:168
electroconvulsive therapy for,
I:111
gabapentin for, III:119
magnetic resonance imaging for,
I:12–13
maintenance on life-support
systems, II:541
medical decision making
dilemmas related to,
II:537–538
parenteral haloperidol for
intramuscular, II:118
intravenous, II:117
paroxetine metabolism in, II:76
prevalence of Parkinson's
disease in, III:158
quazepam for, II:87
risperidone for, III:115–116
SPECT evaluation of depression
in, II:157
stimulants for, I:476
systemic lupus erythematosus
in, III:188–189
tacrine for Alzheimer's disease
in, III:133–136
zolpidem for, III:131–133
Electrocardiography (ECG), II:200
after mesoridazine
administration, II:118
bupropion effects on, II:77, II:78
desipramine effects on, in
children, III:100–101
fluoxetine effects on, II:70
imipramine effects on, III:96
intravenous haloperidol effects
on, III:103–104
lithium effects on, III:112
nefazodone effects on, III:96
paroxetine effects on, II:76

Electrocardiography (ECG)
(continued)
Q-T interval on, II:213–214
risperidone effects on, III:115
sertraline effects on, II:75
terfenadine effects on, III:86,
III:103
venlafaxine effects on, III:95
Electroconvulsive therapy (ECT)
anesthesia and, I:118–123
assessment for, I:112–115
contraindications to, I:104–111
drug treatment and, I:63–65,
I:109–112, I:123–125
eye problems and, I:103
for HIV-infected persons, III:283
for medically ill patients,
II:575–578
case study of, II:575–576
liability issues related to,
II:575–578
safety of, II:575
monitoring during, I:117–118
mortality from, I:134–135
for neuroleptic malignant
syndrome, I:445
for Parkinson's disease, II:460,
III:170–172
pheochromocytoma and, I:108,
I:131–132
physiological response to,
I:100–103
for postpartum psychosis, II:256
pregnancy and, I:622
preoperative orders for, I:115–117
side effects of, I:103, I:133–135
use in systemic lupus
erythematosus, III:208
Electroencephalography (EEG)
ambulatory cassette EEG,
I:182–184
brain electrical activity mapping,
I:21–22, I:180, II:492
drug detection on, I:171–172

electrode placements for,
I:166–167
evoked potentials and, I:177–180
for headache evaluation, I:396
in Huntington's disease, II:492
during hypnosis, II:47–48
in Lennox-Gastaut syndrome,
III:116
limitations of, I:165
neuroleptics and, I:474–475
seizures on, I:164–169
in systemic lupus
erythematosus,
III:196–199, **III:198**
topographic mapping and,
I:173–177
Electromyography (EMG), II:347
Elimination of drugs, III:9,
III:14–18
in cardiac disease, III:28–29
clearance, **III:5**, III:15–16
half-life, **III:5, III:16,** III:16–18
phase I reactions, **III:9,** III:14–15,
III:36
phase II reactions, **III:9,** III:15,
III:36
Empathic changes, I:376–378
"Empty nest syndrome," II:272
Enalapril, interaction with lithium,
III:113
Encainide
metabolism by cytochrome
P_{450}-2D6, **III:83**
use after myocardial infarction,
III:98
Encephalitis, II:157
benign myalgic, III:217, **III:220.**
See also Chronic fatigue
syndrome
subacute, III:268
Encephalopathy
hepatic, II:93
HIV, III:268
multifocal, I:352

related to total-body irradiation, III:435–436
early-delayed, III:435–436
late-delayed, III:436
Endometrial biopsy, II:306
Endometrial hypoplasia, II:275
Endometriosis, II:268–269
definition of, II:268
etiology of, II:268
hormone changes associated with, II:268
hormone suppression of, II:308
infertility due to, II:306, II:308
mood disorders and, II:269
pelvic pain due to, II:268–269
prevalence of, II:268
β-Endorphins
effect on gonadotropin secretion, II:267
in polycystic ovarian disease, II:267–268
relation of hypnosis to, II:49–50
role in premenstrual syndrome, II:262
Enflurane
epileptogenicity of, II:402
interaction with cyclic antidepressants, II:400–401, **II:401**
English Common Law, II:538
Enterovirus, chronic fatigue syndrome and, III:232
Environmental illness (EI), III:347–378
clinical description of persons with, III:355–366
personality profile, **III:358–361**, III:364–366
physical disorders, III:363–364
psychiatric disorders, III:356–363, **III:357–361**
clinical ecologist and, III:348–349
definition of, III:351
diagnosis of, III:351–352

differential diagnosis of, III:349–350
evaluation of patient with diagnosis of, III:366–369, **III:370**
future directions in, III:376–377
history of, III:348
lack of acceptance by mainstream medical community, III:349
prevalence of, III:348
putative causes of, III:351
support groups for people with, III:351, III:355
terminology for, III:347–348
theories of, III:352–353
bipolarity phenomenon, III:353
spreading phenomenon, III:353
switch phenomenon, III:353
total body load concept, III:353
treatment of, III:369–376
behavior modification, III:371–372
case example of difficulty of, III:373–376
by clinical ecologists, III:353–354
for coexisting psychiatric disorders, III:372–373
combination treatment measures, III:373
environmental modifications, III:370–371
psychotherapy, III:369–370
recommendations for, **III:377**
Environmental sensitivity, III:217. *See also* Chronic fatigue syndrome
Enzyme-limited drugs, III:32–33, III:39
Enzyme-linked immunosorbent assay (ELISA), I:251–252, I:269
for HIV infection, III:264

Enzyme-multiplied immunoassay
test, I:153
Eosinophilia, clozapine-induced,
III:108
Ephedrine, II:400
Epidemiologic Catchment Area
(ECA) study, III:223, III:227,
III:266
Epidemiology
of chronic fatigue syndrome,
III:223–229
of cigarette smoking, I:542–543
of hemophilia, I:194–196
of HIV infection, I:245,
III:258–259
of Lyme disease, I:267
of migraine headaches, I:399
of Parkinson's disease, III:158
of psoriasis, I:290
of psychiatric disorders among
persons with mental
retardation, I:508
of sickle cell disease, I:203
of syphilis, I:257
of thalassemia, I:210
Epilepsy. See also Seizures
carbamazepine for, I:75–76
EEG and surgery for, I:164
lithium effects in, I:41–42
nonconvulsive status
epilepticus, I:170
periodic lateralized epileptiform
discharges, I:170
polycystic ovarian disease and,
II:266
SPECT evaluation of, II:156
Epistaxis, fluoxetine-induced, II:73
Epoetin alfa, III:305
Epstein-Barr virus (EBV) infection,
chronic, III:217, III:230–232,
III:238–239, **III:240**. See also
Chronic fatigue syndrome
Erythema chronicum migrans,
I:267, I:270

Erythema multiforme, I:301
Erythromycin
inhibition of cytochrome
P_{450}-3A4 by, **III:85**, III:86
interaction with carbamazepine,
III:123
interaction with terfenadine,
III:86, III:103
interaction with valproate, III:130
Esmolol, II:576, II:577
Esophageal motility testing, III:99
Esophageal spasm, hypnosis for, II:54
Esophagitis, in bone marrow
transplant recipient, III:433
Essential fatty acids, for chronic
fatigue syndrome, III:239,
III:242
Estazolam, II:85–86
cardiac effects of, II:85
cognitive effects of, II:86
compared with flurazepam for
insomnia, II:85
dosage of, II:85
duration of action of, II:85, II:86
formulations of, **III:8**
half-life of, II:85, **III:19**
metabolism of, II:85, **III:9**
respiratory effects of, II:85–86
safety in medically ill patients,
II:85
Estradiol, II:238, II:239, II:269
in endometriosis, II:268
physiological effects of, II:239
Estrogen
antidopaminergic effect of, II:239
conversion of androgens to,
II:239
deficiency of
after bone marrow
transplantation,
III:453–454
at menopause, II:271
mood changes associated
with, II:273

symptoms of, III:453–454
effect on monoamine oxidase
    levels, II:239–240
effect on neurotransmitters, II:239
effect on tardive dyskinesia,
    II:239
effect on tryptophan
    metabolism, II:243
facilitation of serotonergic
    activity by, II:240
malignancies associated with,
    II:245
mechanism of action of, II:239
in oral contraceptives, II:244
physiological effects of, II:239
in polycystic ovarian disease,
    II:268
postpartum blues and, II:251
premenstrual syndrome and,
    II:261
receptors for, II:239
    in brain, II:238
sources of, II:238
Estrogen replacement therapy,
    II:270, II:273–276
after bone marrow
    transplantation, III:456
androgens added to, II:275
for atrophic vaginitis, II:276
breast cancer and, II:274
effect on depression, II:273
to prevent osteoporosis, II:275
progesterone added to, II:274,
    II:275
uterine cancer and, II:274, II:275
for vulvodynia, III:408
Estrone, II:238, II:269
Ethambutol, III:305
Ethanol
    paroxetine interaction with, II:76
    zero-order kinetics and, III:19–20
Ethchlorvynol, use in renal disease,
    III:58–59
Ether, II:389

Ethical issues, II:585–606
    ethics versus laws, II:585–586
    in genetic testing, II:189–190
        for Huntington's disease,
            II:168, II:170–172, II:189
    in medical decision making,
        II:537–538
    in medical-psychiatric practice,
        II:590–605
        autonomy and truth telling,
            II:590–591
        complexity of
            interdisciplinary moral
            relationships, II:600–601
        duty to treat, II:602–604
        justice and loyalty, II:601–602
        manifest versus latent content,
            II:591–599
        refusal of treatment, II:599–600
        self-preservation: physicians'
            rights, II:604–605
    moral theory, II:586–589
        beneficence, II:587–588
        justice, II:588–589
        respect for autonomy, II:587
        rights and duties, II:586–587
        special duties of physicians,
            II:589
    related to advance medical
        treatment directives,
        II:557–559, **II:558**
    related to bone marrow
        transplantation, III:428–430
Ethosuximide, **III:186**
Etoposide, before bone marrow
    transplantation, III:417, III:430
Euphoria, II:423–424
    definition of, II:423–424
    in multiple sclerosis, II:423–424,
        II:425–426
    clinical reports of, **II:425–426**
    management of, II:424
    pathology related to, II:424
    prevalence of, II:424

Event-related potential (ERP)
studies, of hypnosis, II:48
Evoked potentials, I:177–180. *See
also* Electroencephalography
in Huntington's disease, II:492
Executive function deficits after
head injury, III:312
testing for, **III:326–327**
Exercise
for migraine, I:406
for patient with low-back pain,
II:367–368
for premenstrual syndrome,
II:262
to reduce risk of osteoporosis,
II:275
Expanded Disability Status Scale
(EDSS), II:417–419
Extrapyramidal symptoms. *See also*
Parkinsonism; Tardive
dyskinesia
in Alzheimer's disease, II:448,
II:449
buspirone for, II:81, II:83
clozapine for, III:109
drug-induced
buspirone, II:83–84
fluoxetine, II:72, II:74, II:452
fluphenazine decanoate,
II:119–120
haloperidol
depot preparation,
II:119–120
intramuscular, II:118
intravenous, II:117
neuroleptics, II:452
selective serotonin reuptake
inhibitors, III:91–92
in HIV-infected persons,
III:283–285
risperidone and, III:115–116

Facet sprain, II:370
Factitious disorder, I:611

Fagerstrom Tolerance
Questionnaire, I:561–563
Fainting, stress-related, II:204–205
Fairness, II:588–589
False imprisonment, II:569–570,
II:572–574
Families
conflict management for, I:495,
I:500
hemophilia effects on, I:198–199
Huntington's disease in, II:486
intervention models for,
I:495–496
organ transplantation effects on,
I:313
of patients with frontal lobe
dysfunction, I:378–379
sickle cell anemia effects on,
I:205–206
thalassemia effects on,
I:212–213
Family Assessment Device, I:493
Family therapy, I:483–503
for family of patient with
low-back pain, II:368–369
Fanconi's anemia, III:417
Fansidar. *See* Sulfadoxine/
pyrimethamine
Fatherlessness, II:313
Fatigue, III:215
after bone marrow
transplantation, III:434
chemotherapy-induced, III:431
chronic, III:215–250. *See also*
Chronic fatigue syndrome
epidemiology of, III:223
gabapentin-induced, III:120
in multiple sclerosis, II:436–437
"nerve fiber," II:436–437
postconcussional, III:315
psychiatric comorbidity with,
III:215
Fears. *See also* Anxiety
preanesthetic, II:390

preceding ventricular
arrhythmias, II:217
Febricula, III:217. *See also* Chronic
fatigue syndrome
Felbamate, III:116–119
dosage of, III:117
drug interactions with,
III:117–118
antidepressants, III:118
carbamazepine, III:117–118
valproate, III:118
efficacy for seizures, III:117
indications for, III:116
mechanism of action of, III:116
side effects of, III:117–118
Fenoprofen, for low-back pain,
II:357
Fentanyl
awareness related to, II:397–398
interaction with monoamine
oxidase inhibitors, II:399,
II:401
for preanesthetic anxiety, II:394
Fertility drugs, II:307–308
Fever
in chronic fatigue syndrome,
III:221
headaches and, I:417
neuroleptic malignant syndrome
and, I:437
Fibromyalgia, II:373–374, II:379,
III:217, III:234, **III:236.** *See also*
Chronic fatigue syndrome
diagnostic criteria for, II:373–374
major depression and, II:374
myofascial pain syndrome and,
II:374
treatment of, III:241, **III:246–248**
"Fibromyositis," I:418
Filicide, II:257
Financial issues, I:487
Fiorinal, for patient with low-back
pain, II:367
First-order kinetics, III:18–19

First-pass effect, III:2
Flecainide
metabolism by cytochrome
P$_{450}$-2D6, **III:83**
use after myocardial infarction,
III:98
Floating, II:57
Flow-limited drugs, III:32–33, III:39
Fluconazole, III:86
neuropsychiatric side effects of,
III:304
for vulvar candidiasis, III:400,
III:402
Flumazenil, II:90–93
adverse effects of, II:91–92
application to rapid
tranquilization, II:93
approved indications for, II:91
benzodiazepine inhibition by,
II:90, II:91
for benzodiazepine overdose,
II:91–93
delirium after reversal of
sedation for outpatient
procedures due to, II:93
dosage of, II:92
for hepatic encephalopathy, II:93
intravenous solution of, II:90–91
metabolism of, II:91
onset of action of, II:91
for outpatient surgery, II:396–397
pharmacokinetics of, II:91
technique for administration for,
II:92
use in liver disease, II:91
Fluorescence polarization
immunoassay, I:152
Fluorescent treponemal
antibody-absorbed test, I:263
Fluoxetine, II:69–74
achieving steady state of, II:75,
III:17
active metabolite of, II:71, II:73,
III:17, III:36, III:84–85

Fluoxetine (continued)
  cardiac effects of, II:70
    cautions in patients with
      cardiovascular disease,
      II:70
    electrocardiographic findings,
      II:70
    incidence of, II:70
    mechanism of, II:70
    types of, II:70
    "unexpected deaths," II:70
  cytochrome P_{450} inhibition by,
    III:36, III:46, **III:84,**
    III:84–85
  for depression, I:335
  discontinuation of, II:73
  drug interactions with, II:71–73,
    III:87–88
    anesthetics, II:400
    carbamazepine, III:123–124
    clonazepam, III:37
    clozapine, III:108
    desipramine, III:85
    pharmacodynamic
      mechanisms of, II:72–73
    pharmacokinetic mechanisms
      of, II:71–72
    terfenadine, III:86
    warfarin, III:90
  formulations of, **III:8,** III:23
  half-life of, II:73, III:17, III:336
  for head-injured patient, **III:332,**
    III:336
  for HIV-infected persons,
    III:280–281
  for Huntington's disease, **II:496,**
    II:497
  metabolism of, II:70–71
  for Parkinson's disease, II:459
  for patient with low-back pain,
    II:359, II:366
  for postpartum depression, II:254
  for premenstrual syndrome,
    II:264

  protein binding of, II:71, II:72
  selecting for use, II:76–77
  side effects of, I:44–47, I:302,
    II:73–74
    akathisia, III:92
    bleeding diatheses, II:73, III:90
    bradycardia, III:80
    in diabetic patients, II:73
    extrapyramidal symptoms,
      II:72, II:74, II:452
    hematologic effects, III:90–91
    hyponatremia, II:73–74
    seizures, II:73
    sexual dysfunction, II:74
    skin rashes, II:74
    syndrome of inappropriate
      antidiuretic hormone
      secretion, II:74
  use in gastrointestinal disease,
    III:23
  use in liver disease, II:71,
    III:45–46, III:92
  use in renal disease, II:70–71,
    III:54–55, III:66, III:92
  use in systemic lupus
    erythematosus, III:208
Fluphenazine
  formulations of, **III:8**
  for head-injured patient, **III:330**
  for HIV-related mania, III:283
  intramuscular, **II:114**
  metabolism by cytochrome
    P_{450}-2D6, **III:82**
Fluphenazine decanoate, **II:114,**
  II:118–120, II:598
  conversion from oral dose to,
    II:119
  dosage of, II:119
  extrapyramidal effects of,
    II:119–120
  guidelines for administration of,
    II:114, II:119–120
  half-life of, II:118
Fluphenazine enanthate, II:118

Flurazepam, II:84
  active metabolite of, II:87
  ataxia due to, II:87
  cognitive effects of, II:86
  compared with estazolam for
      insomnia, II:85
  formulations of, **III:8**
  half-life of, **III:19**
  metabolism of, **III:9**
  respiratory effects of, II:86
  use in liver disease, III:42
  use in renal disease, **III:56–57**
Flurbiprofen, for low-back pain,
  II:357
Flushing, stress-related, II:202
Fluvoxamine
  drug interactions with, **III:87**
    imipramine, III:86, III:89
    warfarin, III:90
  use in liver disease, III:92
Folic acid
  deficiency of, I:226–229, II:240
    teratogenesis and, II:100
  metabolism of, I:226
  supplementation of, II:100
Follicle-stimulating hormone (FSH),
  II:307
  in bone marrow transplant
    recipients, III:453, III:455
  in human menopausal
    gonadotropin, II:307
  levels at menopause, II:271
  in polycystic ovarian disease,
    II:266–267
Formaldehyde "off-gassing,"
  III:350, III:353
Foscarnet (Foscavir), III:304
Fourteenth Amendment Due
  Process Clause, II:544
Fracture dislocations, II:331
Fragile X syndrome, II:175–177
  genetic testing for, II:175–177
    premutation, II:176–177
  in males versus females, II:176

  mental retardation due to,
    II:175–176
  mode of inheritance for,
    II:176–177, II:179
  prevalence of, II:175
Free association, II:5
Freud, S., II:5, II:41
Frontal lobe syndromes, III:312,
  III:314. *See also* Head injury
  alcoholism and, I:366–367
  assessment for, I:355–364
  attention-deficit hyperactivity
    disorder and, I:365–366
  neurobiology of, I:353–355, I:358
  psychopathology and, I:364–366,
    I:379–381
  reflexes and, I:362–363
  signs of, I:362–363
  treatment of, I:367–379
Fungizone IV. *See* Amphotericin B
Furosemide, use in patient taking
  lithium, II:402

GABA. *See* gamma-Aminobutyric
  acid
Gabapentin, III:119–120
  advantage of, III:119
  for elderly patients, III:119
  side effects of, III:120
  use in liver disease, III:119
  use in renal disease, III:119
Gabbard, G. O., II:4
Gait disturbance
  frontal lobe dysfunction and,
    I:363
  in Huntington's disease, II:486
  in Parkinson's disease, II:448
Galactorrhea, risperidone-induced,
  III:114
Galveston Orientation and Amnesia
  Test (GOAT), **III:320, III:321,**
  III:322, **III:326**
Gamete intrafallopian transfer
  (GIFT), II:308–309

Gamete intrafallopian transfer
(GIFT) *(continued)*
cost of, II:308
delivery rate for, II:309
Ganciclovir, III:304
Gas chromatography/mass
spectrometry, I:155–156
Gastrointestinal disease, I:460,
III:21–26
effect on drug absorption, III:2,
III:3, **III:6,** III:21–22
gastroenteritis in bone marrow
transplant recipients,
III:433
hypnosis for, II:54–55
use of antidepressants in,
III:23–24
use of antipsychotics in, III:22–23
use of anxiolytics in, III:22
use of carbamazepine in, III:25
use of lithium in, III:24–25
use of valproate in, I:77, III:25–26
Gastrointestinal effects
of electroconvulsive therapy,
I:103
of fluoxetine, II:73
of nefazodone, III:96
of zolpidem, III:131
Gate theory of pain, II:371–374
Gay Men's Health Crisis, III:288
Gender effects
on prevalence of fatigue, III:223,
III:228
on prevalence of HIV infection,
III:258–259
on psychopharmacokinetics, III:1
on reactions to infertility
treatment, II:314–316
Gene mapping, II:167
General Health Questionnaire
(GHQ), II:223, II:314
for multiple sclerosis patients,
II:431–432, II:435
Genetic counseling, II:168, II:181

for Huntington's disease,
II:171–172, II:190,
II:502–503
for psychiatric disorders,
II:190–191
Genetic diseases, II:178–184
classification of, II:179–181
definition of, II:178–179
finding disease genes for,
II:181–184
direct approaches, II:181–182
animal models, II:182
reverse genetics, II:181–182
indirect approaches, II:182–184
association studies, II:183
linkage studies, II:184
markers, II:182–183
sib pair method, II:183–184
genotypes, II:181
phenotypes, II:178–180
autosomal dominant, II:179
autosomal recessive, II:179
chromosomal, II:179–180
X-linked, II:179
Genetic screening, II:168
Genetic testing, II:167–191
confidentiality of, II:190
definition of, II:168
ethical issues in, II:168, II:189–190
Huntington's disease, II:168,
II:170–172
helping patients who request,
II:190–191
informed consent for, II:171,
II:189
for inherited diseases of nervous
system, II:169–177
adrenoleukodystrophy, II:177
Alzheimer's disease,
II:173–174
fragile X syndrome, II:175–177
Huntington's disease,
II:169–173, II:482–485
neurofibromatosis, II:175

tuberous sclerosis, II:174–175
prenatal, II:168
rationale for, II:167–168
Genetics
of hemophilia, I:196
of Huntington's disease, II:474
of psychiatric disorders,
    II:185–189
  adoption studies, II:186
  etiologic and genetic
      heterogeneity, II:187–188
  genetic linkage studies,
      II:188–189
  genetic mechanisms,
      II:186–187
  twin studies, II:186
psychopharmacokinetics and,
    III:1
of sickle cell disease, I:203–204
of thalassemia, I:210–213
Genotypes, II:181
Georgia Living Wills Statute, II:552
Germ-free hospital environment,
    III:417, III:443–445
"Giving-up complex," II:211
Glasgow Coma Score (GCS),
    III:320, III:322, **III:326**
Global Assessment Scale (GAS),
    II:81
Glossitis, triazolam-induced, II:89
Glucose-6-phosphate
    dehydrogenase deficiency,
    II:178
Glucuronidation, III:14
  in liver disease, III:37–39
  in renal disease, III:52
Glutamate, in Huntington's disease,
    II:473
Glutamic acid decarboxylase, II:239
Glutathione peroxidase, II:453
Glutethimide, use in renal disease,
    III:58–59
Glyburide, sertraline interaction
    with, II:75

Gold salts, **III:186**
Gonadotropin secretion
  effect of endogenous opioids on,
      II:267
  in polycystic ovarian disease,
      II:265–268
Gonadotropin-releasing hormone
    (GnRH) analogs, II:264
Graded exposure techniques,
    II:391
Graft-versus-host disease (GvHD),
    III:416–419, III:431–432,
    III:437–438
  chronic, III:438, III:451
  clinical features of, III:438
  prevalence after bone marrow
      transplantation, III:437,
      III:438
  prevention of, III:438
Grief
  excess mortality related to,
      II:222–223
  preceding ventricular
      arrhythmias, II:217
Griseofulvin, **III:186**
Group therapy
  for depressed multiple sclerosis
      patients, II:434
  for families, I:497–498
  for HIV-infected persons,
      III:287–288
  for pain management training,
      II:354–355
  for smoking cessation, I:577, I:584
Growth disorders, in bone marrow
    transplant recipients, III:435,
    III:451
Growth hormone, II:83
Guanoxan, **III:82**
Guardianship, II:515, II:517, II:533,
    II:540–541, II:574
  Florida law on, II:517, II:519
  "limited" versus traditional,
      II:518

Gynecomastia,
    risperidone-induced, III:114

Hair pulling, I:296–297
Halazepam
    formulations of, **III:8**
    half-life of, **III:19**
    metabolism of, **III:9**
    use in liver disease, III:42
Half-life, **III:5, III:16,** III:16–18
    apparent volume of distribution
        and, III:17, III:34
    of benzodiazepines, III:18, **III:19,**
        III:284
    calculation of, III:17
    disease effects on, III:18
    of metabolites, III:18, **III:19**
Hallucinations
    anesthetic-induced, II:402
    in Parkinson's disease,
        III:159–160
    postpartum, II:255
    zolpidem-induced, III:133
Haloperidol, II:603
    clinical response related to
        serum level of, II:120
    for delirium, I:332–333
    extrapyramidal effects of, II:81
    first-pass metabolism of, III:2
    formulations of, **III:8**
    for head-injured patient, III:329,
        III:330
    for HIV-infected persons, III:283,
        III:285–286
    for Huntington's disease,
        II:495–497, **II:496**
    interaction with fluoxetine, **III:87**
    interaction with paroxetine, II:76
    intravenous, III:103–104, III:286
    for multiple sclerosis patients,
        II:436
    parenteral, II:116–118
        for agitated patients in
            intensive care, II:116

combined with lorazepam,
    II:124
guidelines for administration
    of, **II:114**
intramuscular, II:117–118
intravenous, II:116–117
for persons with mental
    retardation, I:519
for postoperative agitation and
    delirium, II:404
torsades de pointes induced by,
    III:103–104, III:286
use in liver disease, III:44
use in renal disease, III:53,
    III:60–61
use in respiratory disease, II:124
Haloperidol decanoate, **II:114,**
    II:118–120
    dosage of, II:119
    extrapyramidal effects of,
        II:119–120
    guidelines for administration of,
        II:114, II:119–120
    half-life of, II:118–119
Halothane, II:397
    headaches due to, II:402
Halstead Category Test, II:418
Hamilton Anxiety Scale, III:268
Hamilton Rating Scale for
    Depression, II:126, III:113,
        III:268, III:278, III:323, **III:327**
    for multiple sclerosis patients,
        II:433, II:435
Harvey, W., II:199
Head injury, III:307–340
    attention-deficit hyperactivity
        disorder and, I:365–366,
            III:319, III:322
    brain imaging after, III:311–313,
        III:321, III:325–328
    bupropion-induced seizures in
        patients with, II:79
    classification of severity of,
        III:308–309

clinical interview and
neuropsychiatric mental
status examination after,
III:321, III:322–323
deaths due to, III:307
depression after, III:309–310,
III:311
DSM-IV diagnoses associated
with, **III:309**, III:309–310
history taking for patient with,
III:319–322, **III:320–321**
peritraumatic history,
III:319–322
pretraumatic or premorbid
history, III:319
incidence of, III:307
mild, III:307–340
neuropsychiatric assessment of
patient with, III:318,
III:320–321
neuropsychological testing of
patient with, III:323–325,
III:326–327
clinically driven testing,
III:323–324
forensically driven testing,
III:324
test domains, III:324–325
pathophysiology of, III:310–314
clinical significance of,
III:314
contusions and lacerations,
III:310–312
diffuse axonal injury,
III:310–311, III:313–314
indirect damage, III:312–313
shear damage, III:312–313
personality change after, III:310,
III:312, **III:312**
postconcussional disorder after,
III:314–317, **III:316**
posttraumatic stress disorder
after, III:317–318
prognosis for, III:319, III:321–322

psychotropic medications for
persons with, III:328–340,
III:330–334
antidepressants, III:335–337
antiepileptic drugs, III:337–339
benzodiazepines, III:339
buspirone, III:339–340
dopamine agonists, III:329,
III:335
dopamine antagonists, III:329
lithium, III:337
psychostimulants, III:335
SPECT evaluation of, II:157
types of, III:308
Headache
brain tumors and, I:414
in children, I:420–421
in chronic fatigue syndrome,
III:221
classification of, I:396–419
clinical evaluation of, I:394–396
dental work and, I:418
felbamate-induced, III:117
head trauma and, I:411–412
high cervical disc disease and,
I:418–419
laboratory tests for, I:395–396
migraine
causes of, I:401
in children, I:420–421
cocaine and, I:416–417
depression and, I:404–405
symptoms of, I:398–400
treatment of, I:401–406
postconcussional, III:315
risperidone-induced, III:114
sinus, I:418, I:421
tension
causes of, I:408
diagnosis of, I:407–408
substance abuse and, I:416
treatment of, I:408–409
vascular, I:412–413
"whiplash," I:418

Health maintenance organizations
(HMOs)
brief psychotherapy related to
medical service utilization
in, II:8
limits on reimbursement for
psychotherapy, II:9
Heart rate
morning surge in, II:227
during sexual activity, II:229
Heatstroke, I:435
Hematologic disorders, I:193–232
bone marrow transplantation
for, III:415–460
Hematologic effects
of carbamazepine, I:71–72,
III:120–121
of fluoxetine, III:90–91
of valproate, I:78, III:125–127
of zidovudine, III:283
Hematomas, brain, III:310–311
Hemodialysis, III:51
fluoxetine metabolism in
patients on, II:71
Hemoglobinuria, paroxysmal
nocturnal, III:417
Hemophilia, I:194–203
in children and adolescents,
I:199–200
epidemiology of, I:194–196
family support for, I:198–199
genetics of, I:196
HIV infection and, I:202–203,
III:260
medication for psychiatric
disorders in, I:201
mental health services for, I:194
psychiatric issues related to,
I:200–202
symptoms of, I:195–196
Hepatic blood flow (HBF), III:32–33
in congestive heart failure, III:28
diseases affecting, III:33
Hepatic disease. See Liver disease

Hepatic encephalopathy, II:93
Hepatic metabolism of drugs, III:2,
III:9, **III:9,** III:14–15
in cardiac disease, III:27
in liver disease, III:36–40
Herpesviruses
chronic fatigue syndrome and,
III:231–232
genital herpes infection, I:294
herpes encephalitis, I:171
vulvar herpes simplex virus
(HSV), **III:394,** III:395
vulvar herpes zoster, **III:394,**
III:395
Hexamethylpropyleneamine oxime,
technetium-99m-labeled,
II:146–148, **II:147,** II:492
Hexobarbital, use in renal disease,
III:54–55
Hickman catheter–related
problems, III:436–437
Hidradenitis suppurativa, vulvar,
III:392
Hippocratic Oath, II:589
Hirsutism, II:265, II:268
HIV. See Human immunodeficiency
virus (HIV) infection
Hives, I:288–290
Hivid. See Zalcitabine
Hodgkin's disease, bone marrow
transplantation for, III:419
Homocystinuria, II:180
Homosexuality
children of lesbian women,
II:313
HIV infection and, III:258–260
Homovanillic acid (HVA), tacrine
effects on, III:136
Hormone replacement therapy
after bone marrow
transplantation, III:456
for symptoms of menopause,
II:274–276
Horowitz, M., II:27–33

Hospitalization
  involuntary, II:519–521
  of patient with out-of-control
    behavior, II:603–604
  for postpartum psychosis,
    II:256
  use of hypnosis during,
    II:46–47
Hostility, of new mother toward
  infant, II:248, II:250
Hot flushes, II:269, II:271
Human Ecology Action League
  (HEAL), III:351
Human herpes virus 6, chronic
  fatigue syndrome and,
  III:231–232
Human immunodeficiency virus
  type 1 (HIV-1), III:261
  type 2 (HIV-2), III:261
Human immunodeficiency virus
  (HIV) infection, II:411,
  III:257–290
  AIDS dementia complex,
    I:245–246, I:248, I:254–256,
    III:268–277
    brain imaging in, III:276
    cerebrospinal fluid analysis
      in, III:276
    clinical features of, III:269–270
    diagnosis of, **III:271–274,**
      III:276
    neuropsychological testing
      for, III:276–277
    pathogenesis of, III:274–276
    prevalence and incidence of,
      III:270, III:274
    staging of, III:270, **III:275**
    terminology for, III:268–269
    treatment of, III:286
  assessing immunologic status in,
    III:260
  Centers for Disease Control
    classification system for,
    III:259, III:260

  central nervous system disorders
    in, I:245–247, II:154–155,
    III:271–274
  depression and, III:267–268,
    III:269–270, III:277–278
  epidemiology of, I:245
  hemophilia and, I:202–203, III:260
  incidence of, III:257
  among injecting drug users,
    III:258–260, **III:267,**
    III:269–270, III:289
  laboratory tests for, I:251–252
  manic syndromes and,
    III:279–280
  maternal-to-infant transmission
    of, III:262
  mechanisms of infection and
    virology in, III:261–262
  neuropsychological testing in,
    I:254
  outcome of, III:262
  prevalence of psychiatric
    morbidity in, III:266–268,
    III:269–270
  psychiatric disorders in, I:244,
    I:249–250
  psychiatric evaluation in,
    I:252–254
  psychopharmacologic and
    somatic therapies for,
    III:280–286
    antidepressants, I:255,
      III:280–282
    antimanic drugs, III:283–284
    anxiolytics, III:284
    for delirium, III:285–286
    for dementia, III:286
    electroconvulsive therapy,
      III:283
    neuroleptics, III:284–285
    neuropsychiatric side effects
      of drugs, III:303–305
    stimulants, I:58, III:282–283
  psychotherapy for, III:286–288

Human immunodeficiency virus
(HIV) infection *(continued)*
role of psychiatrist in
management of, III:257–258
search for causative agent in,
III:260–261
among severely mentally ill
patients, III:288
sexual activity of person with,
II:538
sexual counseling about,
I:202–203
shifting demographics of,
III:258–259
SPECT evaluation of, II:154–156
suicidality and, III:268, III:279,
III:287
symptoms and complications of,
I:250–251
syphilis and, I:265–266
testing for, III:262–265
antibody responses, III:263
counseling before and after,
III:265–266
distress related to, III:264–265
enzyme-linked
immunosorbent assay,
III:264
patient's right not to be tested,
II:605
in sperm donors, II:310
treatment of, I:255–257
tuberculosis and, III:289–290
screening for, III:290
Human lymphocyte antigens
(HLAs)
histocompatibility testing for,
III:417
in multiple sclerosis, II:412
Human menopausal gonadotropin,
II:307
cost of, II:307
multiple pregnancies due to,
II:307

ovarian hyperstimulation due to,
II:307
for ovulation induction, II:307
Human papillomavirus (HPV)
infection, III:396
Human T-lymphotropic virus
(HTLV), III:260–261
Hunter, J., II:199
Huntington's disease (HD),
I:351–352, II:471–504
age at onset of, II:169, II:472
clinical course of, II:169,
II:474–475
definition of, II:169, II:471
demographics of, II:471–472
diabetes mellitus and, II:490
differential diagnosis of,
II:492–494, **II:493**
genetic counseling for,
II:171–172, II:190, II:483,
II:502–503
genetic testing for, II:167,
II:169–173, II:482–485
errors in, II:483
ethical issues in, II:168,
II:170–172, II:189,
II:483
exclusion testing, II:485
follow-up after, II:171–172
genetic linkage analysis,
II:170, II:187
implications for psychiatrist,
II:173, II:483–484
as model for testing for other
neuropsychiatric
disorders, II:170
patient examination before,
II:171
patient selection for, II:171
in patients with psychiatric
disorders, II:172
potential benefits of, II:484
results of, II:172, II:484–485
genetics of, II:474

history taking and basic
  examination for, II:485–489
  bedside mental status
    examination, II:487–489
  family history, II:486
  neuropsychological testing,
    II:489
  physical findings, II:486–487,
    II:487
individual and marital therapy
  for, II:498–501, **II:499**
juvenile (Westphal) variant of,
  II:472, II:487
laboratory evaluations in,
  II:489–492
  brain imaging, II:490–491
  electroencephalography, II:492
  PET and SPECT, II:153,
    II:491–492
  routine, II:489–490
management of, II:494–504
medical features of, II:471–475,
  II:472
medications for, II:494–498
  for affective states, II:497
  cautions about drug use,
    II:497–498
  for disease prevention,
    II:494–495
  for psychotic and aggressive
    states, **II:496,** II:496–497
  to suppress movements, II:495
misdiagnosed as Parkinson's
  disease, II:448, II:449
mode of inheritance of, II:169
neurodiagnostic workup for,
  II:485
neuropathology of, II:169, II:472,
  II:490–491
neurophysiology of, II:472–473
pathophysiology of, II:473–474
placement outside family for,
  II:502
prevalence of, II:169, II:471–472

psychiatric features of, **II:476,**
  II:476–485
  alcoholism, II:479–480
  conduct and antisocial
    personality disorders,
    II:477
  dementia and cognition,
    II:480–481
  depression and affective
    syndromes, II:477–478
  in family members, II:482
  personality: apathy and
    irritability, II:478–479
  prevalence of, **II:476,**
    II:476–477
  psychodynamic factors and,
    II:481–482
  schizophrenia, II:478
racial distribution of, II:472
rehabilitation programs for, II:502
respite for caregivers of patients
  with, II:501
sex distribution of, II:471
suicide and, **II:476,** II:480
  prevention of, II:503–504
time to death after diagnosis of,
  II:475
Welfare and Social Security
  benefits for, II:501–502
Huntington's Disease Society of
  America, II:190
Hurler's syndrome, bone marrow
  transplantation for, III:417
Hydralazine, III:27, **III:186**
  lupus induced by, III:184
Hydrazine, **III:186**
Hydrocephalus, I:353
  chronic, I:415
Hydrocodone, for low-back pain,
  II:358
Hydrolysis, III:15
Hydroxychloroquine, III:208
3-Hydroxydiazepam, **III:19**
N-1-Hydroxyethylflurazepam, **III:19**

Hydroxyhaloperidol, II:120
5-Hydroxyindoleacetic acid
    (5-HIAA), tacrine effects on,
    III:136
1-Hydroxymethylmidazolam, **III:19**
9-Hydroxy-risperidone, III:114
5-Hydroxytryptamine. *See* Serotonin
Hydroxyzine, III:434
Hyperammonemia,
    valproate-induced, III:128
Hyperamylasemia,
    valproate-induced, III:128
Hyperarousal, I:60
Hyperbilirubinemia, III:34
Hypercalcemia, lithium-induced,
    III:111–112
Hypercholesterolemia,
    carbamazepine-induced, III:121
Hyperglycemia, after fluoxetine
    discontinuation, II:73
Hyperlipidemia,
    carbamazepine-induced, III:121
Hyperparathyroidism,
    lithium-induced, III:111–112
Hyperprolactinemia,
    risperidone-induced, III:114
Hypersalivation,
    clozapine-induced, III:164
Hypertension
    clozapine-induced, III:107
    electroconvulsive therapy and,
        I:109
    monoamine oxidase
        inhibitor–induced, I:66–67
    stress-related, II:202, II:204
    use of bupropion in, II:78
    venlafaxine-induced, III:94
Hyperthyroidism, II:489
Hyperviscosity syndrome, I:229–230
Hypnosis, II:39–61
    for anxiety reduction, II:43
    for assessment of conversion and
        malingering, II:44–45,
        II:57–58

for asthma, II:53–54
billing for, II:47
for classic "psychosomatic"
    disorders, II:51–55
definition of, II:42
development and utilization of
    hypnotic strategies,
    II:45–46
diverse strategies for, II:60
efficacy for physiological
    disorders, II:39–40
for gastrointestinal disorders,
    II:54–55
goal of medical hypnosis, II:45
history of, II:40–41
in hospital setting, II:46–47
for insomnia, II:58–59
measurement of hypnotic
    responsivity, II:43–45
    diagnostic usefulness, II:44–45
    Hypnotic Induction Profile
        (HIP), II:43–44
    screening procedure as
        "ceremony," II:44
    Stanford Hypnotic
        Susceptibility Scale, II:43
misperceptions about, II:39
to mitigate side effects of cancer
    chemotherapy, II:55–56
naturally occurring altered states
    of awareness and, II:40
neurophysiology of, II:47–49
    cortical event-related
        potentials, II:48
    electroencephalographic
        studies, II:47–48
    laterality of eye movements,
        II:47
other medical applications of,
    II:59, **II:60**
for pain control, II:42, II:46–47,
    II:49–50
    during and after surgery, II:50,
        II:51

compared with acupuncture,
II:49
versus placebo analgesia,
II:49
relation to endorphins,
II:49–50
self-hypnosis, II:46, II:50
patient's "gift" for, II:43, II:61
for phobias, II:56–57
psychobiological process
associated with, II:42
results of, II:60–61
safety of, II:40
for skin disorders, II:51–53
for smoking cessation, I:576
symptom substitution under,
II:40, II:42, II:46
techniques for induction of, II:46
training in, II:61
Hypnotic Induction Profile (HIP),
II:43–45, II:58
Hypnotic phenomena, II:41–43
definition of, II:42
examples of, II:42
Hypnotic trance, II:41–42
Hypnotizability, II:40, II:42–43
of children, II:43
phobic behavior related to, II:56
Hypochondriasis, II:377, III:356,
III:365
Hypoglycemia, III:217
fluoxetine-induced, II:73
headaches and, I:417–418
Hypomania, II:423
Hyponatremia
carbamazepine-induced, I:74–75,
III:122
fluoxetine-induced, II:73–74
risperidone-induced, III:114
Hypothalamic-pituitary function, in
polycystic ovarian disease,
II:265–268
Hypothyroidism
carbamazepine and, III:122

effect on albumin binding of
drugs, III:10
Hysterectomy, II:272
Hysteria, I:178, II:377, **II:493**
effect on short-term dynamic
therapy of stress response
syndromes, II:31, **II:32**
Hysterosalpingography, II:306

Ibuprofen, for low-back pain,
II:357, II:366
ICU psychosis, II:116, III:443
Illness behavior, II:375–376
Illness Behavior Questionnaire,
III:356
Imipramine
for anxiety disorders in
Parkinson's disease
patients, II:460
cardiac effects of, III:96
cardiovascular effects of, II:78
for chest pain in patients with
normal coronary
angiograms, III:99–100
drug interactions with
diltiazem, III:105
fluoxetine, **III:87**, III:89
fluvoxamine, III:86, **III:87,**
III:89
labetalol, III:105
verapamil, III:105
formulations of, **III:8**
for Huntington's disease,
II:497
inhibition of serotonin uptake
by, II:126
metabolism of, III:45, **III:85**
by cytochrome P_{450}-2D6,
III:36, **III:82**
parenteral, **II:115**, II:125–129
dosage of, II:128
for symptoms of benzodiazepine
withdrawal, II:80
use in cardiac disease, III:30

Imipramine *(continued)*
    use in renal disease, III:53,
        III:64–65
    volume of distribution of, III:13
Imipramine-binding sites, II:240
Immune system
    bone marrow transplantation for
        dysfunction of, III:415–460
    chronic fatigue syndrome and,
        III:218, III:232–233
    environmental illness and,
        III:347, III:352–353, III:368
    in HIV infection, III:257–290
Immunochemical methods of drug
        testing, I:152
Immunoglobulin G (IgG)
    chronic fatigue syndrome and,
        III:232–233, III:239, **III:243**
    in multiple sclerosis, II:411, II:414
Immunosuppressive agents,
        I:328–332
    behavioral side effects of, II:417
    before bone marrow
        transplantation, III:417,
        III:430, III:434–435
    for multiple sclerosis, II:417
    for systemic lupus
        erythematosus, III:189,
        III:207–208
Immunotherapy, for environmental
        illness, III:354
Impact-on-Family Scale, I:492–493
Impotence, II:303, II:310
Impulse control problems
    after head injury, III:314
    assessing bone marrow
        transplant candidate for,
        III:423–424
In re Conroy, II:543
In re Jane Doe, II:546–547
In re Karen Ann Quinlan, II:543
In re L.H.R., II:546
In vitro fertilization (IVF),
        II:308–309

bone marrow transplantation
        and, III:456–457
    cost of, II:308
    delivery rate for, II:309
    egg donation for, II:310
    for menopausal woman, II:310
    personalities of women seeking,
        II:309
    psychological impact of failed
        cycle of, II:315
Incompetency, II:516–517,
        II:540–541. *See also* Competency
    determinations
    historical views of, II:517
    incapacity and, II:541
    persons deprived of rights due
        to, II:517
    recent legislation related to, II:517
    standards for assessment of,
        II:541
Infanticide, II:257
Infertility, II:237
    adjustment to stresses of, II:303
    advocacy group related to, II:325
    definition of, II:302
    due to polycystic ovarian
        disease, II:265, II:268
    etiologies of, **II:302,** II:302–303
    marital problems related to,
        II:303
    medical workup for, **II:304,**
        II:304–307
        basal body temperature chart,
            II:305, II:305–306
        endometrial biopsy, II:306
        hysterosalpingography, II:306
        laparoscopy, II:306
        postcoital test, II:306
        postejaculatory urinalysis,
            II:306
        semen analysis, II:306
        transrectal ultrasound, II:306
    prevalence of, II:302
    stigma of, II:303

stresses associated with, II:301,
II:303–307
before evaluation begins,
II:303–304
during medical workup,
II:304–307
Infertility treatment, II:301–325
cost of, II:301
decision to stop, II:313–314
declining provision of, II:320–321
differences between men and
women in emotional
reactions to, II:314–316
explanations for, II:315
greater psychological
symptoms of women,
II:314–315
implications of, II:316
men's distress when there is a
male infertility factor,
II:315
donor insemination for single
women, II:312–313
forms of, II:307–310
donor insemination,
II:309–310
egg donation, II:310
endometriosis treatment,
II:308
gamete intrafallopian transfer,
II:308–309
ovulation induction, II:307–308
surrogacy, II:310
in vitro fertilization, II:308–309
zygote intrafallopian transfer,
II:308–309
helping patients cope with
stresses of, II:323–324
increasing demand for, II:302
informing child of his or her
origin, II:311–312
managing depression in women
undergoing, II:324–325
moral issues in, II:301

psychological implications of
sperm and egg donation,
II:310–312
psychological issues in other
interested parties related
to, II:317–319
children conceived through
technology, II:311–312,
II:317
family, friends, co-workers,
II:317
gamete donors, II:312,
II:317–319
physicians and staffs of
infertility programs,
II:319
religious prohibitions against,
II:311
role for psychiatry in, II:319–325
helping partners reach
consensus, II:322–323
helping patients with decision
making, II:322
psychiatric liaison with
infertility clinic,
II:319–320
screening, II:320–321
Informed consent. *See also* Consent
to treatment
assessing competency for,
II:525–533
for bone marrow
transplantation, III:426–428
for drug testing, I:147
for electroconvulsive therapy,
II:577
exceptions to requirement for,
II:572
failure to obtain, as malpractice,
II:563
for genetic testing, II:171, II:189
information that must be
disclosed for, II:540
laws related to, II:516

Informed consent *(continued)*
    medical information for, II:527,
        II:527
    necessary functional abilities for,
        II:526–527
    "patient's rights" approach to,
        II:542
    "rule of informed consent," II:539
    for treatment of children and
        adolescents, I:458–459
    for treatment of persons with
        mental retardation,
        I:528–529
Informed refusal, II:539, II:542. *See
    also* Refusal of treatment
Innovar. *See* Droperidol-fentanyl
Insemination
    artificial, with donor sperm,
        II:309–310
    in vitro, II:308–309
Insomnia. *See also* Sleep
    disturbances
    benzodiazepine hypnotics for,
        II:84–85
        estazolam, II:85–86
        quazepam, II:86–88
        rebound insomnia and,
            II:89
        selection for medically ill
            patients, II:89–90
        triazolam, II:88–89
    due to postpartum depression,
        II:252, II:253
    felbamate-induced, III:117
    hypnosis for, II:58–59
    risperidone-induced, III:114
    venlafaxine-induced, III:93
    zolpidem for, III:132–133
Insulin therapy, fluoxetine use in
    patient on, II:73
Insurance, I:608–611
Interferon-α, for chronic fatigue
    syndrome, III:241, **III:245**
Interferon alfa-2a, III:305

Interferon beta, for multiple
    sclerosis, II:417
Intermittent explosive disorder,
    II:476
International Bone Marrow
    Transplant Registry (IBMTR),
    III:420
*International Classification of
    Diseases-9*
    postpartum blues in, II:250
    postpartum psychosis in, II:255
International Society for the Study
    of Vulvovaginal Disease,
    III:386, III:403
Interpersonal conflicts, preceding
    ventricular arrhythmias,
    II:217–218
Interstitial cystitis, III:386,
    III:387–388
Interstitial Cystitis Association,
    III:387
Interstitial pneumonitis
    in bone marrow transplant
        recipient, III:451
    carbamazepine-induced,
        III:122
Intracranial pressure elevation, due
    to total-body irradiation, III:435
Intubation, fear of, II:391
Involuntary commitment, II:519–521
    for "dangerousness," II:521
    malpractice claims related to,
        II:573–575
    versus nonconsensual treatment,
        II:519–520
    Rennie v. Klein, II:520
    Rogers v. Okin, II:520
    Winters v. Miller, II:519–520
    Youngberg v. Romeo, II:520
Involutional melancholia, II:272,
    II:274
Iodine-123 (^{123}I), II:142
    amphetamine labeled with
        (IMP), II:146–148, **II:147**

benzamide labeled with (IBZM),
II:158, II:159
clonidine labeled with, II:158
commercial source for, II:146
half-life of, II:146, II:156
inconvenient features of use of,
II:146
ketanserin labeled with, II:158
lysergide labeled with, II:158
MK-801 labeled with, II:158
N1N1N'-trimethyl-N'-(2
hydroxy-3-methyl-5-123
I-iodobenzyl)-1,3-propan-
ediamine 2HCl (HIPDM),
II:156
quinuclindinyl-iodobenzilate
labeled with ([^{123}I]QNB),
II:153, II:159
RO-16-0154 labeled with
(Iomazenil), II:158
Irritability
in Huntington's disease,
II:478–479
postconcussional, III:315
Irritable bowel syndrome, II:55
Isocarboxazid, for Huntington's
disease, II:497
Isoniazid, **III:186**
interaction with valproate,
III:130
neuropsychiatric side effects of,
III:305
Isoproterenol, II:205
Isoquinazepan, **III:186**
Itching, I:293–294, I:304
hypnosis for, II:52–53
vulvar, III:381–382, III:388,
III:398–399. *See also*
Vulvodynia
Itraconazole
cytochrome P$_{450}$ inhibition by,
III:85
neuropsychiatric side effects of,
III:304

*Jefferson v. Griffin Spaulding County
Hospital Authority*, II:546
Justice, II:588–589
loyalty and, II:601–602

Kainic acid, II:474
Kaposi's sarcoma, III:259
Karnofksy score, after bone marrow
transplantation, III:452
Keratosis follicularis, I:299–300
Ketamine, II:402–403
Ketanserin, labeled with iodine-123,
II:158
Ketoconazole
cytochrome P$_{450}$-3A4 inhibition
by, III:36–37, **III:85**, III:86
for environmental illness, III:354
interaction with terfenadine,
III:86
neuropsychiatric side effects of,
III:304
Ketoprofen, for low-back pain,
II:357
Kidney disease. *See* Renal disease
Kindling, III:352
Kirby v. Spivey, II:546
Korsakoff's psychosis, II:157
Kurtzke Scale, II:418–419
Kynurenic acid, in Huntington's
disease, II:473–474

Labetalol, interaction with
imipramine, III:105
Laboratory tests
for AIDS dementia complex,
III:276
certification of laboratories, I:157
for children and adolescents,
I:457–485
for chronic fatigue syndrome,
I:274–275
drug testing, I:150–156
before electroconvulsive therapy,
I:114–115

Laboratory tests *(continued)*
   for environmental illness, III:352,
      III:367, **III:370**
   for folate deficiency, I:228
   for headache evaluation,
      I:395–396
   for HIV infection, I:251–252,
      III:262–265
   liver function tests, III:40
   for Lyme disease, I:269–270
   to measure drug blood
      concentration, III:12, III:18
   for neuroleptic malignant
      syndrome, I:441
   for persons with mental
      retardation, I:511–512
   for porphyrias, I:217–219
   smoking effects on, I:560–561
   for syphilis, I:260–263
   for systemic lupus
      erythematosus, III:195,
      III:197–198
Lacerations, brain, III:310–311
Lactate, pain associated with,
   II:371–372
Laminar-air flow rooms, III:417,
   III:443–445
Lamprene. *See* Clofazimine
Language testing, after head injury,
   III:324, **III:326**
Laparoscopy, II:306
Late luteal phase dysphoric
   disorder (LLPDD), II:257,
   II:258, II:261, II:264–265.
   See also Premenstrual
   syndrome
Laughing, pathological, **II:427,**
   II:427–428
Law of master and servant, II:578
LE cell test, III:195
Learning, under hypnosis, II:42
Legal issues. *See also* Malpractice
   competency determinations,
      II:515–533

consent to treatment, II:525–533,
      II:538–542
living wills and advance medical
      treatment directives,
      II:537–559
malpractice, II:561–581
neuropsychological testing of
      brain-injured patient,
      III:323, III:324
related to bone marrow
      transplantation, III:428–430
related to children and
      adolescents, I:458–459
related to persons with mental
      retardation, I:528–529
right-to-die cases, II:542–548
Legionnaire's disease, III:350
Lennox-Gastaut syndrome, III:116
Lentiviruses, III:261
Lesch-Nyhan syndrome, II:178
Lethal catatonia, I:434–435
Lethargy, in HIV infection, III:270
Leukemia, II:599, II:604–605
   bone marrow transplantation
      for, III:415–460
Leukopenia, use of carbamazepine
   in, III:121
Leuprolide
   for ovulation induction, II:307
   for premenstrual syndrome,
      II:264
Levodopa, I:372
   chorea induced by, **II:493,** II:494
   for head-injured patient, III:329
   "neurodestructive" effect of,
      II:453
Levodopa/carbidopa, II:448, II:456,
   III:154
   controlled-release, II:455
   for Parkinson's disease,
      III:152–153, III:161–162
   psychotoxicity of, III:161–162
   visual hallucinosis induced by,
      III:151

Levonorgestrel, II:244
Lewy bodies disease, III:168
"Liberty interest," II:544
Libido
    androgens and, II:239
        in postmenopausal women,
            II:275, II:276
    effect of menopause on, II:269
    fluoxetine effect on, II:74
    premenstrual, II:259
    progestins and, II:240–241
Lichen planus, **III:392, III:393**
Lichen sclerosus et atrophicus,
    III:390, **III:392,** III:399
Lichen simplex chronicus, II:53,
    III:384, **III:392,** III:398–399
Lidocaine
    metabolism by cytochrome
        P$_{450}$-3A4, III:85
    neurotoxicity of, II:402
    use in cardiac disease patients,
        III:26
Life-support systems, II:541
    durable power of attorney for
        health care and, II:555–556
    living will directives related to,
        II:552–553
    nutrition and hydration systems
        as, II:545, II:547, II:553,
        II:556
    withholding and withdrawal of,
        II:542. *See also* Right-to-die
        cases
Lightheadedness
    nefazodone-induced, III:96
    stress-related, II:205
Linear kinetics, III:18–19
Lipid solubility of drugs, III:12–14
Lipid storage diseases, bone
    marrow transplantation for,
    III:419
Lisinopril, interaction with lithium,
    III:113
Lithium, **II:493,** III:79, III:110–113

cardiac effects of, III:31
diabetes and, I:41
distribution of, III:13
drug interactions with, I:42–44,
    III:112–113
    anesthetics, II:402
    fluoxetine, II:72, II:74
    valproate, III:127–128
EEG detection of, I:171–172
electroconvulsive therapy and,
    I:112
excretion of, III:36
formulations of, **III:8,** III:24
for head-injured patient, **III:333,**
    III:337, III:337
for HIV-infected persons, III:282,
    III:283
for Huntington's disease, II:496,
    II:496
lupus induced by, **III:186**
for multiple sclerosis patients,
    II:436
parathyroid function and,
    III:111–112
parenteral, **II:115,** II:130–132
    advantages of, II:131
    guidelines for administration
        of, **II:115,** II:131
    indications for, II:130–131
    pharmacokinetics of, II:131
    preparations of, II:132
    side effects of, II:131–132
    for thyroid storm, II:131
    toxicity of, II:131
parkinsonism induced by,
    II:452
for persons with mental
    retardation, I:523–524
pregnancy and, I:620–623
for premenstrual syndrome,
    II:264
renal failure and, III:110–111
side effects of, I:39–40, I:298–300,
    III:283

Lithium *(continued)*
    use in cardiac disease, III:27,
        III:31–32, III:112
    use in gastrointestinal disease,
        III:24–25
    use in liver disease, III:33, III:46–47
    use in renal disease, **III:60–61,**
        III:66–67, III:111
    volume of distribution of, III:13
Liver disease, I:45–46, III:32–49. *See
    also* Cirrhosis
    antidepressant use in, III:44–46
        fluoxetine, II:70–71, III:45–46,
            III:92
        sertraline, II:75, III:46
        trazodone, III:45
        tricyclics, III:39, III:41, III:44–45
        venlafaxine, III:94
    antipsychotic drug use in,
        III:43–44
    anxiolytic drug use in, III:42–43
    ascites and, III:35
    benzodiazepine use in, II:122–123
    bupropion use in, II:79
    buspirone use in, II:84
    carbamazepine use in, I:72–73,
        III:47–48
    clonazepam use in, I:80–81
    delirium and, I:325
    felbamate use in, III:49
    flumazenil use in, II:91
    gabapentin use in, III:119
    hepatic encephalopathy, II:93
    hyperbilirubinemia and, III:34
    lithium use in, III:46–47
    midazolam use in, II:122, II:123
    pharmacokinetic effects of, **III:7,**
        III:32–35
        bioavailability, III:32–33, III:39
        drug metabolism, III:36–40,
            III:38
        flow-limited and
            enzyme-limited drugs,
            III:32–33, III:39

    hepatic blood flow and,
        III:32–33
    hepatic clearance, III:39
    preservation of
        glucuronidation
        reaction, III:37–39
    protein binding of drugs,
        III:10, III:34–35
    systemic availability,
        III:39–40
    quazepam use in, II:87
    recommendation for drug
        dosing in, III:40–42
    renal disease and, III:41–42
    tacrine use in, II:96, II:97
    valproate use in, I:77–78,
        III:48–49, III:126, III:128
    zolpidem use in, III:131
Liver extract-folic acid-
    cyanocobalamin (LEFAC), for
    chronic fatigue syndrome,
    III:239, **III:242**
Liver function tests, III:40
Living wills, II:537, II:552–553. *See
    also* Advance medical
    treatment directives
    availability of, II:552
    compared to durable power of
        attorney for health care,
        II:555–556
    Georgia Living Wills Statute,
        II:552
    language required for, II:552
    purpose of, II:552
    requirements for, II:553
    restrictions on, II:553
Locality rule, II:564
Long Q-T syndrome (LQTS),
    II:213–214, II:221
    treatment of, II:214
Loratadine, III:103
Lorazepam, II:20, II:603
    achieving steady state of,
        III:17

for bone marrow transplant
recipient, III:439
clearance of, III:17
formulations of, **III:8**
half-life of, III:17, **III:19,** III:284
for head-injured patient, **III:334,**
III:339
for HIV-infected persons, III:284,
III:286
interaction with fluvoxamine,
III:87
interaction with valproate,
III:127, III:129
intramuscular, III:3
metabolism of, II:122, **III:9,**
III:14–15, III:52
for nausea and vomiting, III:434
onset of action of, III:3
parenteral, **II:114–115,** II:116,
II:122–123
combined with haloperidol,
II:124
intramuscular, II:123
intravenous, II:123
for patient with low-back pain,
II:367
pharmacokinetics of, II:122
for postanesthesia emergence
reactions, II:403
for preanesthetic anxiety,
II:393–394
use in cardiac disease, III:27
use in elderly patients and
children, II:125
use in liver disease, III:39, III:42
use in renal disease, **III:56–57**
volume of distribution of, III:13,
III:17
Loss, II:15
Loss of chance rule, II:579–580
Loss of consciousness (LOC),
III:320
diffuse axonal injury indicated
by, III:313

severity of brain injury based on,
III:308–309
"Low-back loser," II:337, II:377
Low-back pain (LBP), II:331–383
acute, subacute, and chronic,
II:348–349, **II:350**
analgesics for, **II:356–359**
anatomy and physiology of,
II:360, II:370
behavioral mechanisms in
progression from acute to
chronic pain, II:376
conditioned fear model, II:376
muscle reeducation model,
II:376
operant model, II:376
psychophysiological model,
II:376
biopsychosocial model of,
II:332–335
Diagnostic Net, II:332–334,
II:333, II:336, II:339
biopsychosocial phenomenology
of acute versus chronic
pain, II:348–349, **II:350**
causes of, II:339, II:370
chronic disability due to, II:334
chronic pain as psychiatric
disorder, II:377–380
clinical course of, II:332–333
clinical management of,
II:334–351
consultation and referral process
for, II:335–339
patient's perspective, II:337
psychiatrist's perspective,
II:338–339
referring physician's
perspective, II:335, II:337
depression and, II:341, II:366,
II:378–379, II:381–382
economic impact of, II:332, II:334
factors affecting outcome of,
II:332, II:334

Low-back pain (LBP) *(continued)*
  family therapy for, II:368–369
  impact of chronic disability due
      to, II:334, **II:335**
  management of chronic pain,
      II:354–363
    multidisciplinary
        rehabilitation team,
        II:354
    pain management protocol,
        II:362, **II:363**
    pain management training,
        II:354–355, II:360–362
  management of subacute pain,
      II:351–354, **II:353**
    advocating for patient, II:352
    goal-oriented plan, II:352,
        II:353
    objectives for, II:352
  medical psychiatric evaluation
      and management of acute
      pain, II:339–341
  medical psychiatric evaluation
      of chronic pain, II:341–348
    biomechanical, functional,
        and vocational
        assessment, II:347–348
    laboratory examinations, II:347
    pain medicine interview,
        II:343–345
    pain rating charts, II:343,
        II:343
    patient record keeping, **II:343,**
        II:348
    physical examination,
        II:345–346
    questionnaires, II:342–343
    radiography, II:346–347
    reasons for, II:342
    stages of, II:341
    usual practices for, II:341
  myofascial pain syndrome and,
      II:337, II:368, II:370,
      II:372–374

  occupational therapy for, II:348,
      II:368
  physical therapy for, II:367–368
  prevalence of, II:332, II:334
  problems in pharmacotherapy
      for, II:364–367
    benzodiazepine and other
        sedative dependency,
        II:367
    excessive reliance on
        narcotics, II:364–366
    untreated or partially treated
        major depression, II:366
  psychiatric comorbidity with
      chronic pain, II:381–382
  psychiatric disorder and
      psychosocial factors
      affecting outcome of,
      II:332, II:334–335
  "psychiatric" profile of patient
      with, II:337
  psychological factors in chronic
      pain, II:375–376
    external health locus of
        control, II:375
    hysteria, II:375
    illness behavior, II:375–376
    predisposing factors, II:375
    type A personality, II:375
    used to predict treatment
        outcome, II:376
  psychotherapy for, II:369
  risk factors for outcome in
      chronic pain, **II:335**, II:382
  terminology related to, II:370
  treatment along pathway to
      chronicity, II:351, **II:351**
"Low-back schools," II:340
Loxapine, **III:8**
  intramuscular, **II:114**
Lumbar puncture, in systemic
    lupus erythematosus, III:196,
    III:198
Lumbosacral sprain or strain, II:370

Lung cancer, bone marrow
transplantation for, III:419
Lupron. *See* Leuprolide
Lupus
discoid, III:184, III:187
drug-induced, III:184
clinical features of, III:184,
III:187
differentiating from systemic
lupus erythematosus,
III:184
drugs associated with,
III:186
carbamazepine, III:122
chlorpromazine, III:184
hydralazine, III:184
procainamide, III:184
valproate, III:129
laboratory features of, III:184,
III:187
treatment of, III:184
Lupus anticoagulant (LA), III:204
Luteinizing hormone (LH), II:306
in bone marrow transplant
recipients, III:454, III:455
in endometriosis, II:268
in human menopausal
gonadotropin, II:307
in polycystic ovarian disease,
II:266–267
Lyme disease, I:267–271
cause of, I:267
epidemiology of, I:267
laboratory tests for, I:269–270
neuropsychiatric diagnosis in,
I:270–271
symptoms of, I:267–269
treatment of, I:271
Lymphadenopathy, in chronic
fatigue syndrome, III:221
Lymphomas, bone marrow
transplantation for, III:415–460
Lysergide, labeled with iodine-123,
II:159

Macrophages, role in multiple
sclerosis, II:411
Magical beliefs, about death,
II:227–228
Magnesium, for chronic fatigue
syndrome, III:241, **III:243**
Magnetic resonance imaging (MRI)
after head injury, III:313, **III:321,**
III:325–328
after stroke, II:151
in AIDS dementia complex,
III:276
applications of, I:11–12
compared with SPECT, II:141
computed tomography and,
I:8–12
contraindications to, I:11
in dementia, II:152
for elderly persons, I:12–13
to evaluate headache, I:394–395
in HIV infection, II:155
in Huntington's disease,
II:490–491
mechanism of, I:9–10, I:13–14
in multiple sclerosis, II:414–415,
II:419
of spine, II:347
in systemic lupus
erythematosus, II:154,
III:198, III:199–201
Magnetoencephalography, I:22,
I:181
Major histocompatibility complex,
genes associated with multiple
sclerosis, II:412
Malaise, in chronic fatigue
syndrome, III:221
Malignant hyperthermia, I:435,
I:439–440
Malingering, I:208, I:611–612,
II:377
dermatitis artefacta, I:294–296
hypnosis for assessment of,
II:58

Malnutrition
    effect on albumin binding of
        drugs, III:10
    quazepam use in, II:87
Malpractice, II:561–581. *See also*
    Legal issues
    definition of, II:563
    legal principles related to,
        II:561–567
        establishing malpractice,
            II:563–565
        damages, II:566–567
        dereliction or departure
            from standard of
            care, II:563–565
        direct or proximate
            causation, II:566
        duty, II:565
        tort law, II:561–563
    liability related to
        electroconvulsive therapy
            for medically ill patients,
            II:575–578
    potential sources of liability for
        psychiatric consultants,
        II:568–575
        related to consultation
            relationship, II:569–573
        related to involuntary
            commitment, II:573–575
        related to missed diagnosis,
            II:578–580
        loss of chance rule, II:579–580
    standards of care in
        medical-psychiatric
        practice, II:567–569
Malpractice insurance, II:563
Mania
    cerebral blood flow studies in,
        II:158
    due to postpartum psychosis,
        II:255
    versus euphoria, II:423
    HIV-related, III:279–280

    in multiple sclerosis, II:435–436
Manifest and latent content,
        II:591–599
    case studies of, II:593–596
    definitions of, II:592
    determining in medically ill
        patients, II:596–597
    impact on establishing
        diagnosis, II:596
    in patient manifesting
        noncompliance, II:597–599
MAOIs. *See* Monoamine oxidase
    inhibitors
Maprotiline
    for fibromyalgia, **III:247**
    formulations of, **III:8**
    for HIV-infected persons, III:282
    use in renal disease, **III:54–55**
Marfan's syndrome, II:180
Marinol. *See* Dronabinol
Marital therapy, for Huntington's
    disease patients, II:500
Marriage
    effect of childlessness on, II:316
    effect of infertility on, II:303,
        II:316
Martin-Bell syndrome. *See* Fragile X
    syndrome
Masturbation
    premenstrual, II:259
    to provide semen sample for
        analysis, II:307
"Materiality rule," II:540
Maternal-infant bonding, II:251
Mazicon. *See* Flumazenil
Medical care team and families of
    ill children, I:486, I:496–497
Medical decision making dilemmas,
    II:537–538
Medical hypnosis. *See* Hypnosis
"Medical ovariectomy," II:264
Medical service utilization, II:8
Medical-psychiatric units, II:604
Medicare, II:538

Meditation, effect on ventricular arrhythmias, II:225, **II:226**

Medroxyprogesterone
added to estrogen replacement therapy, II:275
for contraception during postpartum psychosis, II:256
for endometriosis, II:308

Melena, fluoxetine-induced, III:90

Memory deficits
alcoholism and, I:366
buspirone and, II:82
in chronic fatigue syndrome, III:221
cigarette smoking and, I:547
electroconvulsive therapy–induced, I:133
estazolam and, II:86
in HIV infection, III:269
midazolam and, I:60
in multiple sclerosis, II:418
postconcussional, III:312, III:315
testing for, III:324–325, **III:326**
triazolam and, II:88
among Vietnam veterans with posttraumatic stress disorder, III:317–318

Menarche, II:241–242
depression after, II:241
emotional responses to, II:237, II:241
among black girls, II:241–242
concealment taboos and, II:242
girls' sources of information about, II:241

Meningitis
aseptic, I:247
cryptococcal, II:154

Meningovascular syphilis, I:259

Menopause, II:269–276
age of, II:269–271
definition of, II:269
depression related to, II:272–274

diagnosis of, II:270–271
dysesthetic vulvodynia after, III:402
estrogen replacement therapy for symptoms of, II:270
factors affecting timing of, II:271
hormone treatment for, II:274–275
medical view of, II:270
mood changes associated with, II:237, II:271–272
nonmedical view of, II:269–270
physiologic symptoms of, II:269
premature, due to total-body irradiation, III:435
psychopathology related to, II:272
psychosocial factors and, II:270
sociocultural impact of, II:273
surgical, II:272
vaginal dryness due to, II:269, II:276
vasomotor symptoms of, II:269, II:271

Mental retardation, I:507–529
assessing bone marrow transplant candidate for, III:423
buspirone to reduce aggression and anxiety in, II:81
drug treatment for, I:518–529
due to fragile X syndrome, II:175–176
epidemiology of psychiatric disorders in, I:508
legal issues related to, I:528–529
psychiatric disorders and, I:509–517
psychiatric evaluation of persons with, I:510–512
valproate for persons with, III:125

Mental status examination
after head injury, **III:321,**
III:322–323
versus competency
determinations, II:522
in Huntington's disease,
II:487–489
standard of care for, II:568
Mental Status Examination in
Neurology, **III:326**
Meperidine, I:61–62
interaction with monoamine
oxidase inhibitors, II:399,
II:401
interaction with selegiline, II:98,
II:400
interaction with tacrine, II:97
Mephenytoin, **III:186**
Meprobamate, use in renal disease,
III:60–61
Mepron. *See* Atovaquone
Mering procedure, III:397
Mesmer, II:40
Mesoridazine, **III:8**
contraindicated for patients with
cardiac conduction defects,
II:118
intramuscular, **II:114,** II:118
Met-enkephalin, in Huntington's
disease, II:473
Metergoline, II:83
Methacholine, II:54
Methadone
interaction with rifampin, III:290
for low-back pain, **II:358,**
II:365–366
Methamphetamine, **III:83**
Methaqualone, use in renal disease,
III:60–61
Methimazole, **III:186**
Methotrexate, III:417, III:435
for multiple sclerosis, II:417
Methoxamine hydrochloride,
II:400

3-Methoxy-4-hydroxyphenylglycol
(MHPG)
in Parkinson's disease, II:450
in polycystic ovarian disease,
II:266
Methoxyphenamine, **III:82**
N-Methyl-D-aspartate (NMDA),
II:473
N-Methyl-D-aspartate (NMDA)
receptors, role in AIDS
dementia complex, III:275
Methylation, III:15
Methyldopa, II:452, **III:186**
Methylphenidate, I:373, I:477, **II:493**
as adjunct to tricyclic
antidepressants, II:129
for bone marrow transplant
recipient, III:440
contraindicated for psychosis,
II:130
formulations of, **III:8**
for head-injured patients,
III:330, III:335
for HIV-infected persons,
III:282–283
intravenous, **II:115,** II:129–130
for Parkinson's disease patients,
II:460
for poststroke depression, III:113
use in cardiac disease, II:129
1-Methyl-4-phenyl-1,2,5,6,
tetrahydropyridine (MPTP),
II:447
Methylprednisolone, for multiple
sclerosis, II:416
Methylthiouracil, **III:186**
Methysergide, **III:186**
Metoclopramide, **II:493,** III:2, III:434
parkinsonism induced by, II:452
Metoprolol, II:216, **III:186**
interaction with fluoxetine,
III:88
metabolism of, **III:82**
Michaelis-Menten kinetics, III:19–20

β2-Microglobulin
  in AIDS dementia complex, III:276
  in renal disorders, III:51
Midazolam, I:59–60
  flumazenil to reverse sedation
    induced by, II:91, II:92
  formulations of, **III:8**
  half-life of, **III:19**
  interaction with cyclosporine,
    III:37
  intramuscular, III:3
  metabolism of, II:122, **III:9**
    by cytochrome P_{450}-3A4,
      III:36, III:85
  for outpatient surgery, II:396
  parenteral, **II:114–115**, II:116,
    II:122–123
    intravenous, II:123
    use in respiratory disease,
      II:124
  patient-controlled, for
    postoperative anxiety,
    II:392
  for postanesthesia emergence
    reactions, II:403
  for preanesthetic anxiety, II:393
  use in liver disease, II:122, II:123,
    III:43
  use in renal disease, **III:58–59**
  volume of distribution of, III:13
Migraine. *See* Headache
Millon Behavioral Health
  Inventory, I:607–608
Mini-Mental State Exam (MMSE),
  II:94, II:96, **II:528**, III:134, III:277
  for head-injured patient, III:322,
    III:326
  in Huntington's disease,
    II:488–489
  in multiple sclerosis, **II:420**
  in Parkinson's disease, II:450
Minnesota Multiphasic Personality
  Inventory (MMPI), II:218,
  III:323, **III:327,** III:356

  for multiple sclerosis patients,
    II:430, II:432
  for patients with low-back pain,
    II:342, II:349, II:375, II:378
MK-801, labeled with iodine-123,
  II:159
Moclobemide, for vulvodynia,
  III:408
Modified Stroop Test, **II:420**
Molindone
  formulations of, **III:8**
  for head-injured patient, **III:331**
  for HIV-infected persons, III:285
Molluscum contagiosum, **III:394,**
  III:396
Monoamine oxidase (MAO), II:239
Monoamine oxidase inhibitors
  (MAOIs), II:129, III:79
  cheese reaction and, II:400
  for depression, II:239
  electroconvulsive therapy and,
    I:109–110
  for head-injured patient, **III:332,**
    III:335–337
  for HIV-infected persons, III:282
  interaction with anesthetics,
    I:61–65, I:109, II:399–400,
    II:401
  interaction with fluoxetine, II:72
  metabolized by cytochrome
    P_{450}-2D6, **III:82**
  for migraine headaches,
    I:403–404
  over-the-counter drugs and,
    I:68–70
  for premenstrual syndrome,
    II:264
  preoperative discontinuance of,
    II:399, II:400
  selegiline, II:98
  side effects of, I:63, I:65–68
  tacrine, II:94, II:97
  use in gastrointestinal disease,
    III:23

Monoamine oxidase inhibitors
  (MAOIs) *(continued)*
  use in renal disease, **III:62–63**
  withdrawal from, I:70–72
Mononucleosis, chronic. *See*
  Chronic fatigue syndrome
Mood disorders. *See also* Bipolar
  disorder; Depression; Mania
  after head injury, III:309–310,
    III:311, III:314, III:315
  associated with HIV infection,
    III:267–268
  cigarette smoking–induced,
    I:544–545
  due to general medical
    condition, III:309–310,
    III:311
  endometriosis and, II:269
  environmental illness and,
    III:356, **III:358–361,** III:372
  folate deficiency–induced,
    I:227
  gabapentin-induced, III:120
  in Huntington's disease, **II:476,**
    II:476–478
  menopause-related, II:271–274
  mental retardation and, I:512–514
  monoamine oxidase levels and,
    II:239
  multiple sclerosis and, II:421–423
  in systemic lupus
    erythematosus, III:188,
    III:191, III:192
Mood stabilizers. *See also* specific
  drugs
  for head-injured persons,
    III:337–339
  use in gastrointestinal disease,
    III:24–26
  use in liver disease, III:46–49
Moral theory, II:586–589. *See also*
  Ethical issues
  beneficence, II:587–588
  justice, II:588–589

respect for autonomy, II:587
  rights and duties, II:586–587
Moricizine, III:98
Morphine sulfate
  for Huntington's disease, II:497
  interaction with monoamine
    oxidase inhibitors, II:399,
    II:401
  interaction with tacrine, II:97
  for low-back pain, **II:358**
  slow-release formula (MS
    Contin), II:366
Motivation, I:601–603, I:606–607
Motor deficits, in HIV infection,
  III:269
Movement disorder, I:520
MRI. *See* Magnetic resonance
  imaging
Mucositis, III:433
Multidimensional Pain Inventory
  (MPI), II:342–343, III:408
Multi-infarct dementia, I:172–173,
  II:153
Multiple Affect Adjective Check
  List (MAACL), II:218
Multiple chemical sensitivity,
  III:347–349, III:351. *See also*
  Environmental illness
Multiple myeloma, bone marrow
  transplantation for, III:419
Multiple sclerosis (MS), II:411–438
  affect and, II:421–423
    bipolar disorder, **II:430–433,**
      II:435–436
    depression, II:423, II:428–435,
      II:430–433
    euphoria, II:423–424,
      II:425–426
    pathological laughing and
      weeping, **II:427,**
      II:427–428
  age at onset of, II:413
  cognitive impairment in,
    II:417–419

therapy and management of,
II:419–421
diagnosis of, II:413–415, **II:414**
cerebrospinal fluid analysis,
II:414
magnetic resonance imaging,
II:414–415, II:419
environmental determinants for,
II:412
industrialized areas, II:412
latitude-related gradient,
II:412
epidemiological studies of,
II:412–413
fatigue in, II:436–437
genetically based risk for, II:412
grading severity of, II:417–419
histopathology of, II:411–412
immune abnormalities in, II:411
major histocompatibility
complex genes associated
with, II:412
natural history of, II:415
prevalence of, II:413
psychological testing in, II:418,
II:420
sex distribution of, II:413
sexuality and, II:437–438
stress and, II:422–423
treatment of, II:415–416
exacerbating-remitting
disease, II:416
relapsing-progressive and
progressive disease,
II:416–417
triggering events for, II:413
Munchausen syndrome, II:594–595
Muscle relaxants
electroconvulsive therapy and,
I:123–125
interaction with lithium,
II:402
Muscle tone and frontal lobe
dysfunction, I:363

Muscular dystrophy, depression in,
II:429
Musculoskeletal disorders, II:331,
II:332. *See also* Low-back pain
Myalgias, chronic fatigue syndrome
and, III:234
Myambutol. *See* Ethambutol
Myelography, spinal, II:347
Myelopathy, associated with HIV
infection, **III:272–273**
Myocardial infarction, I:128–129,
II:201, II:207–208, II:212
β-blockers to prevent ventricular
fibrillation after, II:216
circadian variations and,
II:225–227
depression after, II:223
drug protein binding and, III:10,
III:27
electroconvulsive therapy and,
I:106–107, II:575–578
high levels of stress after,
II:223–224
resuming sexual activity after,
II:230
during sexual activity, II:220
tricyclic antidepressants and,
I:35–36
use of antiarrhythmics after,
III:97–98
Myocardial ischemia, stress-related,
II:220
Myofascial pain syndrome, II:379
diagnostic criteria for, II:373
fibromyalgia and, II:373–374
depression and, II:374
low-back pain and, II:337, II:368,
II:370, II:372–374
mechanisms of, II:374

Naloxone, I:527
effect on hypnotic analgesia,
II:50
Naltrexone, I:527–528

Nancy Beth Cruzan, by Her Parents and Co-Guardians, Lester L. Cruzan, et ux., Petitioners v. Director, Missouri Department of Health, et al., II:542, II:544–546
Naproxen
  for fibromyalgia, **III:247**
  for low-back pain, **II:357**
Naproxen-sodium, for low-back pain, **II:357**
Narcissistic injury, II:16
Narcotics. *See* Opioids
National Bone Marrow Registry (NBMR), III:420
National Marrow Donor Program (NMDP), III:421
National Multiple Sclerosis Society, II:419
National Organ Transplant Act (PL 98-507), III:429
Natural death directive, II:552. *See also* Living wills
Nausea and vomiting
  in bone marrow transplant recipient, III:431, III:433–435
  drug-induced
    felbamate, III:117
    nefazodone, III:96
    venlafaxine, III:93, III:281
    zolpidem, III:131
  habitual reflex vomiting, II:55
  hypnosis for, II:55–56
  medications for, III:434
Needle and intravenous catheter phobia, II:390–391
Nefazodone, III:79, III:95–97
  cytochrome P$_{450}$-3A4 inhibition by, **III:85**, III:86
  cytochrome P$_{450}$-mediated biotransformation of, III:36
  drug interactions with, III:97
  mechanism of action of, III:95

  pharmacology in medical patients, III:97
  side effects of, III:95–97
Negligence, II:563. *See also* Malpractice
Neonaticide, II:257
Nephrotic syndrome, III:10, III:50
Nerve trunk pain, I:419
Nervous exhaustion, III:217. *See also* Chronic fatigue syndrome
Nervousness
  felbamate-induced, III:118
  venlafaxine-induced, III:93
Neural tube defects, III:123
  prenatal diagnosis of, II:101, III:123
  related to antiepileptic drug use in pregnancy, II:99–101, III:123
Neuralgia, III:389
  postherpetic, III:395
  pudendal, III:389–390
Neurasthenia, III:217, III:348. *See also* Chronic fatigue syndrome
Neurobehavioral Rating Scale (NBRS), **III:321**, III:322, **III:327**
Neuroblastoma, bone marrow transplantation for, III:417, III:419
Neurodermatitis, hypnosis for, II:52
Neurofibromatosis, II:175
Neuroleptic malignant syndrome (NMS), II:117–118, II:498
  causes of, I:437–440
  clozapine-induced, III:108–109
  course of, I:436–437
  diagnosis of, I:430–431
  frequency of, I:427
  laboratory tests for, I:441
  neuroleptic treatment after, III:109
  relapse rates in, I:445–446
  risk factors for, I:428–429
  symptoms of, I:429–431

treatment of, I:440–445

Neuroleptics, **II:493**. *See also* specific
  drugs
  active metabolites of, II:120
  for children and adolescents,
    I:471–473
  drug interactions with
    anesthetics, II:401
    bupropion, II:79
    fluoxetine, II:71, II:72
    valproate, III:127–128
  electroencephalographic effects
    of, I:474–475
  formulations of, **III:8**
  for head-injured patient, I:370,
    III:329, **III:330–331**
  for HIV-infected persons,
    III:284–285
  for mania, III:283–284
  for Huntington's disease, II:495,
    II:496, **II:496**, II:498
  metabolism of, **III:9**, III:14
    by cytochrome P$_{450}$-2D6,
      III:82–83
  parenteral, II:113, II:116–120,
    III:22–23
    clinical response related to
      serum levels, II:120
    combined with
      benzodiazepines,
      II:123–125
    guidelines for administration,
      II:114
    intramuscular, II:117–118
    intravenous, II:116–117
    long-acting (depot)
      preparations,
      II:118–120
  for persons with mental
    retardation, I:518–522
  for postoperative agitation and
    delirium, II:404
  for premenstrual syndrome,
    II:263–264

for psychosis in Parkinson's
    disease, III:163–164
  side effects of, I:302–303, I:370,
    I:425–447, I:474,
    I:520–522
    parkinsonism, II:452
    syndrome of inappropriate
      antidiuretic hormone
      secretion, II:74
  use after neuroleptic malignant
    syndrome, III:109
  use in cardiac disease, III:31
  use in gastrointestinal disease,
    III:22–23
  use in liver disease, III:43–44
  use in renal disease, III:53
  use in systemic lupus
    erythematosus, III:207,
    III:208
  withdrawal from, I:522

Neurological examination
  in HIV infection, III:276
  malpractice claim related to lack
    of, II:579–580
  for patient with chronic
    low-back pain, II:345–346

Neuropeptide Y, II:473

Neuropsychological testing, I:254,
    I:608
  in AIDS dementia complex,
    III:276–277
  of bone marrow transplant
    recipients, III:436
  of head-injured patients,
    III:323–325, **III:326–327**
  in Huntington's disease, II:489
  in multiple sclerosis, II:418,
    II:420
  in Parkinson's disease, II:462–463
  of patients with chronic
    low-back pain, II:342,
    II:349, II:375, II:378
  in polycystic ovarian disease,
    II:265

Neuropsychological testing
(continued)
in systemic lupus
erythematosus, III:194,
III:198, III:199
of ventricular arrhythmia
patients, II:218
Neurosyphilis, I:259–260, II:155. See
also Syphilis
asymptomatic, I:259, I:263
parenchymal, I:259–260
Neurotic excoriations, I:296
Neurotransmitters
clozapine effects on, III:164–165
frontal lobe function and,
I:368–369
in Huntington's disease,
II:472–473
in Parkinson's disease, II:450
in polycystic ovarian disease,
II:266–268
sex steroid effects on, II:238,
II:239
tacrine effects on, III:136
Neutropenia,
carbamazepine-induced, III:121
New York's Gay Men's Health
Crisis, III:288
Nicorette, I:566
Nicotine. See also Cigarette smoking
dependence on, I:553–556
drug interactions with, I:552–553
effects of, I:545–556
fading, I:573
fluoxetine interaction with, II:72
protein binding of, III:10
resin complex, I:565–567, I:579,
I:583
withdrawal from, I:554–556,
I:559–560, I:569–570
Nicotine nasal solution, I:568
Nicotine transdermal patch,
I:567–568
Niemann-Pick disease, II:178

Nifedipine, III:85
Night sweats, II:269
Nimodipine, for AIDS dementia
complex, III:275
Nitrazepam
metabolism of, III:90
use in liver disease, III:42
use in renal disease, **III:58–59**
Nitrofurantoin, **III:186**
Nitrous oxide, II:389, II:397
neuropsychiatric effects of,
II:402, II:403
Nizoral. See Ketoconazole
Nociception, II:370–372. See also
Pain perception
soft-tissue sources of, II:374,
II:377
Nociceptive (noxious) stimulus,
II:370–372
Nociceptors, II:371
"No-code" orders, II:546
Noncompliance
of bone marrow transplant
recipient, III:423,
III:431–432, III:439
refusing organ transplant due to,
II:602
Nonlinear kinetics, III:19–20
Nonsteroidal antiinflammatory
drugs (NSAIDs), for low-back
pain, **II:356,** II:365, II:366
Norepinephrine
cardiac, II:213, II:215
coronary vasoconstriction due
to, II:215
desipramine inhibition of uptake
of, II:126
estradiol effects on synthesis of,
II:239
in Parkinson's disease, II:450
in polycystic ovarian disease,
II:266, II:267
role in chronic pain, II:371
role in thermoregulation, II:271

Norethindrone, II:244
Norfluoxetine, II:71, II:73. *See also*
   Fluoxetine
   cytochrome P₄₅₀ inhibition by,
      III:36, III:84, **III:84**
   half-life of, III:17, III:85
Norgestrel, II:244
Norplant. *See* Levonorgestrel
Nortriptyline, I:30, I:403
   for anxiety disorders in
      Parkinson's disease,
      II:460
   drug interactions with
      carbamazepine, III:124
      fluoxetine, **III:87**
      quinidine, III:37
      valproate, III:106
   formulations of, **III:8,** III:23
   for head-injured patient, **III:331,**
      III:336
   for HIV-infected persons, III:281,
      III:282
   for low-back pain, **II:359,**
      II:366
   metabolism of, III:45
      by cytochrome P₄₅₀-2D6,
         III:36, III:37, **III:82**
   for mucous membrane
      dysesthesias, III:390
   for premenstrual syndrome,
      II:264
   for pruritus ani, III:399
   use in cardiac disease, III:30
   use in renal disease, **III:64–65,**
      III:66
   volume of distribution of, III:13
   for vulvodynia, III:408
Nurse-doctor relationship,
   II:600–601
Nurse-patient relationship,
   II:600–601
Nursing Home Reform Act, II:542
Nystatin, for candidiasis, III:354,
   III:362

Obesity, in polycystic ovarian
   disease, II:265, II:267, II:268
Object relations, II:5
Obsessive-compulsive disorder
   buspirone for, II:81
   genetic linkage studies of, II:188
   genetics of, II:185
   intravenous clomipramine for,
      II:125–127
   in women, II:237
Obstructive sleep apnea, II:87
   quazepam use in, II:88
   triazolam use in, II:89
Occupational medicine, III:367
Occupational therapy, for patient
   with low-back pain, II:348, II:368
Olfaction and frontal lobe
   dysfunction, I:357, I:363
Oligospermia, II:306, II:309
Olivopontocerebellar atrophy,
   II:448, III:169
Omnibus Budget Reconciliation Act
   (OBRA) of 1987, II:542
Ondansetron, for psychosis in
   Parkinson's disease, III:169
Open heart surgery, II:390, II:596
Opiate antagonists, I:427–428
Opioids, I:405–406, **II:493**
   after bone marrow
      transplantation,
      III:433–434, III:441
   endogenous, role in
      premenstrual syndrome,
      II:262, II:263
   estrogen effects on, II:239
   as induction agents, I:123
   interaction with carbamazepine,
      III:124
   interaction with monoamine
      oxidase inhibitors, II:399,
      II:401
   for low-back pain, **II:357–358**
   contingencies for use of,
      II:365

Opioids *(continued)*
  for low-back pain
    conversion to longer-acting
      drugs, II:365–366
    detoxification from, II:365
    excessive reliance on, II:355,
      II:364–366
    patient's pain behaviors for
      acquisition of, II:364
    recording use of, II:365
  for outpatient surgery, II:396
  for preanesthetic anxiety, II:393,
    II:394
Oral contraceptives, **II:493, III:186**
  depression related to, II:237,
    II:238, II:242–245
    depressed mood, II:242
    mechanism of, II:243
    susceptibility to, II:242
    twin studies of, II:243
    vitamin B$_6$ deficiency and, II:243
    in women with history of
      depression, II:243
  for endometriosis, II:308
  interaction with carbamazepine,
    II:99, III:124
  interaction with valproate, II:99
  mortality due to, II:244
  for premenstrual syndrome,
    II:263
  prevalence of use of, II:242
  psychiatric side effects of, II:242
  stroke and, II:244
  subarachnoid hemorrhage and,
    II:244
  types of, II:244
    continuous, II:244
    cyclic, II:244
    sequential, II:244
  use by smokers, II:244
  use during breast-feeding, II:244
  use during pregnancy, II:245
  vitamin B$_6$ deficiency and,
    II:243

Oral hypoglycemic agents,
  fluoxetine use in patient on,
  II:73
Orbitofrontal lobe syndromes,
  III:312, III:314
Organ transplantation, III:415. *See
  also* Bone marrow
  transplantation
  addicted patients and, I:318–321
  candidate selection for, I:310–321
  compliance concerns and,
    I:316–318
  lithium use and renal
    transplants, I:40–41
  postoperative care and, I:326–332
  preoperative care and, I:321–326
  psychological adjustment stages
    related to, I:322–323
  quality of life and, I:337–339
  waiting period for, I:323
Organic Aggression Scale (OAS),
  III:321, III:322, **III:327**
Organic mental disorders
  associated with HIV infection,
    III:267, **III:269–270**
  buspirone to reduce aggression
    and anxiety in, II:81
  folate deficiency and, I:227–228
  in organ transplant recipients,
    I:328
  SPECT scanning in, II:150–157
    CNS HIV infection, II:154–156
    CNS lupus, II:153–154
    dementia, II:152–153
    elderly patients with
      depression, II:157
    epilepsy, II:156
    miscellaneous disorders,
      II:157
    stroke, II:150–152
  treatment of, I:332–334
Oropharyngeal ulcers, III:433
Orphenadrine, for parkinsonism,
  II:132

Orthostatic hypotension, I:65–66,
    II:78
    drug-induced
        clozapine, III:107
        imipramine, III:96
        nefazodone, III:96
        risperidone, III:116
    in head-injured patient, III:329
Osteomyelitis, II:339, II:370
Osteoporosis, II:346, II:370
    hormone therapy for prevention
        of, II:275
    menopause and, II:270, II:275
    risk factors for, II:275
Outpatient surgery, II:395–397
    anesthesia for, II:396–397
    increasing use of, II:395–396
    preanesthetic management for,
        II:396
    requirements for discharge after,
        II:397
Ovarian cancer, II:272
    oral contraceptives and, II:245
Ovarian failure,
    chemotherapy-induced,
        III:453–455
Over-the-counter drugs, interaction
    with monoamine oxidase
    inhibitors, I:68–70
Ovulation
    evaluation during infertility
        workup, II:304
    induction of, II:307–308
    infertility due to defects of,
        II:302, II:303
    suppression for premenstrual
        syndrome, II:264
Oxazepam, II:122
    formulations of, III:8
    half-life of, III:19, III:284
    for head-injured patient, III:334,
        III:339
    metabolism of, III:9, III:14–15,
        III:52

use in cardiac disease, III:27
use in liver disease, III:33, III:39,
    III:42
use in renal disease, III:58–59
volume of distribution of, III:13
2-Oxoquazepam, II:86, II:87, III:19
Oxprenolol, II:216, III:186
Oxycodone, for low-back pain,
    II:358
Oxyphenisatin, III:186

P300, I:179
Paced Auditory Serial Addition
    Test, II:420, III:326
Pacemakers, I:130–131
    for vasovagal syncope, II:205
Pacing skills, for low-back pain
    patients, II:361
Pain
    after bone marrow
        transplantation, III:434
    chronic, III:408
    DSM classifications of, II:379–380
    hypnosis for, II:42, II:46–47,
        II:49–50
    low-back, II:331–383
    management of, I:207–210
    modulation of, II:370
    pelvic, due to endometriosis,
        II:268–269
    postoperative, II:403
    psychogenic, II:379–380
    rating charts for, II:343, II:343,
        II:348
    sciatic, II:346
    somatoform pain disorder,
        II:379
    terminology used by pain
        clinicians, II:370
    threshold of, II:370, II:371
    tolerance of, II:370
    vulvodynia, III:381–411
Pain behaviors, II:345
    to acquire medication, II:364

Pain management training,
    II:354–355, II:360–362
    coordinating with physical
        therapy, II:367
    group program for, II:355
    psychiatrist's roles in, II:355
    sequential tasks in, II:355,
        II:360–362
Pain medicine interview, II:343–345
Pain perception, II:370–374
    definition of, II:370
    gate theory of, II:371–374
        algogenic processes and
            interventions, **II:373**
        central factors in chronic pain,
            II:372
        myofascial pain, II:372–374
        peripheral factors in chronic
            pain, **II:361**, II:371–372
Pain prone disorder, II:378
"Pain prone patient," II:378
Pain-tension cycle, II:355,
    II:360–361
Palpitations, stress-related, II:202
Pancreatitis
    clozapine-induced, III:107
    effect on albumin binding of
        drugs, III:10
    effect on drug absorption, III:2
    valproate-induced, III:128
Pancuronium, interaction with
    lithium, II:402
Panic disorder, I:625
    genetic linkage studies of, II:188
    genetics of, II:185
    with hot flushes, II:272
    pregnancy complications and,
        II:246
    valproate for, III:125
    in women, II:237
Paralysis
    with awareness under
        anesthesia, II:398–399
    simulated, II:595

Paranoid disorder, in Huntington's
    disease, II:476
Parathyroid hormone (PTH), in
    patient on lithium, III:111–112
Paratonia, II:448, II:449
Parkinsonism. *See also*
    Extrapyramidal symptoms
    aggravated by tacrine, II:96
    animal model of, II:447
    atypical, clozapine for,
        III:168–169
    compared with Parkinson's
        disease, III:152
    drug-induced, II:447, II:448,
        II:452
        depot neuroleptics, II:120
        fluoxetine, II:74
        selective serotonin reuptake
            inhibitors, III:91
    Huntington's disease and, II:475
    orphenadrine for, II:132
"Parkinsonism plus" syndromes,
    II:448
Parkinson's disease (PD), I:350–352,
    I:372, I:521, II:447–464
    age at onset of, III:158
    anxiety disorders in, II:459
    cognitive impairments in, II:450,
        II:460–464
        aggravated by depression,
            II:461
        clinical evaluation of,
            II:462–463
        combinations of deficits, II:461
        driving performance, II:461
        effect of brain implants on,
            II:463–464
        management of, II:463
        medications and, II:462
        neuropathology, II:460–461
        related to disease stage, II:460
        types of deficits, II:461–462
    compared with parkinsonism,
        III:152

depression in, II:457–460
  contradictions in literature
    about, II:457–458
  diagnosis of, II:458–459
  "on-off" phenomena and,
    II:459, II:462
  prevalence of, II:457–458
  treatment of, II:459–460
dopamine receptor subtypes in,
  II:447
early-onset, II:449
  definition of, II:449
  prevalence of, II:449
  symptoms of, II:449
exacerbated by selective
    serotonin reuptake
    inhibitors, III:91
heterogeneity of, II:448
  biochemical, II:450
history taking for, II:451
misdiagnosis of, II:448–449
neuropathology of, II:450,
  II:460–461
pathophysiology of, III:152
physical examination for, II:451
preclinical phase of, II:451
recent research on, II:447
signs of, II:448
SPECT evaluation of, II:153,
  II:157
staging of, II:451–452
treatment of, II:452–457,
  III:152–156, **III:154–155**
  amantadine, II:454–455, III:156
  anticholinergics, II:454–455,
    III:156
  clozapine, I:54–55, II:456–457,
    III:106, III:164–169
  controlled-release
    levodopa/carbidopa,
    II:455
  dilemma in, III:151
  dopamine agonists,
    II:453–454, III:153

electroconvulsive therapy,
    III:170–172
  levodopa, III:152–153
  management of later-stage
    disease, II:456
  neuroprotective strategies,
    II:453
  selegiline, I:70, II:69, II:97–98,
    II:448, II:453, III:153,
    III:156
use of fluoxetine in, II:74
variably present features of,
  II:450
  autonomic disturbances, II:450
  cognitive impairments, II:450
Parkinson's disease–associated
    psychosis, III:156–176
  differential diagnosis of,
    III:156–158
  differential psychotoxicity of
    antiparkinsonian drugs,
    III:161–162
  epidemiology of, III:158
  phenomenology of, III:158–160
    delusions, III:160
    hallucinations, III:159–160
    sleep disturbances, III:160
  risk factors for, III:158
  treatment of, III:162–176
    adjustment of
      antiparkinsonian drugs,
      III:162–163
    approach to, III:172–175,
      III:173
    case reports of, III:175–176,
      III:177
    clozapine, III:164–169, **III:166**
    electroconvulsive therapy,
      III:170–172
    hospitalization, III:174–175
    ondansetron, III:169
    risperidone, III:169
    typical neuroleptics,
      III:163–164

Parlodel. *See* Bromocriptine
Parnate, I:374
Paroxetine, II:76
    cardiac effects of, II:76
    cytochrome P$_{450}$ inhibition by,
        III:36, III:46, III:84, **III:84,**
        III:280
    drug interactions with, II:76,
        III:88
        valproate, III:130
        warfarin, III:91
    formulations of, **III:8**
    half-life of, II:76, III:17
    for head-injured patient, **III:333,**
        III:336
    for HIV-infected persons, III:280
    limited clinical experience with,
        II:77
    metabolism of, II:76
    for patient with low-back pain,
        II:366
    side effects of, II:76
    use in cardiac disease, III:31
    use in elderly patients, II:76
    use in gastrointestinal disease,
        III:23
    use in liver disease, III:92
    use in renal disease, II:76
Paternalism, II:588, II:593, II:597,
    II:600
Patient Self-Determination Act
    (PSDA), II:537, II:548–552
    concerns in implementation of,
        II:550–551
    documentation requirement of,
        II:550
    education requirement of, II:550
    information requirement of,
        II:549
    nondiscrimination requirement
        of, II:550
    purpose of, II:549, II:551
    role of clinician related to,
        II:551–552

    service providers to which act
        applies, II:549
Patient-controlled analgesia (PCA),
    III:434
Patient's Bill of Rights, II:542
Pediatricians, I:486, I:496–497
Pemoline, I:373–374, **II:493**
    formulations of, **III:8**
    for head-injured patients, III:335
    for HIV-infected persons, III:282
Penicillamine, **III:186**
Penicillin, **III:186**
Pentamidine (Pentam), III:303
Pentazocine, fluoxetine interaction
    with, II:72–73
Pentobarbital, use in renal disease,
    III:54–55
Percocet, II:344
Pergolide, for Parkinson's disease,
    II:453–454, III:153, **III:154**
Pergonal. *See* Human menopausal
    gonadotropin
Perhexiline, **III:83**
Perimenopause, II:269
Perineal pain, III:385, III:389–390
Peritoneal dialysis, III:51
Perphenazine
    formulations of, **III:8**
    for Huntington's disease,
        II:495–497
    interaction with fluoxetine,
        III:87
    intramuscular, **II:114**
    metabolism by cytochrome
        P$_{450}$-2D6, III:36, **III:82**
Personality, II:32–33
    effect on short-term dynamic
        therapy of stress response
        syndromes, II:31–33, **II:32**
    hypnotizability related to, II:40
    importance in medical
        treatment, II:32–33
    of women seeking in vitro
        fertilization, II:309

Personality changes
after brain injury, III:310, III:312,
III:312, III:314
chronic pain related to, II:375
due to general medical
condition, III:310, **III:312**
in Huntington's disease, **II:476,**
II:478–479
Personality disorders
antisocial personality in
Huntington's disease,
II:476, **II:476,** II:477
associated with HIV infection,
III:269–270
borderline personality, II:263
chronic fatigue and, III:235
environmental illness and,
III:356, **III:358–361,**
III:364–366
obsessional personality, II:31,
II:32
schizotypal personality, II:179
PET. *See* Positron-emission
tomography
Petechiae, fluoxetine-induced, III:90
Pharmacokinetics. *See*
Psychopharmacokinetics
Pharyngitis, in chronic fatigue
syndrome, III:221
Phase I reactions, **III:9,** III:14–15, III:36
Phase II reactions, **III:9,** III:15, III:36
Phencyclidine receptor binding,
II:473
Phenelzine, II:98
for head-injured patient, **III:332**
for Huntington's disease, II:497
use in renal disease, **III:62–63**
Phenformin, **III:83**
Phenobarbital
interaction with paroxetine, **III:88**
use in renal disease, **III:54–55**
Phenothiazines
for Huntington's disease,
II:494–495

protein binding of, III:10
use in renal disease, III:53,
III:62–63
Phenotypes, II:178–180
Phentolamine, for chronic pain,
II:371
Phenylbutazone, **III:186**
Phenylethylacetylurea, **III:186**
Phenylketonuria, II:167
neonatal screening for, II:168
Phenytoin, I:520–521, **II:493**
interaction with clozapine, III:108
interaction with fluoxetine, **III:88**
interaction with paroxetine,
III:88
for long Q-T syndrome, II:214
lupus induced by, **III:186**
prophylactic, for patient taking
bupropion, II:79
protein binding of, III:10
withdrawal from, III:119
zero-order kinetics and, III:19–20
Pheochromocytoma,
electroconvulsive therapy and,
I:108, I:131–132
Phobias
hypnosis for, II:56–57
needle and intravenous catheter
phobia, II:390–391
reframing strategy for, II:56–57
treatments for, II:56
in women, II:237
Physical examination
for chronic low-back pain,
II:345–346
for Huntington's disease,
II:486–487, **II:487**
for Parkinson's disease, II:451
standard of care for, II:568–569
Physical therapy, for low-back pain,
II:367–368
acute, II:340
chronic, II:354
subacute, II:352

Physician-nurse relationship,
    II:600–601
Physician-patient relationship, II:39
    chronic fatigue syndrome and,
        III:215, III:239
Physicians' rights to
    self-preservation, II:604–605
Physostigmine
    effect on cerebral blood flow,
        II:150
    in Alzheimer's disease, II:153
    for scopolamine-induced
        postoperative delirium,
        II:404
Pick's disease, I:350–352, II:153,
    II:493
Pimozide
    formulations of, **III:8**
    interaction with fluoxetine, **III:88**
    use in cardiac disease, III:31
Pindolol, for Huntington's disease,
    II:498
Pinworms, III:399
Platelet-activating factor, II:89
Platelets
    drug-induced abnormalities of
        carbamazepine, III:121
        fluoxetine, II:73, III:90
        valproate, III:126–127
    morning surge in aggregation of,
        II:227
Pneumonia
    effect on albumin binding of
        drugs, III:10
    Pneumocystis carinii, III:259
        neuropsychiatric effects of
            drugs used for, III:303
Polacrilex, I:566
Polycystic ovarian disease (PCOD),
    II:265–268
    androgens in, II:265–268
    Briquet's syndrome and, II:266
    clinical features of, II:265
    β-endorphins in, II:267–268

genetics of, II:265
histology of, II:265
inappropriate gonadotropin
    secretion in, II:265–267
neurotransmitters in, II:266–268
pathophysiology of, II:265–266
psychological features of, II:265
sex steroids in, II:268
stress and, II:265–268
temporal lobe epilepsy and,
    II:266
treatment of, II:268
Polycythemia, I:489, **II:493**
Polyserositis, clozapine-induced,
    III:108
Porphyrias, I:213–220
    psychiatric problems and,
        I:215–216
    symptoms of, I:213–217
    treatment of, I:219–220
Positron-emission tomography
    (PET)
    in AIDS dementia complex,
        III:276
    compared with SPECT, II:142
    in dementia, II:152
    future of, II:160
    in Huntington's disease,
        II:491–492
    mechanism of, I:19–20
    in schizophrenia, I:20–21
    in systemic lupus
        erythematosus, II:154,
        III:194, III:202
Postcoital test, II:306
Postconcussional disorder,
    III:307–308, III:314–317, **III:316.**
    See also Head injury
    duration of, III:316–317
    symptoms of, III:315–317
    terminology for, III:315
Postpartum depressions, II:238,
    II:246–254
    blood hormone levels and, II:247

blues, II:250–252
classifications of, II:250–251
clinical features of, II:250
duration of, II:250
factors predisposing to, II:251
hormonal changes and, II:251
prevalence of, II:250
progression to depression,
II:250
psychiatric consultation for,
II:251–252
time of onset of, II:250
compared with depressions
occurring at other times,
II:246, II:247, II:249, II:252
cultural factors and, II:248
economic effects of, II:247
effect on infants and children,
II:247
etiology of, II:247–248
hostility toward infant due to,
II:248
limitations of literature on,
II:249–250
major depression, II:252–254
duration of, II:253
prenatal depression and, II:254
prevalence of, II:252
psychotropic drugs for, II:254
recurrences of, II:253
risk factors for, II:252
screening for, II:253
self-report questionnaires for,
II:252
symptoms of, II:252–254
time of onset of, II:253
undetected, II:253
psychodynamic issues
associated with, II:248
risk factors for, II:249
spectrum of, II:246
thyroid function and, II:248
treatment of, II:249
Postpartum psychosis, II:255–257

associated with birth of girls,
II:256
classifications of, II:255
compared with nonpuerperal
psychosis, II:255
diagnosis of, II:256
incidence of, II:256
murder of infant due to, II:257
obstetric complications and,
II:255
recurrences of, II:256
risk factors for, II:255
symptoms of, II:255
time of onset of, II:255
treatment of, II:256
Posttraumatic stress disorder
(PTSD), II:398
after head injury, III:317–318
zolpidem for, III:131
Postural instability, II:448, II:451
Potassium, II:227
Practolol, **III:186**
Prazepam
active metabolite of, III:3, III:15
formulations of, **III:8**
half-life of, **III:19**
metabolism of, **III:9**
onset of action of, III:3
use in liver disease, III:42
use in renal disease, **III:58–59**
Prednisone
for multiple sclerosis, II:416
for polycystic ovarian disease,
II:268
Preferred provider organizations
(PPOs), II:9
Pregnancy
after bone marrow
transplantation, III:457
antiepileptic drugs in, II:98–101
carbamazepine in, III:123
course of psychiatric illness in,
I:616–617
depression in, I:623–624, II:254

Pregnancy *(continued)*
  depression in
    reduced risk of psychotic
      depression, II:240
  effect of zidovudine on
    maternal-to-infant HIV
    transmission in, III:262
  effects of age and work on, II:246
  effects of oral contraceptive use
    in, II:245
  inability to achieve. *See* Infertility
  lack of psychosocial support
    during, II:246
  men's psychopathology related
    to, II:254
  multiple, related to ovulation-
    inducing drugs, II:307
  postponed, II:245–246
  psychiatric disorders during,
    I:619–626
  psychology of, II:245
  psychotic denial of, II:256
  psychotropic drugs in, I:617
  role of emotional factors in,
    II:237, II:238, II:245–246
  systemic lupus erythematosus
    and, III:206
Premature birth, related to fertility
  drugs, II:308
Premature ejaculation, II:303
Premenstrual syndrome (PMS),
  II:237, II:257–265
  comorbidity with depression,
    II:260
  diagnosis of, II:258–260
    Daily Rating Form, II:259,
      II:261, II:293–300
    Premenstrual Assessment
      Form, II:259, II:287–292
    in DSM-III-R, II:257, II:258
    kinds of premenstrual problems,
      II:258
    limitations of literature on, II:257
    physicians' lack of belief in, II:257

predisposing factors for, II:261
  psychiatric examination for
    woman with, II:261
  referred to by psychotherapy
    patients, II:258
  risk factors for, II:260
  symptoms of, II:259–260
  treatment of, II:261–265
    antidepressants, II:264
    anxiolytics, II:263
    benzodiazepines, II:263, II:264
    diet, II:262
    diuretics, II:263
    exercise, II:262
    neuroleptics, II:263–264
    oral contraceptives, II:263
    ovulation suppression, II:264
    progesterone, II:263
    vitamin B$_6$, II:262–263
  workup for, II:260–261
Prenatal diagnosis, II:168
  of neural tube defects, II:101,
    III:123
Priapism, clozapine-induced, III:107
PRIDE program, II:354
Primidone, **III:186**
Privacy rights, II:543
Procainamide, lupus induced by,
  III:184
Prochlorperazine
  formulations of, **III:8**
  for nausea and vomiting, III:434
Procrit. *See* Epoetin alfa
Profile of Mood States, III:436
Progesterone
  added to estrogen replacement
    therapy, II:274, II:275
  behavioral effects of, II:240
  in brain, II:240
  brain receptors for, II:238
  effect on libido in women,
    II:240–241
  effect on monoamine oxidase
    levels, II:239

in endometriosis, II:268
natural versus synthetic, II:263
in oral contraceptives, II:244
postpartum blues and, II:251
premenstrual syndrome and,
    II:261, II:263
Progressive multifocal
    leukoencephalopathy, II:155
Progressive supranuclear palsy
    (PSP)
    misdiagnosed as Parkinson's
        disease, II:448, II:449
    SPECT evaluation of, II:157
Prokine. *See* Sargramostim
Prolactin, II:240
    buspirone effects on secretion of,
        II:83
    effect on occurrence of hot
        flushes, II:271
    in endometriosis, II:268
    in polycystic ovarian disease,
        II:265, II:268
Propafenone
    drug interactions with, III:106
    metabolism of, **III:82**
Propantheline, III:2
Propofol, I:121–123
Propranolol
    for akathisia, III:92
    drug interactions with
        fluoxetine, II:72
        fluvoxamine, **III:87**
        paroxetine, II:76
    for head-injured patient, I:372,
        III:334
    for Huntington's disease, **II:496,**
        II:497, II:498
    metabolism of, **III:82**
    to prevent ventricular fibrillation
        after myocardial
        infarction, II:215, II:216
    use in HIV-infected persons,
        III:284
    volume of distribution of, III:13

Propylthiouracil, **III:186**
ProSom. *See* Estazolam
Protein binding of drugs, III:9–12
    in cardiac disease, III:29
    dialyzability and, III:51
    diseases affecting, III:10–12,
        III:11
    effect on laboratory
        measurement of
        therapeutic range, III:12
    in liver disease, III:10, III:34–35
    myocardial infarction and,
        III:27
    in renal disease, III:10, III:50
Prothrombin time (PT), III:40
Protriptyline
    formulations of, **III:8**
    for HIV-infected persons, III:281
    metabolism of, III:45
    use in renal disease, **III:64–65**
Provera. *See* Medroxyprogesterone
Pruritus, I:293–294, I:304
    ani, III:385, III:399
    hypnosis for, II:52–53
    vulvae, III:385, III:398–399. *See
        also* Vulvodynia
Pseudotumor cerebri, I:415
Psoriasis, I:290–292
    hypnosis for, II:52
    lithium-induced, I:299
    pruritus and, I:293–294
    trazodone-induced, I:301
    vulvar, **III:392**
Psychiatric-medical units, II:604
Psychoanalytic interventions,
    II:4–5
"Psychodynamic life narratives,"
    II:16–17
Psychodynamic psychotherapy. *See
    also* Brief psychodynamically
    informed therapy
    descriptive formulations for, II:6
    importance of training in, II:4
    new model of, II:5

Psychodynamic psychotherapy
    (continued)
    psychodynamic formulations
        versus psychoanalytic
        interventions, II:4–5
    for understanding of patients,
        II:3–4
Psychopharmacokinetics, III:1–67,
    III:4–5
    absorption, III:1–9, **III:4**
    bioavailability, **III:5**, III:9
    clearance, **III:5**, III:15–16
    disease effects on, **III:6–7**,
        III:20–67
        cardiac disease, III:26–32
        gastrointestinal disease,
            III:21–26
        liver disease, III:32–49
        renal disease, III:41–42,
            III:49–67
    distribution, **III:5**, III:9–14
    drug metabolites, III:3, **III:9**,
        III:15, III:18
    elimination, III:9, **III:9**, III:14–18
    factors influencing, III:1
    half-life, **III:5**, **III:16**, III:16–18,
        III:19
    lipid solubility, III:12–14
    pharmacokinetic models,
        III:18–20
        first-order kinetics, III:18–19
        zero-order kinetics, III:19–20
    protein binding, III:9–12, **III:11**
    steady state, **III:5**
    volume of distribution, **III:5**,
        III:12–14
Psychosis
    assessing bone marrow
        transplant candidate for,
        III:423
    bupropion contraindicated in,
        II:77
    in critical care settings (ICU
        psychosis), II:116
    drug-induced
        buspirone, III:284
        corticosteroids, III:208
        gabapentin, III:120
        genetics of, II:184–185
        in HIV-infected persons,
            III:284–285
        in Huntington's disease, II:476
        ICU, II:116, III:443
        mental retardation and, I:514–515
        methylphenidate
            contraindicated for, II:130
        in organ transplant recipients,
            I:327–328
        parenteral lorazepam-
            haloperidol for agitation
            of, II:124
        in Parkinson's disease,
            III:151–176. See also
            Parkinson's disease–
            associated psychosis
        postpartum, II:255–257
        pregnancy and, I:619–620
        steroid, II:255
        in systemic lupus
            erythematosus, III:191,
            III:192, III:207, III:208
Psychosocial Adjustment to Illness
    Scale, I:493
Psychosocial Assessment of
    Candidates for
    Transplantation, I:311
Psychostimulants. See Stimulants
Psychotherapy. See also
    Psychodynamic psychotherapy
    brief psychodynamically
        informed therapy, II:3–33
    for chronic fatigue syndrome,
        III:241, **III:244**, III:249,
        III:249
    for depressed multiple sclerosis
        patients, II:434
    for environmental illness,
        III:369–370, III:373

for frontal lobe dysfunction,
    I:376
for HIV-infected persons,
    III:286–288
for Huntington's disease,
    II:498–501, **II:499**
for patient with low-back pain,
    II:354, II:369
short-term dynamic therapy of
    stress response
    syndromes, II:27–33
for systemic lupus
    erythematosus, III:206
time-limited dynamic,
    II:18–27
Psychotropic drugs. *See also* specific
    drugs and drug classes
benzodiazepine hypnotics,
    II:84–90
    estazolam, II:85–86
    quazepam, II:86–88
    selection for medically ill
        patients, II:89–90
    triazolam, II:88–89
buspirone, II:80–84
dosage of
    calculating loading dose,
        III:14
    in cardiac disease, III:28–30
    kinetics affecting increases in,
        III:20
    in liver disease, III:40–42
    related to route of
        administration, III:2
    in renal disease, III:51–52
effect on cerebral blood flow,
    II:148
flumazenil, II:90–93
formulations of, **III:8**
for HIV-infected persons,
    III:280–286
for Huntington's disease,
    II:494–498, **II:496**
intramuscular, III:3

measuring blood concentration
    of, III:12, III:18
metabolized by cytochrome
    P$_{450}$-2D6, **III:82–83**
onset of action of, III:3
parenteral, II:113–133, III:3, **III:8,**
    III:22–23
    benzodiazepine-neuroleptic
        combinations, II:123–125
    benzodiazepines, II:120–123
    guidelines for administration
        of, **II:114–115**
    indications for, II:113
    lithium, II:130–132
    neuroleptics, II:113, II:116–120
    stimulants, II:129–130
    tricyclic antidepressants,
        II:125–129
for patients with mild traumatic
    brain injury, III:328–340,
    III:330–334
for premenstrual syndrome,
    II:263–265
second-generation
    antidepressants, II:69–80
    bupropion, II:77–80
    fluoxetine, II:69–74
    paroxetine, II:76
    selection of serotonin
        reuptake inhibitor,
        II:76–77
    sertraline, II:74–75
selegiline, II:97–98
standard of care for treatment
    with, II:564–565
tacrine, II:94–97
use during breast-feeding, II:249,
    II:254
use during pregnancy, II:246
Pudendal neuralgia, III:389–390
Pulmonary disease, I:52, I:132–133
Pulmonary fibrosis, due to
    total-body irradiation, III:435
Pulse, stress and, II:202

Purpura
    fluoxetine-induced, II:73
    psychogenic, I:230–231
Pyrazinamide, III:305
Pyridoxal phosphate, II:243
Pyridoxine deficiency, II:243

Quality of life, I:337–338
Quality of Well-Being Scale, I:338
Quazepam, II:86–88
    active metabolites of, II:87
    ataxia due to, II:87
    contraindications to, II:87–88
    daytime sleepiness with, II:87
    drug interactions with, II:87
    formulations of, III:8
    half-life of, II:87, III:19
    metabolism of, III:9
    pharmacodynamic selectivity of,
        II:87
    pharmacokinetics of, II:86–87
    protein binding of, II:87
    use in medically ill patients,
        II:87
Quinidine
    cytochrome P450 inhibition by,
        III:36, III:37
    interaction with fluoxetine, II:72
    interaction with nortriptyline,
        III:37
    interaction with venlafaxine,
        III:95
    lupus induced by, III:186
    metabolism by cytochrome
        P450-3A4, III:85
    use after myocardial infarction,
        III:98
Quinine, interaction with
    carbamazepine, III:123
Quinolinic acid, in Huntington's
    disease, II:473–474
Quinuclindinyl-iodobenzilate,
    iodine-123-labeled ([123I]QNB),
    II:153, II:159

Quisqualate, in Huntington's
    disease, II:473

Racial effects, on
    psychopharmacokinetics,
    III:1
Radiation accidents, III:417
Radioactive compounds, II:142,
    II:146–148, II:147
Radioimmunoassay, I:153–154
Radiopharmaceuticals, I:16
Ranitidine, III:21
Rapid plasma reagin test, I:260
Raven's Standard Progressive
    matrices, II:420
Recombinant granulocyte
    colony-stimulating factor
    (rG-CSF), III:107
Reflex sympathetic dystrophy
    (RSD), II:371, III:389
Refusal of treatment, II:539. See also
    Consent to treatment; Informed
    consent
    autonomy and, II:599–600
    informing patients of right to,
        II:549
    involuntary commitment and,
        II:519–521
    "liberty interest" and, II:544
    living will directives on,
        II:552–553
    malpractice suits related to,
        II:569–575
    in right-to-die cases, II:542–548
Regression, II:5, II:14
Reimbursement
    for bone marrow
        transplantation, III:420
    for hypnosis, II:47
    for psychotherapy, II:9
Relaxation training
    for esophageal spasm,
        II:54
    for low-back pain, II:360–361

Religious beliefs
    about artificial insemination
        with donor sperm, II:311
    about death, II:227
Renal blood flow (RBF), III:50–51
    in congestive heart failure,
        III:27–28
Renal disease
    liver disease and, III:41–42
    in organ transplant recipients,
        I:40–41
    pharmacokinetic effects of, **III:7,**
        III:49–52, **III:54–65**
        absorption, III:49
        dialysis, III:51
        fluid shifts and protein
            binding, III:10, III:50
    recommendations for drug
        dosing in, III:51–52
    use of antidepressants in, III:53,
        III:54–55, III:66
        fluoxetine, II:70–71, III:66,
            III:92
        nortriptyline, III:66
        paroxetine, II:76
        tricyclics, I:34–35, III:53,
            III:62–65, III:66
        venlafaxine, III:94–95
    use of anxiolytics in, III:52–53
    use of gabapentin in, III:119
    use of lithium in, I:39–40,
        III:60–61, III:66–67,
        III:110–111
    use of zolpidem in, III:131
Renal drug excretion, I:460,
    III:41–42
Rennie v. Klein, II:520
Reproductive endocrinology,
    II:237–276
    endometriosis, II:268–269
    menarche, II:241–242
    menopause, II:269–276
    oral contraceptive depression,
        II:242–245

    polycystic ovarian disease,
        II:265–268
    postpartum depressions,
        II:246–254
        major depression, II:252–254
        postpartum blues, II:250–252
        postpartum psychosis, II:255–257
    pregnancy, II:245–246
    premenstrual syndrome,
        II:257–265
    sex steroids and mood and
        behavior changes,
        II:238–241
Reproductive technologies,
    II:301–325. *See also* Infertility
    treatment
Research Diagnostic Criteria (RDC),
    II:433, II:435
Reserpine, **III:186**
    for Huntington's disease,
        II:495
"Resident's Bill of Rights," II:542
Resolve, Inc., II:325
Respectable minority rule, II:564
Respiratory disease
    buspirone use in, II:82
    estazolam use in, II:86
    parenteral benzodiazepine use
        in, II:124
    quazepam use in, II:88
    triazolam use in, II:89
    zolpidem use in, III:131–132
Respiratory drive and clonazepam,
    I:81
Respite, for caregivers, II:501
Retrovir. *See* Zidovudine
Retroviruses, III:261–262
Rheumatoid arthritis
    cognitive impairment in, III:192,
        III:193
    effect on protein binding of
        drugs, III:10
    environmental illness and,
        III:363

Rifampin (Rifadin, Rimactane)
  interaction with methadone,
    III:290
  neuropsychiatric side effects of,
    III:305
Rights and duties, II:586–587
Rights theory, II:586
Right-to-die cases, II:542–548
  "best interest" standard in, II:543
  constitutional rights applied to,
    II:544
  core factors influencing decision
    making in, II:558, **II:558**
  Cruzan case, II:542, II:544–546
  "jurisdiction of the state"
    approach to, II:545–546
  "liberty interest" in, II:544
  nutrition tubes as "artificial life
    supports," II:547
  in re Conroy, II:543
  in re Jane Doe, II:546–547
  in re Karen Ann Quinlan, II:543
  in re L.H.R., II:546
  State of Georgia v. McAfee, II:547
  "substituted judgment"
    standard in, II:543
Rigidity
  in Alzheimer's disease, II:449
  in Huntington's disease, II:475,
    II:486, II:487
  in Parkinson's disease, II:448,
    II:451
Risperidone, III:79, III:114–116
  active metabolite of, III:114
  for elderly patients, III:115–116
  formulations of, **III:8**
  half-life of, III:114
  for head-injured patient, III:329,
    III:331
  for HIV-infected persons, III:284,
    III:285
  mechanism of action of, III:114
  metabolism by cytochrome
    P$_{450}$-2D6, III:115

for psychosis in Parkinson's
    disease, III:169
  for schizophrenia, III:114
  side effects of, III:114–116
Ritalin. *See* Methylphenidate
Ritual Interview, I:493
Rituals, I:502–503
RO-16-0154, labeled with
    iodine-123 (Iomazenil), II:158
Robots, II:331
Roferon-A. *See* Interferon alfa-2a
Rogers v. Okin, II:520

Salicylate, fluoxetine interaction
    with, II:72
Salsalate, for low-back pain, **II:357**
San Francisco Shanti Project, III:288
Sargramostim, III:305
Scale for the Assessment of Positive
    Symptoms (SAPS), III:159
Schedule for Affective Disorders
    and Schizophrenia (SADS)
  for Huntington's disease
    patients, II:476
  for multiple sclerosis patients,
    II:432–433, II:435
Schilling test, I:224–225
Schizoaffective disorder, associated
    with HIV infection, **III:269**
Schizophrenia, II:493, **II:493**
  associated with HIV infection,
    III:267, **III:269–270**
  brain electrical activity mapping
    in, I:21–22, I:180
  buspirone as adjunctive therapy
    for, II:81
  cerebral blood flow studies in,
    I:14, II:149, II:158
  clozapine for, I:54, III:165
  computed tomography in, I:6
  eye-movement abnormality in,
    II:186
  frontal lobe function in, I:353
  genetic linkage studies of, II:188

genetics of, II:186
in Huntington's disease, **II:476,**
 II:476–478
mental retardation and, I:515
P300 amplitude in, I:179
positron-emission tomography
 in, I:20–21
pregnancy and, I:616
risperidone for, III:114–116
violence and, I:381
Schizotypal personality disorder,
 II:179
School rule, II:564
Sciatica, II:346
Scoliosis, II:370
Scopolamine, postoperative
 delirium due to, II:404
Seborrheic dermatitis, vulvar, **III:392**
Secobarbital, use in renal disease,
 III:54–55
Secondary gain
 chronic pain and, II:377–378
 simulated symptoms and, II:595
Sedation
 due to total-body irradiation,
  III:435
 risperidone-induced, III:114
 venlafaxine-induced, III:93
Sedative-hypnotics, I:525
 benzodiazepines, II:84–90
 dependence of low-back pain
  patient on, II:355, II:367
Seizures. *See also* Epilepsy
 drug-induced
  bupropion, I:49, II:69, II:78–80
  clozapine, III:107
  cyclosporine, I:329–332
  enflurane and cyclic
   antidepressants,
   II:400–401, **II:401**
  flumazenil, II:91–92
  fluoxetine, II:73
  tricyclic antidepressants, II:73,
   II:78, II:79

venlafaxine, III:95
EEG detection of, I:164–169
felbamate for, III:116–117
gabapentin for, III:119
in persons with mental
 retardation, I:516–517
in systemic lupus
 erythematosus, III:191,
 III:196, III:207
Selective Reminding Test, III:318
Selective serotonin reuptake
 inhibitors (SSRIs), II:69,
 III:80–93. *See also* specific drugs
achieving steady state of, III:17
dopamine inhibition by, III:91
drug interactions with, III:86,
 III:87–89, III:336
 carbamazepine, III:336
 clozapine, III:108
 desipramine, III:85
 felbamate, III:118
 selegiline, II:98
 trazodone, III:83
 warfarin, III:90
fluoxetine, II:69–74
half-lives of, III:17
for head-injured patient,
 III:332–333, III:335–336
for HIV-infected persons,
 III:280–282
inhibition of cytochrome
 P$_{450}$-3A4 by, **III:85,** III:86
inhibition of cytochrome
 P$_{450}$-2D6 by, III:36–37,
 III:46, III:83–85, **III:84**
metabolism of, **III:9**
paroxetine, II:76
for patient with low-back pain,
 II:359, II:366
pharmacology in medical
 patients, III:80–93
for postpartum depression,
 II:254
selection of, II:76–77

Selective serotonin reuptake
    inhibitors (SSRIs) *(continued)*
    sertraline, II:74–75
    side effects of, III:80, III:336
        cardiac effects, III:80, III:92–93
        extrapyramidal symptoms,
            III:91–92
        hematologic effects, III:90–91
        surgery in patients on, III:91
        use in cardiac disease, III:30–31,
            III:92–93
        use in gastrointestinal disease,
            III:23
        use in liver disease, III:92
        use in renal disease, III:92
Selegiline, I:70, I:372, II:97–98
    for Alzheimer's disease, II:98
    clinical applications of, II:98
    dosage of, II:98
    drug interactions with, II:98
        meperidine, II:98, II:400
    mechanism of action of, III:153
    neuroprotective effect of, III:153
    for Parkinson's disease, II:69,
        II:98, II:448, II:453, III:153,
        III:154, III:156, III:162
Self psychology, II:5
Self-determination, II:542
    Patient Self-Determination Act,
        II:537, II:548–552
    patient's rights to, II:542
    right-to-die cases and, II:543
Semen analysis, II:306
Seromycin. *See* Cycloserine
Serophene. *See* Clomiphene citrate
Serotonin (5-HT)
    estrogen effects on, II:239, II:240
    imipramine inhibition of uptake
        of, II:126
    inhibition of dopaminergic
        transmission by, II:84
    low mood associated with
        deficiency of, II:243
    nefazodone effects on, III:95

    in Parkinson's disease, II:450
    in polycystic ovarian disease,
        II:266, II:267
    tacrine effects on, III:136
Serotonin syndrome, I:67–68, II:72
Sertraline, II:74–75
    cardiac effects of, II:75
    cytochrome P$_{450}$ inhibition by,
        III:36, III:46, **III:84,**
        III:84–85
    drug interactions with, II:75,
        III:89
        anesthetics, II:400
        desipramine, III:85
        felbamate, III:118
        warfarin, III:90–91
    effect on liver enzymes, II:75
    formulations of, **III:8**
    given at low doses, II:75
    half-life of, II:75, III:17
    for head-injured patient, **III:332,**
        III:336
    for HIV-infected persons, III:280
    metabolism of, **III:85**
    for patient with low-back pain,
        II:359, II:366
    pharmacodynamic differences
        from fluoxetine, II:74–75
    for postpartum depression, II:254
    selecting for use, II:76–77
    side effects of, II:75
    time to reach steady state level
        of, II:75
    use in gastrointestinal disease,
        III:23
    use in liver disease, III:46
Serum creatinine, III:51–52
Serum glutamic–oxaloacetic
        transaminase (SGOT). *See*
        Aspartate aminotransferase
Serum glutamic–pyruvic
        transaminase (SGPT). *See*
        Alanine aminotransferase
7/24 Spatial Recall Test, **II:420**

Severe combined
immunodeficiency disease,
III:416, III:420
Sex hormone–binding globulin
(SHBG), II:268
Sex steroids, mood changes and,
II:238–241
Sexual abuse, II:375
vaginal or rectal discharge due
to, III:399
vulvodynia and, III:407–408
Sexual activity
arrhythmias and, II:229–230
effect of infertility on, II:303
electrocardiographic monitoring
during, II:229
hemodynamic effects of,
II:229
of HIV-positive persons, II:538
during investigation for
infertility, II:307
myocardial infarction and
cardiac arrest during, II:220
postmenopausal sexual function
and, II:275–276
resumption after myocardial
infarction, II:230
Sexual counseling, I:202–203
Sexual dysfunction
after bone marrow
transplantation, III:453–460
chemotherapy-induced,
III:453–455
radiotherapy-induced,
III:454–456
treatment of, III:456–457
dyspareunia, III:385
fluoxetine-induced, II:74
hypoactive sexual desire
disorder in HIV-infected
women, III:268
male, related to infertility, II:303
in multiple sclerosis, II:437–438
nefazodone-induced, III:96

selective serotonin reuptake
inhibitor–induced,
III:336
venlafaxine-induced, III:93–94
Shagreen patches, II:175
"Shamanism," II:4
"Shell shock," II:41
Short bowel syndrome, III:2
Short-term dynamic therapy of
stress response syndromes,
II:27–33
components of, II:27
control process theory, II:28
person schemas theory, II:28
states of mind, II:27–28
content themes for, II:30–31
goal of, II:28
intrapsychic focus of, II:27
in intrusion and denial phases,
II:28–30, **II:29**
number of sessions for, II:27
personality styles and, II:31–33,
II:32
Shriners' hospitals, II:393
Sialorrhea, clozapine-induced,
III:107
Sick-building syndrome, III:349–350
Sickle cell disease, II:178, II:601
bone marrow transplantation
for, III:417, III:419
epidemiology of, I:203
genetics of, I:203–204
pain management for, I:207–210
psychiatric issues in, I:203–210
sickle cell trait and sickle cell
anemia, I:203–204
symptoms of, I:204
Sickness Impact Profile, III:436
Silver acetate gum, I:572
Sinemet. *See* Levodopa/carbidopa
Single parenting, II:312–313
Single photon-emission computed
tomography (SPECT), I:16–19,
II:141–160

Single photon-emission computed
    tomography (SPECT)
    (continued)
    after head injury, **III:321,**
        III:327–328
    in AIDS dementia complex,
        III:276
    cerebral activation procedures
        during, II:149–150
        acetazolamide challenge,
            II:149–150
        behavioral task, II:150
        cognitive tasks, II:149
        motor tasks, II:149
        olfactory memory task, II:150
    clinical applications of, II:141
    compared with other imaging
        modalities, II:141–142
        computed tomography, II:141
        magnetic resonance imaging,
            II:141
        positron emission
            tomography, II:142
    definition of, II:141
    explanation of, II:143–145
        cameras, II:143–144
        collimator, II:144
        computer development of
            images, II:145
        computer display of images,
            II:145
        filters, II:145
        interpretation of scans, II:145
        light, II:143
        photomultipliers, II:144
    future developments in,
        II:159–160
    in Huntington's disease,
        II:491–492
    interpretation of, II:145,
        II:148–149
        consistency of uptake, II:149
        factors affecting cerebral
            blood flow, II:148–149

in major mental illness,
    II:157–159
    alcoholism and substance
        abuse, II:158–159
    depression and cerebral blood
        flow, II:157–158
    schizophrenia, II:158
in organic mental disorders,
    II:150–157
    CNS HIV infection, II:154–156
    CNS lupus, II:153–154
    dementia, II:152–153
    elderly patients with
        depression, II:157
    epilepsy, II:156
    miscellaneous disorders, II:157
    stroke, II:150–152
procedure for, II:142–143
    from clinician's point of view,
        II:142–143
    from patient's point of view,
        II:142
radioactive compounds used for,
    II:142, II:146–148, **II:147,**
        II:159
    gold-195m, II:146
    iodine-123-labeled
        amphetamine (IMP),
        II:146–148
    technetium-99m-labeled
        hexamethylpropyleneamine
        oxime (HMPAO),
        II:146–148
    xenon-133, II:146
in systemic lupus
    erythematosus, **III:198,**
        III:201–202
time required for, II:142
use in organic mental disorders,
    II:150–157
Skin biopsy, in systemic lupus
    erythematosus, III:195
Skin disorders
    carbamazepine-induced, III:122

discoid lupus, III:184, III:187
drug-induced lupus, III:184,
     III:186–187
fluoxetine-induced rash, II:74
hypnosis for, II:51–53
in neurofibromatosis, II:175
psychiatric illness and, I:287–305
rashes caused by fluoxetine, I:47
systemic lupus erythematosus,
     III:183–209
in tuberous sclerosis, II:175
vulvar, III:390–396, **III:392–394**
Sleep
     decreased myocardial infarction
          and sudden death during,
          II:227
     deprivation of
          atrial arrhythmias and, II:206
          postpartum blues and, II:251
     EEG and, I:165–166, I:184
     effect of intravenous
          clomipramine on,
          II:126–127
     effect on ventricular
          arrhythmias, II:224–225
     mechanisms of death occurring
          during, II:228–229
Sleep disturbances. *See also*
     Insomnia
     in bone marrow transplant
          recipient, III:432, III:439
     buspirone-induced, II:82
     in chronic fatigue syndrome,
          III:218, III:221, III:233–234
     due to hot flushes, II:271
     hypnosis for, II:58–59
     obstructive sleep apnea, II:87–89
     in Parkinson's disease, III:160
     related to protected isolation
          environment, III:443
     in systemic lupus
          erythematosus, III:192
     triazolam for, I:336–337

Smoking. *See* Cigarette smoking;
     Nicotine
Social Security benefits, II:538
     for Huntington's disease
          patients, II:501–502
Society for the Right to Die, II:552
Society of Clinical and
     Experimental Hypnosis, II:61
Sodium nitroprusside, III:27
Somatic complaints, I:513, I:611
Somatization disorder
     chronic fatigue and, III:235
     environmental illness and,
          III:356, **III:358–360,** III:372
     polycystic ovarian disease and,
          II:266
     vulvodynia and, III:409
     in women, II:237
Somatoform pain disorder, II:379
Somatostatin
     in Huntington's disease, II:473,
          II:495
     in Parkinson's disease, II:450
Somnolence
     due to total-body irradiation,
          III:435
     gabapentin-induced, III:120
     nefazodone-induced, III:96
Sorcery, death related to, II:227–228
Sotalol, torsades de pointes induced
     by, III:104
"Sperm allergy," II:306
Sperm banking, before bone
     marrow transplantation,
     III:456–457
Sperm donation. *See also* Artificial
     insemination with donor sperm
     donor's anonymity, II:312, II:318
     motivations for, II:318
     payment for, II:317
     psychological issues in donors,
          II:312, II:317–318
     selection and screening of
          donors, II:309–310

Spiegel's eye-roll test, II:43–44, II:47
Spinal cord injuries, II:331
Spinal examination, II:346
Spinal stenosis, II:370
Spironolactone, for premenstrual
    syndrome, II:263
Spondylolisthesis, II:346, II:370
Spondylosis, II:346, II:370
Sporanox. *See* Itraconazole
Sprains, II:331
SSRIs. *See* Selective serotonin
    reuptake inhibitors
Standards of care, II:563–569
    definition of, II:564
    dereliction or departure from,
        II:563–565
    error in judgment or treatment
        failure related to, II:565,
        II:578
    locality rule for, II:564
    in malpractice cases, II:564
    in medical-psychiatric practice,
        II:567–569
        case study of, II:567–568
        related to physical
            examinations, II:567–569
    minimum level of skill and, II:564
    missed diagnoses and, II:578–580
    school rule (respectable minority
        rule) for, II:564
Stanford Hypnotic Susceptibility
    Scale, II:43
Staphylococcal furunculosis,
    III:394, III:396
State of Georgia v. McAfee, II:547
Steady state, **III:5**
    relation to half-life, III:17–18
Stein-Leventhal syndrome. *See*
    Polycystic ovarian disease
Stellate gangliectomy, II:214
Sterility, due to total-body
    irradiation, III:435
Steroid hormones
    morning surge in, II:227

sex steroids
    mood changes and, II:238–241
    in polycystic ovarian disease,
        II:268
Stigma
    of chronic illness and pain, II:337
    of infertility, II:303
Stimulants, I:56–59, I:526–527,
    II:493, III:79, III:113–114
    for attention-deficit
        hyperactivity disorder,
        I:373–374
    cardiac effects of, III:113–114
    for children and adolescents,
        I:475–478
    for depression, I:335–336
    formulations of, **III:8**
    for head-injured patient, I:370,
        III:330, III:335
    for HIV-infected persons,
        III:282–283
    parenteral, **II:115,** II:129–130
    for Parkinson's disease, II:460
    side effects of, I:370, I:373–374,
        I:477
Stomach resection, III:2
Stomatitis, in bone marrow
    transplant recipient, III:433–435
Straight leg raising test, II:346
Streptococcal cellulitis, **III:394,**
    III:396
Streptomycin, **III:186**
Stress
    after myocardial infarction,
        II:223–224
    arrhythmias associated with,
        II:200, II:201, II:205–207
    cardiovascular responses to,
        II:202–207, **II:203**
    cigarette smoking and, I:547–548
    dermatitis and, I:292
    disability and, I:604–605
    effect on protein binding of
        drugs, III:10

of infertility, II:301, II:303–307
  before evaluation begins,
    II:303–304
  during medical workup,
    II:304–307
of infertility treatments
  helping patients cope with,
    II:323–324
  in men versus women,
    II:314–316
management for low-back pain
    patients, II:361–362
multiple sclerosis and, II:422–423
in organ transplant patients,
    I:323–324
polycystic ovarian disease and,
    II:265–268
premenstrual syndrome and,
    II:260, II:261
psoriasis and, I:291
psychological stress testing,
    II:218, **II:219**
sudden cardiac death related to,
    II:199–201, II:210, **II:210,**
    II:216–224
urticaria and, I:288–290
Stress response syndromes
  intrusion and denial phases of,
    II:28–30, **II:29**
  short-term dynamic therapy for,
    II:27–33
Stroke, I:170, I:368
  computed tomographic
    evaluation of, II:151
  in HIV infection, II:155
  oral contraceptives and, II:244
  SPECT evaluation of, II:150–152
Structured Clinical Interview for
    DSM-III-R (SCID), II:344,
    III:323, **III:327**
Structured Interview for DSM-III
    Personality Disorders,
    III:358–361
Subarachnoid hemorrhage, II:244

Substance P
  in Huntington's disease, II:473
  in Parkinson's disease, II:450
Substance use disorders, I:145–160
  assessing bone marrow
    transplant candidate for,
    III:423
  associated with HIV infection,
    III:258–260, **III:267,**
    III:269–270, III:289
  cerebral blood flow studies in,
    II:158–159
  among Huntington's disease
    patients, II:477
  vulvodynia and, III:409
"Substituted judgment" standard,
    II:543
Succinylcholine, II:398
  electroconvulsive therapy and,
    I:123–125
  lithium interaction with, II:402
  tacrine interaction with, II:97
Sudden cardiac death. *See also*
    Arrhythmias
  anthropological studies of,
    II:227–229
    death during sleep, II:228–229
    mechanism of death, II:228
  bereavement and, II:222–223
  circadian variations and,
    II:225–227
  depression and, II:222
  due to ventricular fibrillation,
    II:207–208
  evidence for neural and
    psychological factors in,
    II:207–211
    animal studies, **II:208,**
    II:208–209
    human studies, **II:208,**
    II:209–211, **II:210**
  historical descriptions of,
    II:199
  incidence of, II:201

Sudden cardiac death *(continued)*
  parasympathetic mechanisms in,
      II:211–212
  psychosocial factors related to,
      II:209–210, II:222
  risk factors for, II:201
  role of psychological stress in,
      II:199–201, II:210, **II:210,**
      II:216–224
    acute stress, II:216–222, **II:219,**
      II:221
    chronic stress, II:222–224
    sympathetic neural mechanisms
      in, II:212–216
    catecholamine effects,
      II:215–216
    central and local neural
      pathways, II:212–214
Sudden infant death syndrome
    (SIDS), II:257
Sufentanil
  elimination half-life of, II:396
  for outpatient surgery, II:396
  for preanesthetic anxiety,
      II:394
Suffering, II:39
Suicide, I:292, I:317–318
  among adolescent girls, II:241
  associated with HIV infection,
      III:268, III:279, III:287
  among Huntington's disease
      patients, **II:476,** II:480
  prevention of, II:503–504
  malpractice claim of suicidal
      patient, II:569–573
  among multiple sclerosis
      patients, II:428
Sulfadoxine/pyrimethamine,
    III:303
Sulfonamides, **III:186**
Superoxide dismutase, II:453
Support groups
  for environmental illness, III:351,
      III:355

for families of bone marrow
      transplant recipients,
      III:448
  for interstitial cystitis, III:387
  for systemic lupus
      erythematosus, III:206
  for vulvodynia, III:386
Surgery
  drug-induced bleeding
      tendencies and
      selective serotonin reuptake
      inhibitors, III:91
    valproate, III:126–127
  effect on drug absorption, III:22
  effect on protein binding of
      drugs, III:10
  hypnoanesthesia for, II:50, **II:51**
  outpatient, II:395–397
Surrogate motherhood, II:310, II:312
Swan-Ganz catheters, II:391
Sweating
  stress-related, II:202
  venlafaxine-induced, III:93
Sydenham's chorea, **II:493**
Symbol Digit Modalities Test, **II:420**
Sympathomimetics, drug
      interactions with, **II:401**
Symptom Checklist-90-Revised,
      III:356
Symptom substitution, II:40, II:42,
      II:46
Syncope
  bupropion-induced, II:77
  fatal, II:199
  hysterical, II:204
  vasovagal, II:204–205
Syndrome of inappropriate
      antidiuretic hormone secretion
      (SIADH), II:74
  risperidone-induced, III:114
Syphilis
  cause of, I:257–259
  epidemiology of, I:257
  HIV infection and, I:265–266

laboratory tests for,
    I:260–263
symptoms of, I:258–260
treatment of, I:266–267
    efficacy of, I:264–265
Systemic lupus erythematosus
    (SLE), II:411, II:489, II:493,
    II:493, III:183–209
    autoantibodies in, III:184,
        III:187, III:188, III:195,
        III:197
        search for specific antibodies
           in neuropsychiatric
           lupus, **III:198,**
           III:202–206
    causes of death in, III:189
    central nervous system
        symptoms of, II:153–154
    clinical course of, III:189
    clinical features of, III:183–184,
        III:185, III:187, III:187,
        III:190, III:196
    cognitive impairment in, III:188,
        III:191–194
    diagnosis of, III:188–189
        brain imaging, **III:198,**
           III:199–202
        computed tomography,
           III:199
        magnetic resonance
           imaging, III:199–201
        positron-emission
           tomography, III:194,
           III:202
        single photon-emission
           computed
           tomography,
           III:201–202
        electroencephalogram,
           III:196–199, **III:198**
        issues and problems in,
           III:194–195
        lumbar puncture, III:196,
           III:198

        neuropsychological testing,
           III:194, **III:198,** III:199
        serology and chemistry tests,
           III:195, **III:197–198**
        skin biopsy, III:195
    differential diagnosis of,
        III:184–187, **III:186,** III:193
        discoid lupus, III:184, III:187
        drug-induced lupus, III:184,
           III:186–187
    in elderly persons, III:188–189
    epidemiology of, III:184
    immune abnormalities in, **III:187**
    neuropsychiatric symptoms and
        psychopathology in,
        III:188, III:191–192, **III:192**
    prevalence of, III:184
    prognosis for, III:189
    psychiatric presentations of,
        III:192–193
    psychiatrist's role in, III:191
    support groups for patients
        with, III:206
    treatment of, III:189, III:206–209,
        III:207
        drug therapy for
           neuropsychiatric
           syndromes, III:206–208
        guidelines for, III:208–209
        psychiatric effects of
           medications used for,
           III:208

T lymphocytes, in HIV infection,
    III:259, III:260
Taboo practices, II:227
Tachycardia
    clozapine-induced, III:107
    sinus
        during sexual activity, II:229
        stress-related, II:204
    supraventricular
        drug therapy for, II:205
        stress-related, II:205

Tachycardia *(continued)*
  supraventricular
    triggers for, II:205, II:206
  ventricular
    provoked during
      psychological stress
      testing, II:218–220, **II:219**
    stress-related, II:214
    in children, II:214
Tacrine, II:69, II:94–97, III:79,
    III:133–136
  for Alzheimer's disease, II:69,
    II:94–97
  benefit-to-risk ratio for, II:97
  dosage of, II:95
  drug interactions with, II:96–97
  effects on neurotransmitters,
    III:136
  efficacy of, II:94–96, III:134
  guidelines for termination of,
    III:135
  improvement in attention vs.
    memory due to, III:134–135
  indications for, III:133–134
  mechanism of action of, II:94
  monoamine oxidase–inhibiting
    effect of, II:94, II:97
  patient selection for, III:136
  pharmacokinetics of, II:95
  predicting response to, II:96, III:135
  side effects of, II:96–97,
    III:134–136
    aggravation of parkinsonism,
      II:96
    alanine aminotransferase
      elevation, III:134–136
    hepatotoxicity, II:96
Tardive dyskinesia, I:475, I:520,
    II:263–264
  clinical features of, II:494
  clozapine for, III:109
  compared with Huntington's
    disease, II:493–494
  estrogen effects on, II:239

risperidone for, III:115
Tardive dystonia, clozapine for, III:109
Tartrazine, I:303–304, **III:186**
Technetium-99m (^{99m}Tc), II:142
  generation of, II:147–148
  half-life of, II:147
  hexamethylpropyleneamine
    oxime labeled with
    (HMPAO), II:146–148,
    II:147
Tegretol. *See* Carbamazepine
Temazepam, II:84
  formulations of, **III:8**
  half-life of, **III:19**
  for head-injured patient, **III:334,**
    III:339
  metabolism of, **III:9,** III:15, III:52
  use in cardiac disease, III:27
  use in liver disease, III:39, III:42
Temporal lobe syndromes, III:312,
    III:314
Temporomandibular joint
    syndrome, I:418
Tension, preceding ventricular
    arrhythmias, II:217
Tension headache. *See* Headache
Teratogenicity
  of antiepileptic drugs, II:99–101
  folic acid deficiency and, II:100
Terfenadine, III:102–103
  drug interactions with, III:102–103
    cytochrome P_{450}-3A4
      inhibitors, III:86
    nefazodone, III:97
  metabolism by cytochrome
    P_{450}-3A4, III:85
  overdose of, III:103
Terfenadine carboxylate, III:102–103
Testicular cancer, bone marrow
    transplantation for, III:417–419
Testosterone
  for decreased libido in
    postmenopausal women,
    II:276

levels during perimenopause, II:275
levels in bone marrow transplant recipients, III:453, III:455
Tetrabenazine, for Huntington's disease, II:495
Tetracycline, **III:186**
Thalassemia, I:210–213
bone marrow transplantation for, III:417, III:419, III:420
Theophylline, II:54
interaction with fluvoxamine, **III:87**
interaction with tacrine, II:97
Therapeutic donor insemination (TDI). *See* Artificial insemination with donor sperm
Therapeutic range, III:12
Thiopental, use in renal disease, **III:54–55**
Thioridazine, I:519, II:118
cytochrome P$_{450}$-2D6 inhibition by, III:84
formulations of, **III:8**
metabolism by cytochrome P$_{450}$-2D6, III:36, **III:83**
use in cardiac disease, III:31
Thiothixene, I:519–520, **III:8**
intramuscular, **II:114**
Thrombin, II:216
Thrombocytopenia
carbamazepine-induced, III:121
valproate-induced, III:126
Thromboxane, II:216
Thyroid dysfunction, due to total-body irradiation, III:435
Thyroid function tests
postpartum, II:248
for premenstrual syndrome, II:260
Thyroid-stimulating hormone (TSH), in patient on lithium, III:111
Thyrotoxicosis, II:493, **II:493**

Time distortion, under hypnosis, II:42
Time-limited dynamic psychotherapy (TLDP), II:18–27
application to medically ill patients, II:19
bases of, II:18
case example of, II:20–27
dynamic focus, **II:23**
session 1, II:20–21
session 2, II:21–24
sessions 3 to 6, II:24–25
sessions 7 to 10, II:25–26
sessions 11 to 15, II:26–27
development of, II:18
identification of cyclical maladaptive patterns in, II:19
interpersonal focus of, II:27
number of sessions for, II:19
training in, II:19
transference-countertransference issues in, II:19
treatment manual for, II:18
Timolol, **III:82**
Tinea infections, vulvar, **III:394**
Tolamolol, II:215
Tolazamide, **III:186**
Tolbutamide
interaction with fluoxetine, II:72
interaction with paroxetine, **III:88**
interaction with sertraline, II:75
Torsades de pointes, III:86, III:101–104
astemizole-induced, III:103
intravenous haloperidol–induced, III:103–104, III:286
sotalol-induced, III:104
terfenadine-related, III:102–103
Torts, II:561–563
definition of, II:561
intentional, II:562

Torts *(continued)*
unintentional, II:563
Total lymphoid irradiation, II:417
Total parenteral nutrition (TPN)
for bone marrow transplant
recipient, III:416, III:431
complications related to,
III:436–437
Total-body irradiation (TBI)
before bone marrow
transplantation, III:416,
III:430, III:435–436
gonadal dysfunction due to,
III:454–456
long-term neuropsychological
effects of, III:435–436
toxic acute complications of,
III:435
Tourette's disorder, I:526
Toxoplasmosis, II:154
Trail Making test, **III:326**
Training. *See* Education and training
Trance logic, II:42
Trance state, II:41–42. *See also*
Hypnosis
Transcutaneous electrical nerve
stimulation (TENS), II:368
Transference, II:5, II:32, II:39
developed with medically ill
patients, II:14
in time-limited dynamic
psychotherapy, II:19
Transgenic animals, II:182
Transplantation. *See* Bone marrow
transplantation; Organ
transplantation
Transrectal ultrasound (TRUS),
II:306
Tranylcypromine, I:374, II:98
for head-injured patient, **III:332**
Trauma
effect on albumin binding of
drugs, III:10
head injury, III:307–340

psychiatric disorders as
reactions to, II:15
Trazodone, I:301, II:20, II:46
for depressed Parkinson's
disease patients, II:459
formulations of, **III:8**
for head-injured patient, **III:333,**
III:337
for HIV-infected persons,
III:282
interaction with anesthetics,
II:400
interaction with selective
serotonin reuptake
inhibitors, III:83
for mucous membrane
dysesthesias, III:390
use in cardiac disease, III:30–31
use in liver disease, III:45
Tremor
of drug-induced parkinsonism,
II:452
essential, II:448
gabapentin-induced, III:120
in HIV infection, III:269
in Parkinson's disease, II:448,
II:451
stress-related, II:202
Triazolam, II:84, II:88–89
adverse behavioral reactions to,
II:88
anterograde amnesia induced by,
II:88
cognitive effects of, II:86, II:88
duration of action of, II:88
formulations of, **III:8**
half-life of, II:88, **III:19**
inflammatory reactions to, II:89
interaction with nefazodone, III:97
metabolism of, **III:9**
by cytochrome P_{450}-3A4,
III:36, III:85
motor impairment due to, II:89

for obstructive sleep apnea, II:89
rebound insomnia after use of,
    II:89
use in chronic obstructive
    pulmonary disease, II:89
use in liver disease, III:42–43
use in renal disease, **III:58–59**
withdrawal from, II:89
Trichotillomania, I:296–297
Tricyclic antidepressants. *See*
    Antidepressants, tricyclic
Trifluoperazine, **III:8**
    for Huntington's disease, II:495
    intramuscular, **II:114**
Trifluperidol, **III:82**
Trigger points, II:368, II:373–374
Trihexyphenidyl, for Parkinson's
    disease, II:455, II:462
Triiodothyronine (T3), for
    HIV-infected persons, III:282
Trimethadione, **III:186**
Trimethoprim/sulfamethoxazole,
    III:303
N1N1N'-Trimethyl-n'-(2
    hydroxy-3-methyl-5-123
    I-iodobenzyl)-1,3-propanediamine
    2HCl (HIPDM), II:156
Trimipramine, **III:8**
Trisomy 21, II:179
Truth telling, II:590–591, II:602
Tryptophan
    fluoxetine interaction with,
        II:72
    metabolism of, II:243
Tryptophan oxygenase, II:243
Tuberculosis, HIV infection and,
    III:289–290
Tuberous sclerosis, II:174–175
    clinical features of, II:174–175
    genetic testing for, II:174–175
    prevalence of, II:175
Tumors. *See also* Cancer
    bone marrow transplantation
        for, III:415–460

effect on albumin binding of
    drugs, III:10
Turner syndrome, II:179
Twentieth century disease, III:347.
    See also Environmental illness
Twin studies, II:185
    of multiple sclerosis, II:411
    of oral contraceptive–related
        depression, II:243
Two-compartment model, III:13
Type A personality, II:375
Tyramine-restricted diet, for
    patients on selegiline, II:98

Ultrasound, transrectal (TRUS),
    II:306
United States In Vitro Fertilization
    Registry, II:308
Uremia. *See* Renal disease
Urethral syndrome, III:387–388
Urinalysis, postejaculatory, II:306
Urinary retention, tricyclic
    antidepressant–induced,
    III:281
Urticaria, I:288–290, I:304
Uterine cancer, II:274, II:275
Utilitarianism, II:586

Vacuolar myelopathy, I:247–248
Vaginal dryness, II:269, II:276
Vaginismus, II:303
Valproate, I:76–80, III:79, III:125–130
    benefits of, III:129
    drug interactions with,
        III:127–130
        carbamazepine, III:48–49,
            III:117, III:127,
            III:129–130
        clozapine, III:108
        felbamate, III:118
        fluoxetine, **III:88**
        lorazepam, III:127, III:129
        oral contraceptives, II:99
        paroxetine, **III:88**

Valproate *(continued)*
  drug interactions with
    tricyclic antidepressants,
      III:105–106, III:339
  effects on coagulation, III:126–127
  formulations of, **III:8,** III:25
  for head-injured patient, **III:333,**
    III:338–339
  for HIV-related mania, III:283
  indications for, III:125
  metabolism of, **III:9**
  for multiple sclerosis patients,
    II:436
  neural tube defects related to use
    in pregnancy, II:99, II:100
  protein binding of, III:10–12
  rapid loading of, III:129
  side effects of, III:125–126,
    III:128–129, III:338
  use in gastrointestinal disease,
    III:25–26
  use in liver disease, III:48–49,
    III:126, III:128
  use in systemic lupus
    erythematosus, III:208
  volume of distribution of, III:13
  withdrawal from, III:119
Value theory, II:586
Vasodilators, III:27
Venereal Disease Research
    Laboratory (VDRL) test,
    I:260–264, I:266
Venlafaxine, III:79, III:93–95
  active metabolite of, III:93
  dosage of, III:93
  dosing schedule for, III:94
  drug interactions with, III:95
  formulations of, **III:8**
  half-life of, III:93–95
  for head-injured persons, III:337
  for HIV-infected persons, III:281
  metabolism by cytochrome
    P$_{450}$-2D6, III:95
  protein binding of, III:10, III:93

side effects of, III:93–94, III:281
  use in cardiac disease, III:95
  use in liver disease, III:94
  use in renal disease, III:94–95
Ventricular fibrillation
  animal studies of, II:208–209,
    II:216–217
  in children, II:214
  provoked, II:213
  stress-related, II:200, II:214,
    II:216–218
    affective states associated
      with, II:217
    in cardiac disease patients,
      II:220–221, **II:221**
    prevented by β-blockers, II:216
  sudden death due to, II:207–208,
    II:216
Verapamil
  interaction with carbamazepine,
    III:123
  interaction with imipramine,
    III:105
  for supraventricular tachycardia,
    II:205
Vertebral anatomy, **II:360**
Vertebral fracture, II:370
Vicodin, II:344
Videx. *See* Didanosine
Vietnam veterans, cognitive
    impairment in, III:317–318
Vinblastine, **III:83**
Violence, I:379–381
Viral infections
  chronic fatigue syndrome and,
    III:230–232
  vulvar, **III:394,** III:395–396
Visual blurring,
    nefazodone-induced, III:96
Visual hallucinosis,
    antiparkinsonian
    drug–induced, III:151, III:159–160
Visualization
  hypnotic, II:42, II:45–46

use in cancer patients,
II:55–56
Vitamin B$_6$
deficiency of, II:240, II:243
for premenstrual syndrome,
II:262–263
Vitamin B$_{12}$
deficiency of, I:220–226
metabolism of, I:220–221
Vitamin supplementation, for
environmental illness,
III:354
Volume of distribution, **III:5,**
III:12–14
disease effects on, III:18
half-life and, III:17, III:34
Vomiting. *See* Nausea and vomiting
von Willebrand's factor, valproate
effects on, III:127
Voodoo death, II:211–212, II:227
"Voodoo Death," II:199
VP-16. *See* Etoposide
Vulvodynia, III:381–411
areas of future research on,
III:411
chronicity of, III:382–383
clinical features of, III:382–383
complexity of, III:383–384
definition of, III:382
differential diagnosis of,
III:387–396, **III:401**
cutaneous disorders,
III:390–396, **III:392–394**
candidiasis, III:391, III:395
dermatoses, III:390–391
herpes simplex virus,
III:395
herpes zoster, III:395
human papillomavirus
infection, III:396
molluscum contagiosum,
III:396
staphylococcal
furunculosis, III:396

streptococcal cellulitis,
III:396
endogenous dysesthesias,
III:389–390, III:402
interstitial cystitis and
urethral syndrome,
III:387–388
itching and burning, III:388
iatrogenic factors in, III:397–398
alcohol injections, III:397–398
CO$_2$ laser, III:397
side effects of topical steroids,
III:397
itching in, III:381–382, III:388,
III:398–399
management of, III:405–406,
III:409–411
by dermatologist, III:410
by gynecologist, III:409–410
psychiatric referral,
III:405–406, III:411
surgical therapy, III:404
media attention to, III:386–387
patterns of, III:400, **III:401**
cyclic vulvovaginitis,
III:400–402
dysesthetic vulvodynia,
III:389–390, III:402
vulvar vestibulitis, III:403–405
psychiatric issues related to,
III:406–409
approach to patient,
III:406–407
chronic pain, III:408
medication, III:408–409
primary and secondary gains,
III:407
sexual abuse, III:407–408
somatoform disorders, III:409
substance abuse, III:409
psychological aspects of,
III:384–386
relationship with vaginismus,
III:383

Warfarin
    interaction with carbamazepine,
        III:124
    interaction with fluoxetine, II:72
    interaction with paroxetine, II:76
    interaction with selective
        serotonin reuptake
        inhibitors, **III:87–89,**
        III:90–91
    interaction with sertraline, II:75
Warts, hypnosis for, II:52
Watson-Schwartz test, I:219
Weakness
    in chronic fatigue syndrome,
        III:221
    nefazodone-induced, III:96
Wechsler Adult Intelligence
    Scale—Revised (WAIS-R),
    III:199, III:318, **III:326**
    for multiple sclerosis patients,
        II:418, **II:420**
    for Parkinson's disease patients,
        II:462
Wechsler Memory Scale (WMS),
    III:318
    for multiple sclerosis patients,
        II:420
    for Parkinson's disease patients,
        II:462
Weeping, pathological, **II:427,**
    II:427–428
Weight change
    cigarette smoking and, I:551,
        I:571
    felbamate-induced, III:117
    monoamine oxidase
        inhibitor–induced, I:65
    risperidone-induced, III:114
Welfare benefits, II:501–502
Western blot, I:251–252
"Whiplash" headaches, I:418
Widowers, II:222
Wilson's disease, I:351–352, II:449,
    II:493, **II:493**

Winters v. Miller, II:519–520
Wisconsin Card Sorting Test,
    I:358–359, **III:326**
    for multiple sclerosis patients,
        II:420
    for Parkinson's disease patients,
        II:462
    for schizophrenic patients
        during SPECT imaging,
        II:149, II:158
Wiskott-Aldrich syndrome, III:417
Withdrawal of treatment, II:542,
    II:546. *See also* Refusal of
    treatment; Right-to-die cases
Work and disability, I:598–603,
    I:609–610
"Working through," II:5
"Worried well," III:258, III:287
Wrongful death, II:567

Yeast disease, III:348, III:362
Yohimbine, II:74
Young v. Emory University Hospital,
    II:546
Youngberg v. Romeo, II:520

Zalcitabine, III:303
Zant v. Prevatte, II:546
Zero-order kinetics, III:19–20
Zidovudine, I:254–255, II:156, II:605
    effect on maternal-to-infant HIV
        transmission, III:262
    neuropsychiatric side effects of,
        III:303
    to reduce progression of
        AIDS-dementia complex,
        III:286
Zithromax. *See* Azithromycin
Zolpidem, III:79, III:131–133
    dosage of, III:131
    for elderly persons, III:131–133
    half-life of, III:131
    metabolism of, III:131
    respiratory effects of, III:131–132

side effects of, III:131–133
use in liver disease, III:131
use in renal disease, III:131
Zovirax. *See* Acyclovir

Zygote intrafallopian transfer
(ZIFT), II:308–309
cost of, II:308
delivery rate for, II:309

Contents to Volume 1

Contributors xi

Foreword xvii
    George B. Murray, M.D.

Acknowledgments xix

Introduction xxi
    Alan Stoudemire, M.D.
    Barry S. Fogel, M.D.

Section I
Recent Advances in Diagnosis and Treatment

1 Advances in Neuroimaging Technologies 3
    John M. Morihisa, M.D.

2 Psychopharmacology in the Medically Ill:
   An Update 29
    Alan Stoudemire, M.D.
    Barry S. Fogel, M.D.
    Lawrence R. Gulley, M.D.

3 Anesthetic Management of the High-Risk Medical
   Patient Receiving Electroconvulsive Therapy 99
    Gundy B. Knos, M.D.
    Yung-Fong Sung, M.D.

4 Special Technical Considerations in Laboratory
   Testing for Illicit Drugs 145
    Robert M. Swift, M.D., Ph.D.
    William Griffiths, Ph.D.
    Paul Camara, M.S.

5   Advances in EEG-Based Diagnostic Technologies 163
     M. Eileen McNamara, M.D.

Section II
Specific Syndromes and Disease Categories

6   Psychiatric Aspects of Hematologic Disorders 193
     Elisabeth J. Shakin, M.D.
     Troy L. Thompson II, M.D.

7   Human Immunodeficiency Virus and Other Infectious
     Disorders Affecting the Central Nervous System 243
     Paul Summergrad, M.D.
     Randy S. Glassman, M.D.

8   Dermatology 287
     David G. Folks, M.D.
     F. Cleveland Kinney, M.D., Ph.D.

9   Heart and Liver Transplantation 309
     Anne Marie Riether, M.D.
     J. Wesley Libb, Ph.D.

Section III
Clinical Neuropsychiatry

10   Diagnosis and Management of Patients With Frontal
      Lobe Syndromes 349
      Barry S. Fogel, M.D.
      Paul J. Eslinger, Ph.D.

11   Headache Syndromes 393
      James R. Merikangas, M.D., F.A.C.P.

12   Neuroleptic Malignant Syndrome: Clinical
      Presentation, Pathophysiology, and Treatment 425
      Daniel D. Sewell, M.D.
      Dilip V. Jeste, M.D.

Section IV
Child and Adolescent Medical Psychiatry

13 Psychopharmacology in Medically Ill
    Children and Adolescents 455
    Betty Pfefferbaum, M.D.

14 Family Therapy in the Context of Childhood
    Medical Illness 483
    Jane Jacobs, Ed.D.

15 Pharmacotherapy of Severe Psychiatric
    Disorders in Mentally Retarded Individuals 507
    Carl Feinstein, M.D.
    David Levoy, M.D.

Section V
Special Topics

16 Pharmacological and Behavioral Treatment of Nicotine
    Dependence: Nicotine as a Drug of Abuse 541
    Michael G. Goldstein, M.D.
    Raymond Niaura, Ph.D.
    David B. Abrams, Ph.D.

17 Psychiatric Aspects of Medical Disability 597
    Arthur T. Meyerson, M.D.
    Beryl Lawn, M.D.

18 Psychotropic Drug Use in Pregnancy:
    An Update 615
    Lee S. Cohen, M.D.
    Vicki L. Heller, M.D.
    Jerrold F. Rosenbaum, M.D.

Index 635

Contents to Volume 2

Contributors xi

Foreword xvii
    Stuart C. Yudofsky, M.D.

Acknowledgments xxi

Introduction xxiii
    Alan Stoudemire, M.D.
    Barry S. Fogel, M.D.

Section I
Psychotherapy in Medically Ill Patients

1 Brief Psychodynamically Informed Therapy for
    Medically Ill Patients 3
    Hanna Levenson, Ph.D.
    Robert E. Hales, M.D.

2 Medical Hypnosis 39
    Harold J. Wain, Ph.D.

Section II
Psychopharmacology Updates

3 New Psychotropics in Medically Ill Patients 69
    Barry S. Fogel, M.D.
    Alan Stoudemire, M.D.

4 Parenteral Use of Psychotropic Agents 113
     Alberto B. Santos, M.D.
     Karen E. Beliles, M.D.
     George W. Arana, M.D.

Section III
Diagnostic Neuroradiology

5 SPECT Imaging in Medical Psychiatry 141
     Joseph A. Schwartz, M.D.
     Nancy M. Speed, M.D.

Section IV
Special Topics

6 Testing for Genetic Disorders 167
     Susan E. Folstein, M.D.
     Andrew Warren, M.D.
     O. Colin Stein, Ph.D.

7 Cardiac Arrhythmias and Sudden Cardiac Death 199
     Regis A. de Silva, M.D., F.R.C.P.C.

8 Reproductive Endocrinology 237
     Leslie Hartley Gise, M.D.
     Susan C. Weston, M.D.

9 New Reproductive Technologies 301
     Cheryl F. McCartney, M.D.
     Jennifer Downey, M.D.

10 Low-Back Pain Rehabilitation 331
     Rollin M. Gallagher, M.D.
     Michael Woznicki, M.D.

11 Anesthesia 389
     Carla Rodgers, M.D.

Section V
Neuropsychiatry

12 Multiple Sclerosis: Mood Disorders,
    Cognition, and Psychoneuroimmunology 411
    R. B. Schiffer, M.D.

13 Parkinson's Disease: Recent Developments
    of Psychiatric Interest 447
    Barry S. Fogel, M.D.

14 Psychiatric Disorders in Huntington's Disease 471
    Robert A. Maricle, M.D.

Section VI
Medical-Legal Updates

15 Competency Determinations 515
    Vivian S. Auerbach, Ph.D.
    John D. Banja, Ph.D.

16 Living Wills and Advance Medical
    Treatment Directives 537
    William H. Overman, J.D.

17 Malpractice in Psychiatric Practice 561
    Ronald Schouten, J.D., M.D.

18 Ethics in Medical-Psychiatric Practice 585
    James J. Strain, M.D.
    Rosamond Rhodes, Ph.D.
    Daniel A. Moros, M.D.
    Bernard Baumrin, Ph.D., J.D.

Index 607

Contents to Volume 1 655